Scott S. Iwashita #642

To Judy

CONTRIBUTORS

ROBERT G. ANDREWS, D.D.S. Clinical Professor, University of Southern California School of Dentistry; Attending Staff, Rancho Los Amigos Hospital, Downey, California, Hoag Memorial Hospital, Newport Beach, California.

Injured Anterior Teeth.

SEYMOUR J. CARR, D.M.D. Associate Professor, Division of Oral Surgery, University of California at Los Angeles School of Dentistry; Consultant, Oral Tumor Board, University of California School of Dentistry; Consultant, Oral Surgery, Veterans Administration Hospital, Sepulveda, California.

Psychosedation—Part 4: Pharmacosedation—Inhalation Route
(with Norman Trieger).

DONALD E. COOKSEY, D.D.S. Professor, Section of Oral Surgery, University of Southern California School of Dentistry; Senior Attending Staff, Los Angeles County/University of Southern California Medical Center; Medical Staff, Santa Fe Memorial Hospital and Glendale Hospital.

Acute Oral Lesions.

W. HOWARD DAVIS, D.D.S., F.A.C.D. Clinical Professor, University of Southern California School of Dentistry; Associate Professor, Loma Linda University School of Dentistry; Consultant, Long Beach Veterans Administration Hospital, Long Beach Naval Hospital; Staff, Downey Community Hospital, Long Beach Memorial Hospital, St. Mary's Hospital, Long Beach, California.

Emergency Drugs and Allergy.

PETER A. FOREMAN, B.D.S. (N.Z.) Dental Practitioner specializing in anesthesiology and psychosedation; Postgraduate Instructor, University of Oregon Health Sciences Center, University of California at San Francisco, and University of British Columbia; Former Visiting Professor, Departments of Pharmacology and Human Behavior, University of Southern California School of Dentistry; Former Visiting Professor, Department of Restorative Dentistry, University of British Columbia.

Psychosedation—Part 5: Pharmacosedation—Intravenous Route.

NATHAN FRIEDMAN, D.D.S. Clinical Professor and Chairman, Section of Human Behavior, University of Southern California School of Dentistry, Los Angeles, California.

Psychosedation—Part 2: Iatrosedation.

JOHN M. GREGG, D.D.S., M.S., Ph.D. Professor of Oral and Maxillofacial Surgery, University of North Carolina School of Dentistry. Staff, North Carolina Memorial Hospital, Veterans Administration Hospital, Fayetteville, North Carolina.

Psychosedation—Part 1: The Nature and Control of Pain, Anxiety, and Stress.

JOHN O. HAGEN, D.D.S., M.S., F.A.C.D., F.A.D.S.A. Clinical Associate Professor, Section of Anesthesia and Medicine, University of Southern California School of Dentistry; Senior Attending Staff, Los Angeles County/University of Southern

California Medical Center; Staff, St. John's Hospital, Santa Monica, Santa Monica Hospital, and Marina Mercy Hospital, Marina Del Rey, California.

Psychosedation—Part 3: Pharmacosedation—Oral Route (with Stanley F. Malamed); *Basic Life Support and Parenteral Drug Administration* (with Stanley F. Malamed).

CEDRIC L. HAYDEN, D.M.D. Formerly Head, Department of Anesthesia, Port of Spain Community Hospital, Port of Spain, Trinidad, West Indies; Presently in private practice of dentistry and anesthesia for dentistry.

Monitoring (with Thomas F. Mulkey).

JESS HAYDEN, JR., D.M.D. Ph.D. Clinical Professor, Department of Surgical Dentistry, University of Colorado Medical Center, Denver; Consultant in Pedodontics, Denver General Hospital, Denver, Colorado.

Complications from Local Analgesia.

LEO KORCHIN, B.S., D.D.S., M.S., F.A.C.D. Professor of Oral Surgery and Assistant Dean, University of Puerto Rico School of Dentistry; Attending Oral Surgeon, University Hospital, San Juan, Puerto Rico.

Establishing an Emergency Airway.

GUSTAV O. KRUGER, D.D.S., D.Sc., M.A. Associate Dean, Professor and Chairman, Department of Oral Surgery, Georgetown University School of Dentistry; Chief of Dental Staff, Georgetown University Hospital; Consultant, District of Columbia General Hospital, Veterans Administration Hospitals, Washington, D.C., and Martinsburg, West Virginia.

Maxillofacial Pain (with Donald O. Reynolds).

JOHN J. LYTLE, M.D., D.D.S., F.A.C.D. Clinical Professor and Chairman, Section of Oral and Maxillofacial Surgery, University of Southern California School of Dentistry; Chief of Oral and Maxillofacial Surgery, Department of Dentistry, Los Angeles County/University of Southern California Medical Center, Los Angeles; Chief of Staff, Memorial Hospital of Glendale, Glendale, California.

Cardiovascular and Other Medical Emergencies.

STANLEY F. MALAMED, D.D.S. Assistant Professor, Section of Anesthesia and Medicine, University of Southern California School of Dentistry, Los Angeles, California.

Psychosedation—Part 3: Pharmacosedation, Oral Route (with John O. Hagen); *Basic Life Support and Parenteral Drug Administration* (with John O. Hagen).

FRANK M. McCARTHY, B.S., M.S., M.D., D.D.S., Sc.D., F.A.C.D., F.I.C.D., F.A.D.S.A. Professor and Chairman, Department of Surgical Sciences and Anesthesia and Medicine Section, Assistant Dean for Hospital Affairs, University of Southern California School of Dentistry; Director, Dental Anesthesia Service, Los Angeles County/University of Southern California Medical Center; Guest Lecturer, Loma Linda University School of Dentistry; Consultant, Orthopaedic Hospital of Los Angeles.

Sudden Death. Physical Evaluation and Treatment Modification.

LOWELL E. McKELVEY, D.D.S., B.A., M.S. Professor of Oral Surgery, School of Dentistry, University of Texas, San Antonio, Texas.

Maxillofacial Injuries.

JOHN B. McVEIGH, D.D.S., M.S., F.I.C.D. Coordinator, Oral Surgery Residency Training, Alameda County Hospital, Oakland; Chief, Department of Dentistry,

Providence Hospital, Oakland; Associate Staff, Children's Hospital, Merritt Hospital, and Perralta Hospital, Oakland, California.

General Anesthetic Emergencies and Complications.

THOMAS F. MULKEY, D.D.S. Clinical Associate Professor, University of Southern California School of Dentistry; Senior Attending Staff, Los Angeles County/ University of Southern California Medical Center; Chief, Dental Service, Orthopaedic Hospital of Los Angeles; Attending Staff, Daniel Freeman Memorial Hospital, Inglewood, California.

Monitoring (with Cedric L. Hayden).

HERBERT R. PACKARD, B.S., D.D.S., F.I.C.D., F.A.C.D. Chairman, Department of Dentistry and Oral and Maxillofacial Surgery, Highland General Hospital, Oakland, California; Active Medical Staff, John Muir Hospital, Walnut Creek, California; Consultant, Veterans Administration Hospital, Martinez, California; Courtesy Staff, Mount Diablo Hospital, Concord, California, Samuel Merritt Hospital, Oakland, California.

Hospital Dentistry.

THOMAS W. QUINN, D.M.D. Clinical Professor of Oral and Maxillofacial Surgery, Tufts University School of Dental Medicine, Boston; Director, Department of Dentistry, Chief of Oral Surgery, Carney Hospital, Boston; Chief of Oral Surgery, Quincy City Hospital, Quincy, Massachusetts.

Cardiopulmonary Arrest.

LELAND W. REEVE, D.M.D. Clinical Professor, Departments of Oral Surgery and Anesthesia/Medicine; Lecturer, Post-Graduate Division, University of Southern California School of Dentistry; Senior Attending Staff, Los Angeles County/ University of Southern California Medical Center; Attending Staff, Huntington Memorial Hospital, St. Luke Hospital, Pasadena, California.

Hemorrhage.

DONALD O. REYNOLDS, D.D.S., M.S. Professor of Oral Surgery, Georgetown University School of Dentistry, Georgetown University Hospital; Staff, District of Columbia General Hospital; Consultant, Veterans Administration Hospitals, Washington, D.C., and Martinsburg, West Virginia.

Maxillofacial Pain (with Gustav O. Kruger).

LAWRENCE W. RICHARDSON, D.D.S., M.D. Board of Governors, School of Medicine, Stanford University; Lecturer equivalent to Associate Professor, School of Dentistry, School of Medicine, University of California at Los Angeles; Clinical Assistant Professor, University of Southern California School of Dentistry; Assistant Visiting Attending, University of California at Los Angeles Hospital; Senior Attending Dentist, Los Angeles County/University of Southern California Medical Center, St. John's Hospital, Santa Monica, California.

Physical Diagnosis.

GERALD A. SHEPPARD, B.A., L.L.B. Clinical Assistant Professor, University of Southern California School of Dentistry; Guest Lecturer, University of California at Los Angeles School of Dentistry and Loma Linda University School of Dentistry; Member Los Angeles County Bar Association, State Bar of California, and American Bar Association; Practitioner before the Bar of the United States Supreme Court.

Legal Aspects of Emergencies.

ROBERT SHIRA, D.D.S., D.Sc. (Hon.) Dean Emeritus and Professor of Oral Surgery, Tufts University School of Dental Medicine, Boston, Massachusetts.

Surgical Emergencies

ROBERT BRUCE STEINER, D.M.D., B.S., F.I.C.D. Clinical Associate Professor, University of Southern California School of Dentistry; Senior Attending Staff, Los Angeles County/University of Southern California Medical Center; Chief of Dental Section, Children's Hospital of Los Angeles; Staff, Hollywood Presbyterian Medical Center, St. Joseph's Hospital, Sunset Boulevard Hospital, Hollywood Community Hospital, Hollywood, California.

Drugs: Use and Abuse.

NORMAN TRIEGER, D.M.D., M.D. Professor, Dental Surgery, Albert Einstein College of Medicine, Bronx, New York; Chairman, Department of Dentistry and Oral Surgery, Montefiore Hospital and Medical Center, Bronx, New York.

Psychosedation—Part 4: Pharmacosedation—Inhalation Route
(with Seymour J. Carr).

FOREWORD

In recent years, the incidence of emergencies in dental practice has increased vastly—as has the number of negligence claims arising from them. The dental practitioner, for the benefit of patients and as a matter of his or her own self-interest, is obliged to re-evaluate continually the knowledge of prevention, recognition, and treatment of emergency problems.

The extent of these problems and their obvious importance to the practitioner led the Editor of the *Dental Clinics of North America* to invite me to assemble a symposium on Emergencies, which was published in the November 1965 issue of the Clinics. According to the publisher, this proved to be the most popular issue in the history of that journal; and it was out of print almost since the day of publication.

By definition, an emergency is an unforeseen circumstance calling for immediate action. The latitude of topics consistent with this definition is therefore virtually limitless. For this book, topics of special interest to the general practitioner have been chosen; yet no subject has been slighted in depth of coverage. Some topics that might at first appear to have limited primary appeal to the general practitioner were chosen either because of their increasing importance in dental practice or because of the responsible role that must be assumed by the dental doctor as a medical specialist in civilian disaster relief.

The treatment of life-threatening emergencies is not a cookbook exercise. A basic knowledge of the background of disease is necessary before the clinician can act to prevent, diagnose, or treat. Therefore, well over half of this book deals with prevention and recognition. The prevention of a serious emergency represents the most important service that a health practitioner can provide the patient; yet the necessity for immediate and effective treatment of an existing emergency cannot be minimized. The legal and moral responsibility for effective prevention and prompt treatment rests solely in the hands of the able and informed doctor.

I hope that this book will assist the doctor in fulfilling his or her responsibility to prevent emergencies, when possible, and to treat those that are unavoidable with sound judgment, proper technical knowledge, and dispatch.

FRANK M. McCARTHY

PREFACE TO THE THIRD EDITION

This edition of *Emergencies in Dental Practice* is the most extensively revised since the 1965 symposium in *Dental Clinics of North America*. Use of the book continues to increase equally in both the practicing community and in education. The broad-based *emergency* format appeals to the general practitioner of dentistry, dental specialists, physicians, dental hygienists, and all dental auxiliaries. While the broad definition of *emergency* has been followed, as in previous editions, the bulk of additional material has adhered to the prime purpose of this book, the prevention, recognition, and treatment of life-threatening emergencies, with major emphasis on prevention.*

Topics and authors have been added. The subject of management in pregnancy has been transferred as a separate topic to another chapter. The topic of sudden death has been expanded as a separate chapter, and the chapter on physical evaluation has been greatly expanded with material on the USC physical evaluation system, systems review and treatment modification, physical examination, function tests, and laboratory tests and interpretation. Two chapters have been added to the psychosedation section, one on a basic understanding of pain, anxiety, and stress, and the other on the art and science of human behavior related to psychosedation (iatrosedation). A chapter on hospital dentistry has been added so that the dental health professional will have complete reference material available. Hospitalization of the highly anxious and/or fearful patient or the medical risk patient is sometimes required, and this information is necessary to our general protocol for prevention of life-threatening emergencies.

I have studied 63 constructive critiques of the second edition, and most of the revisions in this new edition respond to those suggestions, including more complete indexing, an outline at the beginning of each chapter, expansion of physical evaluation and treatment modification, improvement of illustrations, and the addition of hospital dentistry and further sedation topics.

Two of the critiques suggested that we adopt a handbook format and list symptoms/signs and emergency procedures by the numbers. While the thought is at first intriguing, I feel that a cookbook approach misses the entire point of prevention. We must first understand disease before we can prevent attendant complications, and, understanding disease, we are then in a position to recognize and treat emergencies that are unavoidable. When managing

---

*I have collected 10 legal definitions of the term *emergency*. Nine definitions are similar to that in the *Foreword* of this book. The tenth defines an emergency as *an unanticipated condition where some immediate action is necessary for the preservation of life or health* (Bergen, R.P.: Legal definition of an emergency. J.A.M.A., 206:2327, 1968). This definition has been applied in determining whether a health practitioner is authorized to render medical care without express consent.

life-threatening emergencies, we do not have the luxury of unlimited time that is available when diagnosing an ignition fault with the aid of an automotive handbook. A cardiac conduction defect requires immediate knowledge, not a knee-jerk response.

The reader is urged to develop familiarity with sudden death, physical evaluation, and treatment modification before proceeding to other topics. The classic systems review has been retained as the ideal vehicle for presenting physical evaluation and treatment modification.

I have been deeply involved in the development of physical evaluation, medicine, anesthesia, and emergency medicine in dentistry since 1956, and I have observed with utter amazement and deep pride the near superhuman efforts of dentistry to upgrade these areas. This has been accomplished in the practicing community by a solid commitment to continuing education and in the predoctoral curriculum by vast program enrichment. Improvements in the predoctoral and continuing education curricula have been greatly enhanced by the ADA Commission on Accreditation through development of comprehensive guidelines for teaching physical evaluation and pain/anxiety control. It is no less than staggering to observe the sophistication of physical evaluation and emergency medicine in dentistry today. The contemporary dental doctor in the United States utilizes a more comprehensive physical evaluation routine than does the average medical practitioner and is better equipped (oxygen, other emergency drugs, and emergency team) to manage medical emergencies than is the average medical office, and I suspect that this situation is also true in other countries. During the past three years in the Greater Los Angeles area, four cardiac arrests in medical offices have been treated successfully by dental practitioners and their emergency teams called in for this purpose.

Is there any act more noble than the saving of a life? It is just as noble to *avoid* mortality or serious morbidity by proper pretreatment physical evaluation and by appropriate modification of dental therapy. It is equally as noble to discover undiagnosed disease, and to refer the patient for proper care, thus adding significantly to longevity. In the past 25 years dental doctors have truly joined the ranks of health professionals by developing expertise in medical areas formerly considered to be peripheral to dental practice but now recognized as an essential part of comprehensive dental care. While technical excellence must never be sacrificed, the role of dentistry has broadened to include psychosedation, health screening, and emergency preparedness. During a time when the credibility and motives of the health professions are under constant scrutiny, dentistry has added immeasurably to its public and professional image by extending its treatment scope in the public interest.

In an attempt to categorize a profusion of topics held together by the common thread *emergency*, this edition continues to be divided into four sections: Prevention of Serious Medical Emergencies; Treatment of Serious Medical Emergencies; Prevention and Treatment of Surgical and Operative Emergencies; and Complementary Topics.

In a book which serves both as a general compendium and as a comparatively narrow reference source, a certain duplication of content must be allowed. Overlap of material has been kept to a minimum consistent with proper understanding and continuity.

FRANK M. McCarthy

CONTENTS

Introduction to Psychosedation

PART 2 TREATMENT OF SERIOUS MEDICAL EMERGENCIES

PART 3   PREVENTION AND TREATMENT OF SURGICAL AND OPERATIVE EMERGENCIES

PART 4   COMPLEMENTARY TOPICS

Chapter 23

GUSTAV O. KRUGER AND DONALD C. REYNOLDS

Chapter 24

DONALD E. COOKSEY

Part 1

PREVENTION OF SERIOUS MEDICAL EMERGENCIES

SUDDEN DEATH

FRANK M. McCARTHY

INTRODUCTION

The ultimate catastrophe in the dental office, death of a patient, requires an in-depth understanding of sudden death.

Until advances were made in external cardiopulmonary resuscitation (ECPR) during the 1960's, sudden and unexpected death remained virtually a statistical observation, not a treatable problem, with the rare exception of open-chest cardiac resuscitation performed during anesthesia and surgery. The nonsurgical mode of ECPR allows the reversal of many deaths which formerly were felt to be final, unexplained, and untreatable.

DEFINITION OF SUDDEN DEATH

There are about two million nonaccidental deaths per year in the United States.[1] Approximately one million of these are relatively sudden (cardiovascular and cerebrovascular diseases). Very nearly 20 per cent of all nonaccidental deaths, or 400,000, are sudden *and* unexpected. The mean age of the victims is 45 years.

Sudden, unexpected death occurs from nonaccidental causes in persons who previously appeared to be in good health and who had no history of

3

disease. By various temporal definitions, sudden death occurs from up to one hour to 24 hours after collapse of the individual. Timing from collapse to death is rather academic since most sudden deaths are *instantaneous*.[2] Cardiovascular disease is the major cause, and almost all sudden deaths occur outside of the hospital.

Persons dying *instantaneously* of coronary artery disease differ to a considerable degree from persons dying *suddenly* of coronary artery disease.[3] They rarely exhibit acute symptoms or signs before death, more than one half die during physical stress, death results from a primary arrhythmia (ventricular fibrillation), and their hearts rarely show an acute lesion (myocardial infarction). A disconcerting number of sudden deaths cannot reasonably be accounted for at necropsy (postmortem examination).

CAUSES OF SUDDEN DEATH

The more common causes of sudden, unexpected death are coronary artery disease, cerebrovascular accidents, myocardiopathies, and cardiac conduction defects. These disorders may or may not have an increased familial incidence.

Doyle's review of the causes of sudden, nontraumatic death is outlined in Table 1–1.[2] Two additional causes of sudden death have recently been suggested. One involves the sudden formation of platelet aggregates in small pulmonary arteries and arterioles, with extreme respiratory distress and death in one to 30 minutes.[4] The other involves a progressive atrioventricular conduction defect in three generations of a large family.[5] Clinical findings included a slow heart rate and episodes of syncope. Progression to complete heart block was usually slow, but occasionally a fulminant course led to sudden death within two to three years. None of these deaths was unexpected.

MECHANISMS OF SUDDEN DEATH

The mechanism of sudden death is usually derangement of heart rhythm. In the hospital cardiac care unit (CCU), sudden death is most fre-

TABLE 1–1 CAUSES OF SUDDEN, NONTRAUMATIC DEATH

CARDIAC	Cor pulmonale
Coronary artery disease	acute
Morgagni-Adams-Stokes syndrome	chronic
Aortic stenosis	Status asthmaticus
Floppy mitral valve syndrome	
Primary myocardial disease	EXTRACARDIAC
Acute myocarditis	Dissecting aneurysm of aorta
Acute pericardial tamponade	Exsanguinating hemorrhage
Coronary embolism	Intracranial hemorrhage
Prolonged Q-T interval syndrome	
Congenital heart disease	MISCELLANEOUS
	Sudden infant death syndrome
PULMONARY	Pokurri disease; Bangungut
Asphyxia ("cafe coronary")	Unexplained

quently the result of ventricular fibrillation. If treatment is immediately instituted, the patient usually survives.

Unconsciousness occurs in healthy young experimental human subjects in an average of 6.8 seconds after occlusion of the cerebral circulation. Syncope is the presenting manifestation of sudden death and *implies circulatory arrest.*[2]

Seventy-five per cent of deaths from acute myocardial infarction (MI) take place during the *first hour*. Hospitalization must be expedited, as must admission to the CCU. One third of all patients with MI are detained in the emergency area for more than three hours until a diagnosis is securely established, thus resulting in a significant number of deaths from preventable cardiac arrest. A normal electrocardiogram (ECG) is perfectly compatible with the presence of an MI that may be fatal within minutes.

HEREDITARY FACTORS

Ten instances have been reported of the occurrence in three generations of sudden, unexpected death associated with stress and attributable to minor anatomical defects of the cardiac conduction system that could predispose to fatal arrhythmias. Pathological examinations were normal except for semiserial conduction studies by the Lev–Shanklin–Laite technique, a method that should be utilized in similar instances of unexplained death in persons with hearts that are grossly normal at necropsy. This type of death is probably far more common than can be proved on the basis of present evidence.

An uncommon type of QT prolongation (see electrocardiographic background in Chapter 4, Monitoring) is heritable and occurs most often in children with congenital deafness or with normal hearing. It is associated with syncopal episodes and sudden death. Asymmetrical sympathetic neural stimulation of the ventricular myocardium may lead to gross changes in the T wave and a prolonged QT interval. Prolongation of the QT interval represents delayed ventricular repolarization and an increase in the susceptibility to ventricular dysrhythmia. In the presence of a prolonged QT interval, premature ventricular contractions (PVCs) may lead to ventricular fibrillation.

If the medical history of a child with or without congenital deafness reveals *frequent syncope*, an ECG to investigate possible QT prolongation would be indicated.

Survival to adulthood by children with heritable QT prolongation indicates the termination of the conduction defect without further risk of sudden death.

With the exceptions of congenital heart disease and heritable conduction defects already covered, heredity has little influence on the development of common varieties of heart disease that can result in sudden, unexpected death. In disorders such as arterial hypertension and rheumatic fever, several genes may influence the disease, but environmental factors are far more important.

ENVIRONMENTAL FACTORS

Respiratory infections kill thousands of people of all ages who have chronic illness, especially old people and those with heart disease. Death rates vastly increase during the winter and in association with cold waves.

The same mortality increase in patients with chronic illness is seen during the summer for almost the entire United States.[6] Deaths from cardiac disease literally soar during hot and humid weather.

When the environmental temperature is at a comfortable level, heat loss at the skin surface occurs primarily by convection and radiation, with some by conduction. If the thermal gradient between the body and the environment becomes too little, or is actually reversed so that the temperature of the environment exceeds that of the body, then heat loss by usual means becomes inadequate or even ceases, and body heat must be lost by evaporation of sweat from the skin surface. If evaporative heat loss is impaired because of humidity, body temperature will rise. For heat loss to occur by evaporation, saturation of the surrounding atmosphere with water (relative humidity) must be less than 100 per cent.

Cardiac output in patients with heart disease is fixed at relatively low maximal levels. Cardiac output at total rest averages 3 to 4.5 liters per minute. In a hot and humid environment with thermal regulatory demands requiring a cardiac output of 20 to 30 liters per minute for any sustained period of time, the diseased heart will fail.

Patients with heart disease must be instructed to avoid hot and humid environments. For some patients with severe heart disease, air-conditioning is essential during dental treatment.

EMOTIONAL FACTORS

Regulatory inhibition of cardiac rate is enhanced by purposeful action and is diminished in situations that appear to be overwhelming and without hope, such as severe dejection or sudden fear. The loss of inhibition provides the death mechanism. Being frightened to death is literally possible.

In a study of 530 out of 817 episodes of acute myocardial infarction, it was possible to determine that 104 (20 per cent) occurred during sleep. Ten patients known to have nocturnal attacks of angina pectoris were monitored during sleep for 12 full nights, 39 episodes of angina pectoris with significant ECG changes being recorded. The dreams involved strenuous exertion, fear, anger, or frustration.

A medicolegal application of the stress response was demonstrated by a $500,000 professional negligence verdict in the hospital general anesthesia death of a 13-year-old male who, it was claimed, was in a state of panic preoperatively and was therefore not a fit candidate for anesthesia or surgery.

The role of emotional stress associated with anesthesia and dentoalveolar surgery has been recognized as a cause of death by leading dental authorities in the United Kingdom.[7, 8] Emotional as well as physical stress is capable of precipitating complications in individuals with heart disease.[9]

It is my opinion that emotional stress is responsible for more deaths related to dental therapy than any other single factor.

AGE AND DEATH

Age at each end of the spectrum strongly influences the incidence of sudden death.

Sudden, unexpected infant deaths occur at a markedly high rate in the 10-day to 16-week age group, leveling off at six months of age.

Sudden, unexpected death rates increase proportionally with age until the middle years, when the rate increases in direct relationship to the diseases of aging. In an analysis of 328 fatally injured drivers, there was no significant correlation between accident responsibility and disease, but the proportion of drivers 60 years of age or older was five times as high among those killed as among those who survived multi-vehicle crashes. The aged had a markedly increased incidence of death from complications of existing disease, such as coronary atherosclerotic heart disease.

Age alone has a marked influence on hospital fatalities. Patients less than 60 years of age average 12 per cent fatalities, and older patients show a steadily increasing fatality percentage up to 50 per cent in the oldest age group. Patients hospitalized in facilities with CCUs have *slightly lower* fatality rates than other patients. Monday admissions substantially exceed fatalities on other days of the week.[10]

INDIVIDUALS AT RISK

The identification of the individual at greatest risk of sudden death merely represents the delineation of his or her coronary risk profile; for example, male sex, relative youth, arterial hypertension, overweight, glucose intolerance, hypercholesterolemia, indolence, and heavy smoking.[2] I hasten to add that hypercholesterolemia may be removed from the preceding profile. Clinicians remain unconvinced that the low fat, low cholesterol, polyunsaturated diets promoted since 1950 have any effect on coronary heart disease. No diet therapy has been shown effective for the prevention or treatment of coronary heart disease, and there is no safe and efficacious drug known for the management of hypercholesterolemia.[11] Low fat diets at least have not been harmful to those following the latest trend, though dogs subsisting on table scraps in such families have commonly developed mange (fat deprivation).

Evidence suggests that fit and active people are spared the complications of coronary artery atherosclerosis. Studies of the Masai indicate that exercise makes even atherosclerotic vessels enlarge so that the capacity of coronary vessels increases despite an increase of atherosclerosis.[11]

If the electrocardiographic pattern of left ventricular hypertrophy (LVH) is added to the usual coronary risk profile, the risk of sudden death increases as much as sixteen-fold between individuals at opposite ends of the risk factor scale.[12]

There are few characteristics associated specifically with a likelihood of sudden death. PVCs are common in the general population, increase in frequency with age, and have little significance in healthy individuals. However, PVCs are universally observed during myocardial infarction and are often a precursor to ventricular fibrillation, and are therefore of prognostic significance in individuals *with* heart disease.[2]

The possibility of impending sudden death should be considered with the appearance of inappropriate bradycardia (heart rate less than 60 beats per minute) or significant PVCs during dental treatment. Sudden death rates among persons over age 30 with PVCs is six times that of persons over age 30 without PVCs.

REVERSAL OF DEATH

Successful reversal of sudden death in the dental office demands immediate and effective treatment before transportation to the hospital. Approximately 70 per cent of patients dying from coronary atherosclerotic heart disease (CAHD) never reach the hospital. Death is frequently instantaneous. About 60 per cent of all sudden deaths occur in patients with CAHD.

According to Jude and Nagel,[13] sudden total circulatory collapse in the operating room can be expected to have a 60 to 75 per cent survival via ECPR; in the cardiac catheterization laboratory, success is 95 to 100 per cent; in the CCU, sudden arrhythmic death can be reversed in 50 to 60 per cent of cases; in the general hospital setting, 8 to 15 per cent are successfully resuscitated.

No reliable statistics are available for successful reversal of the out-of-hospital death (OHD), although fragmentary evidence is disappointing. In a study on delay in the prehospital phase, delay due to inappropriate patient behavior was the most important component. However, 60 to 75 per cent of OHDs occur so rapidly that their prevention by reduction of prehospital delay seems impossible.[14] In another mortality study the median patient delay, from onset of symptoms until hospital arrival, was 5.6 hours.[15] Public education and a vast increase of mobile and other ancillary medical facilities will be necessary in order to significantly further reduce OHDs.

It is interesting to note that the age-adjusted death rate from coronary artery disease declined between 1963 and 1968, while at the same time an epidemic of coronary artery disease has been claimed, based only upon crude death rates. This discrepancy is due to a shift in the age composition of the population. The increase in crude death rates will continue so long as gains in life expectancy result in a bigger population in the older ages, even though there may be a decrease in mortality for every individual age group.[16] There is an approximate five-year time lag in the publication of U.S. government age-adjusted mortality rates.

CARDIAC CARE UNIT

The cardiac care unit (CCU), sometimes known by the more general term intensive care unit (ICU), proliferated vastly in the 1970s. Originally established as a special area where MI patients could be provided with continuous ECG monitoring and specially trained nurses, the typical CCU now requires the use of complex diagnostic, physiologic, and therapeutic procedures. Burch feels that MIs can be treated very well with simple bed-side procedures and therapy. He quotes a 12.3 per cent mortality rate among 253 unselected MI patients treated only by ECG monitoring and close observation in the CCU compared to mortality rates of 13 to 21 per cent in other U.S. institutions. Burch objects to invasive monitoring tech-niques; for example, the placement of catheters to record central venous pressure, systemic venous pressure, capillary wedge pressure, and pulmo-nary or systemic arterial pressure. He feels that the catheters are not only hazardous but are uncomfortable and frightening to many patients, and that they interfere with rest.[17] Since stress increases the number of PVCs in the infarcted heart,[18] it is probable that CCUs will revert to less involved moni-toring for an increasing number of patients. Further, the cost-effectiveness of invasive monitoring is being questioned.

Some hospitals are introducing intermediate cardiac care unit (ICCUs), to which patients at less risk are transferred very early from the CCU and mon-itored in less intensive, less heavily staffed areas, rather than being trans-ferred to general medical wards where nursing coverage may be sparse and monitoring nonexistent. The subacute areas of these ICCUs utilize radio-telemetry to allow early ambulation.

OTHER MORTALITY RATES

We have examined sudden death mortality rates in and out of the hos-pital. For a more comprehensive understanding of death, we will review myocardial infarction related to general anesthesia, general anesthesia mor-tality in the hospital, and general anesthesia mortality in the dental office.

GENERAL ANESTHESIA AND MIs

Patients who have had an MI are at high risk of reinfarction under general anesthesia, 6.6 per cent experiencing another MI during the first postoperative week. There is no relationship between incidence of reinfarc-tion and type or duration of anesthesia, although operations on the thorax and upper abdomen are followed by three times as many reinfarctions as operations at other sites.[19]

Patients who are operated on within three months of infarction have a 37 per cent reinfarction rate. This rate decreases to 16 per cent in patients at three to six months after infarction, and remains at 4 to 5 per cent over six months. Over 50 per cent die as a result of reinfarction.[19]

GENERAL ANESTHESIA MORTALITY

Approximately 15 million general anesthetics are administered yearly in hospitals in the United States. Forty per cent of the anesthetics are ad-

TABLE 1–2 GENERAL ANESTHESIA MORTALITY

Dental offices, U.S.	−1:400,000
Dental offices, South. Calif.	−1:400,000
Dental offices, U.K.	−1:300,000
Large teaching hospitals, U.S.	−1:1500
Suburban hospitals, U.S.	−1:9000
T & A, hospitals, U.S.	−1:40,000

ministered by trained anesthesiologists (MD), 40 per cent by certified registered nurse anesthetists (CRNA), and 20 per cent by other personnel.[20] Approximately five million general anesthetics are administered yearly in dental offices in the United States. Seventy per cent of the anesthetics are administered by trained dental practitioners, 4 per cent by anesthesiologists, 10 per cent by CRNAs, and 16 per cent by other personnel.[21]

Table 1–2 demonstrates the general anesthesia mortality experience in dental offices in the United States[21], Southern California[22], and the United Kingdom.[23] Comparison is made with general anesthesia mortality in large teaching centers[24] and suburban hospitals[25] in the United States. The tonsillectomy and adenoidectomy (T & A) mortality rate of 1:40,000 is quoted, as it is the most favorable report I have discovered in the literature, although the national T & A general anesthesia mortality rate is 1:20,000.[21] The Southern California survey reported a 100 per cent response.

It would appear that general anesthesia in the dental office is at least 10 to 20 times safer than general anesthesia in the hospital. It is improper, however, to make comparisons without stressing the great differences between hospital general anesthesia and dental office general anesthesia. General anesthesia in the dental office is purely elective and is available only to favorable risk patients; duration of anesthesia is comparatively short; the treatment can be terminated instantly in an emergency; operative delays are uncommon; and the anesthetic depth is ultralight, rarely approaching surgical depth with depression or obtundation of protective reflexes.

Mortality greatly increases if the preoperative physical status of the patient is unfavorable, and it increases again for emergencies as compared to elective procedures.[26] In a computerized analysis of postanesthetic deaths, the prime determinants of mortality were considered to be the physical status of the patient and the judgment and skill of the physician.[27] In this same study, which reported an overall general anesthesia mortality of 1.82 per cent, mortality of Class I and Class II physical status patients (favorable risk) was 1.70 per cent, and this despite the fact that 30 per cent of the Class I and Class II patients were emergencies.

DENTAL OFFICE MORTALITY

There are no totally reliable national or regional records of patient deaths in dental and medical offices, and there does not seem to be much chance of accurate surveys being made, except under unusual control circumstances.[22]

Coroner records are unreliable, as the deceased may be certified in the medical office or hospital emergency room and thus not become a coroner's case. National and regional surveys are questionable, as doctors are reluctant to divulge information, and reporting is usually incomplete. Liability insurance records are both privileged and subject to distortions.

In my opinion, based purely upon informed speculation, the average dental doctor will experience one or two patient deaths during his or her practice lifetime, occurring either in the office or within a 24-hour post-treatment period, and there will be an additional known four or five patient deaths occurring within one week of treatment. These deaths are probably unrelated to therapy and occur at random, although treatment stresses may represent contributing factors.

In closing this section on mortality associated with dental therapy, allow me to quote Mark Twain: *There are lies, damned lies, and statistics.* The reader must make the judgment.

SUDDEN DEATH AND TRENDS IN DENTISTRY

A review of current trends in dental care related to mortality or serious morbidity in the office will be limited to medicolegal pressures. In California there is an average of one wrongful death medical lawsuit per month with judgment of one million dollars or more. Wrongful death dental lawsuits in California have reached a top of $300,000 as of this writing and are certain to go higher. Risk-free therapy is impossible, yet the public has been educated by the news media to expect a perfect result as a norm. The reader is referred to Chapter 25 for a comprehensive review of the disturbing legal aspects of the situation.

As patient mortality closely related to dental treatment reaches the point of ultimate catastrophe, we note increases in the following areas: publicity, malpractice charges, malpractice awards, and criminal negligence charges (negligent homicide). These pressures are influencing the dental doctor, consciously or unconsciously, to avoid treatment which might be a basis for a malpractice claim.

In the arena of medical emergencies and possible morbidity or mortality involving the risk patient, local analgesic agents without vasoconstrictors are being arbitrarily chosen, although depth of analgesia may suffer and the risk of toxic overdose is increased; high risk patients are being hospitalized for dental care under general anesthesia, thus subjecting them to enormous risk, while the same procedure could be performed far more safely in the dental office with local analgesia and perhaps sedation for anxiety control; sedation via the inhalation and intravenous routes is being used less commonly for the risk patient in order to avoid possible claims, whereas the risk patient vastly benefits from sedation. Lastly, an increasing number of dental practitioners are flatly refusing to treat the risk patient. All of these alterations in treatment standards work to the distinct detriment of the medically compromised patient.

WHEN YOUR OFFICE PATIENT DIES

When your patient dies in the office, it is a shattering experience not only to the deceased's relatives but also to you and to your office staff. It can be damaging to your professional reputation, it can result in a wrongful death malpractice suit, and it can result in a charge of criminal negligence. Conviction of criminal negligence usually absolves your professional liability insurance carrier of any financial obligation resulting from subsequent malpractice action.[28]

Humane and practical considerations are five in number:[29]

1. Preplan your resuscitative procedures with your office staff. Practice simulated emergencies. If your procedures are not preplanned and rehearsed, you will perhaps treat a life-threatening emergency in a less than adequate manner. Keep your resuscitative kit updated and handy for instant use. If your patient does not survive, despite your prompt and definitive treatment, you will be able to demonstrate that you did everything that could reasonably be expected of you.
2. Take extreme care when informing the next-of-kin of a death. Tell the relative in the privacy of your office that the patient collapsed, that everything possible was done, but to no avail. It is virtually impossible to extend too much grief and sympathy *without admitting liability*. Avoid any statement about the cause of death until you have had time to review and complete your records. Just say *sudden collapse*.
3. Have the patients in your reception room excused, with only *serious emergency* as explanation.
4. Compile a complete record — the patient's appearance, the probable cause of death, and the resuscitative efforts. It is mandatory in most states to report such a death to the coroner's office. Also, certain liability insurance carriers require that they be notified immediately of any event that could result in a claim. Sudden death in the office is a leading cause of large judgments.
5. Guard your reputation. You will have to fend off pointed questions by the deceased's relatives and friends. Silence on your part will intrigue the relatives and fortify suspicions about your possible responsibility. Repeat your shock and grief, offer sincerest sympathy, but simply say that the deceased suddenly collapsed.

Always accompany the patient to the hospital. If you are refused transportation in the emergency vehicle, proceed in another vehicle. Do not remain in the office under any circumstances.

Proper resuscitative efforts, even though ultimately unsuccessful, will usually result in transportation to the hospital while living. Do not discontinue ECPR in the office. It is also possible that the death may be certified by the emergency room physician, thus obviating the need for a coroner's report.

Preparation before the fact is the key in order to weather such a catastrophe in a proper, humane, and practical manner.

PREVENTION OF DEATH

In the general community, success in reducing the incidence of sudden death rests mainly with the individual seeking early medical assistance, with discouraging results to date. For example, despite the biennial physical examinations in the Framingham study, 50 per cent of all subjects who died suddenly had no prior clinical diagnosis of heart disease.[30] The authors concluded that the only road to a substantial reduction of coronary heart disease mortality is prevention of coronary heart disease.

All is not gloom, however. Coronary care ambulances have shown great promise. In one study, highly motivated ambulance personnel were trained so that they achieved a high degree of accuracy in ECG interpretation, and by persistent vigorous ECPR combined with defibrillation were able to salvage seven out of 14 patients, all of whom were subsequently discharged from the hospital.[31]

In the dental community, a high degree of success in the prevention of sudden death during dental treatment can be achieved. Three areas of primary importance include proper physical evaluation before therapy, adequate pain/anxiety control, and knowledgeable treatment of medical emergencies by a team composed of the doctor and assistants.

COMMENT

The incidence of sudden, unexpected death is so high that a significant number of such deaths can and do occur coincidentally in the dental office or soon after treatment. Furthermore, since most primary causes of sudden, unexpected death can be influenced by physical or emotional stress, it is probable that such deaths in the dental office could be secondarily related to treatment stress. This is strong justification for adequate pain/anxiety control for dental patients who are in apparent good heatlh, and is obvious justification for an in-depth grasp of the prevention, recognition, and treatment of life-threatening emergencies.

REFERENCES

1. Vital Statistics Report — Annual Summary for the United States, 1970. Rockville, Maryland, U.S. Public Health Service, 1970, p. 3.
2. Doyle, J. T.: Mechanisms and prevention of sudden death. Mod. Conc. Cardiov. Dis., 45:111–116, 1976.
3. Friedman, M., et al.: Instantaneous and sudden deaths. J.A.M.A., 225:1319–1328, 1973.
4. Editorial: Sudden death — a new syndrome. J.A.M.A., 230:1018, 1974.
5. Lynch, H. T., et al.: Hereditary progressive atrioventricular conduction defect — a new syndrome. J.A.M.A., 225:1465–1470, 1973.
6. Burch, G. E., and Giles, T. D.: The burden of a hot and humid environment on the heart. Mod. Conc. Cardiov. Dis., 39:115–120, 1970.
7. Goldman, V., Los Angeles Times, July 24, 1970.
8. Drummond-Jackson, S. L.: A tragic story. Newsletter SAAD, 2:195, 1974.
9. Hockwald, R. S.: Can emotional stress cause atherosclerosis? J.A.M.A., 218:1308, 1971.
10. Peterson, D. R., et al.: Ischemic heart disease prognosis, a community wide assessment (1966–1969). J.A.M.A., 219:1423–1427, 1972.
11. Mann, G. V.: Diet–heart: end of an era. New Engl. J. Med., 297:644–650, 1977.
12. Kannel, W. B., et al.: Precursors of sudden coronary death. Circulation, 51:606–613, 1975.
13. Jude, J. R., and Nagel, E. L.: Cardiopulmonary resuscitation 1970. Mod. Conc. Cardiov. Dis., 39:133–139, 1970.
14. Gillum, R. F., et al.: Delay in the prehospital phase of acute myocardial infarction. Arch. Intern. Med., 136:649–654, 1976.
15. Feinleib, M., and Davidson, M. J.: Coronary heart disease mortality. J.A.M.A., 222:1129–1134, 1972.
16. Walker, W. J.: Coronary mortality: what is going on. J.A.M.A., 227:1045–1046, 1974.

17. Burch, G. E.: A reappraisal of coronary care units. Resident & Staff Physician, 5:51–54, 1977.
18. Lown, B., and Verrier, R. L.: Neural activity and ventricular fibrillation, New Engl. J. Med., 294:1165–1170, 1976.
19. Tarhan, S., et al.: Myocardial infarction after general anesthesia. J.A.M.A., 220:1451–1454, 1972.
20. Jenkins, M. T.: Anesthesiology. J.A.M.A., 211:282–285, 1970.
21. Driscoll, E. J.: ASOS anesthesia morbidity and mortality survey. J. Oral Surg., 32:733–738, 1974.
22. Lytle, J. J.: Anesthesia morbidity and mortality survey of the Southern California Society of Oral Surgeons. J. Oral Surg., 32:739–744, 1974.
23. Tomlin, P. J.: Death in outpatient dental anesthetic practice. Anaesthesia, 29:551, 1974.
24. Beecher, H. K., and Todd, D. P.: A Study of Deaths Associated with Anesthesia and Surgery. Springfield, Charles C Thomas, 1954, p. 43.
25. Mannix, A. J.: Medicolegal implications of operating room deaths. New York J. Med., 60:683, 1960.
26. Vacanti, C., et al.: A statistical analysis of the relationship of physical status to postoperative mortality in 68,388 cases. Anesth. Analg., 49:564–566, 1970.
27. Marx, G. T., et al.: Computer analysis of postanesthetic deaths. Anesthesiology, 39:54–58, 1973.
28. McCarthy, F. M.: When your office patient dies. In Archer, W. H.: Oral and Maxillofacial Surgery. Philadelphia, W. B. Saunders Co., 1975, pp. 1544–1545.
29. Aarons, E. F.: What if a patient dies in your office. Med. Econ., 195: (Jan. 19), 1970.
30. Gordon, T., and Kannel, W. B.: Premature mortality from coronary heart disease — the Framingham study. J.A.M.A., 215:1617–1625, 1971.
31. Rose, L. B., and Press, E.: Cardiac defibrillation by ambulance attendants. J.A.M.A., 219:63–68, 1972.

2

PHYSICAL EVALUATION AND TREATMENT MODIFICATION

FRANK M. McCARTHY

PHYSICAL EVALUATION

USC PHYSICAL EVALUATION SYSTEM

SYSTEMS REVIEW

PHYSICAL EXAMINATION

PHYSICAL EVALUATION

DEFINITION

Physical evaluation in dentistry consists of the establishment of a basic medical risk factor, without necessarily reaching a definitive diagnosis, prior to dental therapy.[1]

The art and science of physical evaluation utilizes a medical history, which is usually completed by the patient, and applicable physical examination, sometimes assisted by function tests and laboratory tests. On the other hand, physical diagnosis in medicine establishes a medical diagnosis in response to a complaint and usually leads to therapy; the medical history is usually conducted verbally by the health practitioner; and a more complete physical examination may be performed. Physical evaluation and physical diagnosis are markedly similar, differing only in the degree of application of methods for general diagnosis, since medical risk factor orientation alone is the goal of the former.

There follows an outline of the various parts of physical evaluation compared to physical diagnosis:

Physical Evaluation	*Physical Diagnosis*
1. Medical history	1. Medical history
2. Physical examination	2. Physical examination
3. Function tests	3. Function tests
4. X-rays and lab tests	4. X-rays and lab tests
5. Establish physical status	5. Establish diagnosis
6. Modifications to therapy	6. Treat illness
7. Mitigate fears and anxieties	7. Mitigate fears and anxieties

INTRODUCTION

Routine physical evaluation of the patient prior to dental treatment has become a standard of care in the United States during the past 20 years. This has come about because of the increased morbidity and mortality risks with longer dental treatments, the adoption of sophisticated sedation tech-

niques, the increasing numbers of geriatric dental patients, the introduction
of external cardiopulmonary resuscitation, and the normal elevation of
standards for the public good. Proper evaluation is a legal obligation as
well as a moral responsibility. No longer is the casual question, "Are you in
good health?" considered to be an adequate pretreatment evaluation in
dentistry.

Knowledge by the dental practitioner of an effective evaluation technique is desirable because death, serious illness, and minor physical reactions may be directly related to dental treatment. Such complications are
preventable in large part by proper pretreatment evaluation.

In addition, patients consult the dental practitioner five times more frequently than the physician. This represents a marvelous opportunity for
valuable health screening and is a highly significant health service. As one
example, early detection of arterial hypertension usually allows effective
treatment, while late detection after serious damage to target organs (heart,
kidneys, brain), may represent a virtually hopeless treatment situation.

A review of 4785 consecutive medical histories at the Temple University dental clinic revealed that only 877 patients of that group had consulted a physician within the past year, 25 per cent had a chronic illness, 10.8
per cent had more than one medical problem, and 18.5 per cent were taking routine medications.[2]

GOAL OF PHYSICAL EVALUATION

The doctor's goal in evaluation is simply to determine the physical and
emotional ability of a particular patient to tolerate a specific dental procedure in comfort and relative safety. The goal is not to diagnose or treat the
medical problem, although accurate diagnoses will be achieved by the use
of a proper evaluation technique and by experience. We wish to produce
an evaluation factor by which it is determined whether we may proceed
with dental treatment in relative safety or that medical consultation is indicated before treatment.

FUNCTION OF PHYSICIAN

The function of the physician is to reach a diagnosis and treat the medical problem. When any doubt exists regarding the medical status of a
dental patient, the physician should be consulted. The physician is a vital
member of the health team, and will be more than willing to discuss dental
treatment plans as they relate to the specific medical problems of the patient. The dental practitioner has a responsibility to the patient to consult
the physician when indicated and to be guided but not directed by the
advice. The final responsibility to the dental patient cannot be equally
shared by the physician except under unusual circumstances. The practitioner should receive the physician's advice with an open mind, and should
discuss the treatment plan and anticipated problems. Most misunderstand-
ings occur as a result of lack of communication.

In most cases, consultation with the physician will result in little alteration of the treatment plan. In some cases it may be markedly altered, and in the rare instance it may be necessary to delay treatment or postpone it indefinitely. It makes little sense to rehabilitate dentally a patient with terminal cancer, nor does it make better sense to subject a high-risk cardiac patient to prolonged, stress-producing restorative dentistry. The dental doctor must be prepared to justify anything except emergency dental treatment for the high-risk patient.

EVALUATION TECHNIQUE

The evaluation technique described here is designed to be used by all practitioners, regardless of past training or experience. The general practitioner may utilize the health questionnaire only. As experience is gained, and particularly if he or she supplements knowledge by continuing education, the doctor will progress further into full evaluation of the patient. Depending on background and interest in the subject, the general practitioner may readily develop the ability to make a detailed and highly accurate judgment of the patient's physical status. I urge the doctor to reach a tentative conclusion and treatment plan following a *full* history and physical examination *before* calling the physician in consultation, rather than calling the physician at the first mention of a potential health problem. This will give the practitioner experience in evaluation and will prepare him or her to discuss the problem with knowledge and insight.

The medical history that follows can be used by all dental practitioners, regardless of type of practice. The oral surgeon is obligated to make a detailed analysis, particularly when general anesthesia is to be used; yet the general practitioner should not feel that he or she is excused from the obligation of evaluation. The risk of local analgesia or any dental treatment in a particular case may be very high; mortality reports in the general dental office support this recommendation.

MEDICAL HISTORY QUESTIONNAIRE

Synonyms or euphemisms for the medical history in dentistry have included the following terms: health questionnaire, health history, health review, and health analysis. Since the dental practitioner obtains a comprehensive though relatively brief medical history, and since it is commonly more comprehensive than the history obtained in the average medical practice, it is refreshing to observe the present trend to use of the proper term, medical history.

Every dental patient should be required to complete a medical history questionnaire. For a basic, risk-factor evaluation by the experienced practitioner, I suggest the short-form medical history taken from the 1977-78 edition of *Accepted Dental Therapeutics* (Fig. 2–1).[3] It has been kept as brief and as simple as possible in order to facilitate patient accuracy and understanding. Four of the questions apply only to the patient who is to receive general anesthesia or sedation.

HEALTH QUESTIONNAIRE

Date _____

Name _____   Address _____
        Last   First   Middle   Number & Street

City _____   State _____   Zip Code _____   Home & Business Phone _____

Age _____   Sex _____   Height _____   Weight _____   Occupation _____

Married _____   Spouse _____   Single _____

Closest Relative _____   Phone _____

If you are completing this form for another person, what is your relationship to that person?

_____

PLEASE ANSWER EACH QUESTION   CIRCLE

1. Have you been a patient in a hospital during the past 2 years?   Yes   No
2. Have you been under the care of a physician during the past 2 years?   Yes   No
3. Have you taken any kind of medicine or drugs during the past year?   Yes   No
4. Are you allergic to penicillin or any drugs or medicine?   Yes   No
5. Have you ever had any excessive bleeding requiring special treatment?   Yes   No
6. Circle any of the following which you have had:

    heart trouble   jaundice   arthritis
    congenital heart lesions   asthma   stroke
    heart murmur   cough   epilepsy
    high blood pressure   diabetes   psychiatric treatment
    anemia   tuberculosis   sinus trouble
    rheumatic fever   hepatitis

7. (Women) Are you pregnant now?   Yes   No
8. Have you had any other serious illnesses?   Yes   No

    TO BE ANSWERED ONLY BY PATIENTS RECEIVING SEDATION OR GENERAL ANESTHESIA.

9. Have you had anything to eat or drink within the last 4 hours?   Yes   No
10. Are you wearing removable dental applicances?   Yes   No
11. Are you wearing contact lenses?   Yes   No
12. Who is to drive you home today?

    a. Name _____

Reviewed by _____   Signature _____

P1-HQ1

Figure 2–1.   Short-form medical history, taken from the 1977-78 edition of *Accepted Dental Therapeutics.*

HEALTH QUESTIONNAIRE

Date _____

Name _____ Address _____
    Last   First   Middle   Number & Street

City _____ State _____ Zip Code _____ Home & Business Phone _____

Date of Birth _____ Sex _____ Height _____ Weight _____ Occupation _____

Married _____ Spouse _____ Single _____

Closest Relative _____ Phone _____

If you are completing this form for another person, what is your relationship to that person?

_____

In the following questions, circle yes or no, whichever applies. Your answers are for our records only and will be considered confidential.

1. Has there been any change in your general health within the past year .... YES   NO

2. My last physical examination was on _____

3. Are you now under the care of a physician .... YES   NO
   a. If so, what is the condition being treated _____

4. The name and address of my physician is _____
   _____
   _____
   _____

5. Have you had any serious illness or operation .... YES   NO
   a. If so, what was the illness or operation _____

6. Have you been hospitalized or had a serious illness within the past five (5) years .... YES   NO
   a. If so, what was the problem _____

7. Do you have or have you had any of the following diseases or problems.
   a. Rheumatic fever or rheumatic heart disease.. YES   NO
   b. Congenital heart lesions.. YES   NO
   c. Cardiovascular disease (heart trouble, heart attack, coronary insufficiency, coronary occlusion,
      high blood pressure, arteriosclerosis, stroke)... YES   NO
      1) Do you have pain in chest upon exertion .... YES   NO
      2) Are you ever short of breath after mild exercise.................................... YES   NO
      3) Do your ankles swell.. YES   NO
      4) Do you get short of breath when you lie down, or do you require extra pillows when you sleep ... YES   NO
   d. Allergy.. YES   NO
   e. Sinus trouble.. YES   NO
   f. Asthma or hay fever.. YES   NO
   g. Hives or a skin rash .... YES   NO
   h. Fainting spells or seizures... YES   NO
   i. Diabetes... YES   NO
      1) Do you have to urinate (pass water) more than six times a day .... YES   NO
      2) Are you thirsty much of the time .... YES   NO
      3) Does your mouth frequently become dry .... YES   NO
   j. Hepatitis, jaundice or liver disease .... YES   NO
   k. Arthritis... YES   NO
   l. Inflammatory rheumatism (painful swollen joints)... YES   NO
   m. Stomach ulcers .... YES   NO
   n. Kidney trouble .... YES   NO
   o. Tuberculosis .... YES   NO
   p. Do you have a persistent cough or cough up blood... YES   NO
   q. Low blood pressure.. YES   NO
   r. Venereal disease .... YES   NO
   s. Other _____

(over)

Figure 2–2. Long-form medical history, taken from the 1977-78 edition of *Accepted Dental Therapeutics.*

8. Have you had abnormal bleeding associated with previous extractions, surgery, or trauma .... YES   NO
   a. Do you bruise easily .... YES   NO
   b. Have you ever required a blood transfusion.. YES   NO
      If so, explain the circumstances _____

9. Do you have any blood disorder such as anemia.. YES   NO
10. Have you had surgery or x-ray treatment for a tumor, growth, or other condition of your mouth or lips .. YES   NO
11. Are you taking any drug or medicine... YES   NO
    If so, what _____

12. Are you taking any of the following:
    a. Antibiotics or sulfa drugs... YES   NO
    b. Anticoagulants (blood thinners)... YES   NO
    c. Medicine for high blood pressure.. YES   NO
    d. Cortisone (steroids).. YES   NO
    e. Tranquilizers.. YES   NO
    f. Antihistamines .... YES   NO
    g. Aspirin .... YES   NO
    h. Insulin, tolbutamide (Orinase) or similar drug.. YES   NO
    i. Digitalis or drugs for heart trouble .... YES   NO
    j. Nitroglycerin.. YES   NO
    k. Other _____

13. Are you allergic or have you reacted adversely to:
    a. Local anesthetics.. YES   NO
    b. Penicillin or other antibiotics .... YES   NO
    c. Sulfa drugs.. YES   NO
    d. Barbiturates, sedatives, or sleeping pills .... YES   NO
    e. Aspirin.. YES   NO
    f. Iodine .... YES   NO
    g. Codeine or other narcotics... YES   NO
    h. Other _____

14. Have you had any serious trouble associated with any previous dental treatment .... YES   NO
    If so, explain _____

15. Do you have any disease, condition, or problem not listed above that you think I should know about... YES   NO
    If so, explain _____

16. Are you employed in any situation which exposes you regularly to x-rays or other ionizing radiation... YES   NO
17. Are you wearing contact lenses... YES   NO

WOMEN

18. Are you pregnant .... YES   NO
19. Do you have any problems associated with your menstrual period............................... YES   NO

Remarks:

_____
SIGNATURE OF PATIENT

_____
SIGNATURE OF DENTIST

P1-HQ

Figure 2–2. Continued.

The recommended short-form medical history (now slightly modified) was created in 1956 by the six oral surgeons who originally made up the Dental Anesthesia Service, Los Angeles County/University of Southern California Medical Center, and is routinely used in their offices. The dependability of the form is attested to by their having administered a total of over 720,000 office general anesthetics through 1978 with but one contributing general anesthetic mortality (subarachnoid hemorrhage in a patient with polycythemia vera).

The long-form medical history in *Accepted Dental Therapeutics* (Fig. 2–2) is adequate for physical evaluation. It also serves as a reliable teaching aid and as an excellent departure point for physical diagnosis.[4]

A guide to a complete dialogue medical history may be seen in the chapter on *physical diagnosis*. This is a suggested form for physical diagnosis, and will not be considered further in this chapter.

OTHER QUESTIONNAIRES

Other medical history questionnaires are equally applicable. I feel, however, that a questionnaire designed primarily to produce a basic evaluation and risk factor can be entirely *too* detailed, resulting in annoyance to the patient, inattention, and inaccuracies. Some questionnaires are unnecessarily long and confusing to the patient. Although medicolegal considerations tempt the practitioner to utilize a voluminous health questionnaire, in my opinion the accuracy of a brief and simple questionnaire is in the best interests of the patient. I do not think that a highly detailed questionnaire is indicated for most purposes in other than a teaching environment, and I therefore recommend a short-form questionnaire to the experienced practitioner, to be followed by a dialogue history as indicated.

A programmed medical history was introduced in medicine in 1966,[40] followed by a programmed physical examination in 1971.[41] Such complexity is not required for our purposes.

RELIABILITY OF QUESTIONNAIRE

Well controlled surveys have shown that a self-administered medical history is reliable and readily accepted by patients. Although questionnaires are superior to the conventional dialogue history in terms of providing a recorded data base, they have not been shown to be superior with respect to initial diagnostic and therapeutic decisions. It is my feeling that the method of history-taking described in this chapter, a self-administered questionnaire followed by a dialogue history conducted by the practitioner, is the most accurate, least time consuming, and least annoying to the patient of any method to date.

Some practitioners prefer to personally make the queries directly from the questionnaire (or have the assistant do so), feeling that accuracy is enhanced. While this claim is unproven at the moment, the routine is to be recommended if time allows, as it notably improves rapport early in the treatment relationship, and gives the doctor or assistant the opportunity to explain any question that is confusing or appears to be irrelevant.

The relatively unstructured verbal inquiry has been demonstrated to be deficient compared to a structured patient-completed questionnaire.[39]

CHECKING THE QUESTIONNAIRE

It is the policy of the LAC/USC Dental Anesthesia Service to have the new patient complete the medical history questionnaire and other standard records in the reception room, after which the dental assistant reviews the questionnaire with the patient to make certain that it is complete. The patient and assistant sign the dated form, and the practitioner then has proof that the history was taken and is accurate. We do not feel that it is necessary for the doctor or assistant to personally ask the history questions, although this may be done if desired.

TIME LAPSE IN TREATMENT

When the doctor meets the patient in consultation, the medical history is reviewed and evaluation proceeds as indicated. When the patient returns to the office after a period of time, it is my custom to have the assistant ask the patient if he or she has had any health problems or is taking any medication not previously discussed. Such changes are noted on the record and initialed by the assistant. A new questionnaire is not necessary.

DIALOGUE HISTORY

The detailed, follow-up, or dialogue history is verbally conducted by the doctor after reviewing the questionnaire. This includes further specific evaluation of positive information obtained via the preliminary patient-completed form. If the medical history discloses areas for further investigation, and the doctor is unable or unwilling to proceed further, he or she should consult the patient's physician at this time. I do not believe, however, in slavish, automatic medical consultations for potentially serious diseases such as arterial hypertension and coronary heart disease when the doctor is competent through training and experience to make a proper judgment and conduct therapy in an approved manner.

To assist in continuing with a dialogue history, certain broad categories of disease will be reviewed, and questions will be suggested for their evaluation in dentistry. Only the most common relevant diseases will be covered. I have also granted myself a certain license for the purpose of describing the medical background of each disease entity. First we will review the medical consultation and an evaluation system, then proceed to systems review.

MEDICAL CONSULTATION

When indicated by physical evaluation (either abnormal history or physical findings), the dental doctor is responsible for initiating a medical consultation. Slavish, automatic consultation without good cause is *not* called for. Your responsibilities are as follows:

1. Receive the physician's advice with an open mind.
2. Be *prepared* to discuss your treatment plan and anticipated problems.
3. Do not call until after performing a *complete* physical evaluation.
4. You are solely responsible for your treatment plan and treatment risks. Responsibility can rarely be shared with the physician. If you knowingly follow incorrect advice, you are liable. The physician advises but does not direct. It is your responsibility to follow a proper standard of care.

Friction between dental doctor and medical doctor during consultation is not common, but a review of the usual causes is in order, with advice on comportment:

1. Fatigue or bad manners by either party.
2. Lack of communication skills by either party.
3. Inadequate preparation by the dental practitioner.
4. Don't argue — educate. If education of a physician is not possible, remain courteous. An argument solves nothing and is not in the best interests of the patient. Exceptionally improper behavior on the part of the physician which *materially interferes* with proper patient care may be reported to the Grievance Committee of the local medical society, if the physician is a member, or to the State Board of Medical Examiners. This action would very rarely be indicated. Be forgiving—we all have bad days.
5. Accept the physician's advice in good grace, then treat in the patient's best interests.

USC PHYSICAL EVALUATION SYSTEM

INTRODUCTION

The author conceived the University of Southern California School of Dentistry Physical Evaluation System to assist in categorizing dental patients from the standpoint of risk-factor orientation.* The system was introduced as a limited pilot program in 1975, and was adopted school-wide in 1977. Certain sections of narrative are taken from the school manual, and I have further modified the system to make it easily adaptable to the needs of private practice.

The purpose of this system is to quickly and easily place each patient in an appropriate medical-risk category and to thereby provide dental therapy in comfort and relative safety. During the original physical evaluation the patient is placed in one of four physical status classes devised by the

---

*Grateful acknowledgement is made to Dr. Stanley Malamed for his support in expanding methodology, and to the Physical Evaluation Task Force for its invaluable critique of the first draft in 1975. The task force was composed of Drs. Albert Abrams, Arlos Aduddel, Marianne Alessio, Donald Cooksey, Randy Gates, Barbara Mills, Kit Neacy, Thomas Pallasch, and Robert Ziehm.

American Society of Anesthesiologists. The physical status classification then serves as a helpful guide to the level of dental therapy, suggested management, and treatment modification for the medically compromised patient.

ASA Physical Status Classification System

In 1940 the American Society of Anesthesiologists (ASA) conceived this system to classify the physical status of a patient about to undergo general anesthesia and surgery. The system has proved to be so valuable that it is used to classify all patients prior to surgery, manipulation (casting), or diagnostic studies of any kind utilizing any type or combination of anesthesia/sedation modalities.

Table 2–1 shows the ASA system on the left; on the right are general considerations for dental therapy modification. The system is very valuable in determining relative risk prior to dental treatment and the possible need for treatment modification.

Stress Reduction

In Table 2–1 and in the systems review section to follow, stress reduction merely refers to consideration of a psychosedation modality to relieve anxiety, possibly prescribing medication for sleep the night before treatment, limiting treatment to morning hours when functional reserve is at its highest, limiting the duration of treatment, avoiding elective treatment during unusually hot and humid weather, and giving special attention to post-treatment pain/anxiety control. Stress and sudden death walk hand in hand. While stress reduction for the ASA Class I patient is surely in order if indicated, it is of paramount importance for the ASA Class II to IV patients if

TABLE 2–1

ASA Physical Status Classification	Therapy Modification
I. A normal healthy patient	None (stress reduction as indicated).
II. A patient with mild to moderate systemic disease	Possible stress reduction and other modification as indicated
III. A patient with *severe systemic disease* that *limits activity* but is not incapacitating	Possible strict modifications; stress reduction and medical consultation prioritized
IV. A patient with *severe systemic disease* that *limits activity* and is a *constant threat to life*	Minimal emergency care in office; hospitalize for complicated treatment; medical consultation urged
V. A moribund patient not expected to survive 24 hours with or without operation.	Treatment in the hospital is limited to life support only, e.g., airway and hemorrhage management

(An emergency operation is preceded by an E—e.g., E I, E IV, etc.—which is an admission that we do not have the necessary facts to make an accurate estimate of the patient's physical status).

there is the slightest indication. Please see the section on *psychosedation* for further information on pain/anxiety control.

CLASSIFICATION GUIDELINES

Guidelines for ASA classification will be given for relevant diseases under systems review. Brief examples, any *one* of which calls for ASA Class II placement, are as follows: present history of allergic rhinitis (hay fever), history of any drug allergy or hypersensitivity, history of hepatitis B that is currently antigen-positive, history of arrested pulmonary tuberculosis without disability, history of rheumatic fever with heart murmur and no disability, history of heavy smoking with chronic bronchitis, chronic pulmonary emphysema without significant disability, history of corrected congenital heart disease without disability, history of chronic glomerulonephritis or pylonephritis without disability, history of controlled arterial hypertension without disability, history of controlled diabetes mellitus without disability, history of controlled chronic glaucoma, history of possible attitudinal problems with health care (as negative experiences with prior practitioners), and history of behavioral problems with health care (as moderate to extreme anxiety). Many of the preceding diseases or conditions could become Class III or IV, depending upon the history and physical examination. Some doctors drop the patient one class if there are two or more diseases, none of which is disabling; for example, a patient with allergic rhinitis, penicillin allergy, and chronic glomerulonephritis could be placed in ASA Class III rather than Class II. This is a judgment decision and is based upon your perception of physical status related to treatment stresses.

A Class II designation noted on your patient's record is a red flag indicating that special care may be in order. It alerts the doctor and staff to the possible necessity of anxiety control, avoidance of possibly lethal drugs, possible antibiotic prophylaxis to guard against bacterial endocarditis, and so forth. The importance of a Class III or IV designation goes without saying.

It is suggested that the Table 2–2 chart be added as a permanent part of your patient records, and that the appropriate designation be circled during the original physical evaluation. This can be changed up or down as circumstances dictate. For example, a post-MI patient would be considered Class IV at three months, yet probably revert to Class III or even Class II at six months if the disease were no longer considered to be a constant threat to life, or if significant disability did not exist.

TABLE 2–2

ASA Physical Status	*Reason(s) For Status Selection*
Class – I	(Write in)
Class – II	
Class – III	
Class – IV	
(Circle appropriate class)	

In closing this section on the USC Physical Evaluation System, may I emphasize that ASA numbers cannot substitute for knowledge and good judgment. Recommended physical status categories and treatment modifications should not be considered as absolutes but merely as guides. While the guidelines may appear to be inflexible, they should not be considered so. Deviation from the recommendations is often justified and is expected.

SYSTEMS REVIEW

INTRODUCTION

Also known as system review, review of systems, inventory of systems, and systemic review, the traditional method of understanding disease is to study the diseases involving the various body systems; that is, blood, eye, heart, and other systems. By understanding disease, we are able to prevent most emergencies, and, when necessary, treat the rare life-threatening emergency that is unavoidable.

Dentistry is the most disciplined of all the health sciences. We are trained to be utter perfectionists* — witness the horror evoked by an imperfect margin or a retained root tip. Since the treatment of emergencies is admittedly peripheral to dental care (and something we could all do without), we naturally tend to search for a highly disciplined, treat-by-the-numbers approach; for example, if the patient is short of breath, administer oxygen and call the paramedics. Under such circumstances, the patient with hyperventilation syndrome may eventually desist, owing to boredom, fatigue, or muscle cramps, but the patient with advanced pulmonary emphysema may die. We treat chronic pulpitis by understanding the disease and therefore the treatment options; we do not treat symptoms *per se*. In this chapter we shall, therefore, approach prevention and recognition of emergencies by understanding the disease process. Unfortunately, there is no simple by-the-numbers or by-the-symptoms method.

My choice of systems and diseases is of necessity pragmatic. It is limited to those diseases that, in my view, are particularly relevant to oral health care and potential medical emergencies. For serious students of physical evaluation, a textbook of medicine, such as Beeson-McDermott, is recommended. It makes fascinating reading in small doses, is ideal for the insomniac and hypochondriac, and will vastly increase your skills and pleasures in the health sciences.

VIRAL DISEASES

Of general interest to the practitioner is the third most common disease known to man, the common cold (acute coryza). It is caused by at least 88 different viruses and some nonviral agents; immunity to a specific virus exists for one to two years; one is contagious for one to two days before

---

*A perfectionist is one who takes great pains in executing a task, and who produces great pain in all those involved with the task.

symptoms develop and throughout the symptom phase (nasal discharge and sneezing); repeated infections can produce chronic bronchitis and pulmonary emphysema; and the chance of contagion is 10 per cent with close contact.

Of equal general interest under viral diseases is the dental doctor who predicts measles (rubeola) in a young patient by observing Koplik's spots one to four days before the skin rash, and who will thus become known in the neighborhood as a diagnostician akin to Sir William Osler.

Other viral diseases require little comment other than the proper evaluation of residual disability, if any, following poliomyelitis or viral encephalitis. Minor motor disability would indicate ASA Class II designation, as would the patient who is hepatitis B antigen-positive (the doctor and staff requiring masking and double-gloving, and special attention being paid to sterilization).

BACTERIAL DISEASES

Again little comment is called for with this group. The doctor will not be treating patients with active bronchopneumonia, meningitis, or rheumatic fever, and he or she will be evaluating the degree of disability, if any, resulting from these diverse bacterial diseases, placing the patient in ASA Class I to IV as indicated.

One type of bacteria that merits mention is the beta-hemolytic group A streptococcus that causes up to 3 per cent rheumatic fever and 20 per cent glomerulonephritis in infected patients (throat or skin), resulting in dental management concerns. To assist in ASA placement some examples are given:

ASA Class I — history of rheumatic fever, negative for rheumatic heart disease.

ASA Class II — rheumatic heart disease, no disability.

ASA Class III — rheumatic heart disease, congestive heart failure, mild to moderate disability.

ASA Class IV — rheumatic heart disease, severe congestive heart failure, barely ambulatory.

Modification to therapy would include antibiotic prophylaxis with a history of rheumatic heart disease. ASA Class II and III would require any or all stress reduction factors mentioned under *stress reduction* during review of the USC Physical Evaluation System. An ASA Class IV patient is offered emergency office treatment only.

EYE, EAR, NOSE AND THROAT DISEASES

A past history of acute glaucoma (narrow-angle) calls for the avoidance of drugs in dental treatment that can cause dilatation of the pupil, such as atropine, scopolamine, or diazepam (Valium), and thus cause an acute attack. Untreated acute glaucoma results in permanent blindness in two to five days. Chronic glaucoma (open-angle) under medical treatment requires no special therapy modification, though the doctor should be aware that emotional stress may accentuate the disease process, and thus sedation could be considered (Valium is acceptable).

Meniere's disease is caused by dilatation of the cochlear duct at about age 40 to 60, and is marked by recurrent severe vertigo and possibly nausea and vomiting. Utilization of sedation during active episodes of the disease could further handicap the patient.

Acute maxillary sinusitis may result from acute dental infection, and sometimes is misdiagnosed as acute dental pain. Chronic maxillary sinusitis is often of dental origin, estimated at up to 70 per cent of all cases.

Acute pericoronitis associated with a partially erupted mandibular third molar is sometimes misdiagnosed by the medical doctor as acute pharyngitis, acute tonsillitis, or acute peritonsillar abscess.

FOREIGN BODIES — LARYNGEAL, BRONCHIAL, AND ESOPHAGEAL

Dental instruments, devices, and materials may act as foreign bodies, and the outcome can be lethal. The use of a rubber dam may avoid most episodes, but some are totally unavoidable.

Foreign bodies in the larynx and bronchi produce initial coughing and respiratory distress, and possibly complete obstruction of the airway with asphyxia. With a bronchial foreign body, the initial coughing is followed by a "silent" period of hours, months, or years, then obstruction or inflammation occurs, with cough, atelectasis (lung collapse), wheezing, and bronchopneumonia. See Chapters 17 and 19 for treatment of laryngeal and bronchial foreign bodies by the *Heimlich maneuver* and for treatment of laryngeal foreign bodies by *cricothyrotomy* should the Heimlich maneuver fail. Direct laryngoscopy in the hospital could be necessary for either of these types of foreign bodies.

Esophageal foreign bodies cause initial coughing, gagging, and pain, with subsidence of symptoms if the foreign body reaches the stomach. Perforation of the esophagus during passage or by retention of the foreign body in the esophagus may lead to mediastinal infection, which has a 50 per cent mortality rate.

If there is the slightest question of a foreign body, immediate x-rays should be taken to determine location, after which competent medical advice should be followed.

Depending upon circumstances, any one of these three foreign bodies could place the patient temporarily (or permanently) in ASA Class II to V.

BRONCHOPULMONARY DISEASES
Terms

A review of common terms is in order prior to a review of this section.

Dyspnea – shortness of breath, difficult or labored breathing; further subdivided into exertional dyspnea and rest dyspnea; rest dyspnea is characteristic of congestive heart failure, while exertional dyspnea is characteristic of either pulmonary emphysema or congestive heart failure.

Orthopnea — difficulty in breathing except in the upright position (sitting or standing); characteristic of congestive heart failure.

Cough — the most common symptom of respiratory disease, representing inflammation of one or more areas from the oropharynx to the terminal bronchioles; may be dry or productive; a paroxysmal cough suggests bronchial obstruction, such as productive bronchitis, emphysema, tumor, bronchopneumonia, bronchiectasis, lung abscess, or foreign body.

Expectoration — mucoid (white) sputum, tracheobronchitis and bronchial asthma; purulent sputum (yellow or green), bacterial infection; foul-smelling sputum, anaerobic infection, lung abscess; pink, frothy sputum, acute pulmonary edema, characteristic of advanced congestive heart failure.

Wheezing — occurs during *expiration* only, characteristic of bronchial narrowing; forced expiration or expiration after exercise may produce wheezing that is normally absent; the wheezing of bronchial asthma is paroxysmal; localized wheezing indicates local bronchial obstruction.

Chest Pain — the lung and visceral pleura (pleura covering lung surface) are insensitive to pain; the pain of lung disease is due to involvement of parietal pleura (pleura covering chest wall) or the chest wall itself; cardiac pain is usually substernal (precordial), and may radiate.

Hemoptysis — coughing of blood may occur with bronchitis, tuberculosis, tumor, and bronchiectasis; fatal hemorrhage is rare.

Cyanosis — blue skin color due to reduced hemoglobin in blood over 5 gm per 100 ml; normal adult hemoglobin is 12 to 18 gm per 100 ml; in the patient who is severely anemic, cyanosis may not occur even as a terminal sign.

Bronchiectasis

Bronchiectasis is much less common due to the early treatment of pneumonia, pertussis, and tuberculosis. It is caused by chronic dilatation of smaller bronchi and terminal bronchioles, with dependent pooling of pus. There is a very productive, purulent cough; rales and rhonchi are heard over the lung bases on auscultation; diagnosis is by bronchogram, which demonstrates bronchial dilatations.

A rale is a sound produced by air moving through liquid in the bronchus or lung. A rhonchus is a coarse, very loud rale heard over a partially obstructed bronchus.

ASA classification of bronchiectasis will be discussed under functional reserve classification of congestive heart failure. If the disease is particularly active and the body temperature is 101°F or higher, drop to the next lower ASA class (see temperature discussion under Vital Signs). Follow therapy modifications in Table 2–1; for the ASA Class II or III bronchiectatic patient, oxygen therapy during dental treatment is beneficial (such as 3 L/min via nasal cannula).

Pulmonary Emphysema

Heredity and smoking are major causative factors in pulmonary emphysema. There may be a hereditary defect in pulmonary elastic tissue, or the disease may be secondary to chronic bronchial obstruction (acute or chronic bronchitis, bronchial asthma, silicosis).

The pathologic physiology is twofold. First, the lung is made up of millions of tiny air sacs (pulmonary alveoli) where gas exchange occurs — oxygen in, carbon dioxide out. If these pulmonary alveoli were laid flat, they would cover the surface of a tennis court. The healthy individual therefore has the square footage of a tennis court for essential gas exchange. In emphysema the walls (septa) between alveoli break down; hundreds and even thousands of pulmonary alveoli form larger chambers, and the square footage for gas exchange markedly decreases. The individual with moderate emphysema may have the alveolar membrane square footage of one fourth of a tennis court; the person with advanced emphysema has far less. Shortness of breath results. Secondly, the elasticity of the smaller bronchi and terminal bronchioles is impaired. On expiration, the bronchi and bronchioles collapse, and the air in the larger air sacs cannot be expelled. We therefore have a patient with greatly reduced lung tissue for gas exchange, plus trapping of oxygen-deficient waste gases in the lungs.

The characteristics of pulmonary emphysema are:

1.   Diffuse distention and over-aeration of alveoli.
2.   Loss of intra-alveolar septa.
3.   Loss of pulmonary elasticity.
4.   Partial obstruction of smaller bronchi.
5.   Impaired pulmonary function.

Exertional dyspnea and chronic productive cough are the primary symptoms and signs of emphysema. Their onset is insidious and is usually not noticed until the disease is moderately advanced. There are frequent intercurrent respiratory infections (bronchitis, bronchopneumonia), which may prove to be fatal. A barrel chest develops late in the disease; the chest becomes fixed in the inspiratory position. Prolonged, wheezing expirations are noted. Late in the disease, accessory muscles of respiration (shoulders, neck) are used. At this time a chest x-ray will demonstrate overaerated lung fields and a flattened diaphragm from lung expansion in the inspiratory position.

Emphysema can be differentiated from congestive heart failure and bronchial asthma by history and examination.

Function tests such as timed forced expiratory volume, match test, and breath-holding test are discussed under Physical Examination in this chapter. They will allow you to make an accurate estimate of the physical status of your emphysema patient. ASA classification will be reviewed under *functional reserve classification* of congestive heart failure.

Follow therapy modifications in Table 2–1, and stress reduction as indicated. Oxygen therapy is beneficial during dental treatment for the ASA Class II and III emphysema patient (3 L/min via nasal cannula). Respiratory cripples are ASA Class IV (rest dyspnea), and only minimal emergency care should be provided in the office. *Oxygen therapy is not indicated,* unless you are trained in advanced life support and are able to supply 30 per cent oxygen in the inspired air. Patients with advanced emphysema tolerate a very high arterial carbon dioxide tension. When the administration of 100 per cent oxygen lowers the carbon dioxide tension, breathing may cease, and artificial ventilation may be required.

Bronchial Asthma

This is marked by *paroxysmal* attacks of expiratory wheezing, dyspnea, cough, and production of mucoid sputum, and is caused by reversible bronchial constriction (constriction with emphysema is *not* reversible); rales and expiratory wheezing are heard on auscultation. The extrinsic type is responsible for 50 per cent of the cases (allergy; antigen-antibody response), and 50 per cent are intrinsic (response to infection, exercise, irritating inhalants, emotional stress).

Stress during dental treatment is also a factor in the extrinsic type, and many asthmatic episodes in the dental operatory, whether extrinsic or intrinsic in origin, can be rapidly controlled by moving the patient from the operatory, or can be prevented by adequate sedation.

ASA Class II is proper for most asthmatics. Stress reduction is in order. An asthmatic will temporarily become an ASA Class III during an attack. Progression to ASA Class IV is rare (status asthmaticus), but sudden death is remotely possible under these circumstances.

CARDIOVASCULAR DISEASES

Terms

Atrium — one of a pair of smaller cavities of the heart, from which blood passes to the ventricles. The right atrium receives systemic venous blood; the left atrium receives pulmonary venous blood.

Ventricle — one of a pair of larger cavities of the heart, with thick muscular walls. The right ventricle propels blood through the lungs; the left ventricle propels blood through the systemic arterial system.

Paroxysmal nocturnal dyspnea — sudden, severe nocturnal dyspnea occurring in the supine position, characteristic of acute congestive heart failure.

Palpitation — patient awareness of a rapid or irregular heart beat. The term is not pleural, though lay people usually make it so (palpitations).

Edema — accumulation of *intercellular* fluid.

Heart Failure: Pathologic Physiology

The heart is a complex pump that can suffer from disease for years before failing in its function of delivering an adequate supply of blood to body tissues.

The heart fails in three common ways:

1. A portion of heart muscle supplied by a diseased coronary artery may become ischemic (not necrotic) and temporarily lose its contractile ability while the heart still delivers an adequate supply of blood to other body tissues. This is the clinical syndrome of angina pectoris and does not represent systemic failure.

2. With cardiac standstill or ventricular fibrillation (both called cardiac ar-

rest), there is immediate syncope and the patient dies. See Chapter 14, on *cardiopulmonary arrest*.

3. More commonly, the diseased heart loses it ability to effectively pump blood to peripheral tissues, resulting in the slow development of the clinical picture called congestive heart failure.

Failure of circulation occurs when the heart is unable to pump sufficient blood for body needs. The heart may be unable to pump out blood returned to it by the great veins (heart failure), or venous return may be inadequate (peripheral circulatory failure; see Shock in Chapter 16, on *general anesthetic emergencies*).

The clinical picture of heart failure is produced by:

1. Inadequate blood supply to peripheral tissues (forward heart failure).
2. Inadequate venous drainage of peripheral tissues, with accumulation of excess blood in tissues and organs (backward heart failure).

Forward and backward heart failure must occur together, but the signs and symptoms of congestion (backward heart failure) are clinically more evident.

The amounts of blood pumped from the left and right heart are normally identical. When left ventricular output is decreased by disease, right ventricular output overloads the pulmonary vascular bed and the lungs become congested and edematous. This is called left heart failure. When right ventricular output is decreased, the left ventricular output overloads the peripheral vascular bed and there are signs of systemic congestion and edema. This is called right heart failure. Clinically, right and left heart failure usually occur together, but the signs and symptoms of either pulmonary venous congestion (left heart failure) or systemic venous congestion (right heart failure) may predominate. The clinical syndrome of congestive heart failure includes both right and left heart failure.

In patients with *predominant left heart failure*, congestion is mainly in the lungs whereas in patients with *predominant right heart failure*, congestion occurs in the abdominal viscera and lower extremities, observed as peripheral venous distention (jugular vein distention), hepatomegaly (enlarged liver), ascites (fluid in peritoneal cavity, with abdominal distention), and peripheral edema (pitting edema of ankles).[5]

Compensatory mechanisms in heart disease include concentric hypertrophy of the heart (larger contractile cells) and dilatation of the heart (increased fiber length). Both of these mechanisms increase the force of contraction.

The treatment of congestive heart failure includes rest (decreases heart load), diet (bland, low caloric, salt restricted), digitalis, and diuresis (eliminate excess fluids).

Congestive Heart Failure

This is known also as heart failure or cardiac decompensation. The patient with a failing heart represents one of the commonest risks treated in the dental office.

The main symptoms and signs of congestive heart failure (CHF) are dyspnea (shortness of breath) and undue fatigue. For our purposes, evaluation by degree of dyspnea and fatigue is exceptionally accurate.

Other causes of exertional dyspnea include advanced age, debility, poor physical conditioning (indolence), obesity, chronic pulmonary disease, ascites from any cause, advanced pregnancy, and bronchial asthma.

The term *undue fatigue* may appear rather general for specific evaluation application, but it must be remembered that the usual case of chronic congestive heart failure has been developing for months or years before obvious symptoms and signs appear. For months or years the nutritional requirements of the patient's vital organs and skeletal muscles have not been completely satisfied. For months or years the intercostal muscles have labored to move wet, congested lungs. Although this patient may not present with the classic complaints of exertional dyspnea, paroxysmal nocturnal dyspnea, and orthopnea, he or she will tire easily with little exertion, thus making undue fatigue a most important clinical sign in evaluation.

The *clinical picture* of congestive heart failure results from diverse varieties of heart *disease*, such as congenital, rheumatic, and coronary heart disease (ischemic heart disease), arterial hypertension, certain cardiac arrhythmias, pericarditis, myocarditis, endocarditis, and aortic aneurysm. Most of these specific diseases do not require individual discussion with respect to either physical evaluation or emergency treatment. Some will be covered where applicable in Chapter 3, Physical Diagnosis, and the reader may consult a textbook of medicine for detailed background.

EVALUATION OF CHF

Here are some recommended questions in the evaluation of congestive heart failure:

1. Can you carry on your usual normal activities without shortness of breath or undue fatigue?
Comment: Represents a good risk if other points are negative. No point in evaluation is more important than the fact that the functional capacity of the patient allows him or her to carry on normal activities.

There is a marked mortality increase from congestive heart failure and myocardial infarction associated with recent significant life changes, such as recent serious illness, loss of a job, health or marital concerns, and death or divorce of a spouse.[6] Such a history would merit temporarily dropping the patient one ASA physical status classification, as from ASA Class II to III or ASA Class III to IV.

During your queries about dyspnea, specifically inquire into possible dyspnea occurring after *climbing one flight of stairs*. This gives more valuable information than a general inquiry about exertional dyspnea.[7] See also the following functional reserve classification in this section.

2. Can you climb a flight of stairs without resting?
Comment: Good risk if other points are negative. In past years in dentistry this question was virtually the only evaluation by the practitioner prior to inhalation anesthesia. The mortality record was excellent.

3. Do your ankles swell as the day progresses?
Comment: Compensatory mechanism in chronic right heart failure (systemic venous congestion).

4. Have you ever awakened at night short of breath?
Comment: Known as paroxysmal nocturnal dyspnea, a serious symptom; the result of acute left heart failure with pulmonary edema. Consultation with physician advised.

5. Must you remain in a sitting position in order to breathe comfortably?
Comment: Known as orthopnea (the inability to breathe in comparative comfort except in the upright position); a serious symptom; compensatory mechanism to confine

pulmonary edema to the lung bases and to keep ventilatory capacity at a maximum. Consultation recommended.

6. How many pillows do you use for breathing comfort while sleeping?
Comment: Two or three pillows indicate orthopnea.

7. Have you had a recent large weight gain?
Comment: May indicate rapid fluid accumulation and onset of acute failure. This patient will present with swollen ankles and legs and possibly with a distended abdomen. Consultation recommended.

8. Are you taking medication?
Comment: If taking a diuretic, suspect chronic heart failure. If taking digitalis or a digitalis glycoside (Digoxin, Digitoxin, Lanoxin, etc.), you may assume an episode of failure past or present. Digitalis increases the contractile force of the heart whether it is in frank failure or not. See the chapter on *drugs*. If the patient has resumed normal activities since digitalization, and other points are negative, the failure is compensated and the patient is a good risk.

The following functional reserve classification is an aid in determining the current cardiovascular status in cardiac failure cases and is of assistance in dental treatment planning. This classification is also helpful when there is a history of pulmonary disease, such as lung abscess, tuberculosis, emphysema, bronchial asthma, and bronchiectasis.

This classification system has been in use by the Dental Anesthesia Service at LAC/USC Medical Center since 1956. It correlates exactly with the ASA physical status classification system; that is, FR Class 2 becomes ASA Class II, FR Class 3 becomes ASA Class III, and FR Class 4 becomes ASA Class IV for the purpose of categorizing congestive heart failure. The same correlation is correct with respect to dyspnea and undue fatigue for the purpose of ASA classification of the bronchiectatic or emphysematous patient.

Follow Table 2–1 for therapy modification of congestive heart failure; further recommendations follow.

FUNCTIONAL RESERVE CLASSIFICATION (MCCARTHY)

Class 1. No dyspnea or undue fatigue with normal exertion.

Class 2. Mild dyspnea or fatigue with exertion; may rest at the top of a flight of stairs.
Comment: Assuming that other points are negative, both Classes 1 and 2 represent good risks for all dental treatment. If the Class 2 patient is quite apprehensive, consider sedation to reduce emotional and physical stress. See the chapters on *psychosedation*.

Class 3. Dyspnea or undue fatigue with normal activities; comfortable at rest in any position; may have a tendency toward orthopnea, and may have a history of paroxysmal nocturnal dyspnea; rests before reaching the top of a flight of stairs.
Comment: This patient represents a definite risk; consultation is recommended. Sedation during dental treatment is strongly recommended. Keep appointments short; do not carry treatment to the limit of tolerance. Avoid elective treatment during hot and humid weather unless your office is air-conditioned. Cardiac output of 20 to 30 liters per minute (normal resting output varies from 3 to 4.5 liters per minute) may be required by thermal regulatory demands.

Class 4. Dyspnea, orthopnea, and undue fatigue at all times. The patient will rest on numerous occasions when climbing a flight of stairs, if he or she is able to negotiate them at all.
Comment: A serious risk; only emergency dental treatment should be considered. The patient's physician should be in attendance if possible, or at least within call. Oxygen therapy throughout treatment should be considered.

Coronary Heart Disease

Coronary heart disease (CHD) is a clinical entity presenting as either angina pectoris or acute myocardial infarction. It is related entirely to marked narrowing (at least one third of normal) or complete occlusion of a coronary artery lumen. With the rare exception of syphilitic aortitis, the pathologic entity of coronary heart disease or ischemic heart disease is coronary atherosclerosis, thus accounting for the common clinical term of coronary atherosclerotic heart disease (CAHD).

ANGINA PECTORIS

Angina pectoris is also known as paroxysmal cardiac pain and as anginal syndrome. This patient represents a considerably greater risk than the average case of heart failure. There is at least a 30 per cent higher mortality rate than the average. You must remember that the attack can become irreversible, proceeding to acute myocardial infarction and possibly death.

The cause of angina pectoris is temporary lack of oxygen (ischemia) in the heart muscle, related to narrowing of the coronary arteries, increased cardiac output (exertion, excitement, meals), and increased work load (as with rheumatic/valvular heart disease and arterial hypertension).

The patient will have a history of recurrent attacks of precordial (substernal) pain, varying from mild to severe. There is often radiation of pain to the left shoulder or arm; infrequently to the right shoulder and back. The pain often is precipitated by exertion, anger, emotional stress, anxiety, or meals, and usually is relieved by rest in less than 15 minutes. It usually is not the intense, crushing pain of acute myocardial infarction. The patient usually has taken nitroglycerin for relief of pain. Consultation with the patient's physician regarding the planned dental treatment may be desirable.

The history may indicate a recent significant life change (see comment under congestive heart failure), in which event the risk is increased.[6] Certain factors in your dialogue history of angina pectoris are of great discriminatory value: the risk is increased if anginal pain is incompletely relieved by nitroglycerin, if there is a frequent relationship of anginal pain to exertion, and if there is radiation of pain to the left arm.[8] There is real diagnostic value in inquiring into possible precordial pain related to *climbing a flight of stairs*, rather than a general question about chest pain.[7]

ASA Classification of Angina Pectoris

The following classification is recommended. It is modified by the author from the New York Heart Association Classification of Angina Pectoris.

ASA Class II: *Ordinary physical activity does not cause angina.* Angina may occur with *strenuous* or *prolonged* exertion or with sexual relations. Angina may occur with rapid walking, walking uphill, or climbing stairs rapidly, or by walking more than two blocks on the level or climbing more than one flight of stairs at a normal pace.

ASA Class III: *Marked limitation of ordinary physical activity.* Angina may occur by walking one or two blocks on the level or climbing one flight of stairs at a normal pace. Comfortable at rest.

ASA Class IV: *Inability to carry on any physical activity without discomfort*. Angina may be present at rest.

Therapy modification should follow Table 2–1 and *stress reduction* recommendations previously covered, as well as the following protocol.

Recommended Management of the Angina Patient

1. Routine sedation is strongly advised. See the *psychosedation* chapters. These patients do not tolerate emotional stress well.
2. Make every effort to achieve effective local analgesia; use the proper injection technique as outlined in the chapter on *complications from local analgesia*.
3. Premedicate with nitroglycerin sublingually about five minutes before starting local analgesia. Use the patient's supply of nitroglycerin if possible. A significant number of angina patients (estimated at up to 10 per cent) will exhibit a paradoxical reaction to nitroglycerin when taken in a dosage higher than they normally find effective, and an anginal attack will ensue. If the patient is not carrying his or her usual supply, use nitroglycerin in the dosage of .30 mg (1/200 gr). I do not recommend that the higher dosage forms of nitroglycerin, .45 mg (1/150 gr) and .60 mg (1/100 gr), be stocked. The smallest dose of .15 mg (1/400 gr) is rarely utilized. Nitroglycerin should be replaced six months after the bottle is opened, as it deteriorates.
4. Keep the procedure as short as possible, and make every effort to avoid reaching the limit of tolerance.
5. Remember that the average angina patient's risk level is about the same as that of the cardiac patient in Class 3 functional reserve (ASA Class III).
6. If the patient has daily episodes of chest pain, especially associated with meals, exertion, or emotional stress, consider him or her to be a serious risk. Emergency dental treatment only is recommended (ASA Class IV).

Nitroglycerin: Action, Prophylaxis, and Potency

Only one mechanism for increasing oxygen supply to the heart muscle on demand is of significance, and that is augmentation of blood flow in the coronary arteries. The capacity of the normal coronary circulation to *dilate* and maintain flow is so great that even with prolonged hypotension, infarction is rare.[9]

Nitroglycerin (TNG) dramatically improves the regional perfusion of an ischemic portion of heart muscle while not affecting total coronary flow.[10] It also produces general venous dilatation, which results in a decreased cardiac work load. TNG significantly increases exercise tolerance when taken prophylactically.[11] Long-acting nitrites have not proven more effective than TNG, and there is some doubt that they are equally effective.[9] TNG improves the exercise performance of patients with coronary heart disease, markedly decreasing the frequency of arrhythmias.[12]

TNG is unstable when stored or dispensed improperly.[13, 14, 15] In a study by Edelman,[15] loss of potency at 201 days was less than 5 per cent when tablets were stored in amber or clear glass vials; over the same time period up to 30 per cent loss of potency occurred with polystyrene vials, and 72 per cent loss with polystyrene pillboxes; there was up to 90 per cent loss with individual strip packaging (often used in hospital clinics). Nitroglycerin should be stored, dispensed, and maintained in tightly sealed glass vials, and should never be transferred to pillboxes.[16]

Fresh nitroglycerin produces immediate sublingual burning and a greater systemic effect, while aged TNG produces absent or decreased burning and decreased systemic effect. The burning sensation is a practical index of potency.[17]

ACUTE MYOCARDIAL INFARCTION

Acute myocardial infarction is also known as coronary occlusion and coronary thrombosis or as a "coronary." This patient, as with the anginal case, represents at least a 30 per cent greater mortality risk than the average. About 75 per cent of myocardial infarctions are caused by coronary thrombosis. Infarction may develop in the absence of fresh coronary occlusion, and coronary artery thrombosis can occur without necessarily causing infarction. In the first instance, coronary circulation may be so deficient that coagulation necrosis (infarction) occurs without complete occlusion of the coronary artery; in the latter instance, even in the presence of complete coronary artery occlusion, acquired collateral circulation may be sufficient to prevent infarction.

Recently it has been suggested that coronary thrombosis is the result rather than the cause of infarction. However, substantial evidence supports the classical concept of the primary causal role of coronary thrombosis in the pathogenesis of myocardial infarction.[18]

Long-term survival of the post-MI patient is related to the presence of other chronic diseases and to the presence or absence of angina related to exertion, congestive heart failure, and left ventricular hypertrophy (ECG interpretation). Complete clinical and ECG recovery is compatible with survival for 10 to 15 years. Patients with residual CHF following MI usually die within one to five years.

At onset, symptoms of acute myocardial infarction are similar to those of angina pectoris, but the precordial (substernal) pain is not relieved by nitrites or rest, and dyspnea and weakness are common. Most post-infarction patients will be able to supply you with the proper diagnosis during your dialogue history. If they are not aware of a diagnosis, it is easily established by reviewing the history of the heart problem. In addition to the foregoing, there usually will be a history of hospitalization followed by some weeks or months of inactivity at home. Consultation with the physician is desirable prior to treatment planning.

While it is generally accepted that coronary atherosclerotic heart disease is the primary cause of myocardial infarction, a recent explanation for the Prinzmetal type of variant angina pectoris emphasizes the risk factor of emotional stress.[19, 20] Variant angina occurs at rest and without severe fixed coronary stenosis. It is due to coronary arterial spasm,[20] and is relieved by nitroglycerin. Sir William Osler predicted the cause of this variant type in 1910. Paul Dudley White emphasized the basic risk factor related to stress in the highly nervous sensitive individual, and he predicted that this type of coronary artery disease, as opposed to atherosclerosis, may become more common in these stressful days.[19] The proof of coronary arterial spasm related to stress demonstrates the value of sedation for the anginal or post-MI patient.

ASA Classification for Post-Myocardial Infarction Patient. Any documented MI of less than six months duration is automatically ASA Class IV. A post-MI patient beyond six months who has no current history of angina and whose history and physical is otherwise negative is ASA Class II. Utilize the previously recommended ASA classification of angina pectoris for your further classification of the post-MI patient, related to angina and degree of exertion.

It is emphasized that post-MI patients often develop congestive heart failure (CHF). In fact, CHF is one of the common complications of MI during the acute phase, along with shock and cardiac arrest. If your post-MI patient appears to be ASA Class II, yet the CHF functional reserve classification also places him or her in ASA Class II, then drop to ASA Class III.

Therapy modification follows Table 2–1, with emphasis upon stress reduction and the following protocol. No patient is a more likely candidate for sudden death in the dental office than the post-MI patient under stressful treatment.

Epinephrine.   The use of epinephrine in dental local analgesic solutions continues to cause confusion despite the fact that clear guidelines from the New York Heart Association and latterly the American Heart Association (AHA) have existed for almost 30 years. While the subject will be examined in several other areas of this book, let me say now that the AHA states that there is no hazard for a cardiac patient if not more than .04 mg of epinephrine is utilized at a single dental appointment. You may use two 2.0 ml cartridges at a concentration of epinephrine 1:100,000, and four cartridges at 1:200,000. This guideline assumes proper instrumentation and technique, and it applies both to the post-MI and anginal patient. Please see review in Chapter 15, Complications from Local Analgesia, for detailed information.

Recommended Management of the Post-Myocardial Infarction Patient. Routine management of the post-infarction patient exactly duplicates management of the anginal patient, with three exceptions:

1. Routine premedication with nitroglycerin is open to debate, and therefore is not recommended. However, it is definitely recommended if the patient has current episodes of angina pectoris. Dosage forms are the same as in angina.

Recent reports have suggested that TNG might reduce the degree of ischemic injury in some patients during the acute phase of MI.[21] It has not been proven, however, and since TNG can produce severe hypotension (quickly reversed with leg elevation), particularly in patients not in left ventricular failure, it is not recommended as prophylaxis in the post-MI patient at this time.

2. Do not perform any elective dental treatment for the post-infarction patient for at least six months after the attack. It takes that long for these patients to heal and stabilize. The ban on elective dental care includes dental prophylaxis and minor restorative procedures, even though conducted in a hospital dental department and with the attending physician's approval. The post-infarction patient is extremely intolerant of stress early in the recovery period, and the hospital environment does not provide an umbrella of safety to prevent a recurrent infarction or possibly a fatal dysrhythmia.

3. If the patient is taking an anticoagulant (heparin, dicumarol, Coumadin, Hedulin, etc.), and many post-infarction patients do so for a time after the attack, dental treatment during which even mild bleeding may occur should be avoided until his or her status has been discussed with the physician.

Anticoagulant Therapy Post-MI.   At present, exodontia is frequently performed at a prothrombin level of 20 to 30 per cent, so that the anticoagulant will not have to be withdrawn and thus subject the patient to possible recurrent coronary thrombosis. The surgical routine includes the following, as indicated: hemostatic socket dressing, multiple sutures, intraoral pressure dressings, ice packs, avoidance of mouth rinses and drinking straws, and a soft diet for 48 hours. Hospitalization is not necessary in the usual case. Menadione (vitamin K) under the direction of the physician may be necessary if these measures are not effective in controlling bleeding. There is no clinically demonstrable risk of rebound thromboembolism from use of vitamin K. See the chapters on *drugs* and *hemorrhage* for further views.

Anticoagulant therapy may reduce the death rate during the first three years after infarction. Survival rates of anticoagulant treated and untreated post-infarction patients converge after the third year, and by the fifth year there is no difference in survival of treated and untreated groups.

Recent studies show that anticoagulants are effective in lowering morbidity in the first weeks after MI, particularly the incidence of thromboembolic complications in patients at high risk, as those with CHF, marked obesity, and severe varicosities.[22] When close follow-up of the patient cannot be maintained, the risk of hemorrhage may outweigh the possible benefit. Another study has shown no reinfarction risk when anticoagulant therapy is discontinued.[23]

CORONARY ARTERY SURGERY AND THE BYPASS PATIENT

Coronary artery bypass surgery has become increasingly popular, 50,000 operations having been performed in 1974 alone. While both enthusiastic and pessimistic positions are taken, there is no doubt that the procedure improves the quality of life by relieving symptoms.[24] It remains to be firmly established whether coronary bypass operations improve long-term survival.[25]

Several of Corday's conclusions on the status of bypass surgery will be repeated in part for your general information:[24]

1. Coronary bypass surgery relieves angina.
2. Life expectancy appears increased in the subgroups of *impending infarction* and *high-risk lesions* (italics mine).
3. Because the life expectancy of patients with stable angina pectoris is relatively good, coronary bypass should be reserved for those patients with *uncontrollable angina* (italics mine).
4. Because the long-term fate of the saphenous vein or the intrinsic coronary arteries following the bypass is not yet known, the operation *cannot be considered a prophylactic procedure* (italics mine).

ASA physical status classification of the patient who has had coronary bypass surgery would depend upon the history and probable medical consultation. ASA Class II designation would be uncommon but possible, ASA Class III probable, and ASA Class IV possible.

Management of the bypass patient would follow Table 2–1 and the anginal and post-MI recommendations, as indicated. There is no special protocol. If antibiotic prophylaxis is advised by the physician, no harm should be done; such a routine is not a standard of care at this time. There need be no time delay for elective dental care following bypass surgery, subject to the physician's advice.

CARDIAC PACEMAKERS

There are two types of cardiac pacemakers: the fixed-rate type (asynchronous), which stimulates the heart continuously at a predetermined rate, and the demand type (synchronous), which stimulates the heart only when the rate varies from a predetermined norm. Most pacemakers are of the demand type. The fixed-rate pacemaker is less sensitive to disturbance.[26] Electromagnetic radiation can inhibit the normal function of demand-type pacemakers. Simon states that fixed-rate pacemakers are influenced only by very intense electromagnetic fields, and that no precautions are necessary in the dental office other than the avoidance of electrosurgery, or, when necessary, using it for short bursts (one second or less) spaced 10 or more seconds apart.[27] When the demand pacemaker is inhibited by external electromagnetic energy, the unit reverts to a fixed-rate mode; normal operations resume when the patient moves from the electromagnetic field. Improvements in pacemaker circuitry and design have lessened the risk.

No firm guidelines exist at this time for the conduct of dental therapy in the patient with a demand-type pacemaker. Simon's recommendations will be reviewed in part for your information:[27]

1. The type of pacemaker should be recorded in your medical history.
2. The patient's physician should be contacted for guidance.
3. Follow previously reviewed precautions for electrosurgery.
4. If doubt exists, conversion of the demand pacemaker to a fixed-rate mode may be indicated. This is done by placing a strong magnet over the pulse generator.
5. Persons who wear a pacemaker and work near induction casting equipment should be evaluated on an individual basis.
6. Caution should be exercised with pulp testers and ultrasonic cleaners, although they demonstrated no interference in Simon's limited observations.
7. Tensing of the pectoralis major may inhibit pacemakers. The patient should be cautioned to avoid muscle tension of the upper extremities. Convert to fixed-rate mode if necessary.

While no fixed guidelines exist, one fact is beyond question — over one million patients in the United States wear cardiac pacemakers. The dental practitioner should consult the physician and proceed with caution.

Arterial Hypotension

Hypotension, or *low* blood pressure, does not exist in the healthy conscious patient. Life insurance statistics demonstrate that life expecantancy increases as blood pressure decreases. The *ideal* blood pressure is the lowest pressure a person can tolerate without going into shock.

Arterial Hypertension

Arterial hypertension is defined as a measurement that is consistently higher than 140/90 mm Hg. Pressure elevations 30 per cent above normal are not uncommon in the dental office. A borderline measurement should be rechecked several times before the physician is called in consultation.

When the patient has a history of hypertension, you should first investigate the possible existence of heart failure or angina pectoris. It is natural to think of stroke first when confronted with a hypertensive history, but the fact is that 65 per cent of hypertensives die of heart disease, whereas only 20 per cent demonstrate predominantly cerebral symptoms. This is not true of black people, however. They develop hypertension earlier in life, it is frequently more severe, and it results in a higher mortality at a younger age, more commonly from stroke than from coronary heart disease.[28]

The complications of hypertension include the following: congestive heart failure, angina pectoris, myocardial infarction, cerebral hemorrhage, cerebral thrombosis, and kidney failure.

ASA physical status classification is made according to the clinical syndrome resulting from hypertension, and it will be discussed further in the section on blood pressure under *vital signs*. The same is true of treatment modification. Follow Table 2–1.

Other Heart Diseases

Congenital heart disease represents 2 per cent of all adult heart disease. Congenital lesions consist of narrowing of vessels or valves, septal defects between atria or ventricles, and others.

Rheumatic heart disease results from a single or repeated attacks of rheumatic fever which produce deformity of valve cusps and fusion of valve commissures. Deformity or fusion produces valve stenosis or insufficiency or both; the mitral valve is involved in 50 to 60 per cent of cases, the mitral and aortic in 20 per cent, and the aortic alone in 10 per cent. There is a history of rheumatic fever in only 60 per cent of the cases of rheumatic heart disease, so 40 per cent of the cases must develop from subclinical or unrecognized rheumatic fever.

Antibiotic prophylaxis aside (bacterial endocarditis prevention), the common denominator of congenital heart disease and rheumatic heart disease is a pump that will fail from intolerably increased work loads. The patient will most likely develop congestive heart failure, although both angina pectoris and myocardial infarction are possible.

Aortic aneurysm is a localized dilatation of the ascending aorta as the result of syphilitic cardiovascular disease. Complications include aortic valve insufficiency (development of congestive heart failure), occlusion of the coronary artery ostia (development of angina pectoris or myocardial infarction), rupture of the aorta (sudden death), and dissecting aneurysm with rupture.

ASA classification of these three diverse types of heart disease depends upon the clinical picture, and the same is the case for treatment modification. Follow Table 2–1.

CEREBROVASCULAR DISEASES

Terms

Thrombus — an aggregation of blood factors (platelets, fibrin, and cells) causing vascular obstruction at the point of origin.

Embolus — a clot or other plug brought by the blood from another vessel and forced into a smaller one, causing obstruction.

Hemiplegia — paralysis of one side of body.

Quadriplegia — paralysis of all four limbs.

Infarct — an area of coagulation necrosis (cell death) in a tissue due to local ischemia from circulatory obstruction. The *process* of forming an infarct is called infarction.

Hypesthesia — decreased skin sensitivity.

Occlusive Cerebrovascular Disease – General

Degenerative arterial diseases are primarily caused by arteriosclerosis, most marked after age 40, and with strong predisposition related to diabetes mellitus and arterial hypertension. Raised arterial pressure produces accelerated atherosclerosis of major arteries. *Sustained* hypertension causes the normally reversible arteriolar narrowing to become *permanent* as the result of intimal thickening and muscle hypertrophy. The clinical picture of degenerative arterial diseases, whether cardiovascular or cerebrovascular, is that of a weakening of the arterial wall and a gradual narrowing and ultimate occlusion of the artery.

Occlusive cerebrovascular disease is characterized by three distinct clinical stages:

1. Gradual mental deterioration.
2. Dizzy spells, visual defects, transient weakness of face, arm, or leg.
3. Sudden complete hemiplegia (stroke).

Extracranial arteries are commonly involved in occlusive cerebrovascular disease, such as the common carotid bifurcation (origin of internal and external carotids), the vertebral artery, and intrathoracic segments of aortic branches.

Transient Cerebral Ischemia (TCI)

TCI represents a transient, reversible episode of cerebral ischemia (temporary cerebral artery insufficiency) lasting for 10 seconds to one hour, marked by headache, drowsiness, syncope, mental confusion, speech defect, muscle weakness, and focal hypesthesia. These temporary episodes do not constitute a true cerebrovascular accident (CVA) or stroke, but are prodromal only.

When taking the dialogue history of the patient who has already indicated a past history of CVA on the questionnaire, or the older patient with hypertension, inquire of the patient if there have been symptoms and signs that would indicate TCI. Such information is rarely volunteered. The TCI patient is managed in the dental office as if he or she has had an actual stroke, with the exception of treatment timing (see next section).

Cerebrovascular Accident

A stroke is also called cerebrovascular accident, CVA, and cerebral apoplexy. CVA is caused by cerebral hemorrhage, thrombosis, or embolism, and is marked by the sudden onset of neurologic complaints: focal motor (extremity or face weakness), focal hypesthesia (skin numbness), speech defects, vomiting, convulsions, headaches, and nuchal rigidity (neck), with or without recovery.

Early clinical findings may be sudden and devastating, the patient falling to the ground unconscious with hemiplegia, and there are lesser grades of CVA ranging from slight derangement of speech to muscle weakness and memory loss. Loss of consciousness is not necessary.

Occasionally your CVA or TCI patient will be taking an anticoagulant, and this must be considered in your dental treatment planning (see discussion under *myocardial infarction*). While the evidence does not warrant anticoagulation for patients with a completed stroke, it is of value as prophylaxis in recurrent emboli to the brain (as in rheumatic valvular disease), and it may assist the patient with TCI or progressive stroke.[29]

ASA Classification

The ASA classification for a patient with a history of CVA or TCI and otherwise negative history and physical findings would be Class II; a history of TCI as well as CVA would drop the patient to Class III. Modification of dental therapy follows Table 2–1 and the following recommendations.

Recommended Management of the Post-CVA and TCI Patient

1. A medical consultation is desirable if the patient's physical status is doubtful.
2. No elective dental treatment for at least six months after the episode (CVA only).
3. Keep appointments short.
4. Sedation is highly desirable, but should be used with great care and should not be carried to the point of extreme drowsiness or depression. Deep sedation depresses cerebral circulation and can initiate cerebral thrombosis. See the chapters on *psychosedation*.

KIDNEY DISEASES

Glomerulonephritis and Pyelonephritis

Most cases of glomerulonephritis are the result of immunologic reactions (immune complex disease), with antigen or antibody excess directly damaging the kidney. The disease is usually poststreptococcal (beta-hemolytic group A). Complications of the acute phase include CHF (salt and water retention), CHF with hypertension, hypertensive brain damage (convulsions), and kidney failure.

Pyelonephritis is an acute or chronic bacterial urinary tract infection producing nephrosclerosis (kidney scarring) in the final stages that is indistinguishable from late glomerulonephritis. Both diseases may terminate in kidney failure.

Chronic Renal Insufficiency

Chronic kidney failure is treated by diet and fluids (protein limitation), electrolyte replacement, transfusions, extracorporeal dialysis (kidney machine), and kidney transplant.

With dialysis, there is an 87 per cent one-year survival rate, 73 per cent two-year survival, and 60 per cent six-year survival. With kidney transplant, the kidney of a parent or sibling remains functional for one year in 74 per cent of the cases, and for three years in 70 per cent. A cadaver transplant remains functional for one year in 50 per cent of the cases, and for three years in 42 per cent.

Hemodialysis and Kidney Transplant

ASA classification of the patient in chronic kidney failure depends upon the degree of associated complications such as hypertension, anemia, and congestive heart failure. Renal impairment alone would place the patient in ASA Class II, while the addition of CHF would drop the patient to ASA Class III. Follow the recommendations in Table 2–1, with special attention to stress reduction.

Consultation with the physician is advisable, particularly in regard to drugs you may prescribe.[30] Care should be used with aspirin and acetaminophen; phenacetin and the tetracyclines should be strictly avoided; erythromycin, local analgesics, oxacillin, codeine, barbiturates, and benzodiazepines (Valium) are safe.[31] The physician may wish to advise a prophylactic antibiotic before dental therapy for the patient receiving dialysis or the recipient of a kidney transplant.

DIGESTIVE SYSTEM DISEASES

Peptic Ulcer

Peptic ulcer is a benign ulcer occurring in a portion of the digestive tract which is accessible to gastric acid secretions (stomach or duodenum). A duodenal ulcer is five times more common than gastric ulcer, occurs in 10 per cent of all people at some time, and tends to recur; 10 per cent require surgery. A gastric ulcer has the same prognosis.

The history of an active peptic ulcer would place the patient in ASA Class II. Follow Table 2–1 recommendations, with special attention to stress reduction.

Regional Enteritis and Ulcerative Colitis

Regional enteritis (regional ileitis) is a chronic inflammatory disease of the small intestine. It afflicts the young adult as a rule, and is marked by an insidious onset, intermittent diarrhea, and low fever. It may be low grade or fulminating.

Nonspecific ulcerative colitis is a chronic inflammatory disease of the colon afflicting young adults most commonly. It is characterized by bloody diarrhea, cramps, weight loss, and fever. It is usually low grade, but may be fulminating.

ASA designation would be Class II for either disease unless it were in a fulminant stage, in which case Class III or IV would be possible. Follow Table 2–1 modifications, with special attention to stress reduction.

Corticosteroids are often used in treating either disease, and your history should be concerned with dosage and duration. See adrenocortical insufficiency, discussed under *endocrine diseases*.

LIVER DISEASES

Acute Hepatitis

The dental doctor would normally not treat the patient with acute hepatitis A (infectious hepatitis) or acute hepatitis B (serum hepatitis). In the event of emergency care, special attention should be paid to self and staff protection (masking and double-gloving), sterilization to prevent cross-contamination, and post-exposure prophylaxis for self and staff (immune serum globulin for type A and special immune serum globulin for type B).

Chronic Hepatitis

Chronic hepatitis consists of a chronic inflammatory reaction of the liver demonstrated by abnormal liver function tests and illness beyond six months. It may be the result (sequela) of hepatitis A, hepatitis B (the patient remaining antigen-positive), or may be due to drugs.

Alcoholic hepatitis is the most common type, with parenchymal necrosis from alcohol abuse. Heavy drinking is essential; drunkenness is not. The disease may be reversible, depending upon liver function. If prothrombin time is unduly prolonged, the mortality rate is 40 per cent.

The patient may present for dental care with nothing but a positive history, or there may be anorexia (loss of appetite), nausea, hepatomegaly (enlarged liver), jaundice, ascites, debility, and peripheral edema. Liver failure proceeds to coma and death.

Depending upon signs and symptoms and medical consultation, if indicated, ASA classification may range from II to IV. Follow Table 2–1. Special attention should be paid to stress reduction and to possible bleeding tendencies (see chapter on *hemorrhage*).

ENDOCRINE DISEASES

Diabetes Mellitus

Diabetes mellitus is a clinical syndrome of disordered metabolism and *hyperglycemia* (abnormally high blood sugar) due to insulin deficiency *or* reduction of insulin effectiveness. Being familiar with the basic three types of diabetes is of assistance in physical evaluation and treatment modification.

Types of Diabetes

1. Insulinopenic Type I — insulin is reduced or absent.
   a. Insulinopenic Type IA (severe) — juveniles and nonobese adults; insulin production is absent; diet and insulin required in treatment. This type is often "brittle" and difficult to control; can be high risk.
   b. Insulinopenic Type IB (mild to moderate severity) — nonobese adults; insulin production is reduced; treatment by diet and perhaps oral hypoglycemic agent.
2. Insulinoplethoric Type II (mild severity) — obese adults; insulin is normal; treatment by diet. Due to chronic overeating, there is ineffective insulin action, with overdistention of storage depots and reduced ability to clear nutrients; there is sustained beta cell (pancreas) stimulation and *hyperinsulinism*, which induces receptor insensitivity.

The common clinical features of Type I diabetes are:

1. Polydipsia (increased thirst and water intake)
2. Polyuria (increased urine output)
3. Polyphagia (ravenous appetite, with weight loss)

The common clinical features of Type II diabetes are:

1. Peripheral neuropathy (as numbness of soles of feet)
2. Often no symptoms

Diseases commonly associated with diabetes are cataracts, retinopathy, retinal hemorrhage and detachment, lower extremity occlusive vascular disease, renal hypertension, coronary atherosclerosis, cerebral atherosclerosis, and neuropathies. There are two types of diabetic coma: hypoglycemic coma (insulin shock) and hyperglycemic coma (diabetic acidosis).

MANAGEMENT OF DIABETIC

Do not treat the uncontrolled diabetic. The health picture makes the patient a poor candidate for withstanding dental stress, and it has been shown that emotional stress increases glycemia and the tendency to diabetic acidosis and coma.

Most diabetics can give an accurate estimate of their current status, since they commonly test their urine for sugar. If the urine test is negative, shows a trace, or is 1+ for sugar, little problem with dental treatment would be expected. If the patient is doubtful regarding control, question regarding abnormal thirst, abnormal urine output, and weight loss. These are all signs of uncontrolled diabetes. If doubt still exists, a medical consultation is in order. It should be noted that the brittle diabetic cannot readily be controlled by such insulin substitutes as oral Diabinese, Orinase, Dymelor, and DBI. If the patient is taking one of these substitutes, or is controlled by diet alone, you may assume that the disease is not severe.

Since oral hypoglycemic agents have been associated with an increased risk of cardiovascular mortality in maturity-onset diabetics, physicians are relying more on diet in treating such patients.[32] All diabetics must be careful of their diets, some to avoid the need for insulin and others, who require insulin, to avoid hypoglycemia.

There is a marked tendency toward early development of arteriosclerosis in the diabetic, whether controlled or not. In evaluating the diabetic it is well to inquire into possible symptoms of heart failure and angina pectoris. A comprehensive 10-year study of 370 diabetics and 370 matched controls showed the death rate of diabetics to be 2.5 times that of the controls. The excess mortality was accounted for primarily by a higher prevalence of cardiovascular and renal disease, and, secondarily, by the severity of the diabetes as indicated by high insulin dosage (40 units or more daily), onset of the disease before age 45, and recurrent glycosuria, a definition of the "brittle" diabetic.

Frequently the meal before a dental appointment is inadequate or is missed entirely due to apprehension, and in these days of quadrant dentistry it is common to miss another meal or even two after the appointment. If the contemplated dental procedure may result in several meals being missed, I direct the patient to decrease insulin by half on the day of treatment in order to diminish the possibility of insulin shock. An elevated blood sugar for a short period is harmless. Anesthesiologists normally follow this same routine, either reducing insulin dosage at the time of surgery or withholding insulin entirely until the postoperative period.[22]

The brittle diabetic should pay special attention to urine sugar and acetone postoperatively. After considerable stress-producing treatment in such a patient, I recommend that he or she test the urine for sugar and acetone four times a day for four days and report any unusual deviations to the dental doctor and the medical doctor so that remedial action can be taken after consultation.

ASA CLASSIFICATION

The well controlled diabetic without associated additional disease is ASA Class II, the brittle diabetic with severe control problems is Class III; associated diseases such as CHF, MI, etc., may drop the diabetic to Class III or even IV. Follow Table 2–1, with special attention to stress reduction and the recommendations in the preceding paragraphs.

Hypothyroidism

Thyroid hormone affects all cellular metabolism. Hypothyroidism since infancy (cretinism) causes irreversible metabolic and growth changes. Hypothyroid adults under treatment rarely are a management concern in dentistry, even to the extreme of myxedema with slow pulse, brittle hair, dull facies, nonpitting edema of the face, and lethargic behavior. An enlarged tongue could be a technical problem, but these advanced cases are rarely encountered any more. The myxedematous patient may display signs and symptoms of CHF, and is very sensitive to sedatives.

ASA Class II would be correct for most hypothyroids, unless severe disease exists.

Hyperthyroidism

For our purposes, a history of hyperthyroidism should suggest the possibility of heart failure and angina pectoris. In addition, the moderately severe hyperthyroid suffers from tachycardia, sweating, headache, and nervous manifestations which make him or her a poor candidate for usual dental care.

The treated hyperthyroid would be placed in ASA Class II or lower if other significant disease exists. The untreated, severe hyperthyroid should be considered as Class IV temporarily. Follow Table 2–1.

Adrenocortical Insufficiency

The classic example of chronic adrenocortical insufficiency is Addison's disease, a deficiency of hormones concerned with glyconeogenesis (formation of carbohydrates from amino acids and fatty acids) and with mineral metabolism.

Tuberculosis is the cause of Addison's disease in 50 per cent of the cases, and 50 per cent result from idiopathic (cause unknown) atrophy of the adrenal glands. The patient suffers from weakness, anorexia, skin pigmentation, hypotension, and small heart. Treatment is by steroid replacement therapy (cortisone acetate).

Acute adrenocortical insufficiency is an emergency caused by an insufficient supply of adrenocortical hormones. Adrenal crisis may occur following treatment stress or following withdrawal of the hormone, with chronic insufficiency or with normal adrenals that are temporarily insufficient because of suppression due to recent use of a steroid for other purposes.

MANAGEMENT

There has been reported a near fatal adrenal crisis in an adrenalectomized patient for whom dental extractions were performed.[33] The patient had been prepared with 100 mg cortisone the night before surgery and a like dosage immediately before surgery. Profound shock occurred 90 minutes after surgery. You must assume the possibility of adrenal insufficiency if the patient has taken an adrenocortical hormone (cortisone, hydrocortisone, etc.) within the preceding two years. Irreversible shock may occur with such minor stress as a local analgesic injection or a simple dental extraction. You may consult the patient's physician, and he or she may reinstitute the steroid prior to dental treatment or make other arrangements to supplement. In assessing whether or not a steroid is required, I follow the Rule of Twos (McCarthy): if a patient has taken 20 mg of cortisone or equivalent for at least two weeks during the past two years, I assume the possibility of adrenal suppression. Admittedly the Rule of Twos is very conservative and restrictive, but it is safe.

Adrenocorticals are commonly utilized for the following: chronic collagen disorders (rheumatoid arthritis, lupus erythematosus), dermatologic diseases, rheumatic disorders, allergic states, ophthalmic diseases, respiratory diseases, hematologic disorders, neoplastic disorders, pemphigus, and postoperative inflammations.

The patient may be taking an adrenocortical hormone for chronic collagen disorder, such as rheumatoid arthritis, lupus erythematosus (L.E. disease), or other autoimmune diseases. The physician may wish to increase the dosage of the steroid temporarily if extensive dental therapy is planned and where an increased "stress reaction" would possibly be expected.

ASA CLASSIFICATION

ASA placement for the Addison's disease patient would depend upon signs and symptoms, replacement therapy success, and other diseases. It could range from Class II-IV, with possible strict modification of dental therapy in addition to steroid supplementation. ASA status for the uncomplicated patient to which the Rule of Twos applies would be Class II.

DISEASES OF THE BLOOD

Anemia

Anemia is characterized by one of the following:

1. Reduction below normal in the number of erythrocytes (red cells) — megaloblastic, pernicious, folic acid deficiency, aplastic.
2. Reduction in quantity of hemoglobin — iron deficiency, sickle cell.
3. Reduction in volume of packed red cells — bleeding or destruction (hemolytic).

The signs and symptoms of anemia include easy fatigability, dyspnea, pallor, palpitation, angina pectoris, tachycardia, brittle hair, and brittle nails. Normal adult hemoglobin is 12 to 18 gm per 100 ml; anemia is assumed to be significant at a hemoglobin of 9 grams or less. While a patient in renal failure will often tolerate a 5 gram hemoglobin remarkably well, you will elicit a history of exertional dyspnea, easy fatigability, etc.

ASA designation depends upon the type of anemia and signs and symptoms, relying upon the functional reserve classification primarily. With a 9 gram hemoglobin, ASA Class II would be appropriate, while below 9 grams Class III would be considered. Follow Table 2-1 for therapy modification. Stress reduction is in order, and oxygen supplementation during dental treatment can be helpful (as 3 L/min via nasal cannula). As with all anemias, bleeding tendencies during dental treatment must be considered (see chapter on *hemorrhage*).

Sickle Cell Anemia

This disease is covered separately because a crisis can occur during dental treatment. Nine per cent of U.S. blacks and 45 per cent of central African blacks display the sickling phenomenon, a marked insolubility of *reduced* HbS (hemoglobin S). The reduced HbS crystallizes from solution within the red cells into a sickle-shaped crystal. Infarction of the liver, kidney, brain, or long bones may occur with *extremely low oxygen tension* (flying, inhalation sedation, general anesthesia).

It is emphasized that there is a vast difference between sickle cell anemia, where the hemoglobin is all of the sickle type (SS), and the sickling phenomenon or sickle cell trait, where the S hemoglobin is linked with normal hemoglobin (AS).[34] Only one in 600 U.S. blacks has sickle cell anemia, characterized by HbSS, and this patient is our only concern. The sickle cell trait, characterized by HbAS, is a benign condition.[35] Mass screenings for the sickle cell trait have magnified the problem out of proportion since the sickling phenomenon is definitely a nondisease.

The patient with sickle cell anemia will give a history of fever, and pain in the arms, legs, or abdomen since early childhood. Anemia is severe. Scleral icterus (jaundiced white of eye) is common. The disease is disabling due to recurrent crises, with infarction of bones, joints, and organs. Complications include leg ulcers, hematuria (blood in urine), and heart enlargement. Many victims die in childhood from cerebral hemorrhage; some live beyond age 50; progressive renal damage is common (kidney failure).

ASA placement depends upon signs and symptoms, with the bulk of the patients being Class III. Follow Table 2–1 modifications, with special attention to stress reduction. Adequate oxygen delivery to the patient is essential to inhalation sedation, never falling below 30 per cent. Outpatient general anesthesia would represent a formidable endeavor.

Polycythemia Vera

This is caused by an overproduction of red cells, white cells, and platelets, with symptoms resulting from increased blood viscosity, characterized by malaise, fatigue, weakness, florid face, dusky red mucosa, and headache. Complications include GI hemorrhage, cerebral thrombosis, and pulmonary thrombosis. Excessive bleeding during dental treatment is common. Average survival is 13 years.

Most of these patients would be ASA Class III, depending upon history and signs and symptoms. Follow Table 2–1, with possible oxygen during treatment.

Leukemia

Properly falling under diseases of the white blood cells and reticuloendothelial system, leukemia will be considered here for convenience.

There is a proliferation of abnormal white cells in both acute and chronic leukemia, and most signs and symptoms are due to anemia: weakness, malaise, anorexia, pallor, fever, lymph node enlargement, and splenomegaly (enlarged spleen). Remission of up to one to three years is possible in 50 per cent of acute cases, and there is a life expectancy of three to four years in chronic cases with remissions.

Patients would be placed in ASA Class II to IV, as your judgment dictates. The advice under *anemia* applies, with special concern regarding bleeding.

Hodgkin's Disease

Here we see a proliferation of white cells in one or more lymph nodes, spreading to contiguous lymphatic structures. Lymph nodes are enlarged and nontender; there is fever and fatigue, and the disease is marked by exacerbations and remissions. Early treatment of the disease includes chemotherapy and possibly splenectomy. Late treatment is limited to irradiation. Up to 25 per cent of early cases are cured; overall five-year survival is 30 per cent.

ASA classification and treatment modification follow the anemias.

CONVULSIVE DISORDERS

This discussion is modified from the USC Physical Evaluation Manual. Convulsive disorders are characterized by abrupt transient symptoms of a motor, sensory, psychic, or autonomic nature, frequently associated with changes in consciousness. Epilepsy may be of an idiopathic nature (cause unknown) or be symptomatic of pathological states (brain tumor). The onset of idiopathic epilepsy is usually before age 30; onset thereafter usually suggests organic disease. In patients with classic epilepsy, anxiety and fear play a trigger role.

Convulsive disorders are classified as follows:

1. Grand mal epilepsy (major epilepsy) — 50 per cent of epileptics; loss of consciousness occurs and the patient undergoes generalized skeletal muscle contractions for several minutes, regaining consciousness with a headache and weakness. The seizure is usually preceded by a premonitory sign called an "aura," such as a bright light.
2. Petit mal epilepsy (minor epilepsy) — 10 per cent of epileptics; characterized by brief blank periods without falling or convulsions; most common in children. Neither the patient nor observers may be aware of the episode, which may appear as a brief lapse of attention.
3. Other types of epilepsy include Jacksonian (focal convulsions, consciousness retained), psychomotor disturbances (odd focal seizures, possible amnesia), status epilepticus (constant severe seizures that may be fatal), and febrile convulsions (associated with fever, especially in children).

ASA classification ranges from II to IV, depending upon the history of seizure frequency and severity. Grand mal well managed by medication would be Class II; poorly managed by medication — Class III; frequent seizures associated with dental therapy could merit Class IV and possible hospitalization.

Modification of treatment would include strict adherence to stress reduction, and doctor and staff should be prepared to manage a seizure (see Chapter 13, Cardiovascular and Other Medical Emergencies).

PHYSICAL EXAMINATION

INTRODUCTION

The medical history questionnaire, plus the indicated dialogue history, will provide you in most cases with an adequate pretreatment physical evaluation in dentistry. However, no physical evaluation is complete without a physical examination. Measurement and recording of vital signs is the first part of a physical examination, but will be considered after inspection.

INSPECTION

Inspection of the patient represents the most important part of every physical examination. You have been doing this, perhaps without realizing it, since you became a dental health professional.

Train yourself to actually *see* the patient when checking the medical history questionnaire or taking the dialogue history. Several points to observe are:

1. The color of the skin:
   Cyanosis — heart disease, polycythemia.
   Pallor — anemia, fear, tendency toward syncope.
   Flushing — fever, atropine overdosage, apprehension, hyperthyroidism.
   Jaundice — liver disease.
2. The eyes:
   Exophthalmos — hyperthyroidism.
3. The conjunctiva:
   Pallor — anemia.
   Jaundice — liver disease.
4. The hands:
   Tremor — hyperthyroidism, apprehension, hysteria, paralysis agitans, epilepsy, multiple sclerosis, senility.
5. The fingers:
   Clubbing — cardiopulmonary disease.
   Cyanosis of nail beds — cardiopulmonary disease.
6. The neck:
   Jugular vein distention — right heart failure.
7. The ankles:
   Swelling — varicose veins, right heart failure, kidney disease.
8. The respiratory rate, particularly with heart failure:
   Normal adult — 16 to 18 per minute.
   Normal child — 24 to 28 per minute.
9. The abdomen:
   Ascites — hepatic cirrhosis, right heart failure.
10. Appearance, demeanor, attitude, behavior:
    Is the patient in acute distress (pain or dyspnea); acutely anxious, fearful, antagonistic, belligerent; does the patient appear to be reliable and well informed. Any observed deviation from the norm should be recorded.

VITAL SIGNS

While no clear standard of care exists at the present time regarding what vital signs, if any, should be determined prior to dental therapy, it would appear that determination of blood pressure in adults at the initial physical evaluation is approaching a mandatory status. From the standpoint of comprehensive health care, it is urged that the following three vital signs be measured at the original physical evaluation of all patients:

1. Blood pressure
2. Pulse rate and rhythm

3.   Body temperature

It is further urged that the remaining three commonly measured vital signs also be recorded at the initial examination: height, weight, and respiratory rate.

It is also urged that the dental doctor dedicated to comprehensive health care measure and record at least the blood pressure, and preferably pulse rate and body temperature as well, prior to subsequent dental treatment during which medication of any kind is to be administered (includes local analgesia) or during which significant emotional or physical stress may be encountered by the patient.

Blood pressure measurement before inhalation sedation is highly desirable, and it is mandatory before intravenous sedation. See elsewhere in this book for the technical aspects of *vital sign determination* and for information on *psychosedation*.

Blood pressure should be redetermined after a lapse of six months or longer, and both blood pressure and pulse rate are highly desirable in cases of suspected cardiovascular or cerebrovascular disease.

Blood Pressure

You may easily train your assistant to do this as a matter of routine, although you may wish to check personally if the reading is abnormal.

You will be gratified by the number of undiagnosed and often asymptomatic cases of hypertension which this routine will disclose. Your patients will be most appreciative of this health service, but more importantly your alertness can result in the early and effective medical treatment of hypertension, and your own treatment plan may well be altered by the discovery.

The blood pressure varies up to 140/90 mm in the normal adult. Since it may vary as much as 20 to 30 mm over a short period due to exertion or excitement, take several readings when in doubt, and assume that the lowest is normal for that patient.

There is no simple way of estimating by blood pressure measurement alone whether the patient's hypertension is mild or severe. Such an evaluation must depend on the blood pressure and, more important, on the overall evaluation of the patient. A patient who is taking an antihypertensive drug, and who has a history of a stroke and a blood pressure of 160/100, may be a far greater risk under treatment than a patient with untreated essential hypertension, a reading of 190/120, and a total lack of symptoms referable to hypertension. If any doubt exists regarding the propriety of treatment, consult the physician.

ASA Class II is merited for a pressure consistently in the area of 140 to 160/90 to 95, Class III for 160 to 200/95 to 115, and Class IV over 200/115. A systolic pressure consistently over 200 may be considered a medical emergency. Rechecking by the physician away from the dental environment may demonstrate consistently lower pressures, in which event you should adjust the ASA classification and treatment modification. Three or more consecutive recordings above 140/90 justifies a medical consultation. Follow Table 2–1 therapy modifications, with special attention to stress reduction. Patients taking antihypertensive drugs should be protected against abrupt postural changes, as sitting up or standing. Alter the operating chair position slowly so that the cardiovascular system adapts and postural hypotension with syncope does not occur.

Pulse Rate and Rhythm

Bradycardia — heart rate slower than 60 beats per minute.
Tachycardia — heart rate faster than 100 beats per minute.

Pulse considerations are as follows:

1. Pulse rate varies from 60 to 90 per minute in the normal adult, and 80 to 120 per minute in the normal child. In the endurance athlete, the pulse rate may be as low as 50 to 60 per minute. Loss of consciousness usually occurs below a rate of 40 per minute.
   Comment: A rate of less than 60 or more than 110 in the adult should be viewed with suspicion, and usually is sufficient evidence to justify a medical consultation.
2. The pulse rate should be within normal limits and should be both strong and regular.
3. Any irregularity of the pulse, other than a very occasional premature ventricular contraction (extrasystole, dropped beat), is an indication for medical consultation.
   Examples:
   a. Complete irregularity of the pulse (complete arrhythmia, pulsus irregularis perpetuus) usually indicates atrial fibrillation; may or may not be serious in respect to dental treatment.
   b. Pulsus alternans, which is regular alternation in the size or strength of the pulsations, indicates severe myocardial damage.

As was stated in the chapter on *sudden death,* premature ventricular contractions (PVCs, skipped beats) are common in the healthy adult and are of no significance. When noted in the patient with cardiovascular disease (CHF, CAHD, hypertension), PVCs can be significant. Notation of five PVCs or more per minute in a post-MI patient would be grounds for ASA Class IV designation until a medical consultation dictated a lesser designation. This same is true of a pulse rate in the adult consistently over 110 or less than 60 until explained satisfactorily by medical consultation or by circumstances (athlete). Pulsus alternans is an automatic Class IV. Atrial fibrillation could range from Class II to IV, depending upon the cause and signs and symptoms.

Pulse rate or rhythm alone is not a terribly reliable method for ASA classification, the final designation relying on the disease or condition responsible for the abnormal finding. Follow Table 2–1 for appropriate modification.

Temperature

Body temperature ranges from 96.8 to 99.4° F in the healthy individual, with a "normal" of 98.6° F. Actual body temperatures rise above individual setpoints in warm environments or during work and fall below setpoints in cold environments.[36] The variation range is probably wider, pending investigation of larger groups.

Normal rectal or vaginal temperature is 1° F higher than the oral temperature, and the normal axillary temperature is 1° F lower. Oral, nasal, and axillary temperatures are subject to errors by evaporative cooling, and the rectal site is encumbered by thermally inert masses and is influenced by microbial heat production. In fever there is an upward shift of the individual setpoint by depressing action of the pyrogen, for example, bacterial end products.[36] An individual with a low setpoint could have a 2° fever and still demonstrate a 98.8° F measurement, well within the range of "normal," while an individual with a high setpoint could demonstrate an oral temperature of 101.4° F with the same 2° fever.

As can be seen, body temperature is unreliable as to specific numbers, but an elevated temperature speaks volumes in determining the physical status of a patient. Routine measurement of body temperature by the dental practitioner is called for if comprehensive health care is the goal. It is certainly indicated for an obviously ill patient suffering from oral or nonoral systemic infection.

ASA classification based upon body temperature alone is of necessity empiric and is more wisely based upon the specific disease process. The following guidelines are suggested:

ASA Class II — 99.5 to 101°F — cause of elevated temperature should be sought; no elective therapy if signs of respiratory infection; elective treatment otherwise OK, depending upon evaluation of individual patient; use of psychosedation or general anesthesia is a judgment decision; stress reduction and treatment duration limitation indicated.
ASA Class III — 101 to 104°F — medical consultation; emergency dental treatment only.
ASA Class IV — over 104°F — medical emergency.

Height/Weight

Normal weight may vary 10 to 15 per cent above or below standard weight tables. *Any* recent weight gain or loss may be significant in evaluating the physical status prior to dental therapy. Recording height and weight can be very valuable, especially since loose clothing can mask a considerable over-weight problem.

Weight gain may be produced by:

1. Overeating
2. Endocrine dysfunction (hypothyroidism)
3. Edema associated with:
   a. congestive heart failure
   b. hepatic (liver) failure
   c. renal (kidney) insufficiency

Weight loss may be produced by:

1. Dieting
2. GI dysfunction (peptic ulcer, gall bladder disease, etc.)
3. Endocrine dysfunction (hyperthyroidism)
4. Malignancy
5. Neurosis

Consideration should be given to dropping one ASA classification for either gross overweight or gross underweight (wasting). Gross overweight is especially important in classifying the patient with cardiovascular diseases; an angina pectoris patient in ASA Class II would surely be dropped to Class III in this situation. Follow Table 2–1 modifications and stress reduction.

Respiratory Rate

Observe the type, rate, and depth of breathing at rest. Normal for the reasonably apprehensive adult in the dental environment is 16 to 18 per minute; for the child 24 to 28 per minute. Respiratory depth and rhythm are regular. Rate increases 4 per minute for each 1°F temperature elevation.

Respiration in males is primarily diaphragmatic (abdominal); pronounced use of the chest muscles could indicate air hunger. The reverse is true of females, whose breathing is primarily costal (chest); pronounced use of the diaphragm (abdomen) could indicate dyspnea. Use of the accessory muscles of respiration (neck, shoulders) could indicate dyspnea.

Breath odors can be of value. A fetid (foul, putrefactive) breath may be noted with lung abscess or bronchiectasis. An acetone odor (sweet, fruity) could indicate diabetic acidosis and perhaps threatened hyperglycemic coma. The odor of ammonia may indicate uremia (kidney failure). In liver failure the breath may have a musty odor (fetor hepaticus; methyl mercaptan). The odor of alcohol may indicate self-medication on a sedative or compulsive basis, and is good reason for a thorough evaluation of possible anxiety or a drinking problem.

The respiratory rate does not lend itself to ASA physical status classification. A demonstrated hyperventilation syndrome would be designated as ASA Class II, while the Kussmaul breathing of diabetic acidosis (rate — 30 to 40/min) would classify as ASA Class IV and would be considered a medical emergency.

AUSCULTATION OF HEART AND LUNGS

Although it is not mandatory that the dental doctor be experienced in auscultation of the heart and lungs, this examination is well within the standard of practice in dentistry. Many states have dental practice acts which specifically mention physical evaluation as being within dental standards of practice, while in other states its legality may be taken for granted, as the technique can be a necessary adjunct to the safe practice of dentistry.

Stethoscopic examination of the heart and lungs as an aid in physical evaluation may be made with perfect propriety by the dental practitioner who is competent through training and experience. I consider the following guidelines to be essential to this examination:

1. Regardless of the sex or age of the patient, a dental assistant should be present with the patient and doctor throughout the examination. The claim of sexual impropriety by the unbalanced adult or fantasizing child or teenager, even though unsubstantiated, can be extremely damaging to the

doctor's reputation. I am aware of criminal charges being filed in such instances. This same advice is sound when the axilla is examined, as such has been interpreted as a sexual caress.

2. Reasonable justification is essential to the examination; that is, there must be reasonable concern regarding the possibility of cardiovascular or bronchopulmonary disease. Exceptions to this advice include the teaching environment, the patient being examined prior to general anesthesia or admission to the hospital, and the patient for which complete physical evaluation is being performed by the practitioner.

An impression of chronic congestive heart failure gained by the dialogue history may be supported by rales heard over the lung bases on auscultation. A history of possible valvular heart disease may be supported upon auscultation of the heart. It is probable that in the future heart sounds will be analyzed by an office telephone connection with a computer. In a study of 3797 children, no known cases of heart disease were missed by the computer, the false-positive ratio was 5.6 per cent, and the computer picked up eight previously unknown cases of heart disease out of a grand total of 16 for the group.

Auscultation of the heart and lungs has been taught in all advanced oral surgery training programs in the United States for many years. At the University of Southern California a continuing education course in advanced physical diagnosis has been presented to general dental practitioners since 1961. Auscultation has been taught to the predoctoral student and the dental hygiene student at USC since 1976, and the examination has been adopted as a routine for selected patients in the dental clinic since 1978, all predoctoral students participating on a required basis.

Inasmuch as complete physical diagnosis is the next step for meaningful progress in physical evaluation in dentistry, and since such advancement is in the public interest, the following chapter is devoted exclusively to that subject so that the advanced student of physical evaluation will have dental-oriented material available. It is suggested that the reader at least review the material on the significance of heart sounds and breath sounds.

FUNCTION TESTS

Introduction

At the completion of the medical history and applicable physical examination, you may have serious reservations about the functional reserve of a patient with cardiovascular or bronchopulmonary disease. Should the patient be placed in ASA Class II, III, or IV, and what therapy modifications are therefore in order. The Anderson Breath-Holding Test is very valuable in this instance. It serves as a test flight of stairs in the dental office.

The suspicion of bronchopulmonary disease may be very strong, but you need function tests to reinforce your impression of lower airway obstruction (pulmonary emphysema). The Match Test and Timed Forced Expiratory Volume are of great assistance. They may allow an unnecessary medical consultation to be avoided, or may give you valuable information with which to initiate a medical consultation.

Anderson Breath-Holding Test

Technique:

1. The patient takes a deep breath.
2. The patient pinches the nostrils together in order to prevent exhalation; also some patients may inadvertently breathe through the nose.
3. The breath is held as long as is reasonably comfortable, and you time the interval. It is my practice to stop the test at 20 seconds.

Interpretation:

1. The upper limits vary greatly and may be beyond 35 to 45 seconds.
2. 20 seconds or more – excellent
   15 seconds or less — caution
   10 seconds or less — great caution

A test result of 15 seconds or less should be viewed with suspicion, especially if there is evidence of cardiovascular or bronchopulmonary disease. Repeat the test at least once if the result is questionable. An observation of 10 seconds or less would militate against elective therapy and indicate a medical consultation, as an ASA Class IV designation is in order, at least temporarily. Patients with congestive heart failure or emphysema in Class III will usually achieve a test result of 15 seconds.

Match Test

The Match Test is of great value in respiratory system evaluation. The patient attempts to blow out a half-burned match held at 6 inches from the mouth with lips parted wide, not pursed. Failure to pass this test indicates FEV per second (see next test for explanation) in the area of 1 liter (L), or a peak flow rate of under 100 liters per minute,[37] a serious situation. Further evaluation by pulmonary function tests would be in order.

Timed Forced Expiratory Volume

Vital capacity (VC) is the maximum expelled volume of air after a maximum inspiration. Forced vital capacity (FVC) is normally expelled in 3 seconds or less with effort; if the timed expulsion is 5 seconds or more, bronchial obstruction exists (emphysema, asthma, other). You may time the forced expiration in the office. While the use of a spirometer would improve accuracy, it is not necessary to support your impression.

Forced expiratory volume (FEV) is the maximum expelled volume in a timed interval, as 1, 2, 3, 4, or 5 seconds. The expelled volume may be expressed as a percentage of FVC or in liters (L). The following are percentage values for the normal healthy patient:

$$\text{FEV 1 sec, or } FEV_1 = 83\% \text{ of actual VC}$$
$$\text{FEV 2 sec, or } FEV_2 = 97\% \text{ of actual VC}$$
$$\text{FEV 3 sec, or } FEV_3 = 99\% \text{ of actual VC}$$

Here are examples of expelled volume (requiring a spirometer) for the normal healthy patient. In this patient the total lung capacity (TLC) is 5.08 L, the residual volume (RV) is 1.54 L, and the FVC is 3.33 L:

$$FEV_1 = 2.23 \text{ L}$$
$$FEV_2 = 2.84 \text{ L}$$
$$FEV_3 = 3.21 \text{ L}$$

Reduction to 60 to 75 per cent of estimated normal is indicative of obstructive lung disease (emphysema); reduction to 40 to 60 per cent of normal represents a very serious functional loss. The most useful test is FEV_1. Failure to expel 60 per cent of the 3 second FEV in the first second indicates trouble.[37] Examples of risk patients are: high risk — $FEV_1 = 1.64$ L; very high risk — $FEV_1 = 1.20$ L.

Estimate the FEV in your office over a timed interval of 5 seconds. The maximum volume should be expelled in 1 to 2 seconds. If the patient is still expelling significant volume at 5 seconds, and if the medical history is suspicious, a consultation and possible pulmonary function tests would be in order.

Further, if the patient's maximal chest expansion is over one inch, it is unlikely that restrictive disease of the thoracic cage exists.[37]

Double Two-Step Exercise Test

While this test will be performed in the medical office, it is extremely valuable in the diagnosis and prognosis of coronary artery disease. Robb concludes that a nonischemic ECG response to exercise practically excludes coronary disease of a type that will cause premature death, and the exercise test is more reliable than the medical history in the diagnosis of silent coronary disease.[42]

LABORATORY TESTS

For years hospitalized patients have had prior to general anesthesia a minimum laboratory examination consisting of a routine urinalysis and a complete blood count. In dental offices such examinations have never become routine, although a small minority of offices perform a hemoglobin or hematocrit determination and check the urine for sugar. It is doubtful if such routine examinations add significantly to the usual basic evaluation outlined here, although they are a significant public service as a health screen.

Routine health screening is assisted by a microhematocrit (packed cell volume), hemoglobin, and basic urinalysis (sugar and protein), all of which are simple to perform at small cost in the dental office. Urinalysis is cost-effective as a health screen, while the other tests are not considered so by public health authorities for general screening in public clinics. This reasoning does not apply to the dental office.

Regarding urinalysis, a positive result for protein (albumin) would not contraindicate usual dental treatment or even outpatient general anesthesia but would suggest a medical consultation to investigate possible kidney disease. A positive sugar in the patient with diabetes indicates possible control problems, while possible diabetes should be investigated in the event of a negative history.

It is suggested that a hematocrit below 30 per cent or hemoglobin below 10 grams is a contraindication to outpatient general anesthesia.[38] Normal adult hemoglobin is 12 to 18 gm per 100 ml. I consider a hemoglobin of 9 grams or less to be significant and worthy of investigation. A hemoglobin as low as 5 grams will usually be accompanied by exertional dyspnea, tachycardia, palpitation, and undue fatigue.

If you are not performing screening tests in the office, and if you have doubts regarding possible kidney disease, anemia, bleeding tendencies, diabetes, etc., it would be wise to refer the patient to a clinical laboratory, depending upon your background and experience in interpreting such tests, or refer to a physician for appropriate examination, tests, and opinion.

COMMENT

Adequate physical evaluation is the most important method by which the dental practitioner is able to prevent life-threatening emergencies during therapy, and is followed closely in importance by proper stress reduction and other indicated modifications to therapy. You must first be dedicated to prevention, and, understanding the hows and whys of prevention, you will then understand the treatment of extant emergencies, treating appropriately by knowledge of disease, rather than blindly utilizing by-the-numbers, by-the-symptoms cookbook therapy.

REFERENCES

1. McCarthy, F. M.: Physical evaluation. Dent. Clin. North Amer., *17*:191–209, 1973.
2. Halpern, I. L.: Patient's medical status — a factor in dental treatment. Oral Surg., *39*:216–226, 1975.
3. Accepted Dental Therapeutics. Chicago, American Dental Association, 1977–78, p. 9.
4. Ibid, pp. 7–8.
5. Yu, P. N.: Lung water in congestive heart failure. Mod. Conc. Cardiov. Dis., *40*:27–32, 1971.
6. Rahe, R. H., et al.: Recent life changes, myocardial infarction, and abrupt coronary death. Arch. Intern. Med., *133*:221–228, 1974.
7. Hershberg, P. I., et al.: The medical history question as a health screening test. Arch. Intern. Med., *127*:266–272, 1971.
8. Horwitz, L. D.: The diagnostic significance of anginal symptoms. J.A.M.A., *299*:1196–1199, 1974.
9. Lesch, M., and Gorlin, R.: Pharmacological therapy of angina pectoris. Mod. Conc. Cardiov. Dis., *42*:5–10, 1973.
10. Becker, L. C., et al.: Effect of ischemia and antianginal drugs on the distribution of radioactive microspheres in the canine left ventricle. Circ. Res., *28*:263–269, 1971.
11. Medical Letter on Drugs and Therapeutics: Drugs for prophylaxis of angina pectoris, *17*:57–58, 1975.
12. Gey, G. E., et al.: Exertional arrhythmia and nitroglycerin. J.A.M.A., *226*:287–290, 1973.
13. Medical Letter on Drugs and Therapeutics: Disintegration and storage of nitroglycerin tablets, *13*:13–14, 1971.
14. Editorial: Nitroglycerin tablets: loss of potency, J.A.M.A., *216*:878, 1971.
15. Edelman, B. A., et al.: The stability of hypodermic tablets of nitroglycerin packaged in dispensing containers. J. Amer. Pharmaceut. Assoc., *NS11*:30–33, 1971.
16. FDA Drug Bulletin: Nitroglycerin packaging affects potency. February, 1972.
17. Copelan, H. W.: Burning sensation and potency of nitroglycerin sublingually. J.A.M.A., *219*:176–179, 1972.
18. Chandler, A. B.: Relationship of coronary thrombosis to myocardial infarction. Mod. Conc. Dis., *44*:1–5, 1975.
19. White, P. D.: The historical background of angina pectoris. Mod. Conc. Cardiov. Dis., *43*:109–112, 1974.

20. Carleton, R. A., and Johnson, A. D.: Coronary artery spasm. Mod. Conc. Cardiov. Dis., *43*:87–91, 1974.
21. Medical Letter on Drugs and Therapeutics: Nitroglycerin in acute myocardial infarction. *18*:37–38, 1976.
22. Medical Letter on Drugs and Therapeutics: Anticoagulants in myocardial infarction. *16*:17–19, 1974.
23. Michaels, L.: Incidence of thromboembolism after stopping anticoagulant therapy. J.A.M.A., *215*:595–599, 1971.
24. Corday, E.: Status of coronary bypass surgery. J.A.M.A., *231*:1245–1247, 1975.
25. Medical Letter on Drugs and Therapeutics: Coronary arteriography and coronary artery surgery. *18*:57–59, 1976.
26. Rezal, F. R.: Dental treatment of patient with a cardiac pacemaker. Oral Surg., *44*:662–665, 1977.
27. Simon, A. B., et al.: The individual with a pacemaker in the dental environment. J.A.D.A., *91*:1224–1229, 1975.
28. Finnerty, F. A.: Hypertension is different in blacks. J.A.M.A., *216*:1634–1635, 1971.
29. Medical Letter on Drugs and Therapeutics: Anticoagulants in the prevention of strokes caused by occlusive vascular disease. *13*:27–28, 1971.
30. Westbrook, S. D.: Dental management of patients receiving hemodialysis and kidney transplants. J.A.D.A., *96*:464–468, 1978.
31. Heard, E., et al.: The dental patient with renal disease: precautions and guidelines. J.A.D.A., *96*:792–796, 1978.
32. Medical Letter on Drugs and Therapeutics: Some notes on diet in the management of diabetics. *13*:58–59, 1971.
33. Brontsas, M. G., and Seldin, R.: Adrenal crisis after tooth extractions in an adrenalectomized patient: Report of case. J. Oral Surg., *30*:301–302, 1972.
34. Hussey, H. H.: Sicklemia. J.A.M.A., *229*:192, 1974.
35. Bristow, L. R.: The myth of sickle cell trait. Western J. Med., *121*:77–82, 1974.
36. Benzinger, T. H.: What is normal body temperature. J.A.M.A., *218*:603, 1971.
37. Chase, H. F.: To operate or not to operate — what is the risk. Resident & Staff Physician, 65–77, May 1978.
38. Allen, G. D.: Dental Anesthesia and Analgesia. Baltimore, Williams & Wilkins Co., 1972, p. 22.
39. Rothwell, P. S., and Wragg, K. A.: Assessment of the medical status of patients in general dental practice — a comparative survey of a questionnaire and verbal injury. Brit. Dent. J., *133*:252–255, 1972.
40. Slack, W., et al.: A computer-based medical history system, New Engl. J. Med., *274*:194–198, 1966.
41. Kanner, I. F.: The programmed physical examination with or without a computer, J.A.M.A., *215*:1281–1291, 1971.
42. Robb, G. P., and Seltzer, F.: Appraisal of the double two-step exercise test. J.A.M.A., *234*:722–727, 1975.

3

PHYSICAL DIAGNOSIS

LAWRENCE W. RICHARDSON

INTRODUCTION

The chapter on *physical evaluation* dealt primarily with the establishment of a basic medical evaluation in which the risk factor only was determined prior to dental therapy. This chapter will present material covering the subject of physical diagnosis that has general application to dentistry. Some overlap with other chapters must be accepted for clarity.

The serious student will also find that this fundamental, dental oriented approach makes for a simple transition from physical evaluation to a textbook on comprehensive physical diagnosis.

Either the short-form or the long-form medical history illustrated in Chapter 2 can serve as a departure point for physical diagnosis. The dialogue medical history that will be presented here is not a patient-completed questionnaire, but is a suggested outline from which the practitioner can choose pertinent material for investigation.

This chapter encompasses a brief discussion of physical diagnosis with specific reference to signs, symptoms, and pathogenesis of some of the more common or interesting diseases the practitioner may encounter. Emphasis has been placed on changes in organ function.

The patient comes to the health practitioner because he wants a checkup, knows he is ill, or has a variety of fears and is worried. The practitioner's responsibility is threefold: (1) to establish a diagnosis, (2) to treat the illness, and (3) to mitigate the patient's fears and anxieties.

SYMPTOMS AND SIGNS

Disease manifests itself by abnormal sensations and events known as symptoms, and by changes in structure or function known as signs. Symptoms, being subjective, must be described by the patient and obtained in his history. Signs are objective, and are discovered by the examiner by means of physical examination, laboratory tests, and x-ray. The information obtained from the history and physical examination is of value only when one is able to select and correlate the pertinent facts and recognize the clinical picture that they indicate. Abnormal symptoms and signs should be completely investigated. Mistakes are just as often caused by lack of thoroughness as by lack of knowledge. The history of a patient is absolutely essential in making a diagnosis. In some diseases a physical examination is of great importance whereas a laboratory examination is of little value; in other diseases the reverse is true; but in all diseases the history is of great importance. In some diseases the diagnosis is made entirely from the history. In pulmonary tuberculosis, the history of loss of weight and night sweats and afternoon fever may be of greater value than any physical findings. In angina pectoris the diagnosis is often entirely made from the history of pain under the sternum, which radiates to the left arm and is accompanied by a sensation of impending death.

HISTORY TAKING

Taking of a history includes not only taking the patient's medical history but also his or her personal and social history. During the time utilized in obtaining a history, one also strives to develop a good rapport with the patient, and has the opportunity to make a psychological evaluation and to determine the patient's mental status.

First are recorded name, residence, age, sex, race, marital state, nationality, and occupation. Next is obtained the *chief complaint,* which asks for the nature and duration of the symptoms that brought the patient to the practitioner. *Present illness* (analysis of chief complaint) will include detailed information concerning the current symptoms. This should be a logically developed story, accurately describing the time and mode of onset, duration, severity, location, progress, character, and relation to physiologic function. *Past history* should include diseases of childhood, serious illnesses, injuries, previous surgery and hospitalizations, previous radiation therapy, allergies, blood transfusions, familial diseases, medications now being taken, and habits regarding alcohol and tobacco. Following this is the systems review, which is a methodical questioning about each system of the body with specific questions to remind the patient of symptoms. The systems review is shown in Table 3–1.

PHYSICAL EXAMINATION

The five basic procedures used in conducting a general physical examination are indicated below. These are supplemented by special methods for testing neurologic function.

Inspection — looking at the body.

Palpation — feeling the various parts.

Percussion — listening to the sounds produced and noting the degree of resistance encountered when a region is tapped.

TABLE 3-1 SYSTEMS REVIEW

Head: headache, vertigo, lightheadedness, fainting
Eyes: glasses, vision, pain
Ears: hearing, tinnitus, pain, discharge
Nose: head colds, epistaxis, smell
Mouth: salivation, lesions, pain, sense of taste, swallowing, hoarseness, tonsillitis
Neck: stiffness, venous distention, pulsations, swellings
Respiratory: cough, hemoptysis, sputum, night sweats
Cardiac: pain in chest, palpitation, dyspnea, orthopnea, ankle edema
Gastrointestinal: appetite, nausea, vomiting, diarrhea, hematemesis, jaundice, color of stools, abdominal pain
Genitourinary: pain on urination, hematuria, frequency, purulent urine, incontinence, penile discharge
Menses: age at onset, frequency, regularity, duration, pain, amount, date of last period
Neuromuscular: convulsions, paresthesia, weakness, paralysis, incoordination of movements
Weight: amount and any recent change

Auscultation—listening to the sounds produced within the body.

Smell — odors of a disease may be characteristic.

Examination by these methods is performed after the history has been taken. Those parts of the body to which the history has directed suspicion require detailed investigation; however, it is the responsibility of the practioner to give a thorough physical examination. Pathology frequently exists without producing subjective manifestations and is often found incidentally on examination. The form presented in Table 3–2 is recommended as a guide for general physical examination.

SKIN

Inspection of the skin and mucous membranes is the simplest of all procedures. Only with diseases of the skin can one have such a complete view.

Many skin conditions are associated with general systemic disease, whereas others are skin diseases *per se* and belong entirely within the domain of dermatology.

Color. The color of the skin is one of the first characteristics that should be studied. The conjunctiva and sclera of the eye are excellent sites to observe change in color. Extreme pallor of the skin and mucous membranes may be indications of anemia. Abnormal redness can be a sign of polycythemia vera, which is an overproduction of red blood cells. Jaundice, or yellow discoloration, usually indicates infectious hepatitis or obstructive disease of the bile ducts, such as with neoplasms and gallstones. Cyanosis, a bluish color of the skin, is associated with diminished oxygen-carrying capacity of the blood. It may be present with cardiac or pulmonary disease. With Addison's disease (adrenocortical insufficency) there is a bronze-like discoloration of the skin.

Hemorrhage. Subcutaneous bleeding, occurring spontaneously or after minor trauma, is often an indication of a systemic disease. Lesions less than 2 mm. in diameter are referred to as petechiae, from 2 to 5 mm. as

TABLE 3-2 OUTLINE OF PHYSICAL EXAMINATION

1. Vital signs: pulse, blood pressure, respirations, temperature, weight
2. General appearance: stature, posture, nutritional state
3. Skin: color, texture, moisture, turgor, pigmentation, lesions
4. Head: shape, size, distribution of hair
5. Eyes: conjunctivae and sclera; size and shape of pupils; reaction of pupils to light and accommodation; funduscopic examination of retina for hemorrhage, exudate, vessels, and optic disks; vision
6. Ears: external examination for tophi; tympanic membrane examined for inflammation, exudate; auditory acuity
7. Nose: septum, turbinates, polyps
8. Mouth and throat: teeth, tongue, tonsils, lesions, lips
9. Neck: lymph nodes, thyroid, engorgement of veins, abnormal pulsations, masses, midline trachea
10. Chest: contour, symmetry, equal expansion, axillary lymph nodes
11. Lungs: breath sounds, respiratory rate, fremitus, rales, wheezes, friction rub
12. Breasts: size, masses, secretion, pigmentation, tenderness
13. Heart: point of maximal impulse, thrills, pulse rate, heart sounds, murmurs, rhythm
14. Abdomen: contour, scars, dilated veins, rigidity, tenderness, liver, spleen, kidneys, bladder, masses, fluid, inguinal lymph nodes
15. Male genitalia: discharge, lesions, testicular masses, inguinal hernia
16. Female genitalia: inspection of perineum, cervix, bimanual examination of uterus and adnexa, Pap smear.
17. Rectum: hemorrhoids, masses, prostate
18. Extremities: color of palms, clubbing of fingers, cyanosis, joint swelling or deformity, pulses
19. Back: curvature, mobility
20. Nervous system: deep tendon reflexes, pathologic reflexes, cranial nerves, sensory examination

purpuric spots, and larger ones as ecchymosis. If there is enough bleeding to cause a palpable mass, the lesion is a hematoma. Hemorrhage may occur spontaneously with thrombocytopenic purpura, a disease in which the blood platelets are prematurely destroyed in the spleen; leukemias and lymphomas in which there is a deficiency in platelet formation; aplastic anemia; infections with streptococcus or meningococcus; severe liver disease with a decreased production of prothrombin; and in patients who are taking anticoagulant medications such as Coumadin or dicumarol. When subacute bacterial endocarditis is suspected, the conjunctivae should be frequently inspected for the appearance of petechial hemorrhages.

Edema. Edema is a collection of fluid in the subcutaneous tissue. The skin is tense and shiny, and pits on pressure. An impression made on the skin by pressure with the fingers does not immediately disappear after the fingers are removed. Edema may be due to congestive heart failure; liver failure in which there is too little production of blood proteins such as albumin; renal insufficiency, in which blood proteins are lost in the urine; and starvation. A localized area of edema may be due to trauma, infection, or interference with venous blood or lymph flow.

Subcutaneous Emphysema. The presence of air or gas in the subcutaneous tissue gives an edematous appearance. On palpation there is a crackling sensation (crepitation) under the skin. Air blown into the root canal of a tooth, or around the crevicular margins of a tooth preparation; puncture wounds of the trachea or lungs; the rupture of emphysematous blebs of the lungs; or infection of a wound by a gas-producing organism can cause subcutaneous emphysema.

Primary Lesions of the Skin

MACULES.   These are flat, circumscribed changes in skin color, such as with freckles, petechiae, and flat moles.

PAPULES.   These are circumscribed elevations not over a centimeter in size.

NODULES.   These are circumscribed solid lesions in the subcutaneous tissue which may be inflammatory or neoplastic.

WHEALS (HIVES).   These are morphologically papules, sharply circumscribed, and produced by acute edema.

VESICLES.   These are sharply circumscribed, small elevations, containing clear fluid.

BULLAE.   These are large vesicles, greater than 0.5 cm.

PUSTULES.   These are circumscribed lesions containing free pus.

SCALES.   These are loose fragments of an incompletely shed, dead, keratinized layer of skin.

ULCER.   This is a destruction of the skin extending beneath the epidermis. When an ulcer heals, it always leaves a scar.

SCAR (CICATRIX).   This is a permanent skin change formed of fibrous tissue, replacing the normal tissue lost, following damage. A fresh scar may be temporarily accentuated, but with passage of time scars contract and become less evident. When there is progressive hypertrophy, instead of contraction, a keloid forms.

KELOID.   This is a fibrous tissue tumor, arising in predisposed persons, following a break in the skin. Keloids are seen predominantly in Negroes. Surgical incisions in predisposed patients will heal with keloid formation.

Skin eruptions are present with many systemic diseases. Scarlet fever resulting from a hemolytic streptococcal infection presents with fever, sore throat, and a small fine, vividly red macular rash that disappears on pressure. Measles appear as a red macular rash that coalesces to give a blotchy appearance.

Seborrheic Dermatitis (Dandruff).   This is a chronic scaling eruption, usually in hairy areas that are rich in sebaceous glands. Exacerbations may be related to anxiety, whereas hot and humid weather may cause improvement.

Warts (Verrucae).   These are papular lesions that are caused by a viral infection. They are contagious, and when present on a man's face may be readily spread by shaving nicks.

Drug Eruptions.   Drug eruptions may present themselves as almost any cutaneous lesion. They are usually widespread in distribution, because they result from a circulating agent; are rapid in onset; may occur as edema in the form of vesicles, bullae, and hives; and commonly appear as an inflammatory response with itching. The history is very important in making a diagnosis.

Actinic (Senile) Keratosis.   These begin as brownish macules that become papular and keratotic in areas that are chronically exposed to sunlight. Bald-headed men are particularly prone to this lesion. Although these keratoses are related to aging, they are precipitated by sunlight, and so deserve the term actinic.

Squamous Cell Carcinoma. Squamous cell carcinoma of the skin can usually be prevented because it arises from actinic keratoses. They are firm and show little anaplasia; metastases occur late, in contrast to squamous cell carcinoma of the mucous membrane which metastasizes early.

Basal Cell Carcinoma. This tumor develops most frequently on the exposed surfaces of the skin, the face and scalp. There is practically no tendency to metastasis, but the tumor may kill by direct invasion. It begins as a slightly elevated papule that ulcerates, heals over, and then breaks down again. The crusting ulcer develops a smooth, rolled border that represents the tumor cells spreading laterally beneath the skin.

Spider Angioma. This is a central red papule from which superficial fine blood vessels radiate (legs). The lesions are arterial and a pulsation may be felt in the center. The legs will blanch when the center is pressed. They are related to increased estrogen levels and may be present in pregnant women. They are, however, most characteristic for chronic liver disease when there has been parenchymal destruction such as with cirrhosis.

Syphilis. Syphilis is a chronic, systemic infection transmitted by direct and intimate contact with moist infectious lesions of the skin and mucous membranes. Sexual contact is the most common means of infection, but it can be spread through skin abrasions.

A primary lesion, the chancre, develops at the site of inoculation. The chancre is an ulceration of the skin or mucous membrane that heals spontaneously.

Secondary syphilis, occurring about six weeks after the primary lesion, presents as an erythematous macular or papular rash. Superficial painless erosions on the oral mucosa which may be covered with a grayish exudate are mucous patches.

Latent syphilis is that stage of the disease in which there are no clinical signs or symptoms of the infection. Diagnosis is dependent upon serologic testing.

Signs and symptoms of late destructive syphilis occur up to five to 20 years later. Late syphilis of the skin may appear as either small nodules or ulcerating gummas. The gumma begins as a subcutaneous tumor that softens and ruptures, exuding a gummy material. A gumma may produce a painful destructive lesion of the palate and nasal septum. Cardiovascular syphilis is an aortitis, causing either dilatation of the aorta with aortic insufficiency or a saccular aneurysm. Neurosyphilis causes destruction of the posterior roots of the spinal nerves with resulting ataxia, and a psychosis with dementia, hallucinations, memory loss, poor judgment, and gradual change in personality.

Congenital syphilis results from the passage of the spirochete through the placenta from mother to fetus.

WEIGHT

Charts indicating the normal weight for persons of a given height, age, sex and race are useful as guides. Normal weight may vary from 10 to 15 per cent above or below the given standard. Deviation from the average in a normal individual depends upon food intake, energy output, heredity, size of bony framework, temperament, and differences in endocrine gland activity.

Any recent weight gain or loss may be significant. Weight gain, when not caused by overeating, may be due to an endocrine disturbance such as myxedema (hypothyroidism) or edema as in cases of cardiac, hepatic or renal insufficiency.

Weight loss may be an indication of disturbances of digestion, endocrine disorders such as hyperthyroidism, or malignant disease.

TEMPERATURE

The temperature may be normal, subnormal or increased. Body temperature varies to a degree in different persons and from time to time in the same person. Oral temperature above 96.8°F by mouth and below 99.4°F is regarded as normal.

Fever is present if the temperature is over 99.4°F by mouth. It may be caused by infection, inflammation, malignant tumors, disturbance of the heat-regulating mechanism in the basal ganglia as in cerebral hemorrhage, trauma, or hemorrhage.

A chill manifests by a sensation of coldness and shivering, followed by an abrupt rise in temperature. Chills commonly mark the onset of certain infectious diseases, such as pneumonia.

When sweating occurs with a fever there is an abrupt fall in temperature. Chills and sweating are a means for the body to change temperature.

HEAD AND NECK

The size and shape of the head should be noted. In hydrocephalus the large head with the bulging forehead is very striking. In Paget's disease (osteitis deformans) bone changes cause the head to be disproportionately enlarged in relation to the face. The head and face are both enlarged in acromegaly.

In children with hypertrophied adenoid tissue there may be a history of mouth-breathing, frequent colds, and ear infections.

With myxedema the face is swollen, but in contrast to true edema it does not pit on pressure. The skin is coarse and dry, and the hair is dry and scanty.

With hyperthyroidism, exophthalmus (prominence and bulging of the eyes), warm, moist skin, loss of weight, and goiter (enlargement of the thyroid gland) may be present.

Palpation of the neck for enlarged lymph nodes should be carefully performed. Nodes to be examined are the preauricular, mastoid, suboccipital, submandibular areas, anterior and posterior triangles, supra- and infraclavicular fossae, and axillary. Inflammation of the mouth, particularly a mandibular third molar pericoronitis, or tonsillitis may produce swelling and tenderness of the submandibular nodes. Metastatic tumor from cancer of the mouth, tongue, nasopharynx, oral pharynx, hypopharynx, or thyroid gland may first be diagnosed from a biopsy of a discrete hard node. Lymphoma may first present as a nontender, firm, discrete, multiple lymph node enlargement. Other causes are infectious mononucleosis, leukemia, syphilis, and tuberculous lesions.

Rigidity of the neck (nuchal rigidity) is seen in meningitis. There is a boardlike rigidity of the neck, and the body can be raised from a reclining position by lifting the head.

EYES

The eyes give significant information about a patient and provide clues to the diagnosis of systemic disease. Ptosis (drooping) of the upper lids can result from paralysis of the oculomotor nerve. There is marked feebleness of the upper eyelid in myasthenia gravis. In Bell's palsy with facial paralysis of the orbicularis oculi, the individual is unable to close the eye on the affected side. The eyelids are markedly swollen and the eyes nearly closed in angioedema or edema of nephritis, thyrotoxicosis, myxedema, diabetes, anemia, and acute sinusitis. There is usually protrusion of the eyeballs (exophathalmos) in hyperthyroidism.

Glaucoma is an increase in intraocular pressure causing the eyeball to feel hard. Symptoms include pain, often severe and extending over the head, clouding of the cornea, dilatation of the pupil, and reduction of vision.

Cataract is an opacity of the lens usually coming on in later life causing a decrease and blurring of vision.

The conjunctiva is stained yellow in jaundice. Petechiae commonly appear in the conjunctiva with bacterial endocarditis, leukemia, and aplastic anemia.

Examination of the retina with an ophthalmoscope can disclose (1) papilledema or choked disc, a sign of increased intracranial pressure; (2) arteriosclerosis, readily recognized by narrowing of arterioles at certain points; (3) hypertension demonstrated by a nicking of the retinal veins where they are crossed by arterioles, a condition in which the vein appears to taper down or stop abruptly on either side of the arteriole; (4) diabetic retinopathy associated with arteriosclerosis; and (5) optic atrophy.

CHEST

For convenience in describing the surface anatomy of the chest, imaginary lines are drawn. The midclavicular line is drawn through the middle of the clavicle. On the sides of the chest the anterior axillary line is drawn downward from the origin of the anterior axillary fold.

Inspection and palpation of the chest often reveals much information, such as the barrel-shaped chest often seen with emphysema, enlargement of the axillary lymph nodes as seen with carcinoma of the breast, Hodgkin's disease or other lymphomas, leukemia, and infections of the hand or arm. Carcinoma of the breast is a stony hard mass with distortion of the breast and retraction of the nipple.

Kyphosis is an abnormal curvature of the spine with a dorsal prominence; scoliosis is a lateral curvature of the spine.

Auscultation of the lungs and radiographic examination are the most important methods of detecting pulmonary disease. Auscultation, or listening to the lungs with a stethoscope, can tell much about pathology only after one is completely familiar with the normal sounds. Rales are pathologic sounds produced during inspiration or expiration by the passage of air through any liquids present in the bronchi or lungs. Rhonchi are coarse rales caused by partial obstruction of large bronchi. These rales are usually heard in inflammation of the mucous membranes of the bronchi, and are due to the tenacious mucus that partially occludes the bronchus. Moist rales are not continuous but are short, crackling sounds. Fremitus is a palpatory examination of the lungs produced by placing the hands symmetrically upon the chest and asking the patient to speak. The spoken voice sets up a resonance in the lungs and chest wall which can be felt by the hands. The vocal fremitus is produced by vibrations produced in the larynx passing down the bronchi so that the lungs and chest wall vibrate. Abnormally increased fremitus is produced with a solid lung, as with consolidation, pneumonia, atelectasis, and when there is solid lung tissue between the bronchus and chest wall. Decreased fremitus is produced when there is an abnormal medium between the hand and bronchus such as with pleural thickening, pleural effusion, and bronchial obstruction.

A pleural friction rub is a rasping, harsh, rough sound heard during both inspiration and expiration, usually fairly localized, produced by friction of the movements of roughened visceral pleura over parietal pleura. The pleural friction rub is present with acute fibrinous pleurisy.

Kussmaul breathing is a tachypnea (increase in respiratory rate to as high as 30 to 40 per minute) which may be present with uncontrolled diabetes mellitus caused by acidosis and build-up of CO_2. The respirations are also increased in depth.

The hyperventilation syndrome is rapid breathing caused by an altered emotional state. The hyperventilation causes a lowering of the blood CO_2 with a resulting respiratory alkalosis, which may lead to paresthesia around the mouth and fingers and tetany. Cramps in the arms and legs are present.

Bronchiectasis. A dilatation of the small bronchi with sacculation results in pooling of secretions and chronic inflammation. The patient gives a history of coughing up large amounts of sputum in the morning owing to the overnight collecting of the exudate. Diminished breath and voice sounds are present with moist rales. Clubbing of the fingers is usually pronounced.

Pleural Effusion. Pleural effusion is the accumulation of an exudate in the pleural cavity between the visceral and parietal pleura. There are decreased fremitus and breath sounds, the area is dull to percussion, and there are probably no rales. The exudate is usually due to neoplasm or infection.

Atelectasis. All or part of a lung is deflated owing to impaired inflow from an airway obstruction such as tumor, foreign body, or exudate. Because there is no air in the lungs, there are diminished fremitus, absence of breath sounds, no rales, and dullness on percussion.

Pneumothorax. Air enters the pleural cavity, causing all or part of the lung to collapse. The lung is compressed by air in the pleural space. Adhesions of the lung to the thoracic wall prevent complete collapse. There are no breath sounds or rales, fremitus is diminished, and hyperresonance (tympany) occurs on percussion. Pneumothorax is usually caused by rupture of an emphysematous bleb or by trauma.

Pneumonia. Pneumonia is an acute infectious disease of the lungs. The patient has cough, fever, malaise, rust-colored sputum coughed up from the lungs, and chest pain caused by pleuritis. Breathing will be difficult not only because of the pain but because of the decreased vital capacity of the diseased parenchyma. Fremitus will be increased owing to consolidation of lung tissue. Rales will be heard, and there may be a pleural friction rub. Bronchopneumonia is inflammation of the terminal bronchioles distributed throughout the lungs, whereas lobar pneumonia is an infection involving all of one or more lobes of the lungs.

Bronchial Asthma. Bronchial asthma is an allergic disease characterized by expiratory dyspnea and expiratory wheezing. There is a contraction of the smooth muscle around the medium-sized bronchi, causing increased resistance to the flow of air. There are also edema and swelling of the mucous lining and production of mucus. The airways are smaller during expiration than inspiration owing to the difference in intrathoracic pressure; consequently the patient has more difficulty during expiration. With decreased oxygenation of the blood, the patient may become cyanotic; with decreased elimination of CO_2, somnolence and narcosis may develop.

Emphysema. Emphysema is a degenerative disease that usually occurs after the age of 50. The alveolar septa break down, resulting in formation of sacs. The supporting elastic fibers do not support small airways, so the airways will collapse on expiration to give complete obstruction. Progressive dyspnea is the predominant symptom; secondary infections are inevitable. Cyanosis results with clubbing of fingers. With obstruction to air passage on expiration and trapping of air in the lungs, the chest form becomes larger and larger. These patients develop a barrel chest with a large increase in anteroposterior diameter. On expiration, a little positive pressure on the airway will tend to prevent collapsing of the small airways. This positive pressure gives a pursed-lip expiration. On auscultation, breath sounds will be faint owing to decreased exchange of gas, and rales are usually present.

Tumor of the Lung. The majority of primary tumors of the lung arise from the epithelial lining of the bronchus. These bronchogenic carcinomas are usually of the squamous cell type. Metastatic tumors may be from the breast, stomach, pancreas, thyroid, kidney, prostate, uterus, or sarcoma, especially of bone. These tumors may occur as a single circumscribed mass or in an infiltrative form. Lymphomas may appear in multiple nodular or infiltrative form. Symptoms include a cough, which may be productive of blood-tinged sputum, hemoptysis (bleeding from the lungs); dyspnea when a large bronchus is obstructed; secondary infection; pleural effusion from extension of the tumor into the pleura; bronchial obstruction, causing atelectasis of the lung; and mediastinal obstruction with compression of the superior vena cava, resulting in decreased venous return from the face, neck and arms with edema. Generalized malaise, weight loss, and pain are also present.

Pulmonary Edema. Pulmonary edema, sometimes referred to as cardiac asthma, is acute congestion of the pulmonary vascular bed because of left-sided heart failure and decreased ability of the heart to pump blood. This usually occurs in patients with left ventricular failure caused by hypertension, lesions of the aortic valve, or myocardial disease such as myocardial infarction. The patient may have extreme dyspnea and a feeling of suffocation; if this occurs at night, the term paroxysmal noctural dyspnea is applied. Large quantities of pinkish, frothy sputum are coughed up. Rales may be so prominent as to obscure breath and heart sounds.

Pulmonary Embolism and Infarction. Pulmonary embolism is the lodging of any foreign material in a branch of a pulmonary artery, impairing blood flow. Embolism by clot is a complication in patients recovering from surgical operations; fat emboli occur as a result of injury to bones; a thrombus in the right atrium in long-standing heart disease, or valvular vegetation in a right heart chamber in acute or subacute bacterial endocarditis, may form emboli. Pain is a result of regional pleuritis, and the patient complains of a feeling of suffocation and tightness across the chest. Dyspnea is extreme. Blood pressure drops suddenly. Collapse and death may result.

Pleural Friction Rub. A pleural friction rub is a rasping, harsh, rough sound heard during both inspiration and expiration, usually fairly well localized, produced by friction of the movement of roughened visceral pleura over parietal pleura. Pleural friction rub is pathognomonic of acute fibrinous pleurisy.

HEART

Diseases of the heart, like diseases of other organs and tissues, can be categorized by the pathology present:

1. Inflammatory — endocarditis, myocarditis, pericarditis.
2. Neoplastic — tumors.
3. Degenerative — atherosclerotic, congestive heart failure, defect in the conduction system, hypertensive heart disease.
4. Congenital.
5. Hereditary.
6. Abnormal immune response — Rheumatic heart disease.
7. Trauma.
8. Metabolic.
9. Toxic.

In beginning the examination of the heart, the gross anatomy of the normal heart and the manner in which it is projected against the chest wall should be kept in mind.

On inspection and palpation of the heart we look first for the point of maximal impulse (PMI). This impulse that we see and feel on the normal chest wall is the impulse, not of the apex, but of the left ventricle proximal to the apex. The movements of the heart during systole push the heart against the chest wall.

Systole is the contraction of the heart that forces the blood from the ventricles into the systemic and pulmonary circulations, whereas diastole is the period in which the cardiac muscle is relaxing, allowing for filling of the ventricles. The PMI is normally located at the fifth intercostal space at the left midclavicular line. In valvular disease, and in congestive heart failure when there has been marked enlargement of the ventricles, the PMI will be displaced to the left and downward, indicating left ventricular hypertrophy (LVH).

Heart sounds is the term applied to the sounds caused by movements of the heart valves. The first sound is due to the sudden closing of the mitral and tricuspid valves, the valves between the ventricles and atria, when the heart contracts during systole. As the ventricles contract, the pressure within them moves the blood to close these valves and open the aortic and pulmonic valves. The second sound follows the first by a short pause, and is caused by the sudden closing of the aortic and pulmonic valves at the end of systole. This is the beginning of diastole when the ventricles are relaxed and the increased blood pressure in the systemic and pulmonary arteries close the valves.

Murmurs are extra sounds heard over the heart. Many murmurs indicate valvular or other defects within the heart, whereas some systolic murmurs are unimportant and do not imply the presence of a heart lesion. Murmurs are due to eddies formed in the bloodstream owing to a disturbance of the normal streamlined blood flow. Murmurs are either systolic or diastolic in time, occurring with either systole or diastole. They are also designated according to the valve area where they are best heard. A pathologic process may deform the leaflets so that complete closure does not take place, resulting in insufficiency or regurgitation of blood through the valve, in turn resulting in a murmur. Depending on the valve involved, the blood during systole flows backward from a contracting ventricle to a relaxing atrium (mitral or tricuspid insufficiency) or, during diastole, from the aorta or pulmonary artery into a relaxing ventricle (aortic or pulmonic insufficiency). Scarring of the valve leaflets prevents them from opening properly and causes the orifice to be narrowed. Scarring of the leaflets of the mitral valve prevents the normal flow of blood during diastole from the left atrium to the left ventricle — mitral stenosis. A diastolic murmur is heard. Narrowing (stenosis) of the aortic or pulmonic orifice, diminishing blood flow during systole from the ventricles into the aortic or pulmonic arteries, is aortic or pulmonic stenosis, causing a systolic murmur. If a chamber of the heart becomes dilated, the leaflets of one of its valves may fail to close completely, causing a relative insufficiency. The murmur produced by each valvular lesion is usually heard loudest over the valve area and has its own area of distribution. The mitral valve area is located in the fifth left intercostal space, the pulmonary valve area in the second left intercostal space, the aortic valve area at the right second rib and in the right second intercostal space, and the tricuspid area over the sternum at the junction of the corpus sterni with the xiphoid process (See Fig. 3–1). A systolic murmur is produced when a greater than usual amount of blood passes through an orifice, such as in anemia, hyperthyroidism, and after extreme exercise. Murmurs are also heard from abnormal communication between heart chambers or vessels, such as with a patent ductus arteriosus.

As blood passes through constrictions, the vibrations produced are not only heard as murmurs but may be felt as thrills. In aortic stenosis, a systolic thrill may be felt over the precordium with its maximum intensity at the aortic area.

Figure 3–1. Areas where the heart valves are best heard. A, Aortic valve area; P, pulmonic valve area; T, tricuspid valve area; M, mitral valve area.

Pulse

The average pulse rate in normal adults in the dental environment is 60 to 90 heart beats per minute. The pulse represents ventricular systole with the ejection of blood from the ventricles into the systemic and pulmonary circulations. The electrical impulse that starts the normal heart beat begins at the sino-atrial (S–A) node and spreads through the atrial musculature, causing it to contract. From the atria it extends to the atrioventricular (A–V) node, then along the bundle of His and its branches to the Purkinje fibers, through which it is distributed to the ventricular musculature. This conduction of the impulse can be measured on the ECG; in other words, the ECG represents the electrical activity of the heart. Normally the pulse rate is decreased during sleep and increased during excitement and exercise.

Cardiac Dysrhythmias or Arrhythmias

Dysrhythmias or arrhythmias can occur in the absence of detectable structural disease of the heart. Dysrhythmias can be irregularities of the heartbeat, disturbances of rate, or disturbances of conduction. Dysrhythmias frequently are caused by (1) a pathologic process in the myocardium, such as myocardial infarction, ischemia, rheumatic heart disease, or myocarditis; (2) a sudden drop in blood volume due to hemorrhage; (3) endocrine disturbances, such as thyrotoxicosis or pheochromocytoma; (4) drug toxicity, such as with digitalis; (5) fever and infections; (6) tumor; (7) rapid development of severe hypoxemia (decreased oxygen content) or hypercapnia (increased carbon dioxide); and (8) electrolyte disturbance.

CIRCULATORY DERANGEMENTS ASSOCIATED WITH DYSRHYTHMIAS

With a tachycardia of 160 or more beats per minute or a bradycardia of 40 or less beats per minute, cardiac output can be severely decreased, as stroke volume can not adequately compensate for this alteration in rate. With tachycardia there may be insufficient time for diastolic filling, resulting in too little blood in the ventricle for expulsion during ventricular contraction.

The atria should be considered booster pumps which augment ventricular filling. In many dysrhythmias the normal temporal sequence between atrial and ventricular systole is lost, and effective atrial contraction does not occur. The loss of the atrial booster pump can result in a lowering of cardiac output by as much as 40 per cent.

Coronary blood flow occurs predominantly during diastole, and since the total number of seconds of diastole per minute is reduced with tachycardia, a rapid heart rate can precipitate myocardial ischemia.

In ventricular fibrillation the myocardium contracts in such an irregular and chaotic manner that there is no coordinated contraction with sufficient pressure to propel blood forward.

SPECIFIC DISORDERS OF RATE AND RHYTHM

Paroxymal tachycardia may be auricular, A–V nodal, or ventricular in origin.

Sinus Tachycardia. Sinus tachycardia is an abnormally rapid heart rate, over 100 beats per minute, arising at the normal S–A pacemaker. Causes of sinus tachycardia include stimulation during light anesthesia, hypoxia, hypertension, exercise, anxiety, fever, anemia and thyrotoxicosis.

Atrial Tachycardia. Atrial tachycardia is a common cardiac arrhythmia with a rate of 150 to 300 per minute, arising from an ectopic focus in the atrium.

Atrial Fibrillation. During atrial fibrillation the atria does not contract as a whole. There are many small areas of muscle tissue stimulated at various times. The effect is to obliterate any effective contraction of the atria and to bombard the A–V node and ventricles with a very rapid and irregular series of impulses. The ventricles contract rapidly and with gross irregularity. With the absence of atrial contractions mural thrombi (clots) form in the atria. This patient then becomes subject to the hazard of embolism. Atrial fibrillation is present in a high percentage of patients with rheumatic or coronary heart disease.

Ventricular Tachycardia. Ventricular tachycardia is described as repeated ventricular premature beats occurring at a rapid rate. This premature discharge of impulses originates in the ventricular musculature. The ventricular musculature becomes hyperirritable and gives off an impulse which passes over the ventricle by abnormal pathways. It frequently occurs within a few days following the occurrence of a myocardial infarction.

Ventricular Fibrillation. Ventricular fibrillation is a result of a completely haphazard spread of impulses over the conduction network of the ventricle, causing a disorganized and inefficient contraction of the ventricular musculature with resulting circulatory failure.

Bradycardia. Bradycardia is a slowing of the heart rate and is caused by (1) increased vagal tone, as in sinus bradycardia, or (2) a block in the conduction system. With a block in the conduction system, sudden cessation of circulation often causes syncopal attacks (Stokes–Adams attacks). An A–V block can be caused by a myocardial infarction. With a block in the conduction system, the atria maintain their normal rhythm whereas the ventricles contract much slower. Treatment is by implantation of a pacemaker.

CONGESTIVE HEART FAILURE

The failure of adequate circulation, or cardiac decompensation, is a condition in which the cardiac output is too low for the metabolic needs of the body and too low in relation to the venous return. The heart loses its ability to effectively pump blood to peripheral tissues, resulting in the slow development of the clinical picture called congestive heart failure.

Two theories have evolved: forward failure and backward failure. The former holds that because of myocardial weakness cardiac output becomes incapable of meeting the metabolic demands of the body. Blood flow through the kidneys is reduced, resulting in retention of electrolytes and water in the body. The backward failure theory contends incomplete emptying of the heart due to myocardial weakness results in dilatation of the chambers and increase in intracardiac pressure. With increased intracardiac pressure there is decreased filling of the heart, with increased venous pressure and venous stasis. The venous stasis causes impaired renal function with retention of electrolytes and water; and increased pressure in the capillaries causes loss of fluid into the tissue. The retention of electrolytes and fluid is the most important factor in congestive heart failure.

The symptoms and signs of congestive heart failure are based on the accumulation of fluid. Dyspnea, or shortness of breath, is due to fluid within the lungs preventing adequate ventilation. Ankle edema and enlargement of the liver are present. The neck veins (jugular) are distended and prominent. Ascites is the accumulation of fluid within the abdomen.

Treatment is to reduce the excess fluids by the use of diuretics, and to strengthen the cardiac muscle.

CORONARY HEART DISEASE

Heart disease resulting from coronary atherosclerosis is frequent in many patients beyond middle life. Localized narrowing of the coronary blood vessels reduces the blood flow causing an imbalance between the oxygen requirements of the myocardium and the oxygen supply.

Angina pectoris is a syndrome of paroxysmal cardiac pain, substernal in nature. This pain may radiate to the left shoulder and arm, and infrequently to the right shoulder, back, neck, and jaw. Angina pectoris is caused by a temporary lack of oxygen in the myocardium to meet the present needs; consequently the pain is often precipitated by exercise and emotional stress. Relief is obtained by reducing or stopping activity and by the use of coronary vasodilators.

Myocardial infarction is necrosis (death) of the myocardium caused by coronary artery occlusion, embolism in a coronary vessel, or prolonged myocardial ischemia where there is continued diminished blood flow. The necrotic myocardium can no longer contract. Death may result from diminished cardiac output (shock), massive congestive heart failure with pulmonary edema, destruction of the impulse conduction in the myocardium resulting in ventricular fibrillation, or rupture of the necrotic myocardium. The usual symptoms are agonizing crushing substernal pain, dyspnea, and peripheral circulatory failure with fall of blood pressure. The patient's skin becomes cold, clammy, grayish, and cyanotic with perspiration. With lack of blood to the brain the patient becomes confused and unresponsive. Renal shutdown occurs with prolonged shock. Treatment is directed toward relief of pain, reduction of pulmonary edema, relief of shock, oxygenation of the cardiac muscle, and rest.

HYPERTENSIVE HEART DISEASE

Blood pressure is dependent upon the following factors: (1) the cardiac output from the left ventricle into the systemic circulation, (2) elastic recoil of the aorta and large arteries, which propels the blood down the arterial tree during diastole, (3) the peripheral resistance of the arterioles, (4) the volume and viscosity of the blood.

During ventricular contraction (the period of maximum ejection) blood enters the circulation more rapidly than it escapes from the arterioles. As a consequence, the volume of blood in the reservoir increases; potential energy is stored in walls of the vessels, and the blood pressure rises to a maximum — the systolic pressure. During the phase of cardiac relaxation, the rate of arterial drainage exceeds the blood that enters and the pressure falls to a minimum — the diastolic pressure. The normal systolic pressure ranges up to 140; the normal diastolic pressure ranges up to 90.

Hypertensive heart disease is applied to cases that show ventricular hypertrophy caused by increased peripheral hypertension. Peripheral resistance of the blood vessels is increased by decreased elasticity of the vessels, degenerative changes in the intima of the vessels, and deposition of atherosclerotic plaques and calcium. The left ventricle must hypertrophy in order to exert enough force to eject sufficient blood for the body demands against this increased resistance. As a result there may be cardiac failure caused by an insufficient coronary blood supply to meet the demand of the hypertrophied myocardium; cerebral hemorrhage, because the cerebral arterioles cannot tolerate the increased pressure; or renal disease.

ARTERIOSCLEROSIS

Arteriosclerosis is a degenerative condition in which the walls of the arteries become thickened, narrowing the lumen and decreasing the amount of blood flow through the vessel. This increase in peripheral resistance and decreased blood flow leads to coronary insufficiency, hypertension, and secondary hypertensive heart disease.

RHEUMATIC HEART DISEASE

Rheumatic fever is an inflammatory complication that may follow group A beta-hemolyic streptococcal infection. The basic lesion is degeneration of fibrinoid, which is a substance resembling fibrin. These areas of fibrinoid degeneration when surrounded by inflammatory cells are referred to as Aschoff nodules. Aschoff nodules are found in the heart and joints. This entire disease process may be attributed to a breakdown in the immune mechanism and represent a disease of hypersensitivity. Rheumatic fever is a leading cause of chronic illness, invalidism, and death in children; the morbidity is very high due to the residual effects on the heart. The major clinical manifestations are pathognomonic: migratory polyarthritis, chorea, carditis, subcutaneous nodules, erythematous nonpruritic skin rash.

The larger joints (ankles, knees, hips, wrists, elbows, and shoulders) are involved, often in succession. The joint becomes swollen, hot, red, and tender to touch. Active and passive motion is painful.

Specific cardiac lesions are:

1. Acute pericarditis with a serofibrinous exudate between the epicardium and pericardium. This infiltrate contains leukocytes.
2. Myocarditis consists of Aschoff nodules and fibrinoid necrosis in the connective tissue between the muscle fibers. The action of the muscle fibers is severely limited, and cardiac failure can result.
3. Endocarditis is the result of lesions of verrucae composed of fibrin and blood cells along the borders of the valves and chordae. As these lesions heal they may resolve completely or the lesion may undergo organization and scarring, causing valve leaflets to fuse together to narrow an orifice (stenosis). The valve most often affected is the mitral valve. With mitral stenosis, a diastolic murmur is heard during diastole as blood is passing through the stenosed mitral valve from the left atrium to the left ventricle. Lesions on the chordae may cause shortening of the chordae, preventing a valve from closing completely; may cause a dilatation of the valve ring; and may cause destruction of valve substance, all resulting in an insufficiency of the valve. With mitral insufficiency, a systolic murmer will be heard when blood passes in a reverse manner from the contracting left ventricle into the relaxed atria during systole.

Chorea is a disorder of the central nervous system characterized by purposeless movements and muscular weakness. The attacks are recurrent and often prolonged but eventually recovery is complete.

In the skin rheumatic nodules occur near large joints. They are freely movable firm masses, and are large areas of fibrinoid necrosis with inflammatory infiltrate.

SUBACUTE BACTERIAL ENDOCARDITIS

This is a prolonged, febrile, often fatal disease resulting from streptococcal or other infection of a heart valve or a prosthetic valve. Bacterial infection is established on a valve which has been previously damaged by rheumatic fever or congenital heart disease. Roughening of the endocardial surface predisposes to implanation of the bacteria, which are carried to the heart in the blood stream.

Symptoms include fever, chills, sweating, weakness, malaise, heart failure, and paralysis.

Petechial hemorrhages may be visible on the mucosal surfaces, especially the conjunctiva of the lower eyelid or, less frequently, on the skin covering any part of the body.

The bacterial vegetations on the heart valves are friable, and fragments are broken off by the current of blood passing over them. The usual cause of death is embolism of a bacterial vegetation to the brain, heart, or other organ or progressive, intractable cardiac decompensation (failure).

SHOCK

Circulatory failure, or shock, can be either central, when the heart fails to pump a sufficient amount of blood, or peripheral (hypovolemic shock), when there is an acute reduction in the circulating volume. Hypovolemic shock can be due to blood loss caused by a laceration, bleeding ulcer, crushing injury, ruptured spleen, or ectopic pregnancy; it can result from plasma loss, as with a burn or peritonitis, or a water loss, such as from vomiting and diarrhea.

The classic diagnostic signs of shock are a drop in blood pressure, rapid heart rate, pulse feeble and brief in duration, sweating in the axilla, upper lip, forehead, and palmar region, skin coldness, skin color changes, and coma or vagueness of response in the patient.

SYNCOPE

Syncope is caused by a decrease in the vascular motor tone. The circulatory failure is brief and does not become irreversible, and the individual will recover by being left alone in a horizontal position. The blood vessels have become relaxed, the total blood volume remains the same but is distributed over a greater vascular capacity. The individual becomes light-headed and faints because the cerebral circulation has not been adequate. The most effective therapy is not with the head between the knees but rather the Trendelenburg position, with the individual prone or supine and the legs raised.

ABDOMEN

Abdominal examination is best performed with the patient lying on his back on a table or firm bed. For the purpose of describing and localizing lesions in various parts of the abdomen it is usually divided into nine regions. Two vertical lines on each side extend upward from a point midway between the anterosuperior spine of the ilium and midline; and two horizontal lines, one crossing the abdomen at the lower level of the tenth costal cartilages and the lower horizontal line at the level of the anterosuperior iliac spines. The upper third is divided into epigastrium and right and left hypochondria; the middle third, into umbilical region and right and left lumbar regions; and the lower third into hypogastrium and right and left iliac regions (See Fig. 3–2).

Figure 3–2. Regions of the abdomen. (1) Epigastric; (2) umbilical; (3) pubic; (4) right and left hypochondriac; (5) right and left lumbar; (6) right and left iliac.

Inspection and palpation are the two primary methods of physical examination of the abdomen.

One looks for abnormal general contour, pulsations, local prominence, cutaneous lesions, dilated veins, and abnormalities of the umbilicus.

Two of the most common causes of generalized abdominal enlargements are ascites and ovarian cyst. Ascites is the accumulation of fluid within the abdomen and may be due to cardiac failure, cirrhosis of the liver, nephrosis, and tumors of abominal organs.

A pulsation of the epigastrium is seen in aneurysm of the abdominal aorta.

Palpation of the abdomen in the normal individual yields nothing tangible.

Acute Peritonitis.   Acute peritonitis is a suppurative process caused by spread of infection to the peritoneum from a diseased intra-abdominal organ. The most common causes are acute appendicitis, acute cholecystitis, salpingitis, perforation of peptic ulcer, perforation of the intestinal wall such as from diverticulitis, ulcerative colitis, cancer, or necrosis of bowel wall from impairment of its circualtion as with mesenteric thrombosis or volvulus. Pain is usually present at the site of the underlying lesion. Involuntary rigidity of the abdominal wall is present in the region of the lesion. When especially severe it may cause the patient to lie with knees drawn up, to relieve tension on the irritated muscles. Fever, rapid pulse, increased respiration, nausea, and vomiting may also be present. Rebound tenderness, which is pain experienced momentarily when pressure is released after withdrawing the palpating hand, is often present.

Gastritis.   Gastritis is the most common of all gastrointestinal diseases and is commonly due to an overindulgence in food or alcohol, excessive amounts of aspirin, or food poisoning. The usual symptoms are of epigastric discomfort and tenderness, nausea, vomiting, and diarrhea.

Peptic Ulcer.   Peptic ulcer occurs in the tissues of the stomach and the first section of the duodenum (beginning of the small intestine), the tissues of which are exposed to the hydrochloric acid present in the gastric juice. The depth of the ulcer varies from a shallow erosion confined to the mucosa to a full thickness destruction of the wall with perforation into the peritoneal cavity. Symptoms are heartburn, belching, intolerance to certain foods, vague diffuse abdominal discomfort, and periodic relief of discomfort by the ingestion of alkalis and bland foods. The complications of peptic disease are hemorrhage, perforation with secondary peritonitis from food and gastric secretions emptying into the peritoneum, and obstruction.

Appendicitis.   Appendicitis is an inflammation of the vermiform appendix. It can be caused by various infectious processes or by obstruction. When the appendix becomes obstructed, for example, by a fecalith, pressure within the lumen of the appendix causes inflammation and edema, obstruction of venous return, and impairment of arterial flow, which leads to gangrene, necrosis, and perforation. Abscess or peritonitis can occur. The first symptom in an otherwise well individual is abdominal pain; this is followed by anorexia, nausea, or vomiting. When inflammation occurs in the adjacent peritoneum the pain shifts to the right lower quadrant of the abdomen causing tenderness, spasm of the muscles, and rebound tenderness.

LIVER

If the lower border of the liver extends below its normal level, it can be located by palpation. Hepatic enlargement is present if the lower border is felt below the costal margin in the right hypochondrium. Hepatic enlargement can be caused by fatty infiltration, congestive heart failure when there is impairment of return blood flow (right heart failure), hepatitis, cirrhosis, neoplasm, biliary tract obstruction, and parasitic infestation.

Jaundice.   Jaundice, the term applied to the yellow pigmentation of the tissues of the skin and mucous membranes, is associated with an increase in the bilirubin content of the plasma. Jaundice results from one of three general situations: (1) when bilirubin is presented to a normal liver at a rate which exceeds the ability of the liver to conjugate and excrete the pigment into the biliary system (prehepatic jaundice), (2) when the liver cells are functionally impaired and cannot conjugate and excrete a normal amount of bilirubin presented to them (hepatic jaundice), and (3) when the free flow of conjugated bilirubin through the biliary system is impaired (posthepatic jaundice).

In prehepatic jaundice resulting from a hemolytic disease, the fundamental abnormalitiy is an increased rate of destruction of red cells, an overproduction of bilirubin. The plasma bilirubin is mainly of the indirect type (unconjugated). Since the bilirubin present in the plasma is in the insoluble form as free bilirubin, it is not filtered by the kidneys.

In hepatocellular disease both unconjugated and conjugated bilirubins are increased in the plasma.

In posthepatic jaundice the fundamental defect is in the passage of conjugated bilirubin through the biliary system. In hepatocellular disease and with obstruction of the bile passage, conjugated bilirubin will be regurgitated into the plasma and excreted in the urine, resulting in dark urine. Since there are decreased or no bilirubin by-products in the gastrointestinal tract, the stools will be clay colored.

Hepatitis B.   Hepatitis B is an acute systemic viral infection that affects the liver. There are degeneration and necrosis of the liver parenchymal cells with proliferation and swelling of the reticuloendothelium. The symptoms are fever, headache, anorexia, weakness, nausea, vomiting, indigestion, and abdominal pain. Jaundice appears and is accompanied by bilirubin in the urine (dark urine) and clay-colored stools. The more severe cases can lead to liver failure with development of central nervous system changes, somnolence, disorientation, delirium, convulsions, and coma. The liver can no longer metabolize alcohol and any intake may cause further destruction of the parenchymal cells and relapse.

Transmission of the virus is via the fecal-oral route, the parenteral route resulting from transfusions, or the use of nonsterile instruments, and there is some evidence that suggests transmission can occur through saliva.

The hepatitis carrier becomes the greatest obstacle to the control of the disease. It is generally assumed that those who retain the hepatitis antigen in their blood are potentially infective, although this risk is extremely slight. The antigen appears during the incubation period of the disease and is most often cleared from the blood by three months after recovery; however, some patients may remain antigen-positive for years. The identification of non-A and non-B hepatitis viruses has introduced even greater doubt regarding the hepatitis B "carrier" state.

Cirrhosis.   Cirrhosis is a diffuse fibrosis that destroys the normal lobular architecture of the liver and causes degeneration and necrosis of the parenchymal cells. As the cirrhotic process advances, signs of liver failure and portal hypertension appear. Blood can no longer pass through the liver to the vena cava; consequently, alternate venous return develops in the form of esophageal and abdominal varices. As liver cells fail to function, serum albumin, prothrombin, and fibrinogen levels fall, detoxification decreases, bilirubin builds up and is not conjugated, glycogen storage decreases, and there is a breakdown in protein, carbohydrate, and lipid metabolism. Blood coagulation will be decreased owing to a deficiency of prothrombin and other clotting factors. Patients may have massive bleeding from esophageal varices. The clinical signs of cirrhosis include jaundice, edema, pleural effusion and ascites due to low levels of plasma proteins and increased venous pressure, spider nevi, palmar erythema, gynecomastia, low grade fever, nausea, vomiting, diarrhea, and abdominal pain. The liver becomes enlarged, the skin has a grayish hue, and there is a sickeningly sweet odor to the breath. The patient has a wasted appearance, and develops a flapping tremor and other neurologic changes.

The common types of cirrhosis are:

1. Laennecs's cirrhosis, caused by malnutrition or chronic alcoholism, or both.
2. Postnecrotic cirrhosis, usually a sequela to hepatic necrosis following hepatitis.
3. Biliary cirrhosis, which develops as a result of prolonged obstruction of the extrahepatic bile ducts, and usually has a relatively benign course for a

number of years, during which there are few clinical or laboratory signs of hepatocellular failure.

4. Cardiac cirrhosis, which results from passive congestion of the liver with blood secondary to heart failure. Engorgement of the sinusoids with blood results in atrophy and degeneration of the parenchymal cells.

Carcinoma.   Primary carcinoma of the liver may arise from either the parenchymal cells or the intrahepatic bile duct epithelium. Cirrhosis appears to be an important predisposing factor.

Metastatic neoplasms occur at least 20 times as frequently as primary carcinoma; hepatic metastases are found in approximately one third of all malignancies. Metastasizing cells gain easy access to the liver because of its double circulation — hepatic arterial and portal venous. Gastrointestinal, pancreatic, breast, uterine, ovarian and renal carcinomas often metastasize to the liver first. Clinical signs include cachexia, abdominal pain, jaundice, and ascites as well as enlarged liver.

Kidneys

In diseases of the kidneys the most significant findings are often those discovered in examination of blood and urine.

Nephrotic Syndrome (Nephrosis).   This is a degenerative, noninflammatory lesion confined to the tubules; it may occur with a number of pathologic lesions. Clinically the patient has severe proteinuria (loss of albumin in the urine), low serum protein, secondary edema with pleural effusion, and probably no elevation of blood pressure. This may occur with the nephrotic stage of glomerulonephritis, renal vein thrombosis, diabetic glomerulonephrosclerosis, lupus erythematosus, and multiple myeloma.

Pyelonephritis.   Pyelonephritis, either acute or chronic, is an infectious process of the kidneys. It is more common in females, and the usual infecting agent is the colon bacillus. The clinical signs and symptoms are fever, chills, lumbar pain, pain on urination with increased frequency, and moderate to extreme tenderness in the costovertebral angle. Long-standing disease causes damage to the parenchyma and impaired kidney function. Uremia, serious hypertension, and renal failure may result. Hypertension caused by impaired function is due to renal vascular damage. The urine is loaded with white blood cells and bacteria.

Kidney Stones.   Renal stones may exist for years without causing symptoms, but, when they descend to the ureter, extreme pain (renal colic) will be felt in the lower quadrant of the abdomen and flank. Gross hematuria (blood in the urine) and urgency caused by reflex bladder irritation are present. Calcium stones occur with hyperparathyroidism, prolonged immobilization, high milk intake, and idiopathic hypercalcinuria. Uric acid stones may be present with gout.

Renal Failure.   Renal failure is the impaired ability of the kidneys to clear the blood of metabolites. Urea, creatine, and other nonprotein nitrogens build up in the blood, leading to uremia. The signs and symptoms of uremia are a yellowish-brown discoloration of the skin, pallor resulting from anemia, pruritis, purpura secondary to increased capillary permeability, urea frost on the skin, depression of erythropoiesis, hypertension with secondary heart failure, Kussmaul breathing (deep respirations with slight tachypnea) secondary to a metabolic acidosis, anorexia, nausea, and eventual onset of coma.

Renal failure can occur whenever the kidneys are damaged, such as with malignant hypertension, fulminating pyelonephritis, shock associated with circulatory failure, the degenerative stage of the nephrotic syndrome, or a toxic insult.

Diabetes Mellitus.   Diabetes mellitus is a disorder of carbohydrate metabolism caused by an absolute or relative insulin deficiency. Insulin deficiency leads to inability of the body to transfer glucose into the cells, with resultant hyperglycemia (excessive glucose in the blood) and glycosuria (glucose in the urine). Owing to lack of utilization of glucose, fatty acids and proteins are metabolized to ketone bodies to supply the energy needs of the body. As ketone bodies are acids, metabolic acidosis results. The glycosuria causes diuresis and resultant dehydration. Diabetic coma is due to the effects of acidosis, ketosis, and dehydration on the central nervous system.

Vascular lesions are present; atherosclerosis, arteriosclerosis, calcification of the vessels, and decrease in capillary lumen size occur. These lesions cause the individual to have an increased incidence of coronary artery insufficiency, cerebrovascular accidents, impaired renal function, and gangrene of the toes and feet.

Considering diabetes as an imbalance between ingested carbohydrates and available body insulin, therapy is directed toward dietary restriction and augmentation of insulin effects. Insulin administration does check the hyperglycemia and ketosis but has no influence on the progress of the degenerative disease of the blood vessels.

The more uncontrolled the disease, the more susceptible the individual is to infection. Infections also have a disastrous effect on diabetes, readily changing a controlled state to an uncontrolled state.

Symptoms of the disease are polyuria, polydipsia, polyphagia, dry hot skin, and an emaciated appearance.

THYROID

The function of the thyroid gland is to produce a hormone which is capable of stimulating the rate of metabolism of the tissues, according to the needs of the body.

Hypothyroidism.   Hypothyroidism may be either primary, owing to thyroid gland failure, or secondary, owing to lack of thyroid stimulating hormone from the pituitary gland. Primary hypothyroidism dating from birth is known as cretinism and is a result of genetic defects or a deficiency of iodine. The clinical picture is that of a dwarfed, stocky, somewhat overweight, mentally retarded child, with eyes set apart owing to failure of naso-orbital development, coarse features, thick lips, and protruding tongue. Myxedema characterizes hypothyroidism in the adult. The clinical picture shows a typical facies with a dull uninterested expression and puggy eyelids; alopecia of the outer third of the eyebrows is characteristic, as are dry and rough skin, coarse, brittle, and dry hair, hoarse speech, slowing of mental and physical activity, and poor muscle tone. The relaxation time of the deep tendon reflexes is prolonged.

Hyperthyroidism.   Also known as Graves' disease, this condition results from diffuse hyperplasia of the thyroid gland. Enlargement of the gland is called goiter. There is a peculiar involvement of bulbar tissue which begins with edema of the loose connective tissue, followed by a proliferative fibrosis. This edema and fibrosis lead to displacement of the eye bulb forward, known as exophthalmos. The patient also suffers from the following: fine tremor of the extended fingers and tongue; increased nervousness, irritability, and emotional instability; sweating; hyperkinesis; loss of weight and strength without loss of appetite; intolerance to heat; warm, moist skin; increased metabolic rate; and cardiac findings which include a wide pulse pressure between the systolic and diastolic pressures, tachycardia or atrial fibrillation, frequent systolic murmur, and heart failure. These individuals have soft, silky hair.

Adrenal Cortex

The adrenal cortex produces three types of hormones, all steroids. The glucocorticoids promote gluconeogenesis, which brings about the destruction of protein and its conversion to carbohydrate. The amino acids are diverted toward carbohydrate metabolism at the expense of protein synthesis. The mineralocorticoids cause urinary retention of sodium and water and increased urinary output of potassium and phosphorus The sex hormones, estrogen, progesterone and androgens, contribute to the development of secondary sex characteristics, play some part in skeletal maturation, and promote protein synthesis.

Hypofunction may exist as a primary problem of the cortex known as Addison's disease or secondary to hypopituitarism and lack of cortical stimulating hormones of the pituitary gland. The most common cause of primary progressive adrenal cortical destruction is adrenal tuberculosis. Clinical signs and symptoms are a bronze darkening of the skin due to deposition of melanin, weakness, hypotension, weight loss, anorexia, and hypoglycemia due to lack of glucocorticoids.

Hyperfunction due to bilateral adrenal cortical hyperplasia or adrenal tumor is known as Cushing's syndrome. Clinical signs and symptoms are weight gain, hirsutism, amenorrhea, redistribution of fat producing the characteristic "moon" facies, supraclavicular fat pads, obesity of the trunk and thin extremities, hypertension, muscular weakness due to breakdown of proteins, some evidence of masculinization in females. There is generalized osteoporosis due to increased gluconeogenesis with a breakdown of proteins to carbohydrates. Fractures are seen, with greatest frequency in the vertebra, and the lamina dura around the teeth is often missing. Diabetes may occur. There is a generalized atherosclerosis, well advanced in relation to age.

Parathyroids

Hyperparathyroidism.   This is a disease in which excessive parathormone is produced, causing symptoms of the skeletal, muscular, gastrointestinal and renal systems. Excessive parathormone is produced by an adenoma, carcinoma, or hyperplasia of the parathyroid glands. This hormone stimulates osteoclastic activity, causing osteoporosis. Spontaneous fracture may occur. As a result of mobilization of the calcium and phosphates from bone, renal stones will form; the calcium passing into the gastrointestinal tract causes nausea, vomiting, anorexia, and gastric and duodenal ulcers. Muscle weakness and decreased muscle tone result from the increased circulating calcium.

HEMATOLOGY

ANEMIA

Anemia is a condition caused by an insufficient amount of erythrocytes with a resulting decrease in the total oxygen carrying capacity. Anemia can be a result of a loss of blood inside or outside the body, a failure to manufacture erythrocytes, or a shortened red cell life span, the disease known as hemolytic anemia.

Sickle Cell Anemia. Sickle cell anemia, a hemolytic anemia hereditary in nature, is found only in blacks and is a result of the manufacture of abnormal hemoglobin. The anomaly is inherited as a mendelian dominant characteristic in which each parent having the "trait" transfers the abnormal gene to his or her offspring. The erythrocytes instead of being concentric assume the shape of a half-moon (sickle) when the hemoglobin is in the reduced state. Thus, if a person with the disease is temporarily deficient in oxygen, such as during a plane trip or under general anesthesia, many cells will assume the crescentic form. In the homozygous state the erythrocytes contain sufficient abnormal hemoglobin to bring about sickling within the physiologic range of oxygen tensions. Because of this shape the viscosity of the blood and the mechanical fragility of the erythrocytes are significantly increased, and hemolysis results. Also the sickleshaped cells become enmeshed, forming a mass and causing thrombotic episodes. Because there are many erythrocytes in the sinusoids of the spleen, a splenic thrombotic episode will be very painful, suggesting an abdominal emergency. These individuals have chronic hemolytic anemia, develop thrombosis, infarction, and necrosis in the lungs, spleen, and nervous system, are jaundiced and weak, and often have episodes of aching pain in the joints; x-ray examination of the skull shows a "hair-on-end" appearance of the marrow due to the demand for erythrocyte production.

Iron Deficiency Anemia. Lack of iron can be a result of insufficient iron in the diet or impaired absorption but is usually caused by a chronic loss of blood. Excessive menstruation and occult bleeding from the gastrointestinal tract are common causes. The symptoms are those common to all chronic anemias and may include a variety of vague gastrointestinal complaints such as anorexia, sore tongue, dysphagia, and neuralgic pains.

Pernicious Anemia. Pernicious anemia is a disorder brought about by the body's failure to manufacture erythrocytes. It is a familial disease, occurring usually in middle life. A lack of gastric acid in the stomach prevents absorption of Vitamin B_{12} and folic acid. These vitamins act as coenzymes at different stages in the synthesis of nucleoproteins within the hemoglobin. Neurological abnormalities are also present, since these vitamins are also necessary for the synthesis of proteins within the central nervous system. Individuals with this disease may experience tingling and numbness.

Leukemia. Leukemia is a progressive, malignant disorder characterized by abnormal proliferation of white blood cells and their precursors. This is in contrast to the benign, controlled proliferation that occurs after hemorrhage and during infection. The circulating cells are immature and have deranged serum proteins, thus greatly diminishing their antibody-making capability. Control of infection is a continuous problem in leukemia victims. Because of the massive amounts of tumor cells within the bone marrow, there is a decrease in thrombocytes, causing these individuals to be subjected to abnormal bleeding. The signs and symptoms include great fatigue, weakness, fever, bone pain, purpura, nose bleeds, severe anemia, and chronic periodontitis. Death usually results from an uncontrolled infection or from bleeding within the brain.

LYMPH NODES

The functions of the lymph nodes are to afford mechanical filtration for the lymph stream, removing cellular debris, foreign particles, and bacteria, and to serve as the site of formation of lymphocytes and antibodies.

Enlargement of nodes can be due to the following disorders: suppurative infections such as streptococcus or staphylococcus; antigenic challenge in serum sickness or systemic lupus erythematosus; granuloma formation in such diseases as tuberculosis, syphilis, histoplasmosis, and sarcoid; metastases of malignant disease such as carcinoma; congenital abnormalities as with a lymphangioma; or primary tumors, including Hodgkins disease, lymphosarcoma, and chronic lymphocytic leukemia. Nodes to be examined for enlargement are the cervical, post-auricular, supraclavicular, axillary, ulnar, and inguinal.

COMA

Coma is a prolonged state of unconsciousness in which there is no response to outside stimuli — the patient cannot be roused. When a comatose patient is first seen, certain therapeutic measures take precedence over diagnostic procedures. The comatose patient must have a clear airway; bleeding must be stopped if trauma has occurred, and adequate circulation must be ensured. Coma may occur with any lesion that damages the central reticular formation.

A few of the common causes of coma follow.

Cerebrovascular Accident (Stroke). Cerebral hemorrhage is bleeding directly into the brain; the most common cause is hypertension associated with degenerative changes in the vessel walls. Hypertensive cerebral hemorrhage usually occurs in late middle life, whereas hemorrhage occurring during the first half of adult life is likely to be from a congenital vascular abnormality such as an aneurysm or angioma. The site of hemorrhage is occupied by a red clot, and the surrounding tissues are compressed and may be edematous. Later, if the victim survives, the clot is absorbed and is replaced by a neuroglial scar. A neurological deficit results depending upon the area of the brain where the neural tissue has been destroyed and replaced with scar tissue. The onset is always sudden. Usually the patient complains of a sudden severe headache, may vomit, becomes dazed, and loses consciousness.

Drug Poisoining.   In coma caused by drug poisoning the respirations are slow, and circulatory failure may develop, with a fall in blood pressure. The history is very significant. Narcotic and barbiturate drugs in excessive amounts cause coma.

Head Injury.   Concussion causes temporary unconsciousness lasting a few minutes after trauma. Coma that lasts longer than a few hours is usually a sign of contusion of the brain with cerebral edema or intracranial bleeding. Besides loss of consciousness, other signs of epidural or subdural hematoma are nausea, projectile vomiting, rise in blood pressure, slowing of the pulse, paralysis, fixed, dilated pupils, and slow, irregular breathing. In skull fracture the nose and ears are examined for blood or cerebrospinal fluid loss.

EPILEPSY

Epileptic convulsions result from a paroxysmal discharge of abnormal electrical impulses in some part of the brain. These discharges are likely to be repetitive. The first motor manifestation of the convulsion is a phase of tonic (sustained) spasm of the muscles which is usually symmetrical on both sides of the body. Owing to spasm of the respiratory muscles, breathing ceases during the tonic phase, which usually lasts less than half a minute. Progressive cyanosis occurs during the arrest of respiration but passes off when respirations are re-established. Repeated episodes of cyanosis will result in gradual deterioration of brain function and mentality.

In the second, or clonic, phase, the sustained contraction of the muscles give way to sharp, short, interrupted jerking movements. During the clonic phase the tongue may be bitten, foaming at the mouth may occur, and the individual is incontinent. Toward the end of the clonic phase the intervals between the muscular contractions become longer and the jerking motions finally cease. The individual remains in coma for a variable time, and on recovering consciousness sleeps for several hours.

The convulsion often begins with an aura, or warning of the attack. This is a symptom produced at the beginning of the epileptic discharge and perceived by the individual before consciousness is lost. Since the focus of origin of the attack may be situated in a variety of localities within the brain there is a corresponding variety of auras, which can take the form of a complex mental state, an emotion such as fear, or a hallucination in the sphere of one of the senses such as smell, taste, vision or hearing, or an abnormal feeling referred to some part of the body.

Consciousness is usually lost immediately after the aura.

HEADACHE

The principal pain-sensitive structures within the skull are the large blood vessels, and there is abundant evidence that many headaches are initiated by the effect of pressure or traction on these intracranial vessels. The most common causes are space-occupying lesions, such as a tumor or hematoma, meningeal irritation, such as with an inflammatory exudate, and hypertension. Pain in the head can also be referred from the eye, nasal sinuses, temporomandibular joint, thoracic or abdominal viscera or can be psychogenic.

CEREBRAL ISCHEMIA

There is a group of disorders in which the symptoms are due to insufficiency of the blood supply to the brain. The commonest of these is atheroma of the arteries supplying the brain. Infarction of the brain may occur as a result of the narrowing of an artery by atheroma without its complete occlusion or as the result of its occlusion by thrombosis or embolism.

Since the cerebral circulation depends directly upon the adequacy of the blood pressure, a fall in pressure from any cause, such as myocardial infarction, paroxysmal arrhythmia, or peripheral circulatory failure may render temporarily inadequate the circulation through a narrowed atheromatous vessel.

Mental symptoms are common and include reduction in intellectual capacity, impairment of memory especially for recent events, emotional instability, and attacks of confusion.

Cerebral embolism is a variety of ischemic cerebral disease in which the ischemia develops acutely as the result of some substance being carried in the circulation to lodge in one or more of the cerebral vessels. Embolism can be due to atheroma from an extracranial vessel, a blood clot from a paralyzed left atrium as a result of atrial fibrillation or mitral stenosis, or an infected vegetation breaking off from the aortic or mitral valve in subacute bacterial endocarditis.

HYDROCEPHALUS

Hydrocephalus is enlargement of the head occurring before birth or in early infancy and caused by an excess of cerebrospinal fluid under increased pressure. It is due to an obstruction to the circulation of the cerebrospinal fluid which prevents proper absorption of the fluid into the blood. These children are mentally defective, owing to compression and atrophy of the brain.

MULTIPLE SCLEROSIS

Multiple sclerosis is characterized by widespread occurrence of patches of demyelination of the nerve tracts within the central nervous system. The demyelination is followed by gliosis (scarring). There is a tendency for remissions and relapses, so that the course of the disease may be prolonged for years. Symptoms include blurred vision, double vision, numbness of some part of the body, weakness of a limb, and euphoria with a characteristic sense of mental and physical well being.

MENINGITIS

Acute meningitis is an infection of the pia mater and arachnoid which inevitably involves the subarachnoid space and the cerebrospinal fluid. It may be due to a fracture of the skull, extension to the meninges of a pyogenic infection from one of the nasal sinuses, the middle ear, or mastoid, or spread of infection through the blood stream which may be secondary to a focal infection such as with pneumonia, osteomyelitis, enteric infection or a bacteremia, as with meningococcal meningitis.

The subarachnoid space of the brain and spinal cord becomes filled with a greenish-yellow pus and the cerebrospinal fluid is under increased pressure and loaded with white cells. Cervical rigidity due to spasm of the extensor muscles of the neck is always present; delirium is common in the early stages. The patient also has headache, fever, increased pulse rate, drowsiness, and stupor. Convulsions are common in children. Coma occurs in later stages.

RHEUMATOID ARTHRITIS

Rheumatoid arthritis is a chronic systemic disease in which there are inflammatory changes in the joints causing characteristic deformities. There is chronic inflammation, edema, proliferation of capillaries, and infiltration of inflammatory cells which may progress to the formation of granulation tissue and fibrosis. The layers of granulation tissue covering each surface of the joint interdigitate with their opposing layers to form fibrous adhesions and ankylosis. The clinical manifestations of joint inflammation are pain, swelling, redness, heat, and deformity. Subcutaneous nodules are frequently found near tendon sheaths, and an arteritis may be found in the synovial membrane, muscles, heart, and other organs.

DEGENERATIVE JOINT DISEASE

Degenerative joint disease, also known as osteoarthritis, is a disease related to the physiologic process of aging in which there is degeneration of the articular cartilage and hypertrophy of adjacent bone. There are no systemic manifestations. Pain is present when the joints are used and subsides with rest. Stiffness results from prolonged rest in a fixed position and disappears after resuming activity. The enlarged joints, when present, feel hard and knobby, unlike the soft, fluctuant swelling in rheumatoid arthritis.

CONCLUSION

It is not the intent of this abbreviated discussion of disease processes and significant symptoms and signs to prepare the reader to be an astute diagnostician but merely to familiarize him or her with the method of approach to disease.

Sir William Osler stated: "To study the phenomena of disease without books is to sail an uncharted sea, while to study books without patients is not to go to sea at all. . ."

The dental health professional interested in furthering his or her knowledge of physical evaluation/physical diagnosis and dental treatment modification is invited to become thoroughly familiar with chapters 1 to 3. If more detailed information is desired, proceed to textbooks of medicine, physical diagnosis, and physicial examination, and participate in advanced physical diagnosis continuing education courses.

If you feel that dental patients are not sufficiently medically compromised to provide experience for you, per the Osler quotation, it is suggested that you look again. There is a wealth of relevant clinical material in the dental office for the diligent observer. Once you learn to recognize and evaluate disease, you will be staggered by the large percentage of ASA physical status Class II and III patients who merit proper evaluation and modification to dental therapy, yet whom you otherwise have classified as healthy, normal patients prior to your development of expertise in physical evaluation/physical diagnosis (see chapter on *physical evaluation* regarding ASA classification). Interest, dedication, the powers of observation, and experience are the keys to further development.

REFERENCES

1. Bates, B.: A Guide to Physical Examination. 1st ed., Philadelphia, J. B. Lippincott Co., 1974.
2. Beeson, P. B., and McDermott, W.: Textbook of Medicine. 14th ed., Philadelphia, W. B. Saunders Co., 1975.
3. DeGowin, E. L., and DeGowin, R. L.: Bedside Diagnostic Examination. 3rd ed., New York, Macmillan Publishing Co., Inc., 1976.
4. Delp, M. H., and Manning, R. T.: Major's Physical Diagnosis. 8th ed., Philadelphia, W. B. Saunders Co., 1975.
5. Dineen, J. J.: What constitutes appropriate training in physical diagnosis and medicine for oral surgeons. J. Oral Surg., 33:740–742, 1975.
6. Laskin, D. L., and Lemke, G. W.: Teaching of physical diagnosis to dental students and oral surgery residents. J. Oral Surg., 33:736–739, 1975.
7. Trieger, N., and Goldblatt, L.: The art of history taking, J. Oral Surg., 36:118–124, 1978.

MONITORING

THOMAS F. MULKEY
and CEDRIC L. HAYDEN

INTRODUCTION

Consciously or unconsciously, every practitioner evaluates the patient before, during, and after each operation and procedure. As Adriani informs us, "The term monitoring refers to the overall surveillance of the patient by methods employing the senses of touch, sight, hearing or smell or by means of devices which operate chemically, physically or electronically to measure the adequacy of the various physiological functions."[1]

This chapter will first review all direct observation monitoring that applies to conscious-patient sedation or ultralight general anesthesia in the office. The same monitoring background is also vital with respect to the conduct of a high-risk case or in the treatment of an emergency. The general practitioner is invited to carefully review this chapter.

Later we will cover biomedical and mechanical monitoring, some of which is impractical at this time for office use. Yet, some applications can be made at present in the occasional case, and, as enormous strides are being made in instrument design, we feel that the information should be made available. In this section the general dental practitioner will find the following of greatest interest and most possible application: the "fail-safe" style of gas pressure monitor for the anesthesia or sedation machine, the electronic pulse monitor, and the monaural stethoscope for breath sounds, heart sounds, and blood pressure. The cardioscope is also of interest, as is the general discussion of the more common cardiac arrhythmias.

Monitoring of vital signs is a necessary function during all dental therapy, regardless of the anesthesia utilized. *The degree of surveillance is in direct relation to the degree of pain/anxiety control,* and therefore it varies from the totally unmedicated patient through local analgesia alone, the conscious-patient sedation techniques, ultralight outpatient general anesthesia, and hospital-type, surgical depth general anesthesia in which an endotracheal tube can be tolerated for restorative dentistry or the peritoneum can be incised. *The degree of surveillance also increases with an emergency or with serious disease.*

If we analyze the definition of conscious-patient sedation, we observe:

Conscious — awake to one's own existence, sensations; cognition, having the mental faculties awake.
Sedation — that which causes one to be sedate.
Sedate — calm, quiet or composed, sober, undisturbed by passion or emotion.

To transpose these definitions to a patient about to receive treatment, we have a patient who has received a chemical substance by the oral, inhalation, or intravenous route which has rendered him calm, composed, and undisturbed by his emotions, yet able to respond knowledgeably to question or command, and without depression of protective reflexes.

Analyzing the term ultralight general anesthesia we observe:

Ultra — beyond the ordinary
Light — of small amount, force or intensity.
General anesthesia — general insensibility to pain, with loss of consciousness.

To transpose, we have a patient who is generally insensitive to pain, but of exceedingly small intensity; a patient who is unconscious with no significant muscle relaxation and whose protective reflexes, such as lash, lid, gag, laryngeal, and cough, are depressed either not at all or only momentarily.

Monitoring is in a state of change in dentistry, and few standards can be recognized at the present time. In an attempt to clarify the situation, Table 4–1 shows our estimate of present minimal application of various monitoring techniques. It is assumed that the patient is in excellent health, that there are no emergency problems, and that a routine physical evaluation with blood pressure, pulse, and temperature has been performed. Additional monitoring modalities would be applied as indicated in an emergency or for the high-risk patient.

Direct observational techniques for monitoring the patient are inspec-

TABLE 4-1

	Preop Temp. & Resp.	Preop B.P. & Pulse	Periodic B.P. & Pulse	Continuous B.S. & H.S.	Continuous B.P. & Pulse	Card.
Unmedicated	No—D	No—D	No	No	No	No
Local analgesia only	No—D	No—D	No	No	No	No
Conscious-patient oral sedation	No—D	No—D	No	No	No	No
Conscious-patient inhalation sedation	No—D	No—D	No	No	No	No
Conscious-patient intravenous sedation	No—D	Yes	No—D	No	No	No
Ultralight general anesthesia	Yes	Yes	D	D	Opt.	Opt.
Surgical depth general anesthesia	Yes	Yes	Yes	Yes	Yes	Opt.

B.P. = blood pressure.   D = desirable.
B.S. = breath sounds   Opt. = optional.
H.S. = heart sounds.   Card. = cardioscope.

tion, palpation, auscultation, and percussion. The physiological functions that lend themselves to monitoring and are significant in determining the well being of the patient at any time during anesthesia include those of three organ systems: the central nervous system, the respiratory system, and the cardiovascular system.

The early Egyptian physicians were familiar with the concept of inspection. And one Victorian physician-turned-author, Sir Arthur Conan Doyle, created an unsurpassed detective with tremendous powers of inspection and analysis, Sherlock Holmes. The literary character is said to be based upon an actual physician whose uncanny powers of observation had greatly impressed the young physician Doyle. Although the ancients, including Hippocrates, had some conception of auscultation, this method of diagnosis did not become important until the discovery of the stethoscope by Laennec in the early nineteenth century. Today's anesthetist will sometimes percuss the abdomen to see if the anesthetic gas or air has been forced into the stomach, thereby distending it, or he will use palpation when feeling the pulse.

From the beginning, however, inspection was one of the most important methods used for the assessment of patient health, and it remains so today. It is easily the most significant patient evaluation technique used by health practitioners. By using the main methods of physical diagnosis, the surgeon/anesthetist and the general dental practitioner may monitor patients with great safety.

A brief anatomical description of the three main organ systems mentioned above might be appropriate at this time. The central nervous system pertains to the brain, spinal cord, and the many afferent and efferent nerve fibers that carry the impulses from the sensory surfaces to the reflex centers and back, thus giving us the reflex actions which we monitor. The respiratory system, as referred to in this chapter, includes the nose, pharynx, trachea, lungs, thorax, and respiratory muscles, including the diaphragm and intercostals. These components interact to move the oxygen into the system and waste carbon dioxide out of the body. The cardiovascular system includes the heart, the various categories of vessels, and the blood, functioning together as a transport system for oxygen and carbon dioxide within the body.

At this time we wish to consider the various signs to be assessed by the doctor and his team of trained auxiliary personnel. By using the information received from monitoring the three systems by direct observation, he can give the patient safe, comfortable dental care. In succeeding pages we will introduce the electronic and mechanical devices that have been developed and that are capable of second-to-second monitoring of many vital functions simultaneously.

DIRECT OBSERVATION MONITORING

Central Nervous System

The reflex actions of the central nervous system indicate the degree to which a particular physiological function has been affected during an emergency, conscious-patient sedation, or general anesthesia.

Reflex actions of the eye, including those of the lash, lid, and pupil, are examples of reflex activity that can be evaluated continuously by the team during a procedure in order to determine the physiological status of the patient.

Starting with the structures that are anatomically most superficial, we encounter the lash reflex. This is the blinking of the eye that occurs whenever the upper or lower eyelash is stroked gently with the finger. This stroking is a very weak stimulus, and for this reason the reflex is lost early in the induction phase of anesthesia. Many dentistry procedures that are not particularly painful may be performed when this reflex is still present. For example, suturing of a mucosal incision at the end of a surgical procedure may be completed while this reflex is present. However, elevating a mucoperiosteal flap might not be possible when this reflex is active. The lid reflex is the next we encounter, and this occurs when the eyelid loses its ability to close voluntarily after it has been opened. This reflex is usually seen with the patient in a surgical plane of anesthesia when one is using an intravenous barbiturate. Coordinated movement of the eyeballs when the lids are lifted together is usually seen during the lighter stages of dental anesthesia. It will disappear as the anesthesia deepens.

The pupil of the eye also offers many varied signs to determine the depth of anesthesia. The reaction of the pupil to light in the unpremedicated patient is a sign that may be interpreted very accurately. If the patient has lost the pupillary reaction to light, then he is in a *deeper plane of anesthesia than is usually needed for dental procedures*. The pupil size is another indication of depth of anesthesia. It becomes smaller with increasing depth and is usually constricted in the late surgical plane of anesthesia. Painful stimulation during light anesthesia will cause a dilatation of the pupil. Dilated pupils may indicate either light anesthesia or very deep anesthesia and anoxia. As an indication of adequacy of cerebral oxygenation, *pupillary constriction and dilatation is one of the more reliable signs that we have.*

Muscle activity and response to stimulation is another means of determining the status of the central nervous system during anesthesia. Muscle control diminishes as the anesthesia deepens and relaxation increases. Muscle activity is a result of muscle tone and will, of course, vary with the age, physical status, and muscular development of the patient. Usually the unpremedicated patient will respond to a painful stimulation in a light plane of general anesthesia by movement away from the point of stimulation, or by movement of an extremity. These responses, which may not interfere with a relatively short procedure, are frequently seen in dental ambulatory anesthesia. Such movements would not be acceptable in an abdominal procedure, but they would not present a problem in the short dental procedure. Another reflex muscular activity used in determining the depth of anesthesia is that of swallowing. In barbiturate anesthesia we see depression of the swallowing reflex following the induction phase and continuing throughout most of the surgical plane of anesthesia, with a return as the anesthesia lightens.

In summary, observation of the reflex activity reveals the degree of depression or stimulation and provides essential information in a simple and expeditious manner when properly interpreted and correlated with other data.

Respiratory System

Oxygen is the most important single factor in life. An adult body reserves only about 1 liter of oxygen, which is used up at the rate of 200 to 300 cc. per minute under resting circumstances and at a much faster rate during muscular activity. The elimination of the waste product, carbon dioxide (CO_2), is also of great importance. The respiratory system provides the first step in ensuring that adequate oxygen is available for the needs of the body and the means for the final elimination of the carbon dioxide.

In monitoring the respiratory system we are constantly aware of the movement of the chest and abdomen. We are able to observe, and if necessary feel, if they are moving in a rhythmical manner. We can check the amplitude of each inspiration and expiration. We are also able to observe the movement of the reservoir bag on the anesthesia or sedation machine as another means of evaluating the respiration rate, rhythm, and amplitude (Fig. 4–1). We are able to evaluate the events that occur, such as the deep sigh and transient apnea frequently seen on induction of general anesthesia with an intravenous barbiturate. The increase in the rate of respiration becomes very apparent as the anesthetic plane lightens and the patient reacts to a painful stimulus. Conversely, as the anesthetic plane deepens and the respiratory rate decreases, we are able to detect these signs and withhold the anesthetic agent and assist respiration if necessary until the return of the rhythmical breathing seen in the surgical plane of barbiturate anesthesia.

Observation of the thoracic and abdominal movements during anesthesia quickly reveals any abnormal pattern, such as jerking of the diaphragm and heaving of the chest, during partial or complete obstruction, allowing this pattern to be corrected.

We are able to hear the movement of air in the nose and mouth as it

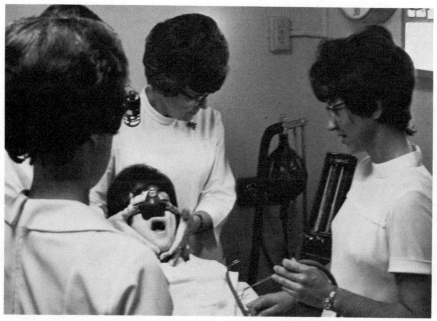

Figure 4–1 The anesthesia assistant can monitor the rate and amplitude of each inspiration and expiration by observing the reservoir bag on the anesthesia machine.

passes to and from the lungs (Fig. 4–2). Other sounds, also detectable during the anesthesia, make us aware of the minute-to-minute function of the respiratory system. These may include the gurgling sound from the passage of air over mucus or blood that has seeped past the pharyngeal partition, or the snoring as the tongue falls back in the oral pharynx and partially occludes the airway. The wheezing associated with bronchial constriction or the high-pitched crowing that may indicate partial laryngeal obstruction can easily be heard and quickly corrected.

Cardiovascular System

The second step in ensuring that the body has sufficient oxygen is having an adequate means of delivering oxygen to the cells. This is the major function of the cardiovascular system. Means available to monitor the cardiovascular system clinically include observation of the pulse rate, blood pressure, color of the skin, mucous membrane, and blood in the surgical field.

Monitoring the pulse is easily accomplished by palpating the radial, carotid, facial, or superficial temporal arteries. These are all within easy reach of the doctor or some member of the team. The strength and character of the pulse can be determined as well as the rate and rhythm. We will see an increase in the normal adult pulse rate during the induction stage, but the rate will usually return to near normal during the maintenance of ultralight anesthesia. The pulse rate will increase in response to painful stimuli, a carbon dioxide excess, and oxygen lack.

Palpation of the pulse may also reveal some of the more common arrhythmias encountered, such as premature beat and sinus arrhythmia, secondary to the patient's respiratory pattern; there are other arrhythmias which may only be detected through the use of the electrocardiograph, and these will be discussed later in the chapter.

The blood pressure must be taken prior to the intravenous administration of any medication for conscious-patient sedation or general anesthesia. Blood pressure is a function of heart action and vascular resistance. Any direct or indirect physiological, psychological or pharmacological action may have an effect on the blood pressure. The initial measurement will serve as a screening device for hypertension, as a preoperative evaluation, and as a baseline which we can compare with readings taken intraoperatively, at the completion of the procedure, or in the event of an emergency. The blood pressure will follow the pulse during the induction stages of anesthesia. It will rise with stimulation and return to the preanesthetic level during the maintenance of ultralight levels of anesthesia. Deeper planes of anesthesia will cause a lowering of the blood pressure and light planes an increase. It will also increase during episodes of hypoxia and carbon dioxide accumulation. There is little chance of misinterpreting the cause of a rise in blood pressure; movement of the extremities will often be seen during light anesthesia, and the blood pressure will be elevated. When hypoxia or carbon dioxide retention is the factor causing an increased blood pressure, there will be no movement of the extemities.

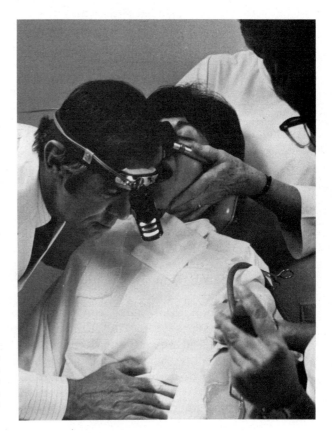

Figure 4-2 The doctor can hear the movement of air in the nose and mouth as it passes to and from the lungs. He is also able to feel the movement of the abdomen and chest in evaluating the respiratory system.

From the color of the skin, mucous membrane, or the blood in the surgical field, we can gain much valuable information. Well-oxygenated blood will appear bright red in the wound, and as the oxygen content diminishes the blood will become a darker red. The color of the mucous membrane can give us an indication of the degree of oxygenation of the blood. The well-oxygenated mucosa will have a healthy pink color. Mucosa with decreased arterial oxygen values appears bluish or dusky. Normal blood contains about 12 to 18 gm. of hemoglobin per 100 ml. Lunsgaard found that the capillary blood must contain approximately 5 gm. of reduced hemoglobin per 100 ml. before cyanosis will appear.[2] Because of this finding, a patient with a low hemoglobin value will not appear dusky or cyanotic in the early stages of hypoxia.

THE SURGEON/ANESTHETIST AND THE ANESTHESIA TEAM CONCEPT

Throughout the section on direct observation monitoring of the patient during general anesthesia, reference was made to the surgeon/anesthetist and the anesthesia team. This concept has been endorsed by the Council on Dental Therapeutics of the American Dental Association, as evidenced by the following statement from the 37th edition of Accepted Dental Therapeutics:

General anesthetics for the ambulatory dental patient can be effectively administered by a qualified team, which may be supervised by the surgeon providing he is thoroughly trained in general anesthesia. Utilization of a separate trained anesthetist is also encouraged. The safety of the patient is paramount and, regardless of the method used, the physical status of the patient must be continuously monitored to assure this safety.[3]

Utilizing this technique, which has been mentioned by Hubbell and Krogh,[4] and described by Hagen and McCarthy,[5] one can observe carefully and constantly the physical status of the patient. Each member of the team has a specific function with regards to monitoring during the anesthetic as well as during an emergency, as described by Hagen and McCarthy.[6] The anesthesia assistant has the primary function of maintaining a patent airway and monitoring the rate, character, and amplitude of the respirations. This is accomplished by maintaining the mandible in a proper position and observing the movement of the patient's chest, abdomen, and the reservoir bag attached to the anesthesia machine. This assistant is also able to monitor the pulse and report any irregularities to the surgeon.

The surgical assistant has the primary function of keeping the field free of blood and mucus which would tend to interfere with the normal respiratory pattern. From her position, she is able to aid in the monitoring of respiration, color, pulse, and blood pressure (Fig. 4–3).

The surgeon has the ultimate responsibility for the patient undergoing any surgical procedure, whether in an office or hospital environment. Because of his background the surgeon/anesthetist is well qualified to train his team in monitoring techniques. Use of a highly qualified team under the supervision of the surgeon will enhance patient safety during the anesthetic. Patient safety, as stated by the Council on Dental Therapeutics,[7]

Figure 4–3 The surgical assistant has the primary function of keeping the field free from blood and mucus, and from her position she is able to monitor respiration, color, pulse rate, and blood pressure.

must be the paramount issue. In like manner, it is the responsibility of the general practitioner to train his or her assistants in observation monitoring so that they may act as a smoothly functioning team both in routine treatment and in the treatment of emergencies.

BIOMEDICAL ELECTRONIC AND MECHANICAL MONITORING

In most instances, the individual to be evaluated is immediately adjacent to the evaluator. However, we are now at a point when it is possible to place men in space, in the caverns of the earth, or in the depths of the sea. For various reasons, it has been necessary to measure the physiological functions of these explorers. One spelunker spent six months alone underground in a cave to ascertain the effect of such isolation on the human body. He was monitored by hardwire connections to the surface. The astronauts provide another example of long-distance monitoring; they, of course, are monitored by telemetry. Through the use of these advanced electronic and mechanical monitors it is possible not only to monitor individuals who are very distant from the evaluator but also to follow equally well the vital signs of a patient a few steps away in the recovery room, or immediately at hand in the dental operatory. As the science of physiological monitoring advances, the practitioner should find himself using more and more of these aids to supplement the information supplied him by direct observation of the patient. Legal considerations may make it prudent to use the instruments the industry makes available to us. A recent large judgment against an anesthesiologist who failed to monitor the patient's pulse, with untoward consequences, is a case in point.

Hospital dental patients treated under general anesthesia (and likewise some restorative office cases) may often require a treatment duration of four to six hours, or more. Keeping patients anesthetized for such an amount of time creates physiological and biochemical problems not ordinarily seen in shorter anesthetic procedures. An increased level of patient monitoring, including lab tests, may be indicated in some of these cases. Also, use of supplemental aids for monitoring the anesthetized patient assumes increasing importance with the advent of four-, six-, and eight-handed dentistry, in which time and motion efficiency experts have urged the practitioner to train his eyes on the operative area, often to the relative exclusion of the "whole" patient. Although constant visual observation of the patient's general physiological state can be partially delegated to other members of the team, use of supplemental monitoring aids will be important, particularly when the doctor is training a new team or orienting a new team member. Many dental offices will in the course of one day administer general anesthestics to more patients than the local community hospital, and each individual treated must be evaluated in some manner preoperatively, as well as during the procedure and throughout the postoperative period. To a large degree, biomedical electronic monitoring can supplement the technique of direct observation, though not replace it. As stated by the ADA Council of Therapeutics, "the safety of the patient is paramount and, regardless of the method used, the physical status of the patient must be continuously monitored to assure this safety."[8]

Our attention will now turn to various types of monitors commercially available to the practitioner.

A number of these products are listed at the end of this chapter for ease in contacting representative manufacturers. Most types of products are manufactured by several competitive companies, and the prospective purchaser may be wise to contact several suppliers prior to purchase, rather than limiting himself to the manufacturers mentioned in this chapter. It should be noted that the instruments mentioned in these pages may not always be identical to the ones illustrated but will be generally similar to them in nature. Some monitors mentioned are used with anesthetic techniques not commonly used by the general practitioner. Other monitors are of equal value to the general practitioner and the surgeon. Understandably, this presentation includes only a very few of the many monitoring devices available. For more information, the reader is referred to the current literature or to trade journals dealing with biomedical electronic monitors.[9]

TEMPERATURE MONITORING

Temperature monitoring and evaluation are important to any patient receiving an intravenous anesthetic. Temperature variations from "normal" can be a result of many different factors; for example, dehydration, infection, exercise, diet, and so forth. The basal metabolic rate is increased 7 per cent for each 1° F increase in the body temperature. This becomes significant when a patient, with a temperature of 103° F, receives an ultralight general anesthesia for the removal of an infected tooth. There has been an increase of 30 per cent in the basal metabolic rate, necessitating a demand for 30 per cent more oxygen. Temperature monitoring is also important in order to ascertain large fluctuations in body temperature. It is unlikely that extreme temperature variations will occur during the shorter dental procedures, such as those performed in oral surgery offices. However, with the increased use of general anesthetics in restorative dentistry, procedures taking several hours or more are not uncommon, and the possibility of significant temperature variations should be considered. Should any change occur, it would usually be a decrease in body temperature (hypothermia), which can be easily controlled by warming the room and covering the patient with blankets. Although significant cooling must occur in the adult before any marked decrease in respiration will occur, such decrease has been noted during prolonged anesthesia. In rare instances, the temperature may increase under general anesthesia (malignant hyperthermia), a condition which seems to be related more to the type of anesthetic given than to the length of procedure or any other consideration known to us. Significantly for dental anesthetics, this condition is not noted with nitrous oxide–oxygen anesthesia, although it has been seen with Fluothane and other anesthetics often used in dental surgery.[10] Malignant hyperthermia is a life-threatening situation of which every anesthesia team member should be aware.

Oral Thermometer

The most generally used method to monitor oral temperature is the glass-mercury thermometer, which is placed sublingually for three to five minutes and read from the scale. An improvement in this technique has been made by the availability of sterile disposable plastic sheaths (TEMP-AWAY),[9A]* which come individually packaged. (Fig. 4–4).

A second and more recent improvement in taking oral temperatures is the use of a system of chemical mixtures* (TEMPRA-DOT),[9B] which melt and recrystallize at a very specific temperature (Fig. 4–5). As the mixture recrystallizes it changes color. The temperature is read on a scale to the last recrystalized dot. The system is disposable and comes sterile and ready for use. The temperature may be read after the system has been in the sublingual area only 30 seconds.

Electronic Thermometer

The third method is by electronic thermometers,[9C] which are used for the continuous monitoring of patients under anesthesia as well as in the

---

*Superscript letters refer to the Manufacturers' List found at the end of this chapter.

TEMP-AWAY Thermometer Sheaths. A single patient thermometer system.

Note: Rectal TEMP-AWAY Sheaths are pre-lubricated.

1 Shake down a Security Bulb Thermometer in the usual way. The B-D thermometer has a tab top. You can shake more vigorously.

2 Insert the thermometer tip into the the preformed opening. You'll find this opening on the end where the written instructions are printed. Push the thermometer in until you feel a "spongy" resistant feeling.

3 Grasp package as shown. Then with thumb and forefinger of each hand, twist package with each hand twisting in the opposite direction. The package will tear at the dotted line.

4 As you twist, pull paper away from the tab top of the thermometer. The paper will slide off, leaving the TEMP-AWAY Sheath covering the thermometer shaft.

5 The remaining paper on the plastic sheath is your handle to place the thermometer in the patient's mouth in the usual way.

6 After temperature is taken, remove sheath by pulling the paper handle toward the thermometer tip while twisting slightly. The sheath will reverse, turning itself inside-out and encapsulating most contamination.

7 Dispose of the sheath in your usual way. Reversed, the TEMP-AWAY Sheath also helps protect housekeeping personnel from cross-contamination.

8 Read temperature in the usual way.

Note: When thermometers are used to take temperatures from patient to patient (not being a single-patient thermometer system) the thermometer must be disinfected prior to each patient use.

BECTON-DICKINSON
Rutherford, New Jersey 07070
Division of Becton, Dickinson and Company
In Canada: Becton, Dickinson and Co. Canada Ltd. Mississauga, Ontario

B-D and TEMP-AWAY are trademarks of Becton, Dickinson and Company
Printed in U.S.A. TWC/76-2001-2

Figure 4–4

New Tempa-DOT™
single use oral thermometer

☐ fast

☐ accurate

☐ easy to read

☐ unbreakable

☐ free from cross-infection risks

☐ no shaking down

☐ no after-use washing

☐ no sterilizing

☐ completely disposable

**Revolutionize
temperature taking
...just 3 simple steps**

ready... aim... fire...

Simply break handle seal at
the score mark by bending
it up and down. Pull thermometer straight out
toward you without twisting
or side-to-side motion.

Insert sensor end of the
Tempa-DOT Thermometer
under either side of tongue,
well back alongside the
frenum. Have patient hold
the stem with teeth, press
tongue down on it, and keep
mouth closed for a mini-
mum of 30 seconds.

Remove from mouth and
read temperature—the last
dot that "fires" to dark
green. Discard the Tempa-
DOT Thermometer. (This
example shows a temperature
of 98.6°F.)

Faster, easier, safer, accurate, and
economical...with no risk of cross-
infection or reinfection because the
Tempa-DOT Thermometer is a
single-use instrument.

Figure 4–5

**Here's the Tempa-DOT
Single Use Oral Thermometer
that can revolutionize temperature
taking in your hospital**

Organon provides an extended in-service
program with members of the nursing
staff to assure complete understanding of
the Tempa-DOT Thermometer and the
technique of using it.

Your Organon Hospital Specialist will be
glad to demonstrate the Tempa-DOT
Thermometer and arrange for its evaluation in accordance with whatever evaluation procedures are used in your hospital.

Figure 4–6

recovery room (Fig 4–6). Any change of more than one half to one degree above the initial stabilized temperature should be observed carefully and cooling procedures instituted if the patient becomes hyperpyrexic. A newer technique for taking temperature that may be of interest in dental anesthesia records the temperature of the ear canal. This location has the advantage of being removed from the oral cavity, but without the difficulties of placing a temperature probe esophageally or rectally.

RESPIRATORY SYSTEM MONITORING

One of the more common anesthetic emergencies is that of hypoxia. It is insidious in that it may be difficult to recognize in the earliest stages. Monitoring of the gas exchange can provide significant information about the pulmonary status. When using an anesthesia or sedation machine to deliver medical gases one may obtain efficient guarding of the oxygen supply by installing an oxygen pressure monitor on the oxygen delivery line or anesthesia machine. When the oxygen pressure drops to dangerous levels, the battery-powered monitor will sound an alarm and flash a red light. This battery-powered device operates independently of the gas pressures and will give an alarm signal when oxygen pressures drop. Unfortunately, when the batteries deteriorate the device will become inoperative. It should be checked each morning to ensure that the audible and visual alarms are functional. It is advisable to check tank pressures of oxygen and nitrous oxide at the same time to ensure a safe supply for the day. A second type of gas pressure monitor is a whistle alarm,[9D] an accessory installed in the an-

Figure 4–7

esthesia machine. If the oxygen supply pressure falls to a predetermined level, a whistle will sound. The device is self-checking, in that any time the oxygen pressure rises from near zero to its normal value, a brief "peep" attests that the alarm is functioning. A small reservoir stores enough oxygen to blow the whistle for at least five seconds. No other source of power is required. An anesthesia machine is often equipped with a device that will cut off the flow of all other gases and vapors when the oxygen supply pressure drops below a predetermined level. This minimizes the chance of delivering a hypoxic mixture to the breathing circuit. The reduced flow of fresh gas may also alert the doctor to the depletion of the oxygen supply, but the alarms described above are probably more reliable. One unwise monitoring practice that is to be avoided is "sniffing" gas flows to determine that the proper anesthetic mixtures are being delivered. This can lead to dependence upon inhalation anesthetics.

Carbon Dioxide Analyzer

An extremely useful monitoring tool is the carbon dioxide analyzer, or capnograph[9E] (Fig. 4–7). Expiratory carbon dioxide is measured by this instrument. The adapter lead is easily inserted into the airway tubing at some readily accessible point close to the patient's airway. It may be used in conjunction with an endotracheal tube, a nasopharyngeal tube, or a nasal or full-face mask. An increase in the amount of expired carbon dioxide may indicate hypoventilation and relative hypoxia. Hyperventilation will cause a decrease in the amount of CO_2 recorded. In the event of cardiac arrest, perfusion of blood to the lungs will cease, thus stopping the excretion of carbon dioxide from the lungs, and the CO_2 analyzer will indicate zero per cent carbon dioxide. A zero per cent indication might also be seen in the event of an airway obstruction; if this occurs, immediate action is indicated. Medical Gas analyzers $9E_2$ (Fig. 4–8) are available that not only will monitor CO_2 but, by using interchangeable pickup heads, will measure nitrous oxide or halothane also.

Figure 4–8

Oxygen Alarm Monitor

It is technically quite easy to continuously monitor the percentage of oxygen in the gases being delivered to the anesthetized patient. An oxygen alarm[9F] monitor may be placed in line between the anesthesia machine and the patient (Fig. 4–9). The monitor will sense any amount of oxygen from 0 to 100 per cent and an audio-visual alarm system is activated when the partial pressure of oxygen falls below a preset limit. The alarm is battery operated, less than six inches long, and weighs less than three pounds. It can be calibrated on room air or 100 per cent oxygen and is extremely accurate.

Figure 4–9

Spirometer

Various instruments are available to monitor respiratory rate, tidal volume (amount of air passing in or out of the lungs during each breath), and minute volume (amount of air passing in or out of the lungs in one minute). Tidal and minute volume values are probably of greater importance to the doctor than is respiratory rate. A person breathing at a "normal" respiratory rate is not necessarily inspiring the amount of oxygen necessary to prevent hypoxia. A person with normal tidal and minute volumes is likely to have adequate gas exchange.

Oximeter

Although gas percentages are easily ascertained in the respiratory gas flow, modern technology is providing simple and inexpensive methods of measuring arterial blood gas saturations. This more direct but noninvasive method of measuring the physiological status of patients deserves at least academic attention. An oximeter[9G] measures the arterial oxygen saturation by colorimetric changes in the arterial circulation of the pinna of the ear (Fig. 4–10). This spectrophotometric instrument is about 16 inches in its greatest dimension and weighs about 37 pounds. Operating independently of skin color and unaffected by motion, it continuously measures arterial oxygen saturation without the necessity of calibration or mathematical manipulation of the readout. Oxygenated hemoglobin absorbs one light spectrum and reduced hemoglobin another. When the loosely fitting earpiece is attached (without skin penetration) a light beam is transmitted through the ear and picked up on the other side by the sensor. Alteration in light intensities at eight different wave lengths is instantly interpreted by the instrument as per

Figure 4–10

cent oxygen saturation. A patient with a satisfactory arterial oxygen saturation is unlikely to suffer the ill effects of hypoxia.

When facilities permit, as on a Hospital Dental Service, micro-blood samples may be taken and quickly processed in a nearby clinical laboratory to determine blood tensions of oxygen and carbon dioxide, the pH, the concentration of electrolytes, and other serum chemistries that can give important information on the status of the patient.

TRACE GASES

Though not of importance to the health of the patient, one should be aware that health personnel who are exposed to trace concentrations of anesthestic gases over long periods of time during multiple exposure might be at some physical risk. The technology is available to measure and monitor anesthetic trace gases in the dental operatory utilizing gas chromatography and infrared spectrometry; scavenging systems can be installed to eliminate the possible problem.

CARDIOVASCULAR SYSTEM MONITORING

The status of the cardiovascular system is of enormous importance during general anesthesia and, fortunately, is easily monitored at a number of anatomical points with many different types of monitors. A few of these methods will be presented now.

Figure 4–11 Pulse monitor. Showing finger tip pickup and earlobe/ nostril pickup (lower left). Acoustic signal is heard from speaker (upper left). Pulse rate per minute is read on the dial, as a light beneath the dial flashes with each pulse beat.

The pulse is probably the easiest physiological sign to monitor in the dental outpatient. Hands and fingers are completely exposed for the application of the pulse monitor. Few if any patients find terror in the application and use of a pulse monitoring device, particularly if its action and function are briefly described as similar to the photoelectric cells often found on elevator doors which respond to interruption of a light beam. In the case of the pulse monitor[9H], the photoelectric beam is interrupted by the blood flow through the finger following each heartbeat, creating a visual and/or audible signal (Fig. 4–11). Available models include a lightweight portable monitor powered by a rechargeable battery. Optional pickups will clip onto a toe, nostril, or earlobe, in addition to the fingertip. Advanced models will portray a visible waveform on the oscilloscopic screen, count the pulse automatically, and emit an audible signal with each heartbeat.

Monaural Stethoscope and Cardiac Audio Monitor

The heart may be monitored effectively by a stethoscope placed just below the trachea in the suprasternal or pretracheal position. In this position, the stethoscope will transmit both cardiac and breath sounds. These are of great interest, and the intensity, rate, rhythmicity and quality provide much information. It is quite convenient to monitor the heart sounds with the use of a custom-fitted ear mold[9I] connected to the chest piece by 5 or 6 feet of lightweight plastic tubing (Figs. 4–12 and 4–13). Should one find the tubing restrictive to motion, the stethoscope may be connected to a microphone pick-up and amplifier and broadcast into the room. This has the advantage of allowing every member of the team to be conscious of the patient's cardiac tones; the doctor is free to move unencumbered by any connection to the patient.

Figure 4–12   Precordial stethoscope with custom-fitted ear mold.

Figure 4–13 Cardiac audio monitor. Microphone (lower left) amplifies heart sounds picked up by stethoscope (lower right). Stethoscope is inexpensively made from heavy pipe fitting. Weight keeps stethoscope in position on the chest.

Esophageal Stethoscope

In some cases it may be difficult to hear satisfactory heart sounds with the precordial or suprasternal stethoscope. An alternative would be the esophageal stethoscope, particularly with the patient who has been intubated (Fig. 4–14). The esophageal stethoscope may be quickly placed by the oral or nasal route. This provides optimum cardiac and pulmonic tones. When a nasal route

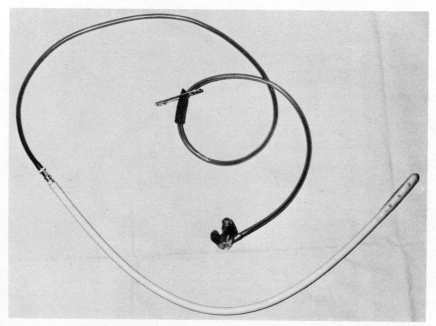

Figure 4–14   Esophageal stethoscope with custom earpiece.

of insertion is chosen, the main precaution to be observed is the prevention of bleeding. A well-lubricated esophageal stethoscope will usually cause no problem if inserted gently. However, children in their teens and younger may have hypertrophic adenoid tissue which can be easily traumatized. Some adults may have friable blood vessels in the anterior portion of the nostril, but adenoid tissue is greatly diminished after adolescence and unlikely to be a problem. Should one nostril seem occluded, perhaps from a deviated septum, the esophageal stethoscope can often be inserted easily in the other nostril.

Oscilloscopes

The oscilloscope is widely and commonly used to give a visual representation of various parameters, including but not limited to the electrocardiograph (ECG), pulse rate, respiratory rate, blood pressure, and electroencephalograph (EEG). All these wave forms may be presented simultaneously on some models, or individually at the discretion of the operator in others. It is probably unwise to use the ECG mode as the sole measure of cardiac activity, as it provides no direct information on the vital characteristics of cardiac output. If the patient is healthy, and has no history of cardiac disease, one might find that monitoring the pulse and blood pressure would do more to avoid unexpected and untoward complications. The ECG will, of course, provide early detection of arrhythmias, and the alert clinician will remember that PVCs are a possible precursor to ventricular fibrillation. The oscilloscope is connected to the patient by painless, easily attached adhesive electrodes.

ECG displays are available in several types. The conventional "bouncing ball" is familiar to most. In this instance, the bright spot moves across the screen from left to right, vanishing at the right only to reappear again at the left. A second type of display is the "moving window" wherein a pattern of steady brightness fills the entire width of the screen, and moves from right to left. Current information enters the screen on the right edge. This is a "non-fade" display, as is the "erase bar" depiction. The "erase bar" also has full screen width and steady brightness but the pattern does not move as a whole. Instead, a narrow gap in the ECG moves across the screen from left to right. Fresh data are found at the left of the gap, and information is erased at the right edge of the gap. Various optional features are available with non-fade displays, such as the "freeze" or "hold" feature. With this tool, one may hold the display on the screen for an indefinite period of time in order to study the ECG. Trend-plotting is available on some models, where the sweep speed is very slow, and a number of cardiac contractions will be represented on the screen at one time. A "cascade" non-fade display allows a number of sweeps of the oscilloscope to be preserved on the screen for a period of time. The sweeps are depicted one above another, on different channels, providing a "cascade."

Monitors are also available which will store physiological information in a solid state memory and give an "instant replay" when desired; in other models a tracing can be "frozen" on the screen, moved to a different channel, and compared with the new tracings flowing across the oscilloscope screen on the original channel. The conventional bouncing ball display will probably meet the needs of most practitioners treating dental patients on an outpatient basis.

Recorders: Telephone ECG Systems

In many instances, for diagnostic or legal purposes, it will be desirable to make hard-copy or permanent records of physiological signs. In these cases it is easy to connect the monitors to recorders and inscribe tracings on paper. This tracing might be filed with the patient's chart for future reference, or shown to a consultant for diagnosis. If one wishes to record an entire lengthy procedure, it might be advisable to use a trend recorder, which is a paper recorder used at very slow speed; a two-hour procedure would be recorded on perhaps two inches of paper.

ECG signals can be transmitted across the phone lines from the patient to the appropriate receiver. Many individuals wearing pacemakers are monitored at regular intervals in this manner to ascertain that the pacemaker is functioning properly. This tool could be available to the dental office; it would be useful for requesting immediate interpretation of questionable tracings during an anesthetic. Preanesthetic and postanesthetic tracings might be transmitted for evaluation by a consultant.

Automatic Blood Pressure Monitor

Blood pressure is most commonly measured by means of a blood pressure cuff applied to the upper arm, though the upper thigh can be used with good results if the situation requires it. During a procedure blood pressures are often taken on a regular time schedule of every five minutes by trained ancillary personnel. Although this is a quick and efficient method, increased reliability can be obtained by use of an automatic indirect blood pressure monitor. This machine, which uses a conventionally applied cuff about the arm, will display at any desired time interval from one to 15 minutes the usual indirect blood pressure measurement, both systolic and diastolic. After the cuff has been placed on the patient's arm and the time interval has been selected, blood pressures will be automatically taken and displayed in lighted numerals depicting millimeters of mercury. The lighted numerals can be easily read by all team members and will be held on the display board for reference until the next automatic reading. The machine does not forget to take the readings in moments of stress. The information has high credibility, as it is taken in a uniform, objective "machine" manner.

The maxillofacial surgeon or other individual concerned with team treatment of patients with traumatic injuries will probably be exposed to invasive techniques of blood pressure monitoring. One fairly common technique involves the cannulation of the radial artery with a percutaneous indwelling 20 gauge Teflon catheter. This can be connected to a transducer to allow beat by beat oscilloscopic display of the pulse contour for determining blood pressure and heart rate. Determination of stroke volume can be made; arterial blood samples can be obtained for blood gas analysis. Alternatively, the same catheter could be connected to a pressure infusor and simple aneroid manometer to provide a cheap, simple, and reliable measure of the blood pressure. Samples could also be drawn. The major disadvantage is that no hard copy record would be available.

Perometer

Measurement of fluid and blood volume is an important consideration when monitoring the cardiovascular system. It is possible for blood loss from some dental procedures, notably oral surgery and periodontal surgery, to exceed one or more units of blood (a unit of blood is equivalent to 500 ml).[11] Though this is not necessarily a significant loss for the healthy adult patient, some patients cannot afford such blood loss, and occasionally a postoperative transfusion is indicated. Methods of evaluating the amount of blood loss include measuring the blood in suction bottles and estimating the blood contained in wet and dry sponges and drapes, gowns, and gloves. Sponges of a known weight, containing only blood and no saline or irrigating solution, may be weighed to determine the amount of blood contained in them. A more satisfactory method for determining blood loss involves use of a "perometer."[9J] This is essentially a washing machine, complete with a spin dryer, and containing a colorimetric device for the measurement of hemoglobin. The hemoglobinometer is set to the known presurgical hemoglobin values of the patient, as determined by the routine preoperative hemoglobin laboratory test. As the operation progresses, all fluid and blood-stained articles are placed in the machine. The blood-laden water from the washing machine is constantly circulated through the hemoglobinometer, and the amount of blood loss in liters or fractions of a liter is read out on a dial. By this technique the doctor may be apprised of the amount of blood loss on a frequent basis, and the blood lost may be replaced precisely by transfusion if indicated.

Doppler

An extremely sensitive and accurate method for indirect, noninvasive blood pressure monitoring is provided by the ultrasonic Doppler flow detector.[9K] This instrument is used for making difficult systolic pressure measurements, and can detect systolic pressures as low as 10 millimeters of mercury. The Doppler probe consists of two crystals, one of which sends a beam of ultrasound energy into the skin, while the other receives the reflected waves. These reflected waves come from underlying tissue and from the moving red cells. Since the underlying tissue is stationary, the frequency of waves reflected from it is exactly the same as the frequency of the transmitted waves. However, the reflected waves from anything in motion (blood) are of a different frequency owing to the Doppler effect. What one hears from the speaker is the frequency difference between the transmitted and received waves. Because of the random velocity of the blood cells, the sound is not a pure tone, but a hissing noise. The pitch of this noise is proportional to the velocity of the moving blood.

To use the Doppler in instances when an ordinary stethoscope will not function, one simply applies an ordinary blood pressure cuff above the elbow. The flat Doppler probe is placed over the radial artery before the cuff is inflated. The cuff is inflated above the systolic pressure and then deflated. A pulsing flow sound is heard during that portion of the cardiac cycle that represents systole. Diastolic pressures are not easily measured with this device.

CENTRAL STATION MONITORING

The greatest utilization of biomedical electronic and mechanical monitoring is found in the intensive care and cardiac care units. Here patients with cardiac disease not only are under the constant observation of trained ancillary personnel but are also connected to electronic and mechanical instruments which determine their physiologic state from minute to minute. This monitoring is made easier by use of a console that will receive information from the various individual instruments. The information is registered on the display area of the console for easy viewing. Parameters such as pulse rate, ECG, blood pressure, temperature, and respiration can be followed. Many of the instruments are of modular design to permit rapid replacement of a defective instrument. Closed circuit television is also being used to monitor the patient visually and to assist in prevention of problems which can only be detected by direct observation.

Computers are being used by many hospitals to monitor patients in intensive care and cardiac care units, as well as in the operating rooms. The computer is programmed to scan the sensors on a group of subjects in sequence. If abnormal data are received from one patient, a signal will immediately alert hospital personnel, start emergency equipment, or provide other programmed services. The computer is also being used as a diagnostic and treatment aid. The day is rapidly approaching when simple automatic corrective procedures will be instituted when the physiological event exceeds preset limits; for example, a computer may be programmed to give blood when the arterial pressure is low. Computers are also good for automatic measurement acquisition, display, storage, retrieval, and charting of information for medical records.

ELECTROCARDIOGRAPHY

As was mentioned earlier in the text, the electrocardioscope may be used as an aid in monitoring the cardiovascular system during ultralight general anesthesia. In utilizing the electrocardioscope and electrocardiogram to monitor the conduction system of the heart, we are most interested in recognition of the normal and abnormal rate and rhythm patterns. We are also interested in what clinical significance these patterns will have and how they affect the administration of a safe anesthetic to our patients. It is not our desire or our need to go into the subtleties of electrocardiologic diagnosis or treatment of these abnormalities. Our purpose for inclusion of this material is to make the members of the team aware of another aid that may be of assistance in monitoring selected patients during general anesthesia.

As interpretation of the information provided by the ECG is less obvious than that provided by other monitoring devices discussed in this chapter, additional explanatory material will be presented.

The electrocardioscope is differentiated from the electrocardiogram in that the latter provides a permanent electrocardiographic record on paper, whereas the former presents to the observer only a transient tracing on the oscilloscope screen. As continual monitoring of the patient by the electrocardiogram would be impractical, the electrocardioscope is commonly used for routine continuous monitoring, and a permanent record is made of only the more important tracings noted.

Electrophysiology

Whenever muscle activity occurs, electrical activity must also occur, and this is what is recorded by the ECG. The inside of any muscle cell carries a negative charge and the outside of the cell a positive one. The resting polarized cell has no potential difference between any two points of the cell. At a point of stimulation the cell potential drops to zero because the cell membrane becomes electrically permeable and the charges on the two sides neutralize each other. A wave of excitation is then created, which spreads over the muscle cell, producing a potential difference between any two points on the cell until the entire surface of the muscle has lost its positive charge and is depolarized.

Since the heart is a pump made up of muscle cells, when one point is stimulated the wave of propagation spreads until the entire surface loses its positive charge and becomes depolarized. The normal pathway for this wave of propagation is formation of the impulses in the sinoatrial (S-A) node, lying in the wall of the right atrium near the mouth of the superior vena cava. It spreads over the wall of the atrium to the atrioventricular (A-V) node near the coronary sinus. From here it spreads toward the ventricle through the A-V bundle of His to the left and right conduction bundles passing down the septum. The wave reaches the Purkinje fibers under the endocardium and spreads outward through the myocardium to the epicardium, reaching the apex first, then the lateral wall of the right and left ventricles and base of the heart, where it terminates.

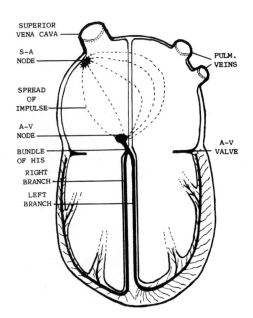

SUPERIOR VENA CAVA

S-A NODE

PULM. VEINS

SPREAD OF IMPULSE

A-V NODE

A-V VALVE

BUNDLE OF HIS

RIGHT BRANCH

LEFT BRANCH

Figure 4–15 Electrical excitation of heart. Normal pathway of impulses from S-A node to myocardium. (Hopkins, H. U.: Leopold's Principles and Methods of Physical Diagnosis. 3rd ed. Philadelphia, W. B. Saunders Co., 1965.)

From early fetal life until death this electrical stimulation and subsequent beating of the heart continues automatically and rhythmically. Interruptions of this usual rhythm are referred to as dysrhythmias or arrhythmias. They are important clinically because they can produce important clinical symptoms, disability, and death. The clinical significance of some rhythm disturbances has been misappraised and has led to needless disability.

As was mentioned earlier in the chapter, the ECG is the means by which many of the arrhythmias can be recognized. In order to recognize the abnormal, we must first be able to recognize the normal. Certain standards have been developed and accepted in the use of the ECG. These standards include the placement of electrodes and the paper which receives the tracing of the cardiac activity.

Leads

Because the total potential developed in the heart at any one time can be expressed as a vector, the form of any ECG tracing obtained will depend to a great extent on the placement of the electrodes. The voltage recorded is the difference between the voltage at these two points. Using the principles of the equilateral triangle as suggested by Einthoven, the three standard limb leads evolved. The difference in potential between the right and left arms is called lead I, that between the right arm and left leg lead II, and that between the left arm and left leg lead III. These are called bipolar leads because they record the difference between the two potentials.

There are also unipolar leads which record the actual potential and not the difference between the two potentials. Greater sensitivity is obtainable with the unipolar leads, and for that reason they are used more for diagnostic purposes than in surgery, where drapes and activity about the patient make these leads difficult to use.

Paper

ECG paper is standardized, and when a direct record is made the various intervals and amplitudes can be easily measured by inspection or with calipers for evaluation of the tracing and diagnosis of the patient's cardiac condition. The standard machine moves the paper at a rate of 25 mm per second. Each small box enclosed by faint vertical lines on the paper represents 0.04 second. Each large box of five small horizontal boxes represents 0.2 second and is enclosed by the heavy vertical lines. Each vertical large box is 5 mm tall (Fig. 4–16). One millivolt equals 10 mm or two large vertical boxes. When using the electrocardioscope as a monitoring device, one finds that these measurements are not as readily apparent as tracings on paper. If precise values are desired, the cardioscope is connected to a direct writer and a tracing is made on ECG paper.

Normal Electrocardiogram

When we take an ECG on an individual with a normal, healthy heart, certain definite deflections occur in the tracing. Each of these deflections

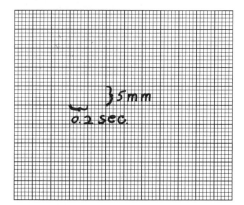

Figure 4–16   Electrocardiogram paper.

indicates certain actions of the heart. Because the cause of the deflections was unknown originally, the developer of the device, Einthoven, ascribed to them the letters P,Q,R,S, and T. The first wave of the complex, the P wave, is caused by the depolarization of the atria when the stimulus starting in the S-A node passes over them. The atria actually contract right after the beginning of the P wave. Then there is an interval of little or no deflection. This is followed by another group of deflections called the QRS complex. This group of deflections is caused by the depolarization which occurs as the impulse from the AV node passes over the ventricular musculature. Following the QRS group, there is another period of little or no potential which is called the S-T interval. This is followed by the T wave, which is caused by the repolarization of the

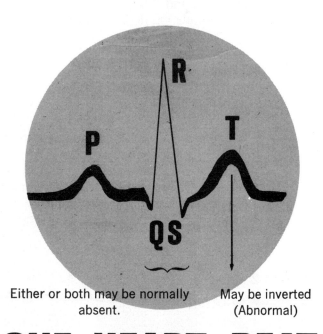

Figure 4–17   Normal ECG complex. (Figures 4–17 through 4–27 are taken from the arrhythmia chart prepared in cooperation with Walter S. Graf, M.D., and The Daniel Freeman Hospital, Inglewood, California, by Dallon Instruments, a Division of International Rectifier Corp., El Segundo, California.)

Either or both may be normally absent.

May be inverted (Abnormal)

ONE HEART BEAT

Figure 4–18 Normal ECG tracing – lead II.

ventricles. As has been previously discussed, it is possible to take tracings from a number of different leads (12 or more) by placing the electrodes at various points on the body. For monitoring purposes one lead is selected to monitor throughout the entire case. The best lead for monitoring during anesthesia, according to Wylie,[12] is lead II (Fig. 4–18).

PHYSIOLOGICAL SINUS RHYTHM AND ARRHYTHMIAS

The usual discharge of impulses from the S-A node is between 60 and 100 times a minute. Below 60 times a minute is termed bradycardia and above 100 times a minute is termed tachycardia.

Sinus Arrhythmia (Fig. 4–19)

Sinus arrhythmia is the name given to the minor benign changes associated with respiration. The heart rate increases during the early part of the inspiration and slows during expiration. It is attributed to varying degrees of vagal stimulation and disappears when the breath is held or under general anesthesia. It is not a disease process and seldom causes any untoward clinical symptoms

Sinus Tachycardia (Fig. 4–20)

Sinus tachycardia is an abnormally rapid heart rate, over 100 beats per minute, arising at the normal S-A pacemaker. Causes of sinus tachycardia include stimulation during very light anesthesia, hypoxia, hypotension, exercise, anxiety, fever, and anemia. Sinus tachycardia may or may not be of clinical significance and is not, in itself, indicative of cardiac disease. If severe or prolonged, the tachycardia may lead to cardiac failure.

SINUS ARRHYTHMIA
Figure 4–19 Sinus arrhythmia tracing.

SINUS TACHYCARDIA (Rate over 100 / min.)

Figure 4–20   Sinus tachycardia tracing.

Sinus Bradycardia (Fig. 4–21)

Sinus bradycardia is a slow sinus rhythm of less than 60 beats per minute. It is frequently seen in highly trained athletes, probably owing to an increase in vagal tone. Other causes of increased vagal tone include hypotension secondary to hemorrhage and pressure on the eyeballs or carotid sinus. Cyclopropane and halothane anesthesia can also induce sinus bradycardia.

PATHOLOGICAL ARRHYTHMIAS

Premature Contractions

Any region of the heart can prematurely discharge the impulse for contraction with the resultant atrial, nodal, or ventricular premature beat. The exact origin of the premature beat is discernible only after viewing the ECG. Atrial and nodal premature beats are often seen during anesthesia and surgery. The QRS is normal and the prematurities apparently have no special significance. Premature ventricular contractions will be discussed later.

Paroxysmal Tachycardia

Paroxysmal tachycardia is a term applied to attacks of rapid heart action in which ventricular contraction responds to regular impulses arising in a focus removed from the S-A node. The ectopic focus may be in the atria, the A-V node, or the ventricles. The heart rate is 100 beats per minute or more. The paroxysm begins suddenly, may last for minutes or days, and ends abruptly. The beats are absolutely regular. Vagal stimulation may change the rate or stop the paroxysm completely.

SINUS BRADYCARDIA (Rate less than 60 / min.)

Figure 4–21   Sinus bradycardia tracing.

Figure 4-22 Atrial tachycardia tracing.

ATRIAL TACHYCARDIA ✪

Atrial Tachycardia (Fig. 4-22)

Atrial tachycardia is a common cardiac arrhythmia. The rate is 150 to 300 beats per minute with the ventricles responding to each atrial beat. The rapid heart rate tends to make the patient dyspneic and weak owing to decreased arterial blood pressure. The ECG shows a rapid succession of abnormal P waves that are deformed because of the fact that the contraction commences in a focus removed from the S-A node. The QRS complexes are equally rapid but regular and normal in form. The paroxysm may stop abruptly, either spontaneously or with vagal stimulation. There is no temporary slowing with this arrhythmia, in contrast to sinus tachycardia. Atrial tachycardia either will resume slow normal contractions with treatment or it will be unaltered. Syncope is not uncommon during an attack. Clinically, most patients have no organic heart disease and the arrhythmia is purely functional.

Atrial Flutter (Fig. 4-23)

In atrial flutter the atria are contracting at a rate of 230 to 360 times a minute and therefore 230 to 360 P waves are observed on the ECG tracing. The ventricles cannot respond to every impulse, so that there is usually either a 2:1, 3:1, or 4:1 block between the atria and the ventricles, resulting in a ventricular rate of one half, one third, or one fourth the atrial rate. The ECG shows characteristic sawtooth arrangements of the P waves. The P-R interval is absent and the ventricular rate may be regular or irregular.

Atrial Fibrillation (Fig. 4-24)

During atrial fibrillation the atria do not contract as a whole. Small areas of the muscle tissue are stimulated at various times so that there are no true P waves. However, there is usually sufficient potential developed so that we see small "f" (or fibrillary) waves appearing in the tracing. As the impulses reach the A-V node, it is stimulated. It sends its impulse to the bundle of His; if the bundle of His is not in a refractory period, the impulse is transmitted to the

ATRIAL FLUTTER with ✪
4:1 block

Figure 4-23 Atrial flutter with 4:1 block tracing.

Rapid ATRIAL FIBRILLATION

Figure 4–24 Atrial fibrillation tracing.

ventricles, and this gives a normal QRS and T complex. The QRS and T complexes are unevenly spaced owing to irregularity of the ventricular rate. Usually only one of every four impulses excites the ventricles, so the ventricular rate is one fourth that of the atria. Atrial fibrillation is seen in coronary atherosclerotic heart disease and many other heart diseases and also may be observed in a clinically normal heart.

Premature Ventricular Contractions (PVCs)

As was mentioned earlier, because of the possibility of premature discharge of the impulse, contractions can originate in the ventricular musculature. These contractions may occur in normal healthy persons during excitement, breath-holding, anxiety, fatigue, and smoking, as well as during anesthesia with hypoxia and elevated CO_2 content in the bloodstream.

In PVCs some point in the ventricle becomes hyperirritable and gives off an impulse which passes over the ventricle by an abnormal pathway. When this occurs we ·see an *abnormal QRS complex*. It is wide, slurred, and notched. The T wave is in the opposite direction from the QRS. There is no P wave preceding a PVC. When impulses from ventricular foci occur regularly with every second beat, the arrhythmia is known as bigeminy; with every third beat, trigeminy. There is also a compensatory pause which assists in the recognition of the PVC. The explanation of the compensatory pause is as follows:

In the beat preceding the PVC, the impulse begins in the S-A node, giving rise to the P wave. This impulse then strikes the A-V node and gives rise to QRS and T complexes. Then, before the atrium can stimulate the ventricle again, the ventricular premature contraction occurs with its abnormal QRS and T complex. When the S-A node now gives off its next impulse, a P wave results. Although the A-V node is stimulated and gives off an impulse, the ventricle is in a refractory period and cannot respond to this stimulus. Therefore, there is a pause until the next impulse leaves the S-A node and reaches the ventricle which reacts and gives the normal QRS and T complex.

A common cause of PVCs is the excessive use of the drug digitalis. The patient may notice a "thumping in the chest" or a "flip-flop heart." An occasional PVC may be innocuous. However, they must be looked upon as *potential precursors of impending ventricular tachycardia and ventricular fibrillation*. Premature ventricular contractions are considered dangerous when they occur in runs of two or more, fall on the T wave, *occur more fre-*

VENTRICULAR TACHYCARDIA ⭐

Figure 4–25 Ventricular tachycardia tracing.

quently than five per minute, or are multifocal as indicated by different shapes to the abnormal QRS complexes.

Experience has shown that placing the patient on 100 per cent oxygen and temporarily terminating the procedure will eliminate the PVCs which are occasionally seen during surgical stimulation in light planes of anesthesia or in episodes of hypoxia. If the abnormal QRS complexes persist, 50 mg of lidocaine is administered intravenously over a one-minute period. Lidocaine should not be used when there is a history of pre-existing complete heart block, since it may cause ventricular arrest.

Ventricular Tachycardia (Fig. 4–25)

Ventricular tachycardia may be described as repeated ventricular premature beats characterized by the aforementioned changes in the QRS and T complex. The rate will usually be from 180 to 250 per minute with a rapid onset. This condition is strongly suggestive of cardiac disease in patients in whom it has not been precipitated by the use of digitalis or other drugs. It sometimes precedes ventricular fibrillation.

Ventricular Fibrillation (Fig. 4–26)

Ventricular fibrillation, the result of a completely haphazard spread of the impulse over the conduction network, causes disorganized and inefficient contraction of the ventricular musculature with resulting circulatory failure. If not corrected immediately, fibrillation will result in death. It may be the terminal event in coronary artery disease or in other forms of heart failure. It will, however, occasionally occur in a healthy patient following minor myocardial infarction, after electric shock, or during general anesthesia in which cyclopropane or halothane has been used, particularly when they have been used with epinephrine.

VENTRICULAR FIBRILLATION ⭐

Figure 4–26 Ventricular fibrillation tracing (terminal).

AGONAL (terminal) RHYTHM ✪

Figure 4–27 Agonal (terminal) rhythm.

Cardiac Standstill

This may be primary or follow ventricular fibrillation. The impulses are no longer functional, and we obtain the agonal rhythm on the cardioscope or ECG tracing (Fig. 4–27). Death is immediate.

Improvements in instrumentation have transformed the electrocardioscope from a bulky, somewhat awkward device into a compact, portable instrument, which is suitable for use in the dental office. There are certain problems encountered when using the instrument on the patient undergoing ultralight general anesthesia.

The major problem associated with its use on patients receiving ultralight general anesthesia is the distortion of the tracing that is caused by the movement of the patient or slight shifting of the electrodes. The lightly anesthetized patient may respond to a stimulus by extremity movement, and this will cause considerable distortion of the tracing as it moves across the screen. However, with training and experience, team members will quickly be able to differentiate these distortions from arrhythmias which may occur during treatment. Other distortions occasionally seen in dental offices are those caused by the use of x-ray equipment in the area and by a drop in the line voltage common to large medical-dental buildings. These problems have been partially corrected by the use of electronic filters, but as reported by Arbeit et al.[13], these filters may further distort the tracing, and any abnormality detected on the scope must be checked by the ECG tracing taken directly from the patient and not through the filtered cardioscope.

DISCUSSION OF COMBINED MONITORING SYSTEMS

An individual may choose one or several biomedical monitors to supplement the essential direct observation of the patient by himself and other members of the team.* After visual inspection of the patient, a precordial or suprasternal stethoscope is placed. The sounds are transmitted to the ear of the anesthetist via five or six feet of plastic tubing. The anesthetist wears a custom-molded earpiece for sustained comfort. A blood pressure cuff is placed on the patient's arm, and the finger monitor is taped to a finger of the same arm. When used, the electrocardiograph leads of an oscilloscope are connected to the patient, using adhesive electrodes. The carbon dioxide

---

*A hypothetical monitoring system with multiple tools is presented here to demonstrate coordination of many monitoring devices.

analyzer lead is inserted in the anesthesia tubing system near the patient's airway. An electric temperature lead is placed at a convenient point, such as the ear canal. The audio signal of the finger pulse monitor is tuned to a convenient level and the oscilloscope situated so that the visual wave can be easily seen. The number of pulse beats per minute can be seen and heard on the monitor. The oximeter is placed on the ear to monitor arterial blood oxygen. When the blood pressure is to be checked, the cuff is inflated, either manually or with a semiautomatic valve that needs only the touch of a finger or foot to inflate the cuff. As the cuff is inflated above the systolic blood pressure, the audiovisual pulse signals cease owing to the lack of circulation in the lower arm and finger. When the cuff pressure is deflated to the systolic pressure and circulation again reaches the finger pulse monitor, the audio signal is heard, and the pulse wave forms are seen. At this moment the doctor may glance at the conspicuously mounted blood pressure dial to check the systolic pressure. Should it prove difficult to obtain, the Doppler could be used to double-check the systolic pressure. The heart and breath sounds are monitored constantly via the stethoscope and monaural earpiece. If it is desirable to broadcast these sounds to the dental operatory at large, the plastic tubing from the chest piece is connected to a cardiac audio-monitor, which will amplify the heart sounds and enable the entire team to be conscious of the respiratory and cardiac status of the patient. If tidal volume needs to be known, a respirometer can be attached to the expiratory breathing tube. When desired, the oscilloscope is switched from the finger pulse lead to the ECG lead and the electrocardioscopic tracing is seen on the screen, together with an audible "beep" at each heartbeat. The oscilloscope may be connected to a paper writer recorder if a permanent tracing is desired. The CO_2 analyzer indicates the carbon dioxide output of each breath; this, too, is often traced on paper by a recorder — usually a trend recorder operating at a very slow paper speed to conserve paper. The electric thermometer constantly displays the body temperature. A "fail-safe" warning system guards the medical gas supply pressure, and the oxygen alarm monitor follows the percentage of oxygen being delivered.

Desirable variations in this procedure might include the use of an automatic indirect blood pressure monitor to record systolic and diastolic pressure in an automatically activated visual display. A small computer could be used to coordinate all this physiological information by monitoring, alarming, displaying, and printing anesthesia records.

Ploss System

While the doctor is using his sense of sight primarily in the operative field, his auditory sense is available for acoustical monitoring. An interesting and economical system has been developed by Ploss,[14] which allows continuous acoustic monitoring of the patient (Fig. 4-28). A lightweight rubber stethoscope pickup is placed over the brachial artery under the blood pressure cuff. The precordial or pretracheal stethoscope is placed on the chest, and the two stethoscopes are connected to the Ploss Automatic Switch Valve[L]. This valve is activated by cuff inflation pressures to exclude heart and lung sounds while the blood pressure is being determined by auscultation. Imme-

Figure 4–28   Ploss automatic switch valve (center). As the blood pressure cuff (1) is inflated by the squeeze bulb (2), Korotkoff sounds are heard through the rubber acoustic pickup (3) which would be positioned over the brachial artery. These sounds are transmitted to the earpiece (4) and the blood pressure is read on the aneroid manometer (5). As the blood pressure cuff is deflated, the heart sounds are heard from the precordial stethoscope (6).

diately upon cuff deflation, the valve automatically switches back to the heart and lung sounds. The valve can be used with conventional sphygmomanometer squeeze bulbs or operated by the Side-Kick^D semi-automatic blood pressure cuff inflator. With this system, heart, breath, and pulse sounds may be evaluated acoustically and with a minimum of detraction from the operative procedure. Use of the automatic switch valve described above frees the operator's hand for other duties. If this extreme efficiency is not necessary, a simple plastic or metal three-way valve may be used to channel the sounds manually with equally good acoustic results.

As most vital signs are taken relative to time, it is helpful to have a large electric clock with a sweep second hand prominently located for timing the various measurements.

An anesthesia record detailing the treatment rendered and the vital signs during the procedure is of importance in recapitulating cases at any later date.

SUMMARY AND CONCLUSIONS

Consideration has been given to various methods of evaluating the patient under general anesthesia. These include the fundamental principles of patient observation as well as monitoring by biomedical electronic and mechanical methods. Every doctor is, by virtue of training and experience, almost instinctively aware of the significance of many physiological signs observed visually and by auscultation, palpation, and percussion. Increased awareness of the patient's status can come through the use of one or more of the commercial monitors available.

Both the general practitioner and the surgeon in practice today have dedicated a number of years to the study of basic and applied science. Their knowledge of these sciences, together with the manual dexterity innate in every dental practitioner, predisposes to make them apt students of the art of anesthesia. They are highly trained and skilled individuals. Those interested in the administration of office and hospital anesthetics utilizing the monitoring techniques discussed in this chapter should find that a period of time spent in a formal course of anesthesia training will rapidly equip them to render a highly desirable service to their patients. During such training, and in later years of practice, it is hoped that some of the concepts presented in this text may be of value.

Acknowledgement

Electrocardiogram tracings used in this chapter are published with the permission of Dallon Instruments of El Segundo, California.

REFERENCES

1. Adriani, J.: Techniques and Procedures of Anesthesia. Springfield, Ill., Charles C Thomas, 1964, p. 60.
2. Best, C. H., and Taylor, N. B.: The Physiological Basis of Medical Practice. 4th ed., Baltimore, Williams & Wilkins Company, 1945, p. 373.
3. General anesthesia. *In* Accepted Dental Therapeutics, 37th ed. Chicago, American Dental Association, 1977, p. 118.
4. Hubbell, A. O., and Krogh, H. W.: Management of intravenous anesthesia to control recovery time. J. Oral Surg. Oral Med. Oral Pathol., 9:403, 1956.
5. Hagen, J. O., and McCarthy, F. M.: General anesthesia for the ambulatory patient: The anesthetic team. J. South. California Dent. Assoc., 37:244, 1969.
6. *Ibid.*
7. *Op. cit.*, General anesthesia.
8. *Ibid.*
9. See the manufacturers' list of instruments at the end of this chapter.
10. Quinn, J. R., Spatz, S., Shensa, D. R., and Esway, J. K.: Malignant hyperthermia during an oral surgical procedure; report of a case. J. Oral Surg., 27:266, 1969.
11. Gores, R. J., Royer, R. Q., and Mann, F. D.: Blood loss during operation for multiple extractions with alveoplasty and oral surgical procedures. J. Oral Surg., 13:299, 1955.
12. Wylie, W. D., and Churchill-Davidson, H. C.: A Practice of Anesthesia. 2nd ed., Chicago, Year Book, 1966, pp. 465–483.
13. Arbeit, S. R., Rubin, I. L., and Gross, H.: Dangers in interpreting the electrocardiogram from the oscilloscope monitor. J.A.M.A., 211:253, 1970.
14. Ploss, R. E.: Simple constant monitoring system. Anesthesiology, 16:466, 1955.

MANUFACTURERS' LIST

A. Temp-Away:

Becton-Dickinson
Division of Becton, Dickinson and
Company
Rutherford, New Jersey 07070

B. Tempra-Dot:

Organon Pharmaceuticals
A Division of Organon Inc.
West Orange, New Jersey, 07052

C. Electronic Thermometer:

Yellow Springs Instrument Co., Inc.
Box 279
Yellow Springs, Ohio 45387

D. Fail-Safe:
   Ohio Side Kick:

Ohio Medical Products
P. O. Box 7550
Madison, Wisconsin 53707

E_1 Capnograph:

Beckman Instrument Co.
2500 Harbor Blvd.
Fullerton, California 92634

E_2 Capnograph:

Corpul Metrix Inc.
6415 S. W. Canyon Court Suite 50
Portland, Oregon 97221

F. Oxygen Alarm Monitor:

Teledyne Analytical Instruments
333 West Mission Drive
San Gabriel, California 91776

G. Blood Gas Oximeter:

Hewlett-Packard
175 Wyman Street
Waltham, Mass. 02173

H. Pulse Monitor:

San-Ei Instrument Co., Ltd.
1-89, Kashiwagi, Shinjuku
Tokyo, Japan

I. Custom Monaural Ear-Mold:

Royale Laboratories
1238 E. Broadway
Glendale, California 91205

J. Perometer:

Particle Data Incorporated
P. O. Box 265
Elmhurst, Illinois 60126

K. Doppler:

Parks Electronic Laboratory
P. O. Box B.B.
Beavertown, Oregon 97005

L. Ploss System:

3M Company, Medical Products Division
3M Center
St. Paul, Minnesota 55101

5

DRUGS: USE AND ABUSE

ROBERT BRUCE STEINER

INTRODUCTION

For those who have been exposed to the first and second editions, this introduction is repetitive, but it is also, I'm sorry to say, apropos! Things change and yet somehow remain basically the same. Greed and profound lack of respect and concern for fellow man is still the vanguard, creed, or philosophy (you choose) of a small group of manufacturers and retailers who, like the poor, it appears will always be with us.

The Food and Drug Administration (FDA), until lately a flickering candle of light on the horizon, has grown into a powerful beam searching into some of the darker recesses of the pharmaceutical industry. Unfortunately, it appears that its zeal and exuberance are overflowing (as is the case with most government entities) in certain questionable areas (as, for example, in the prohibitions on saccharin) but, nonetheless, some control is badly needed.

"For many years a vast system of medical empiricism, sustained by popular credulity and the sanction of government, has prevailed in this country to the serious detriment of the public health and morals.

"The increase of empiricism and of patent medicines within [this century] is an evil over which the friends of science and humanity can never cease to mourn."

A new and timely warning concerning our contemporary "medical specialists" on television? Hardly; this excerpt is taken from House Report No. 52, 30th Congress (2nd Session), 1849.

"Americans are now paying the greatest price they have ever paid for worthless nostrums, ineffectual and potentially dangerous devices, treatments given by unqualified practitioners, food fads, and un-needed diet supplements and other alluring products or services that make misleading promises of cure or end to pain.

"It is incredible that a wealthy nation, priding itself on enlightenment and its thirst for progress should pay such a heavy penalty for ignorance or lack of adequate enforcement."

More verbose and of a larger scope, but the basic theme and tenets are exactly the same. Is this another editorial from the nineteenth century? No, it is an excerpt from the report of the Williams Subcommittee, U.S. Senate, 89th Congress (1st Session), 1965.[61] It specifies, exemplifies, illuminates, and enumerates the odds we face and the progress we've made.

When you finish perusing this chapter you will probably be aware that it is basically negative in tone and content. Before becoming critical of this approach and comfortably certain of your ability to resist the medical hucksters, consider what they are offering: promises of a life free from worries, pain, insomnia, tension, constipation, tired blood, wrinkles, halitosis, weak teeth, body odor, and pimples. Goebbels' theory of conversion of the masses to a preplanned line of thought by continual, monotonous repetition of the big lie mesmerized not only the ignorant and uninformed but also the educated, many with IQ's near and in the genius category.

Dental practitioners are not immune. Because ours is a healing art, we have been trained and suffused with the desire to cure disease and/or alleviate suffering, and we may be more prone to succumb to these blandishments than are our lay brothers. It should not be our role to preach or foster distrust or disillusionment in our patients, but to leaven the euphoria with common sense and to substitute hard facts for wishful thoughts.

There is a moral, ethical, and legal responsibility we must accept with our diplomas — that of analyzing, dissecting, and then accepting or discarding the claims that come not only from Madison Avenue but also from our well-intentioned, but not always well-informed, detail persons. By virtue of didactic education and clinical practice, we know that quackery still flourishes, but that fluoridation is an explosive issue; that *some* drugs are really miraculous, but that *all* are protoplasmic poisons. But do our patients know this?

Do they know that of the approximately 400 new drug products which appear on counter shelves every year, roughly 20 are new compounds whereas the others represent new salts of the same drug, minor changes in structure (such as the exchange of one halogen [Cl] for another [Br]), and mixtures of old brand names? I doubt it!

It is still the popular lay concept that drugs will cure or alleviate almost any misery with great speed and complete safety, and many of us are guilty of subscribing to and encouraging this attitude. Aspirin and its prototypes relieve headache and hangover, antibiotics easily destroy bacteria, and tranquilizers reduce nervous tension. But this supposedly simple and safe alkali-neutralizes-acid kind of drug action is so rare as to be almost nonexistent. Aspirin can cause rash, asthma, and fatal allergic reactions in some persons. Antibiotics produce a swarm of serious disorders. And tranquilizers often give rise to a series of unwanted effects which range from muscular dysfunction to liver malfunctions.

It is an old medical axiom that the use of any drug is a carefully calculated risk. The lack of understanding by the general public that drug action is not simple, that totally unforeseen results can occur with the administration of any medicine, and that newly discovered drugs may have hidden and exotic toxicities which are not revealed until they are widely used, recently led our nation to the brink of what one writer has termed "drug hysteria." We emerged from this state of near-panic with some more federal laws, several scores of lawsuits, and a new anxiety named "drug safety."

Since 1938 no new medicinal agent has been marketed unless the Food and Drug Administration was satisfied that the compound was relatively safe when used according to directions. "Relatively safe" drugs appear to be the best that we can ever hope for. The Surgeon General of the United States has used the phrases "relatively quite safe," and "relatively completely safe." These terms reflect his considered opinion and post a warning that there is a calculated risk involved in the use of any drug or chemical compound.[8]

There is a general tendency to underestimate the toxicity of drugs. Diverse reasons are advanced to explain this phenomenon: overwhelming advertising, in which the patient invariably experiences a pleasing result from taking "medicine"; aesthetic design of both pill and package; natural optimism of the average human; difficulty in recognizing certain types of toxicity because of obscure symptoms; and reluctance of drug manufacturers to list apparent or potential toxic effects of a product.

Broad statistics on episodes of serious toxicity or deaths from drug reactions are either not available or nonexistent. This fact in no way leavens the magnitude of the problem. A significant clue is the sheer abundance of articles relating to toxicity in the medical and allied literature. If this seems undismaying, a survey made in one of our largest teaching medical centers revealed *that toxic reaction to drugs constituted the greatest single cause of hospitalization in the medical service of that institution.*

The avalanches of new products and concomitant advertising, plus the pressures from patients and salesmen alike, pose a problem of primary concern in the study of pharmacology and chemotherapy. The multiplicity of "Siamese" compounds that emerge in the wake of a new and unique drug, especially one which opens fresh vistas or approaches to the control of disease, is certainly an understandable, if not always meritorious, aspect of the free enterprise system, in which failure to compete may mean failure to exist.

Each pharmaceutical company feels that in order to remain competitive in a highly competitive field, it must produce a related or similar product. The end result of this is a spray of congeners which many times yield confusion and frustration to even the most perceptive of our colleagues in the dental, medical, and pharmaceutical professions.

One of the paradoxes of modern chemotherapy is that in our preoccupation with the formulation or discovery of new drugs we seem to forget that their safe and effective use rests ultimately on the practitioners' understanding of current pharmacologic concepts.

Drug intoxication as a topic or an entity must necessarily deal not only with the chemical or agent and its inherent properties but also with the existing state of health of the patient for whom it is prescribed. If a drug is to be used intelligently and safely for the prevention, treatment, or diagnosis of disease, it is imperative that the clinician have information or experience regarding its physiologic effects on both the healthy and the diseased organism.

One basic consideration or rule of thumb which may pre-empt all others is that the existing degree of irritability of the patient's central nervous system determines the amount or dosage of the drug prescribed for that patient. Conditions which *increase* irritability are fear, pain, fever, thyrotoxicosis, alcoholism, excessive musculature, and toxic phenomena → high BMR or higher doses. Conditions which *decrease* irritability are shock, hypothyroidism (myxedema), Addison's disease, senility, and asthenic or wasting diseases → low BMR or lower doses.

Other predominant factors in the choice and dosage of a drug if it is to be safely employed for therapy are race, sex, weight, temperament, environment, route and time of administration, heredity, allergy, and, of course, age.

Race

Orientals are ordinarily more sensitive to depressant drugs, and deeply pigmented races are much less sensitive than others to the mydriatic action of locally applied sympathomimetic amines. In the same vein, it would be futile to accept these or similar observations as more than a guide in attempting to adjust dosage or evaluate inherent sensitivity or toxicity because of, or on account of, specific racial background.

Sex

There are some indications that the sexes respond differently in quantitative terms to drugs, but according to most clinicians if these differences really exist they are slight and in the main relatively unimportant. Nevertheless, it is inadvisable to give the same dosage to a diminutive female as you would to a husky male, other things being equal. It is just the "other things" — temperament, environment, etc.—that matter, however. Of course, in the pregnant female, one has to consider the potential harmfulness of some drugs to the fetus when given in full dosage to the mother, or the toxic effect on the nursing infant through drugs excreted in the milk.

Weight

Empirical clinical practice proceeds on the assumption that it is only common sense to give smaller doses of potent drugs to emaciated, lethargic, or underdeveloped patients than to our corpulent citizens. Drugs are habitually researched and tested on the basis of dosage per kilogram of body weight, and we have been cozened into believing that this is the proper "scientific" approach. However, there is little real justification for the rigid acceptance of such a practice. The imponderables of the relationship of weight to blood volume, individual metabolism, and the inequalities in fat content in individuals of the same weight make a good case for a flexible approach in interpreting a patient's needs when weight is the only factor in determining drug dosage and toxicity.

Temperament

The firmly based clinical impression that individuals respond differently to drugs according to "temperamental makeup" is a dogma embraced by a large majority of practitioners and prescribers of medicines. Easily excited, unstable, neurotic people appear prone to react excessively, although sometimes their state of hyperexcitement and apprehension necessitates the use, in them, of stronger than normal premedication and therapeutic dosage of an appropriate agent.

Environment

Socioeconomic stress and strain are environmental factors that presumably may affect responses to certain types of drugs. Worry, undernourishment, and low resistance are indigenous to low income groups; therefore patients in this category may exhibit other than normal responses to the usual quantitative dosage prescribed.

Climate, humidity, and altitude may affect drug selection and application in many respects, some of which are not yet documented. But it is fairly well accepted that relative oxygen deprivation, from whatever cause, increases sensitivity to a great variety and number of agents.

Route of Administration

The way in which a drug is administered may have a profound influence on the effects achieved. Many agents are not reliable or efficacious when taken orally. Conversely, other agents cannot or should not be injected parenterally. Others must be inhaled to be useful. The astute therapist should have a thorough knowledge of a drug's assimilation before maximum benefit and avoidance of toxicity can be obtained from its use.

Time of Administration

The response expected from a drug after administration is modified favorably or unfavorably by the *time* of administration. Body physiology changes with time and activity, a consideration which determines the most propitious moment for the ingestion or application of the agent selected to impart the desired alteration or alleviation of a pathologic entity.

Heredity

Heredity can make the same drug a boon to one patient and a poison to another. Although knowledge of genetic factors is still rather primitive, the potential reactor can often be identified, too. Wide variations in the rate and pattern of drug metabolism are often accounted for by genetically determined enzyme systems. Half of the population are either fast or slow metabolizers of isoniazid, a drug widely used in the treatment of tuberculosis. This difference has definitely been proved to be inheritable, according to Dr. Bert LaDu of the New York University School of Medicine. Dicumarol is another drug in which dosage varies considerably because of other genetic factors. One 73-year-old man had to take 20 times the "normal" dose before the drug was effective.[29]

Allergy

Allergy has been defined as immunity gone wrong. Immunity relates to those processes in which the introduction of a foreign substance into the organism causes no clinically evident reaction.

For over 50 years histamine has been implicated in anaphylaxis. Recently other substances (SRS, kinins, and serotonin) have been indicated to help share the blame. One reason for enlarging the list of culprits is that antihistamine drugs are completely ineffective in some cases of allergy or altered acquired immunologic response.

Because of the rampant confusion and the differences in approach and treatment, the practical importance of distinguishing toxicity from true allergy is undebatable in these days of greatly expanded drug therapy. In dealing with a toxic or side effect, a simple reduction of the dose may relieve or eradicate untoward symptoms or problems and allow the important or desired therapeutic effect of the drug to be retained. In dealing with an allergy, dose size is almost totally unrelated to the magnitude of the effect, and the drug must be immediately and completely withdrawn and not repeated. The differential diagnosis of allergy from toxicity and idiosyncrasy in obscure cases depends on these factors when a drug is suspect:

1. If reducing the dose reduces or eliminates the symptoms, it is toxicity.
2. If the phenomena in question arise with the initial dose, it is probably idiosyncrasy.
3. If ensuing normal doses produce redness, rash, or hives on the skin, rather sudden edema of the limbs, face or trachea, asthma, or gastrointestinal cramps, it is allergy.

CBC studies are helpful to confirm a suspected allergy in that they usually show less than 30 round cells and an increase in eosinophils.

A better understanding of allergic phenomena and new techniques and drugs to interdict or negate the detrimental effects are in trial at this writing. (See Chapter 12 for a complete coverage of this entity.)

Age

Although drug dosage in infants and children is usually determined by Young's modulus or a similar body weight-age formula, dosage in the elderly is modified as a precautionary measure because the absorptive, distributive, metabolic, and excretionary functions of geriatric patients are often altered appreciably and can be widely divergent from the norm.

Pediatrics. Children are not miniature adults! Their reactions to and tolerance of drugs are often uniquely pediatric. It is poor practice to halve the adult dose because the intended recipient is half the adult size!

Children, especially infants, have underdeveloped livers and enzyme systems—the principal areas for drug detoxification. An immature physiology cannot cope with some agents except in minimal amounts. Evidence suggests permanent damage to growth or maturation of specific organs and systems.

Modell has repeatedly warned that the younger the child, the more striking the problem. Fortunately the dental clinician seldom deals with infants, happily avoiding most of these problems. However, antibiotics, sedatives, and analgesics, three entities common in pedodontic practice, are categories in which child response may differ grossly from adult response.

Intensive or pervasive evaluation and identification of abnormalities, congenital or acquired, and prior and/or current pathosis will dictate the degree of need and influence the dose. The most accurate method of determining normal dosage which is basic for successful therapy is based on the exterior epithelial area of the child's body—ordinarily difficult to measure. A safe and rapid method, using weight and surface area data, is this formula: $0.7 \times$ weight $+ 10 = \%$ of adult dosage.

Lastly, in situations in which exactness is mandatory, the agent must be injected even though psychically traumatic and distasteful for all. Refusal to swallow, spitting, and vomiting make the oral route precarious and the ingested quantity unknown. Rectal suppositories or liquids are also unpleasant and unreliable, frequently precipitating instant bowel movements or uneven and faulty absorption.

Geriatrics. Geriatrics is a fairly new term with many connotations, depending on one's viewpoint. The very word is paramount to some, and anathema to others. Suffice it to say here that it is accepted to mean those citizens (more than 10 per cent of our population) who are past the age of 65. Elderly people often present real problems for business and industry, their families, and their doctors. This appears to be a cruel and tragic simplification of a complex situation, but the premise is true, the people are here, and they must be dealt with. The rather archaic attitudes of industry regarding the usefulness of those over 65 are hopefully about to change. If one considers that the very nature of our efforts in all the healing arts is guaranteed to perpetuate the geriatric scene, it may generate more incentive to cope with the special problems indigenous to it. The usual geriatric patient has a major flaw—it may be physiologic, psychologic, or economic. Regardless of the source, it will affect his attitude toward you and the proposed therapy. Since drugs occupy or encompass a part of virtually all treatment plans and a patient's attitude may have a profound influence on his reactions to these drugs, we have returned full circle to our topic.

Besides his questionable response to the routine dental medicines, synergism, interaction, incompatibility, and additive and cumulative effects are always major considerations in the treatment program of a geriatric patient. It is rare to encounter an aged individual without a systemic malfunction requiring not just one but a planned regimen of drugs to regulate or maintain near-normal or adequate body physiology. Arthritis, hypertension, arteriosclerosis, angina, edema, emphysema, glaucoma, cataracts, menopause, prostatitis—some of these are part and parcel of the everyday existence of most senior citizens.

Steroids, salicylates, thiazides, digitalis, hypotensives, anticoagulants, tranquilizers, insulin, antibiotics, ointments—the roster is endless! The aged learn to live with discomfort, pain, and pills.

A dialogue history with special emphasis on prescription drugs is mandatory before therapy of any kind is attempted. Consultation with the patient's physician may be desirable.

The chart on drug interactions at the end of this chapter precludes a repetitive listing at this point.

Before leaving this topic, two important points are pertinent:

1. It is not unusual for an elderly person to have an ambiguous reaction to drugs (i.e., excitement from barbiturates or scopolamine). If anticipated, surprise will not be an unsettling or damaging factor, and restorative, supportive, or resuscitative therapy will be instituted without doubt or delay.

2. The elderly are perfect "pigeons" for over-the-counter panaceas, and this is not difficult to understand. Disillusioned and/or disappointed with a lack of efficacy or speed in the standard prescription remedies, they turn, often in desperation, to patent potions for relief. Most of these miracle compounds are ordinary, many are frauds, and some are dangerous.

A list of nonprescription remedies, their chemical formulae, and their frequency of use are a very important part of a geriatric patient's history. "To be forewarned is to be forearmed" is not a foolish cliché!

Pregnancy

Unnecessary or excessive medication of the pregnant patient should be stringently avoided. It is known that the fetus is incapable of metabolizing or detoxifying certain drugs that are nevertheless safe and effective in the mother. This is primarily due to immature liver and enzyme function. Most drugs will pass the placental barrier, especially the lipid soluble drugs (includes most anesthetics), and many of their effects are not yet fully known. (Only those drugs over 1000 molecular weight are immune.)

The agent ingested by the mother may directly affect the fetus (or its metabolites may be toxic) according to its distribution to or affinity for fetal tissue, or it may exert an indirect effect by interfering with metabolic processes in the mother. This results in the transmission of potentially toxic metabolites from mother to fetus or embryo. Organogenesis is a factor during the first trimester only.

Congenital malformations occur most readily during the stages of early cellular differentiation (10 to 15 days after conception). Phocomelia (thalidomide), narcotic addiction (heroin), and tooth discoloration (tetracyclines) are but three common and dramatic malformations among many that are known or thought to occur. Teratogenetics, the science of drug-induced birth defects, must be ever in mind when planning treatment for the pregnant patient. Only those agents known to be safe are considered, and all medications should be kept to that minimum required for effective therapy. Seventy-five per cent of all spontaneous abortions occur before the sixteenth week; the second trimester is the safest time for anesthetics and surgery.

But therapeutic nihilism arising from fear of jeopardizing the intrauterine patient by maternal medication is unjustified. In fact, there are times during pregnancy when the withholding of a drug would cause a much more serious consequence than the possible adverse effects to either the mother or child. It is an intolerable judgment if fear of adverse effects to the offspring deprives the mother of drugs that could be essential to her well-being and even to the successful outcome of the pregnancy itself.

Analgesics.   Narcotic and non-narcotic analgesics all cross the placenta. The narcotics (especially morphine and heroin) may cause addiction in utero, and severe respiratory depression, miosis, and withdrawal symptoms at birth. Codeine is safe.

Hypnotics.   Barbiturates yield a level in the fetus of up to 70 per cent of maternal level, but unless the mother suffers derangement of physiology during a general anesthetic or overdose of oral medication, there is no evidence of induced abortion or congenital malformations with this class of drugs.

Antibiotics.   The penicillin family is safe in every area unless severe allergy rears its ugly head. Erythromycin is blameless too, but all other commonly used antimicrobials are either irrevocably harmful or restricted to certain periods during the pregnancy. Included are sulphonamides, the tetracycline family, streptomycin, lincomycin, Clindamycin, and Novobiocin. Consultation with the obstetrician is mandatory if severe or unyielding dental infection exists.

Antihistamines.   Diphenhydramine and chlorpheniramine are known to be inert in the fetus and may be prescribed with safety. Diphenhydramine may also be useful as an antinauseant and mild soporific, two areas in pregnancy that frequently need alteration and medication.

Antacids.   All aluminum salts containing antacids (Amphojel, Phosphaljel, Maalox) cannot cross the placenta; therefore, they are not a toxic factor. Kaopectate falls in the same category.

Tranquilizers.   Many of this class are known to be dangerous, and others are highly suspect. Chlordiazepoxide (diazepam is thought to be similar in action) passes the barrier 100 per cent, and, although teratogenicity has not been proved, these drugs should be used with caution during the first trimester.

Chloral hydrate and the barbiturates ought to be given first consideration when sedation of the pregnant patient is desirable or mandatory.

Local Analgesics.   Local analgesics, especially the aniline series, are not restricted when proper techniques (aspiration, etc.) are employed.

As an addendum to this general classification, I believe a listing of specific drugs that the dentist may use, or at least be interested in, is essential for the complete protection of our unborn children. The medication or agent is listed along with its adverse effects in Table 5–1, taken from Martin's Hazards of Medication, a textbook of infinite worth.

DRUGS IN LACTATING MOTHERS

Drugs administered during lactation follow a similar pattern of action and distribution as in pregnancy, with some startling exceptions. Morphine and codeine do not occur in milk at all, while other narcotics appear in sufficient strength to sedate the nursing infant.

ASA appears in moderate amounts. To negate any possible interactions, the mother should take the tablet just prior to nursing.

Barbital is completely absent, but NaP shows intraces (mgm), and phenobarbital may be present in high enough concentration to cause enzyme induction in the infant's immature liver.

Oxacillin is the only common antibiotic that does not appear in the milk, while penicillin in even trace amounts could precipitate sensitivity reactions in later life. Erythromycin is relatively innocuous, and it is often the drug of choice in most dental infections.

Diazepam may cause a noticeable sedative effect on the child, which could impair feeding.

Local anesthetics are generally innocuous.

As a general rule, all drugs that cause central nervous system depression are suspect until proved innocent, except ethanol, whose ingestion, unless gross, is not contraindicated. Analgesics, hypnotics, and tranquilizers, along with general anesthetics, fall in this class. *The dose is directly related to the effect.* Minimal effective amount for the shortest possible time is the paramount rule.

Teratogenicity is and should be a frightening word! The general welfare of the embryo, fetus, and neonate (along with the mother) must be the prime concern of every prescriber of medicine or chemotherapy. Since this topic is substantial enough for a tome of its own, only those drugs of a dangerous nature and those that can be prescribed and used with safety are mentioned. Many of the newer compounds are missing because insufficient data are available. Others are missing because they have no real place in the dental armamentarium.

When in doubt – don't!

Chronic Illness

All the previous factors are important and unavoidably pertinent in the treatment or therapy plans for our patients, but none more so than in the state of chronic illness. Here is probably the classic challenge to our therapeutic acumen. How best to approach the debilitated patient, whose well-being depends on a balanced regimen of drugs to maintain an acceptable plateau of health and well-being? The ever-burgeoning hordes of people whose function and comfort depend on delicately balanced programs of chemotherapy have every right to expect that their precarious existence will not be jeopardized by careless or ignorant administration of agents which disturb this balance or are incompatible with those drugs already in use.

DRUG DEFINITIONS

The following definitions may help dispel some of the foggy notions concerning all drugs.

TABLE 5–1 LIST OF MEDICATIONS AND ADVERSE EFFECTS
(FROM MARTIN, HAZARDS OF MEDICATION)

Drugs	Adverse Effects
Acetophenetidin	Methemoglobinemia
Alphaprodine (Nisentil)	Fetal respiratory depression
Anesthetics (Volatile)	Depressed fetal respiration
Androgens	Advanced bone age; clitoral enlargement; labial fusion; masculinization
Barbiturates	Depressed respiration
Bromides	Neonatal skin eruptions (bromoderma)
Chloral hydrate (large doses)	Fetal death
Chloramphenicol (Chloromycetin)	Fetal death; gray syndrome
Chlorpromazine	Neonatal jaundice; mortality; prolonged extra-pyramidal signs
Cortisone	Cleft palate
Ether	Neonatal apnea
Ganglionic blocking agents	Neonatal ileus
Iodides	Goiter
Lysergic acid diethylamide (LSD)	Chromosomal damage; stunted offspring
Mepivacaine (Carbocaine)	Fetal bradycardia; neonatal depression
Methadone	Fetal respiratory depression
Morphine	Initial neonatal addiction; respiratory depression; neonatal death
Nicotine (smoking)	Small neonates
Nitrofurantoin (Furadantin)	Fetal hemolysis
Nitrous oxide (anesthetic)	Inhibits fetal respiratory movement
Novobiocin (Albamycin)	Hyperbilirubinemia
Oral progestogens (Norlutin, Lutocylol, Pranone, Progestoral)	Clitoral enlargement; labial fusion; masculinization
Phenobarbital (in excess)	Neonatal hemorrhage and death
Phenylbutazone (Butazolidin)	Neonatal goiter
Potassium iodide	Cyanosis; goiter; mental retardation; respiratory distress
Reserpine	Nasal block; respiratory obstruction
Salicylates (aspirin)	Neonatal bleeding; severe hypoglycemia
Streptomycin	Hearing loss; micromelia; multiple skeletal anomalies; 8th nerve damage
Sulfonamides (long-acting)	Kernicterus; hyperbilirubinemia; acute liver atrophy; anemia
Tetracyclines	Discolored teeth, inhibited bone growth, micromelia; syndactyly
Thalidomide	Hearing defects; phocomelia; death
Thiazides (Chlorothiazide, Methychlothiazide, etc.)	Neonatal death; thrombocytopenia
Vitamin A (large doses)	Cleft palate; congenital anomalies; eye damage; syndactyly
Vitamin D (large doses)	Hypercalcemia; mental retardation
Vitamin K Analogues (large doses)	Hyperbilirubinemia; kernicterus

Psychological dependence (habituation) is an altered psychic or mental state in which a drug and its effects on the conditions associated with its use assume undue importance (almost necessity) for the maintenance of an optimal state of comfort and well-being (tobacco, coffee, sweets, etc.).

Physical dependence (biological craving) is an altered physiological state created by repeated use which necessitates the continued administration to prevent a stereotyped syndrome (withdrawal) which results in objective illness (days to weeks) (narcotics, phenothiazines, tricyclics, amphetamines, and alcohol).

Addiction is a behavioral pattern of compulsive drug use characterized by both *physical* and *psychological* dependence so strong that the addict's whole existence revolves around the procurement and ingestion of the drug, and all of life's normal pursuits are excluded or relegated to an inferior level.

Tolerance (tachyphylaxis) is a reduced physiologic response to a given dose of the agent in question, necessitating larger doses, sometimes to the toxic level, to obtain the effects observed with the original or average dose.

Rebound phenomenon is an exaggerated, negative, or unwanted effect due to increasing tolerance from larger and repetitive doses, resulting not only in ineffectiveness but also in an aberrant increase in the symptoms or complaint, for the reversal of which the original therapy was designed or prescribed.

SELECTION OF DRUGS FOR DISCUSSION

It will soon be apparent to those who read on that many basic drugs and proprietary compounds are not mentioned in the following pages. There has been no conscious intent to exclude or to malign some products or to promote or subsidize others, except in cases where a preponderant number of those colleagues or texts consulted dictated such tactics or opinions. Nor has there been a conscious attempt to impress the reader with a presumptuous knowledge of the intricacies of molecular chemistry and body physiology, which admittedly are not within the author's purview.

With these limitations always in mind, and ever aware of the infinite scope of the subject, the reader should evaluate this chapter as nothing more than a list of commonly prescribed drugs, some of the conditions or situations which modify their actions, and the toxic manifestations which arise or may be encountered when they are used separately or together in the treatment of our patients.

CARDIOVASCULAR DRUGS

The increase in life expectancy of the average patient, while eminently desirable and the certain goal of the healing arts, creates a host of problems which demand perceptiveness and alertness on the part of the practitioner. Nowhere are these problems more pertinent than in the therapy for cardiovascular diseases. There are drugs which stimulate the myocardium; there are others which depress the myocardium. Hypertension is controlled by agents which decrease the blood pressure; hypotension is treated with agents which elevate the blood pressure. Other compounds or chemicals are administered to influence the cardiovascular system by indirect or remote actions; for example, the diuretics, nitrites, and atropine. The clinician is embroiled in these problems because many drugs employed in everyday dental office practice are incompatible, interfere with, or increase the toxicity of the agents used by the physician to control cardiovascular disease.

The *digitalis glycosides* are universally administered to patients to combat myocardial insufficiency or congestive heart failure. Digitalis, digitoxin, digoxin, ouabain, and cedilanid are the generic names for this group of drugs, all of which are naturally occurring and not yet synthesized. The details and ramifications of their actions are hardly within the scope of this chapter, but the necessity of a cautious approach in the application of the drugs required for ordinary dental treatment on the digitalized patient is worthy of comment and consideration.

Digitalis is itself a highly toxic drug which requires intensive care and regulation in determining the proper dosage. The therapeutic dose and the toxic dose are, in many cases, very close. Potassium ion depletion is common in digitalized patients, and gives rise to paroxysmal atrial tachycardia and heart block. Diabetics receiving insulin plus glucose are often low in K ion and therefore hard to control or stabilize. Thyroidectomized persons using thyroxin for maintenance therapy must be alert to possible toxic complications.

Some drugs used frequently in dental treatment which can increase the toxicity of digitalis are atropine, steroids, and the adrenergic agents. Atropine can be dangerous through excessive vagal depression yielding undesirable bouts of tachycardia. Steroids often exert untoward influences which, although vague and difficult to discern, are distressing and sometimes dangerous to digitalis users. The adrenergic drugs, especially epinephrine and ephedrine, sensitize the myocardium, and in combination with digitalis, which has already increased cardiac muscle tone in its host, may precipitate arrhythmias or a fatal ventricular fibrillation. Endogenous epinephrine, released into the cardiovascular system as a direct result of stimuli from painful or psychically traumatic dental procedures, can and does elicit the same toxic phenomena.

Occasionally it becomes mandatory to depress the cardiac muscle tone in certain abnormal states such as arrhythmias and chronic tachycardias. Quinidine, procainamide, and potassium chloride are the agents of choice for this purpose. These drugs exhibit many toxic manifestations of their own which are primarily the concern of the physician, but preparations or dental procedures which are depressant or hypotensive in nature should be approached with caution or avoided. Also, many arrhythmias are worsened by anxiety, which, if severe enough, may negate the therapeutic effect of these agents.

Hypertensive patients are controlled or treated with the rauwolfia alkaloids (reserpine and deserpidine), barbiturates, ganglionic-blocking compounds, and, occasionally, tranquilizers. The barbiturates and tranquilizers are mentioned elsewhere, as are the rauwolfias. The ganglionic-blocking drugs are a potent group employed only in severe hypertensives and used cautiously in deference to their often extreme potency and toxicity. Ansolysen, Veriloid, Apresoline, and Ecolid are the proprietary or familiar names of the more popular of these agents.

Usurping the ganglionic blockers when possible, because of lower toxicity, fewer side effects, and less labile doses, guanethidine (Ismelin) and methyldopa (Aldomet) are more desirable antihypertensives. With a mode of action resembling rauwolfia (because they interfere with the natural catecholamines) but differing in approach (storage and displacement), they are still prone to produce postural hypotension and interactions with other depressors to the extent that a cauldron of trouble awaits the unwary.

Clonidine HCl (Catapres), a fairly new anti-hypertensive, acts differently from any existing drug in this category because it acts centrally on the brain to reduce or suppress sympathetic output. In other respects it is similar to methyldopa (interactions, etc.).

Propranolol (Inderal) is a beta adrenergic receptor blocking agent and as such is enjoying increasing usage in various cardiopathies. After initial employment for prophylaxis of paroxysmal atrial tachycardia and other arrhythmias, some patients suffering from hypertrophic aortic stenosis, angina pectoris, and hypertension are being treated with this potent agent. Regardless of the questionable nature of this form of therapy it behooves all clinicians to be aware of the dangers involved when treating anyone who is currently taking this drug.

Inderal's action prevents the heart from responding to sympathetic stimulation and circulating catecholamines and could precipitate asthmatic attacks in susceptible individuals. All this is germane to the stress inherent or generated in the performance of our profession (daily tasks). Inderal's appearance on a history form should indicate to the doctor that he or she is dealing with a risk patient, thereby provoking a conservative or cautious appraisal of the treatment plan. Isoproterenol is the drug of choice in overcoming beta adrenergic blockade.

Consultation with the physician may be advisable when patients on any "blood pressure medicine" report for dental treatment.

Chronic hypotension is seldom a serious situation except when associated with a definite pathologic state, such as myxedema or Addison's disease. Sudden acute hypotension, of course, is dangerous. It usually results from a toxic response to a drug or a traumatic experience (shock) and must be treated with a vasopressor or similar analeptic. Adrenalin, Phenylephrine, Ephedrine, Vasoxyl, Aramine, Wyamine, and Levophed are the trade names of commonly used vasopressors.

The knowledgeable therapist employs sympathomimetic amines only when it is certain that hypotension is due largely to vasomotor paralysis and not oligemia. Otherwise, serious toxic effects such as acute tubular necrosis (ATN) of the kidneys may result. Also he differentiates between the two distinct vascular actions and the cardiac action, and whether direct rather than indirect agents are appropriate.

Selection of the best one for a particular circulatory problem is easily done in the textbooks, but clinically it is a guessing game. Circulatory measurements and the comprehensive physiologic and pharmacologic data necessary for exactness are seldom available at the instant of decision.

All the currently used adrenergics share five actions but differ quantitatively to a great degree in their amplification: vascular excitatory for alpha receptors which cause constriction; vascular inhibitory for beta receptors which cause dilatation; cardiac excitatory; metabolic excitatory; and CNS excitatory. The variance in strength or propensity for each or all of these five actions should govern the selection of the pressor agent. Some agents act indirectly by releasing vessel and end plate stores of norepinephrine; others act directly on the receptors; and still others have both indirect and direct actions or manifestations.

Indirect alpha — Tyramine, Amphetamine, nasal decongestants (Naphazoline, Oxymetazoline, Phenylpropanolamine)
Direct alpha — Phenylephrine, Methoxamine

Direct beta — Isoproterenol
Indirect and direct alpha — Ephedrine, Metaraminol, Mephentermine
Direct alpha and beta — epinephrine and norepinephrine

Since cocaine prevents release of norepinephrine from vessel sites and effector organs whereas reserpine acts by depleting them, an indirectly acting agent would be useless in restoring vascular tonus or integrity.

In the whole sphere of pharmacotherapeutics, no area of greater controversy exists than that covered by the vasopressors. Each clinician or author invariably adopts a favorite drug, confers on it powers that others fail to perceive, and defends his pet vigorously, often demeaning others in the process.

These sympathomimetic agents are all very potent and can produce serious toxicities of their own, such as acute anxiety, pulmonary edema, and cardiac arrhythmias, including fibrillation. The hazard of these aforementioned toxic responses is grossly magnified for those patients who need emergency vasopressor therapy and are already afflicted with hyperthyroidism, arteriosclerosis, or one of the cardiopathies.

Diuretics

Diuretics are the most prominent indirect agents in the treatment of myocardial insufficiencies. These drugs increase urine flow and promote excretion of Na ions in the kidneys, thereby relieving the edema which is pathognomonic of congestive heart failure. The early diuretics displayed varied and numerous toxic effects, but only the thiazides will be considered here, because chlorothiazide (Diuril) and its congeners are first choice for the majority of patients, while furosemide and ethracrynic acid are more specific and limited in use. These drugs are potent, yet low in direct toxicity. *However, they exert a hypotensive effect which can be markedly enhanced if combined with other such agents.* This factor is of particular interest when IV barbiturates, synergistic with chlorothiazide, are considered for sedation or anesthesia in the dental treatment of such a patient.

Nitrites and Nitrates

These drugs could be considered to have both a direct and indirect effect on the myocardium. Nitroglycerin, amyl nitrite, and Peritrate are most commonly prescribed. Isordil is a long acting form. Their primary use is in the relief of pain in patients suffering from angina pectoris. Nitrites accomplish this feat by relaxing the smooth or involuntary muscle in the walls of certain hollow structures, especially the coronary arteries and veins, thereby increasing the blood flow to the hypoxic myocardium. (Controversy exists over the exact mechanism or mode of action.) This sudden rush of blood perfuses the oxygen-starved cardiac tissues and relieves the pain. Since the appearance of these drugs is not uncommon in the dental office, the symptoms of nitrite intoxication should be listed. Usually precipitated only after large or overdoses, they are throbbing headache, flushing of the face, palpitation, and fainting.

Heparin and the Coumarins

As the number of patients with cardiac and vascular disorders increases, anticoagulants assume a larger role in the scheme of things. This group of drugs is important to the clinician in that they are a factor in the total therapy picture. Allergic responses to heparin, Coumadin, and Dicumarol are extremely rare, and toxicity occurs only with overdose. Compatibility with dental drugs is not a problem, but vitamin K and its analogs will negate the therapeutic effect of the coumarins. Conversely, K can control the toxic effects if or when overdosage creates a problem.

ANALGESIC DRUGS

Relief of pain is one of the great objectives in the healing arts. Drugs whose predominant action is pain relief are termed analgesics, and are loosely divided into three categories: addictive, nonaddictive, and speculatory.* The addictive analgesics are narcotics, whether natural or synthetic, and their use is regulated by the Harrison Act.

ADDICTIVE

Pharmacologic studies have proved that a basic similarity exists among all the narcotic drugs, and because of its great potency, morphine is still used as a standard of comparison for this group.

Morphine

The chief alkaloid of opium, this analgesic has many and various uses in control of pain, reduction of metabolic rate, abolishment of fear and anxiety, relieving pulmonary edema, and eradication of the cough reflex. Despite its many virtues, morphine is a dangerous and extremely toxic drug, and it behooves the practitioner to be thoroughly familiar with its pharmacology. The chief effects are exerted on the central nervous system, the respiratory system, and the gastrointestinal tract.

CNS. Morphine produces profound analgesia and, in large doses, sleep. In addition there are euphoria, emotional placidity, and easing or lessening of muscular tremors. These desirable characteristics are chiefly responsible for addiction, which leads progressively to toxic overdose and dangerous alteration of body physiology.

Respiration. Morphine exerts a powerful depressing effect on the respiratory center in the brain (medulla), causing a diminution of both respiratory rate and volume. This depression can occur even in very small doses, and could be significant in patients with respiratory ailments such as emphysema, bronchiectasis, and the pneumoconioses. Bronchial constriction may occur in asthmatics, sometimes to a lethal degree.

*Author's relative designation.

Gastrointestinal Tract. Morphine constricts the sphincters of the gastrointestinal tract, increases muscle tone in the bowel (spasm), causing constipation, and irritates the chemoreceptor trigger zone in the medulla, which results in nausea and vomiting.

Delay in gastric emptying due to spasm of the pyloric sphincter is a dangerous factor when administration of general anesthetics is contemplated.

Morphine increases intracranial pressure and is contraindicated in patients with head injuries. Hyperglycemia often follows morphine injection and could be toxic to advanced diabetics.

Since this drug is detoxicated in the liver, patients with cirrhosis may experience a prolonged effect. It should be used with caution during pregnancy because morphine readily passes the placental barrier and may have a profound effect on fetal respiration. Hypothyroidism, Addison's disease, anemia, and severe debilitation are other disease states in which narcotics can exert a deleterious or toxic effect in normal dosages.

Acute morphine toxicity presents the following picture and, with few exceptions, exhibits the general diagnostic signs common to all forms of CNS poisoning from natural or synthetic narcotic drugs: irregular mixed stimulation and depression of the central nervous system with selective depression of the respiratory center; slow, shallow or sighing respiration, with unconsciousness, cyanosis, and pupilloconstriction (Argyll Robertson pupil). As depression deepens, and respirations slow and become less adequate, there is a gradual onset of prostration with loss of reflexes and muscular relaxation. The skin becomes pale, cold, and moist, and the pupils dilate; the heartbeat may be slow at first, but later it becomes irregular, rapid, and weak, and the blood pressure drops. There may be convulsions just before paralysis and death.

An interesting study in 1977 has shown that combining dextroamphetamines with morphine sulfate increases potency and euphoria and decreases toxicity.

Dilaudid

An oxidation product of morphine, hydromorphone, exhibits all the properties, bad and good, of the parent drug, except that it may be used in much smaller doses (2 to 4 mg) to gain analgesia, and has considerably less effect on the gastrointestinal tract.

Codeine

This alkaloid of opium is widely prescribed by clinicians, and as such is an important pain remedy. It depresses respiration less than morphine, but has a better antitussive effect, causes less constipation but more nausea, and elicts little, if any, spasm of the gastrointestinal tract.

The analgesic effect of codeine is roughly one-sixth that of morphine, and it fails to produce progressive sedation with increasing doses. This factor, together with a lack of euphoria (except in Percodan), lessens the chances of addiction to codeine. Its greatly reduced toxicity when compared with morphine makes it a much safer drug for nursing or pregnant patients, diabetics, and patients with chronic respiratory ailments, head injuries, and cirrhosis. However, cerebral and cord hyperirritability are more pronounced with codeine, so that before coma supervenes, there may be delirium, and after coma, convulsions. Empirin Compound, Phenaphen, Fiorinal, etc., all depend on codeine for their practical analgesic effect.

Percodan

Percodan is a favorite analgesic of many clinicians, but they should be aware that it contains APC and oxycodone in the HCl and terepthalate salts and is not yet cleared for use in pregnant patients. Oxycodone is derived from thebain, one of the original opium alkaloids, and chemically is considered to be stronger and longer acting than plain codeine, which it closely resembles. Dosage varies, with 1 tablet (containing approximately 5 mg of oxycodone, ASA 224 mg, phenacetin 160 mg and caffeine 32 mg) prescribed q 4 to 6 h and doubled if necessary.

Synalgos DC

This is another analgesic compound which is avidly promoted as superior to codeine sulfate in relief of pain. Synalgos DC is formulated with drocode (dihydrocodeine ¼ gr [16 mg]), promethazine 6.25 mg and APC — it has yet to be cleared for teratogeneity, which negates its value in pregnancy.

It appears to be more potent than plain codeine or its compounds and, as such, probably deserves a trial for a spot in your armamentarium against pain. Dosage is one capsule q 4 h and doubled if necessary in resistant pain syndrome.

Meperidine (Demerol)

A synthetic narcotic which is most popular, this analgesic is not as toxic as morphine, nor is it nearly as potent, ranging from one tenth to one eighth as effective in comparative doses.

Despite conflicting reports, most clinicians consider it equal to morphine as a depressant of respiration, but, since it is a bronchodilator (considered controversial — it would be more correct to say it is not a constrictor as in MS), it should be safer for use on asthmatic patients. Its gastrointestinal activity is similar to morphine but exerted to a lesser degree. It has little effect on the motility of the bowel; therefore, constipation is not a problem.

Demerol appears to be more closely related to atropine than to morphine, because in addition to its analgesic effect it has parasympatholytic actions such as dryness of the mouth, flushing of the face and cervical areas, and bronchodilatation. The pupil of the eye is not affected by Demerol.

This drug is rapidly and almost completely destroyed by the liver; therefore, its use in patients with hepatic disease demands caution and close observation.

Anileridine (Leritine)

This synthetic drug is related to meperidine but is reported to be more potent. It has similar toxic effects, so when administered, the same rules of caution observed with meperidine should prevail.

Phenazocine (Prinadol)

A synthetic analog which earlier showed great promise by being four times as active as morphine, has, in later trials, failed to offer any significant advantages because its addictive and toxic effects are very similar to morphine. However, there is less nausea, and this factor may be an important consideration in certain patients.

Alphaprodine (Nisentil)

This wholly synthetic analgesic compound appears to be more potent than Demerol with less respiratory depression and more rapid onset, usually within five minutes. Its action is of short duration — one to two hours — and this is a paramount consideration in the ambulatory dental patient. It produces negligible euphoria and little sedation, so the average patient remains alert and aware of his surroundings. Nisentil causes fewer side effects and is generally *less toxic* than Demerol.

Fentanyl (Sublimaze)

Fentanyl (Sublimaze) is another synthetic (piperidine) analgesic of great potency, rapid onset (three to eight minutes), and short duration (one-half to one hour, depending on the route of administration). It very much resembles Nisentil in its basic nature and actions, and as such offers a choice.

It is being touted for a secondary effect which is also important — the relief of postanesthetic emergence delirium. If true, this may supersede its primary function. There is a surplus of good narcotic analgesics. There is a dearth of good agents to combat delirium without undue depression.

Methadone (Dolophine)

This synthetic analgesic most closely resembles morphine in potency for pain relief, but has less emetic and constipating actions. Sedation and euphoria are slight, thus limiting its use in preanesthetic medication. Respiratory depression is comparable with morphine, but methadone is less addictive and less toxic. Considering the above factors, methadone is ordinarily confined to use as an analgesic for treatment of severe or traumatic pain.

Methadone is addictive — a narcotic in the true sense as we know it. But it replaces the craving for heroin and morphine and allows the user to work and function normally. In addition, it is inexpensive, requires but one dose per day to alleviate an addict's suffering, and causes much less derangement of normal physiology. Although controversial at this time, methadone, as a controlled substitute for more dangerous drugs, is gaining momentum as the newest weapon in the programs for rehabilitation of addicts.

Hycodan, Numorphan, Metopon, and Pantopon are all morphine congeners with similar uses and toxicity, but without significant advantages and differences which would recommend their general substitution for morphine except in selected cases.

Nalorphine (Nalline); Levallorphan (Lorfan); Naloxone (Narcan); Naltrexone

Although derivatives of certain opiate drugs, Nalline and Lorfan antagonize practically all of the effects of morphine and the other narcotic compounds. Similar in every way, they may be used interchangeably. There are no known differences or specific advantages of one as compared with the other, and employment of either is a matter of personal choice.

The antidotal effects of these agents is thought to be due to competitive inhibition with replacement of potent drugs by a weak compound having higher affinity for the receptor. Nonetheless, they are effective and predictable, and have a wide range of use in negating the action of *all the narcotic drugs*.

However, the appearance of naloxone (Narcan) several years ago has rendered all this information academic. Its superiority is unquestioned for two reasons: it is basically nontoxic and it has no narcotic properties; therefore, if a patient's depression is misdiagnosed (i.e., hypnotic rather than narcotic in origin), Narcan, unlike Lorfan and Nalline, will not act as a narcotic and increase the depression to a lethal degree.

Naloxone (Narcan) dosage is 0.4 mg repeated every two or three minutes. If three doses fail to initiate improvement, the depression is other than narcotic.

It is only effective for two hours and an overdosage of some narcotics may persist for six or more hours, so the patient must not be permitted to leave the office until tests (Gestalt and others) assure CNS depression is eradicated.

Naltrexone, just released, appears to be even better in that it is more potent and much longer lasting (up to 48 hours). It is also non-agonistic except for slight pupillary dysfunction.[58]

NONADDICTIVE

This classification or group encompasses the drugs most frequently used by both professional and lay people. Consumption of salicylates and their congeners is so vast that the quantity must be calculated in tons (6500 tons of aspirin per year alone) rather than grains or grams. This phenomenon is credible and easily explained for the following reasons — effectiveness, wide range of use or application, availability, general low cost, and low toxicity.

In addition to their analgesic properties, many drugs in this group are also antipyretic, anti-inflammatory, antirheumatic, and uricosuric in action.

Salicylates

These analgesic compounds are those preparations related to salicylic acid, and include acetylsalicylic acid, sodium salicylate, and salicylamide.

The mechanism for the therapeutic actions of the salicylates is not well understood and less well explained, except for the uricosuric effect. This particular action increases the excretion of uric acid by inhibition of its resorption by the tubules of the kidneys.

Although the salicylates are considered remarkably safe drugs, they can produce severe adverse effects and even death. They are especially toxic to children, being the chief cause of poisoning in youngsters under three and etiologic in 16 per cent of the cases through 15 years of age. All coal tar analgesics are toxic to the CNS, and in continuous large dosages produce "salicylism," a condition characterized by tinnitus, vertigo, severe headache, and mental confusion. Salicylism, undiagnosed or untreated, progresses to a serious salicylate intoxication, recognized by the symptoms of hyperpnea, gastrointestinal irritation and bleeding, disturbances in the acid-base balance, and petechial hemorrhage. It is thought that the hemorrhagic tendency may result from interference with the formation of prothrombin and also from interference with release of ADP, which provides the "glue" in the clumping of platelets in rouleaux formation. ASA has recently been indicted as a causative factor in permanent alteration of albumin's molecular structure, and in vitro acetylation of gamma globulin, some hormones, and DNA. If widespread, these effects could be disastrous to the body's elemental functions.

Finally, some individuals exhibit true allergies to the salicylates and show anaphylactic reactions, usually of the urticarial or asthmatic type, following even the smallest doses of these drugs. A recent unexpected and startling report revealed that nearly 20 per cent of severely ill asthmatic patients in a famed respiratory disease hospital had aspirin intolerance.[29] Patients' claims to aspirin allergy are not to be ignored or denigrated. Fatalities, although rare, have been reported.

Aniline Derivatives

Acetophenetidin (phenacetin) is more widely used and less toxic than acetanilid, but has been replaced in popularity by N-acetyl-p-aminophenol (acetaminophen), which promises certain advantages over both of these drugs, especially in pediatric use. More and more pharmaceutical houses are dropping phenacetin from their formulation and most pharmacists consider this a wise decision. There is a paucity of studies or literature in support of either additive or potentiating effect of APC compounds over pure ASA (acetylsalicylic acid, aspirin).

Although serious toxic reactions rarely occur, acetanilid and acetophenetidin have a proclivity or potential for producing hemolytic anemia, acidosis, and methemoglobinemia following prolonged usage. At present, acetominophen (Percogesic, Tylenol) appears to be innocent of these toxic effects, and is enjoying increased employment as an analgesic in adult and pediatric therapy. As another plus, it does not irritate gastric mucosa.

The aniline derivatives are effective analgesics and antipyretics, but lack uricosuric and antirheumatic actions, and have yet to demonstrate any superiority to the generally less toxic salicylates.

Excedrin

This is a lavishly promoted "extra strength" compound about which at present there is a dearth of available reliable evidence regarding potency or toxicity. The formula is interesting: 190 mg of ASA, 130 mg of salicylamide, 90 mg of acetaminophen, and 60 mg of caffeine. "Assuming that one equates acetaminophen as being roughly as potent as aspirin, two tablets of Excedrin would contain the equivalent of 560 mg of aspirin (less than the amount in two USP tablets)." Presumably then, the "extra strength" is accounted for by the 260 mg of salicylamide. This premise is questionable, however, because salicylamide, in such a subtherapeutic dose, probably has little, if any, therapeutic value! The "extra strength pain reliever" appears to be possibly as effective as but certainly not more effective than two USP aspirin tablets.[27] Available reports (admittedly scattered and inconclusive) give us little reason to believe that Excedrin produces increased analgesic effect without a corresponding increase in toxicity. Multiple-ingredient medicines should be suspect until proved innocent, because if these products cause toxic or allergic problems, who can name the culprit?

Lately there is an increasing tendency to question the necessity or desirability of adding anilines to salicylates to form analgesic compounds. Recent studies lend support of those clinicians who claim that aspirin alone is as efficacious as and less toxic than any non-narcotic compound of which it forms a part.

Many knowledgeable investigators insist that 10 grains of aspirin at one time is sufficient to gain the maximum analgesic effect obtainable with non-narcotic drugs, and that higher doses or additive compounds are relatively useless for most patients.

The presence of caffeine in most of the proprietary mixtures mentioned above is "justified" on the basis that the cerebral effects of caffeine may relieve the tensions which contribute to certain kinds of headaches. It also may elevate the mood in some individuals.

Indomethacin (Indocin)

Promoted primarily for the treatment of gouty arthritis, Indocin has anti-inflammatory, antipyretic, and analgesic properties. Prescribed also for patients with rheumatoid arthritis, osteoarthritis, and spondylitis, it has enjoyed moderate success.

Although Indocin has been advocated by some for temporomandibular joint problems, its toxic effects — severe headache, peptic ulcer, and hematologic disorders — should suggest that its advocates look for safer medication.

Pyrazolone Compounds

This group includes aminopyrine and phenylbutazone, which exhibit analgesic, antipyretic and antiarthralgic properties but possess no significant advantage over other less toxic analgesic drugs.

Aminopyrine (Pyramidon) has little value in the dental armamentarium, and its use has led to the development of agranulocytosis in a significant number of patients.

Phenylbutazone (Butazolidin) is a newer pyrazolone derivative which is extensively used in the treatment of arthritis and other joint diseases. Although effective, it is much too toxic for general therapy and should be confined to special cases which do not respond to other medication. Its toxic manifestations include skin rashes, gastrointestinal irritation and ulceration, generalized hypersensitivity, bone marrow depression, hemorrhagic tendency, and jaundice.

Butazolidin has uncommon application in dentistry, but the practitioner should be aware of its nature when prescribing for patients who are taking this drug.

Ibuprofen

Ibuprofen (Motrin) is a new non-steroidal *anti-inflammatory agent*. It is derived from phenylalkanoic acid, which so far has produced a family of drugs which, although not yet released (except for Ibuprofen), are considered to be a possibly important breakthrough in the therapy for collagen diseases.

It should be employed only in the treatment of rheumatoid and osteoarthritis victims who do not respond to ASA mainly because its analgesic and antipyretic properties are considered weak.

Fortunately, serious untoward effects so far are rare and although mainly confined to the GI tract, there is less GI bleeding than with ASA. Despite a difference in chemical formulae, there is a similar antigenic determinant; therefore it is not safe to prescribe it for those patients allergic to ASA (dosage 400 mg TID).

A comparative study at Georgetown University (Cooper, Needle and Kruger, J. Oral Surg. 35, Nov. 1977) presented the rather surprising conclusion that Ibuprofen not only is more potent than ASA but has greater efficacy without any notable increase in adverse effects. They suggest additional clinical studies to confirm these results.

Propoxyphene (Darvon)

This synthetic drug, a derivative of methadone, has enjoyed exceptional growth in popularity since introduction, but its potency as an analgesic is conjectural and has been warmly debated by members of the health professions. Ideally it is supposed to approximate codeine in analgesic effect without the depression and respiratory and gastrointestinal side effects.

Although its allergenic potential is low (occasional skin rash), the manufacturer lists these adverse effects: dizziness, headache, sedation, somnolence, paradoxical excitement and insomnia and gastrointestinal disturbance (nausea, vomiting, abdominal pain, and constipation). The clinical picture of overdose parallels that of the true narcotics, plus the added distress of convulsions. Propoxyphene can be abused. Cases of tolerance and addiction are increasingly reported. Addicts discovered that the Darvon part of the compound capsule was in the form of a small pure pill: by splitting several capsules, enough pure Darvon was available for a "high" by intravenous injection. Recent revision by the manufacturer distributes the propoxyphene evenly through the powder, thereby negating this problem. Narcan is indicated and effective in cases of overdose or poisoning.

Propoxyphene is evidently synergized by APC, which is an integral part of Darvon Compound 65. It is also marketed with aspirin and called Darvon ASA.

Because of the instability factor with the hydrochloride salt when formulated as a powder, Lilly has discovered the napsylate salt (propoxyphene napsylate), which is more stable. However, because it lacks the molecular weight, a 100 mg dose of the napsylate salt is required to supply the amount of propoxyphene equivalent (in activity or potency) to that present in 65 mg of the hydrochloride salt. Darvon N is the designation of the new formula with 50 mg of propoxyphene napsylate, while Darvon N ASA has 325 mg of aspirin added. Darvocet–N and Darvocet–N 100 are the same new form with acetaminophen (325 mg and 650 mg respectively) replacing the ASA or APC in the compound.

In March, 1977, propoxyphene was placed in Schedule IV of the Controlled Substances Act. Drugs in this schedule are defined as those that "may lead to limited physical or psychological dependence."

Since it is structurally related or an analog of methadone and has been abused with resultant psychic and physical dependence (low grade) and tolerance, the F.D.A. has changed its classification. This is no way demeans the drug. Most agents which affect the CNS in any way may fall into this category.

Ethoheptazine (Zactane; Zactirin)

Another synthetic related to meperidine, Zactirin occupies the same spectrum as Darvon in the analgesic group of drugs. It is also relatively free from gastrointestinal side effects and respiratory depression, but Zactirin's potency is yet to be satisfactorily determined and must be evaluated by the clinician. Toxicity is minimal, and significant allergenic tendencies have not been reported.

The standard preparation includes APC or ASA in its formula, a factor that should be considered when prescribing this agent. Zactirin is combined with meprobamate to form a compound labeled Equagesic, which has properties and actions common to both drugs. It should have some value in dental office practice.

Measurin, Contac, et al.

Increasing emphasis, desirability, and somewhat garish publicity have pushed time acting or sustained release drug forms to the forefront, especially in the analgesic and cold tablet class. This type of packaging usually encompasses a towering quantity of a drug to be released in measured doses at measured intervals. This controlled action is predetermined by fractioning into sized particles and/or enteric coatings.

Knowing the vagaries of the gastrointestinal tract and the quality control of some manufacturers, prudence should dictate the policy in every instance.

SPECULATORY

The richest plum in the drug orchard, sought by all and as yet unplucked, is a potent analgesic which lacks habituating and addicting powers and does not depress respiration or other vital CNS functions.

There are four recent arrivals on the scene and several more hovering in the wings, all of which showed promise in this direction but are now considered controversial. Because they are new, and also because two of them hint of great merit, they will be discussed in detail. These drugs are labeled speculatory because, although three qualify as potent analgesics without addiction dangers, each has peculiarities which limit usage to specific situations and not general therapy for the average patient.

Methotrimeprazine (Levoprome)

A phenothiazine compound, Levoprome is also a potent non-narcotic analgesic. About half as strong as morphine on a milligram basis, it appears to cause less respiratory depression and finds its greatest use in relieving pain in acute and chronic conditions for those patients confined to bed, in traction, or recovering from major surgery.

Precautions. Like other new drugs, it must be considered to have teratogenetic potential until proved otherwise and thus should be restricted in pregnant patients. Since it has strong sedative effects, operation of autos or complicated machinery following its use is forbidden.

Adverse Reactions. These are numerous and often serious: disorientation, blurred vision, nasal congestion, dry mouth, difficult micturition, and intense pain at the site of injection, plus the usual extrapyramidal syndromes associated with phenothiazines.

Contraindications. Severe orthostatic hypotension which may last for 12 to 16 hours after the initial dose, along with the necessity for deep and painful IM injection (there is no oral form, and subcutaneous instillation causes irritation), practically cancels its value in dentistry.

Levoprome's only feasible use might be for postoperative pain in a major oral surgical case in which the patient is confined to bed and/or allergic to other strong analgesics.

Dosage. The usual dose is 20 mg IM, repeated every four to six hours.

Carbamazepine (Tegretol)

Another phenothiazine type with potent and specific action on pain, Tegretol is an extremely dangerous drug that must not be prescribed as a routine analgesic. Thorough familiarization with the adverse effects and precautionary measures is vital and may be obtained from the Physicians' Drug Reference or current texts on pharmacology.

Although Tegretol has been used in Europe since approximately 1962, its first appearance in American pharmacies occurred in 1968.

A tricyclic compound originally ticketed as an anticonvulsant (as Ponstel was classed as an anti-inflammatory), Tegretol soon exhibited its ability to eradicate the crushing pain of tic douloureux. Since no drug had ever been able to approach, much less achieve, this goal and still enable the patient to ambulate and retain his senses, this compound was hailed far and wide as the "answer." Then came the deluge of reports on side effects and the sobering second thoughts which invariably follow in the wake of a new "miracle" drug.

A CBC and platelet estimate should precede initial therapy and be repeated once a week for the first month, every two weeks for the second and third months, and at monthly intervals as long as the drug is employed. Variants from the norm at any time dictate immediate discontinuance.

Tegretol is remarkably effective, and initial relief is evident in 24 to 48 hours. In approximately 68 per cent of patients with severe symptoms, pain is virtually abolished, although this may take 10 to 14 days. Therapy has been extended for more than two years in some victims before remission is obtained. However, attempts to reduce dosage to the necessary minimum should be a continuing goal, no matter how long therapy is planned or needed. It can be used in conjunction with Dilantin in severe cases.

Evidence suggests that its mode of action is the inhibition of synaptic transmission with the spinal trigeminal nucleus. It is very useful in controlling psychomotor epilepsy — grand mal also responds.

Precautions.   The benefit-risk ratio should be an ever-present guide or criterion in evaluation of the patient's welfare, especially in those with cardiac disease, hepatic pathosis or dysfunction, and borderline psychosis. Appropriate liver function tests are essential in long-term therapy.

Adverse Reactions.   The minor side effects are nausea, dizziness, and drowsiness, which are transient and readily disappear when therapy is suspended. But patients should be made aware of the early signs of hematologic toxicity, such as fever, sore throat, mouth ulcers, and petechial or purpuric hemorrhage in the mucosa or skin. These symptoms precede or warn of the onset of agranulocytosis, thrombocytopenia, and leukopenia. Continued aggravation of the bone marrow could precipitate aplastic anemia with fatal results. Tegretol must never be used concurrently with MAO inhibitors because it is chemically related to Tofranil (a tricyclic) and interacts in the same severe way.

The multiplicity of the side effects and their extensive ramifications require constant vigilance and perception on the part of the prescriber and awareness and discipline on the part of the user.

Dosage.   One hundred milligrams twice a day initially, increasing to 400 to 800 mg. in divided doses every 24 hours if necessary. As stated above, the dosage should be minimized or discontinued at the earliest feasible time, and close control is mandatory (visual and laboratory examinations) for the patient's welfare.

Mefenamic Acid (Ponstel)

I am not convinced that Ponstel belongs in this list, but because of its nature, a thorough airing is desirable. It is a fairly simple compound, but is unique in that it differs from all other agents used in the management of pain. According to the manufacturer, clinical trials have demonstrated that Ponstel is effective in relieving pain from bursitis, backache, sprains, toothache and dental surgery.

Ponstel was originally introduced as an anti-inflammatory agent. Now it is promoted as an analgesic. Distribution of this drug in the United Kingdom has provided most of the experience and data available. An estimated 25 million capsules have been prescribed there.

Precautions.   Ponstel should be administered with caution to patients with abnormal renal function or inflammatory disease of the gastrointestinal tract. If rash occurs, the drug should be promptly withdrawn. Acute exacerbations have been reported in asthmatics following administration of Ponstel. Caution and prudence are mandatory.

Adverse Reactions.   In controlled clinical studies of Ponstel at analgesic doses of up to 150 mg per day, associated side effects were relatively mild and infrequent. Complaints are dose related, being more frequent with higher doses.

In 3205 observations on 1985 subjects over periods of from one to 238 days, the most frequently reported side reactions were (in descending order) drowsiness, nausea, dizziness, nervousness, headache, and gastrointestinal tract discomfort. Upper gastrointestinal tract side effects can be appreciably reduced by taking medication during meals.[43]

As with the administration of any new drug, it is recommended that hematopoietic, renal, and hepatic function studies be done when extended usage is anticipated.

Contraindications.   Like other anti-inflammatory agents, Ponstel is not indicated for use in patients with intestinal ulcerations. However, in double-blind comparison with aspirin, Ponstel appears to be less liable to cause gastrointestinal bleeding. The prescribing of Ponstel to pregnant women and those of child-bearing potential is at present contraindicated. This drug should not be given to children under 14 years of age, because the pediatric dose is yet to be established.

Warning.   If diarrhea occurs, Ponstel should be *promptly* discontinued. The patient so affected is usually unable to tolerate the drug thereafter.

Dosage.   The recommended oral regimen for adults is 500 mg as an initial dose, followed by 250 mg every six hours as needed. Ponstel is indicated for short-term administration *not exceeding one week of therapy*. The margin of safety plummets with higher doses and longer administration.

At this writing Ponstel is still therapeutically controversial. Such an opinion should not be misconstrued as denigrating to this compound. It is certainly premature to make judgments before more data are available.

The original clinical studies of its efficacy were watered down by later FDA trials. These double-blind studies place the drug in the same spectrum as ASA or slightly better.

Consultation with colleagues and pharmacists has revealed a divergence of attitudes but no passionate commitments for either the positive or the negative position in evaluating Ponstel.

Those who report success (and some are enthusiastic) tend to initiate therapy immediately and prescribe the recommended dosage regularly at six-hour intervals through the time period when pain is normally expected. Others have not obtained the results so glowingly reported in the introductory pamphlet.

Pentazocine (Talwin)

Listed in the second edition as a speculatory drug, Talwin has certainly earned its place in the arena of pain control.

Medical people are, for the most part, grudging in their acceptance of a new drug, especially one that has been long sought or desperately needed.

This reluctance is partly engendered by past disappointment with similar panaceas and partly by the awareness of the responsibility shouldered by every doctor who treats patients with new, little-known, and potent medicines. This seemingly stodgy attitude usually works for the patient's benefit in the long run.

Despite the doubts of some and the reluctance of others, Talwin emerges as a highly impressive drug. It is the first really potent non-narcotic, non-phenothiazine analgesic that is relatively safe for ambulatory patients (does not produce severe postural hypotension) and for long-term therapy (drug tolerance does not develop). It has been used in some patients continuously for more than 300 days and discontinued abruptly without withdrawal or untoward symptoms of any kind.

Other advantages of Talwin may be listed as follows: (1) It has a wide range of use in mild, moderate, or severe pain from almost any source. (2) It is not tachyphylactic. (3) It is well tolerated systemically and locally. (4) It is rapid acting and long lasting in effect. (5) It has good shelf life and is free of narcotic controls.

Talwin's only unique and serious disadvantage stems from its secondary role as a weak narcotic antagonist. Because of this, Nalline and Lorfan are useless in combating overdosages and respiratory depression. If the latter occurs, it was treated with oxygen and Ritalin (methylphenidate), a central nervous system stimulant which is not nearly as effective as an antagonist. Narcan is effective and is the drug of choice.

Precautions. Although teratogenetic or embryotoxic effects have not been seen in extensive animal tests or reported in humans, Talwin, like all new drugs, should be given with caution to pregnant women until more data are available.

Since dizziness, sedation, and euphoria are not uncommon, regardless of dosage, ambulatory patients should be warned not to operate machinery, drive automobiles or unnecessarily expose themselves to hazards. This precaution is especially applicable to the unaccompanied dental patient who has probably driven himself to the dental office and intends to return to work after his appointment.

Conditions which result in reduced respiratory capacity from any cause will ordinarily preclude or minimize the use of Talwin. Asthma, pneumoconiosis, lung infections, obstructions, regular therapy with other depressant drugs, and cardiac disease are all capable of interfering with normal or adequate gaseous exchange in the lungs.

Because most drugs are detoxified and eliminated by the liver and kidneys in that order, Talwin should be used with care in patients who suffer from impaired hepatic or renal function.

Narcotic addicts or patients who are "on" morphine at the time should not be given Talwin by the clinician; otherwise withdrawal symptoms may result with their concomitant hazards.

There are a few other precautions which lie mainly in the province of the physician and need not be mentioned here.

Adverse Effects.   Nausea is the most frequent adverse effect and respiratory depression the most serious, although apnea is not a problem even with large doses.

According to The Medical Letter, "when given in equianalgesic doses, pentazocine produces as much sedation, grogginess, dizziness, nausea, vomiting, sweating and other minor subjective complaints as do morphine and other narcotics."

Contraindications.   Like other potent analgesics, Talwin should not be used on patients with head injuries, increased intracranial pressure, or brain pathology until a clearance has been given by the neurosurgeon. It can cloud the central nervous system symptoms and make diagnosis difficult or misleading.

Dosage.   The average parenteral dose is 30 mg, either IV or IM or subcutaneously, and may be repeated every three to four hours. Some patients require up to 60 mg (single dose) for relief, but in this range psychotomimetic reactions are possible and have occurred. The usual oral dose is 50 mg. Talwin is not recommended for children under 12 years of age because of insufficient data on this group.

HYPNOTIC DRUGS

Hypnotics encompass a large field of different drugs which can produce a state of depression of the CNS resembling natural sleep. In smaller divided doses, these same drugs, for the most part, induce a state of drowsiness, and in this capacity they are classified as sedatives. The practical difference between a hypnotic drug and an anesthetic drug is in degree of CNS depression, i.e., dosage. A therapeutic dose of a hypnotic produces sleep from which the patient can be roused, whereas an increased dose of the same agent results in an anesthetic state from which the patient cannot be roused until the drug has been metabolized. The anesthetic dose, with the possible exception of the ultra-short barbiturates, is dangerously close to the toxic and/or lethal dose. Some hypnotics are also listed as tranquilizers more out of deference to common acceptance than accuracy.

Over the past decade the concepts of the use of hypnotics and sedative tranquilizers have changed greatly owing to the intense interest in this field which has generated much useful information.

The indications, selection, and alternative regimens and contraindications are manifest, and primary nervous disorders and sleep disorders such as sleep apnea, nocturnal myoclonus, and circadian rhythm changes call for specific, not empiric, management.

The etiology needs to be determined (for example, depression, anxiety, alcoholism, tension tolerance) and a clear-cut diagnosis or plan developed before any patient is introduced to these drugs, *most* of which create dependency, interact with other drugs, are potent and expensive, and have numerous, often toxic, side effects.

Dr. Robert DuPont, director of N.I.D.A., conservatively estimates that sleeping pills are responsible for at least 5000 deaths and more than 25,000 trips to hospital emergency rooms each year.

The barbiturates, along with Doriden, Noludar, Placidyl, and Quaalude, are the chief offenders and should not be prescribed for the average dental patient. It is much wiser to prescribe one of the benzodiazepines, which are more effective, safer, and ordinarily do not cause the "hangover" feeling common with the other drugs.

Barbiturates

Eminently the most popular and, according to most investigators, the safest hypnotics are the barbiturates, a series of closely related compounds formed by combining urea and malonic acid. This happy marriage yields barbituric acid, which is modified by appropriate substitutions in position 5 of the molecule to produce the familiar drugs of this large group.

The barbiturates differ mainly in varying duration of action or rate of metabolism, thereby establishing their classification as ultra-short, short, intermediate, and long acting (Table 5-2).

Although toxic addiction (from large and protracted dosage) does occur, urticaria or allergic responses and neurologic changes are rare in normal therapy.

Acute toxicity from overdose of barbiturates is manifested primarily as depression of respiration to decreasing levels until cessation ensues. In some agitated, feverish, or elderly patients, barbiturates can evoke an ambiguous or contrary response and stimulate or excite these individuals to a state of delirium (hyperexcitability).

Probably the greatest hazard in the general use of barbiturates is their propensity for synergism with a multitude of other common drugs. Alcohol, reserpine, and antihistamines all intensify the action of barbiturates. When ingested together, sudden, unexpected, and severe depression may result.

Porphyria, a rare disorder involving excessive respiratory pigment, hematoporphyria, must always be considered in any discussion of toxicity. Ingestion of any barbiturate by a patient afflicted with this disorder will ordinarily yield drastic and/or fatal results.

Antidotal measures in the treatment of barbiturate poisoning no longer include convulsant drugs. Mild stimulants, good oxygenation, and maintenance of fluid and electrolyte balance are the accepted remedies for barbiturate intoxication. Analeptic drugs may only intensify the toxic effect or exchange one set of symptoms for another equally dangerous syndrome.

Physostigmine is usually effective and is the drug of choice for barbiturate antagonism.

Chloral Hydrate

Chloral hydrate is a desirable hypnotic, especially for elderly patients, and children, because it gives quick, relatively short sedation without the sequelae that often follow barbiturate ingestion. It is a central depressant, inducing calm, then sleep, without marked respiratory and cardiovascular depression.

Although a gastric irritant forbidden for use in patients with peptic and duodenal ulcers, its toxicity is relatively low in all other respects.

Chloral hydrate, its reputation somewhat tarnished (or enhanced, as the case may be) owing to its storied use by bartenders as a "Mickey Finn," is

TABLE 5–2 CLASSIFICATION, STRUCTURE, AND DOSAGE OF COMMONLY USED BARBITURATES

Duration of Action	Names	Substituents in Position 5	Hypnotic Doses
Ultra-short (IV Anesthetics)	Thiopental° (Pentothal)	Ethyl 1-Methylbutyl	
	Thiamylal° (Surital)	Allyl 1-Methylbutyl	
	Methohexital† (Brevital)		
	Hexobarbital‡ (Evipal)	Methyl, Cyclohexenyl	
Short	Secobarbital (Seconal)	Allyl 1-Methylbutyl	
			0.1–0.2 gm
Intermediate	Pentobarbital (Nembutal)	Ethyl 1-Methylbutyl	0.1 gm
	Butabarbital (Butisol)	Ethyl Sec-butyl	
			0.1–0.2 gm
	Amobarbital (Amytal)	Ethyl Iscamyl	0.05–0.2 gm
Long	Phenobarbital (Luminal)	Ethyl, Phenyl	0.1–0.2 gm
	Barbital (Veronal)	Ethyl, Ethyl	0.3–0.5 gm

°Thiobarbiturate.
†Oxybarbiturate.
‡A CH₃ group attached to the nitrogen.

nevertheless a valuable adjunct in the premedication of those persons who are overly sensitive or allergic to the barbiturates. Dosage is 75 mg per kg on a curve to a maximum of 1500 mg at 50 kg.

Paraldehyde

An excellent sedative, paraldehyde produces moderately prolonged sleep (eight to 12 hours) with little or no medullary or motor depression. It is a powerful CNS depressant, resembling alcohol in effect; but, despite this potency, it has a wide margin of safety when properly prescribed. This attribute (low toxicity) in combination with paraldehyde's powerful effect would enhance its value tremendously except for one thing — a strong, offensive odor which is disagreeable to the vast majority of patients.

Bromides

These compounds (NaBr and KBr), while formerly popular as sedatives and hypnotics, are now rarely prescribed by professionals. However, bromides deserve mention and consideration because they frequently appear as the principal ingredients in proprietary, over-the-counter, nonprescription sleeping pills. Cumulative in the body, these drugs are often highly toxic, causing a condition known as "bromism." This syndrome is characterized by signs of chronic motor and sensory depression and mental aberrations. Dermatitis is another common toxic symptom.

It is difficult to defend the use of such potentially dangerous drugs when superior agents are readily available.

Ethanol

Appropriately or not, many texts list this drug as a hypnotic. Each researcher should be exhorted to experiment with ethanol in the potion which suits him best and then form his own conclusions. Its toxic manifestations should be common knowledge and need no explanation. Intravenous ethanol can and has been used as a supplemental anesthetic for alcoholic patients. Despite its soothing powers on many citizens, alcohol can be a nightmare for others.

It is a sedative and a hypnotic, and in high doses (P.O. or I.V.) it can be an anesthetic.

Ethanol has additive effects on all CNS depressants and potentiates (more than doubles the action of) the barbiturates (especially Nembutal, Seconal, Butisol, Doriden, and Quaalude!) These are known to be deadly when taken with alcohol—there may be others, not yet defined, with similar action.

In addition, it induces the sulfonylureas (Diabinese, Orinase, Tolbutamide) by speeding up their metabolism approximately 50 per cent; increases the absorption of diazepam; and should not be used in conjunction with the phenothiazines, which inhibit alcohol dehydrogenase (the enzyme responsible for the reduction of C_2H_5OH into acetaldehyde and other metabolites), thereby prolonging and intensifying its negative or depressant action. Alcohol is a direct myocardial toxin, and cardiomyopathy is a clinical entity which affects approximately 1 per cent of the adult population in the U.S.A.

Higher Alcohols

This group is represented by three widely publicized, but otherwise undistinguished, drugs: methylparafynol (Dormison), ethylchlorvynol (Placidyl), and phenaglycodol (Ultran).

Generally speaking, they are weakly sedative in action, producing drowsiness in therapeutic doses.

Toxicity is negligible, but some cases of hepatic damage from Dormison have been reported.

Piperidinediones

This group of supposedly mild hypnotics is similar in effect to the short-acting barbiturates, but the mechanism of their action is less well understood and the toxic potential may in some cases be extreme.

Glutethimide (Doriden) frequently causes skin rash and fever, and psychosis and addiction have been reported after prolonged use. It is one of the most lethal drugs in the formulary because abusers do not respond to any known antagonistic, analeptic, or antidotal measures (physostigmine et al.)

Methyprylon (Nodular) may precipitate headache, nausea, and vertigo. Addiction is possible after long-term therapy.

Thalidomide (Kevadon), although never marketed in the United States, deserves mention if for no other reason than its reputation. Most of the professional and lay population are familiar with its toxic manifestations. Phocomelia and other bizarre birth defects are dreadful proof of the dangerous potential of this drug.

TRANQUILIZERS

Tranquilizing drugs are assuming ever greater importance in the practice of the healing arts. These agents can suppress anxiety and modify disturbed behavior in doses which are not profoundly hypnotic. Such characteristics would seem to be eminently desirable in the armamentarium of an office practice. But the sprawling range of potency, multiple actions, overlapping vague responses, plural potentiation, exotic and often severe ancillary effects, and the complex pharmacologic interrelationships among this class of drugs demand a prudent and restrictive approach to dental or medical use. This group may be said to have conceived and nourished that new and blooming specialty iatrogenics.

Tranquilizers act with multiple sites in the CNS, producing sedation, antipruritic activity, antiemetic activity, antihistamine activity, antiserotonin activity, alpha-adrenergic activity, adrenergic potentiation, and analgesia. They can control spasms and convulsions. There are almost 200 drugs which claim to qualify, and the combinations are myriad and bewildering.

It is assumed that any classification will be controversial and even provocative to some, but should be conciliatory, flexible, not too specific, and biphasic for all.

The two phases consist of an arbitrary major-moderate-minor division to denote strength and potency: a chemical or pharmacal grouping to enumerate related drugs whose actions are basically similar. This method is more resilient than perfect, but it offers a catalog as a guide from which drugs for specific needs may be selected. The rauwolfa alkaloids, butyrophenones, and phenothiazines as a class, regardless of individual differences, are proclaimed major tranquilizers. The benzodiazepines fall essentially into the moderate slot with the diphenylmethanes. The large, varied minor group encompasses carbamides, ureides, and higher alcohols.

MAJOR TRANQUILIZERS

Rauwolfias

The Rauwolfia alkaloids are reserpine (Serpasil), deserpidine (Harmonyl), rescinnamine (Moderil), syrosingopine (Singoserp), serpentina (Raudixin), and alseroxylon (Rauwiloid). Although relatively low in direct toxicity, they must be considered major tranquilizers, not only because of potency but also because of their indirect, delayed and long-lasting mode of action. Their pharmacology is complex and needs to be elucidated. They act as antihypertensives indirectly by depleting norepinephrine, epinephrine, and dopamine in vascular storage sites and as tranquilizers by releasing various amines from the brain and some peripheral tissues to depress the CNS. The threat of synergism is always present when hypnotics and other depressants are prescribed for patients "on" the rauwolfias. There are also numerous annoying autonomic side effects: miosis, bradycardia, and increased gastrointestinal activity (which creates an incompatibility with ulcer victims). Nasal stuffiness from mucosal edema rates high on the nuisance list and promotes overuse of decongestant sprays. The most pertinent hazard is the occasional development of severe, sometimes unyielding hypotension during a general anesthetic or IV sedation period.

Butyrophenones

The butyrophenones, relatively new but surging in popularity under the pseudonym "neuroleptic," are clamoring for attention and getting it. What initially seemed a breakthrough is, after close inspection, hardly more than a widening of the present horizon.

Haloperidol (Haldol) and droperidol (Inapsine), although matching the potency and increasing the versatility of the other major tranquilizers, also share their drawbacks.

Toxicity is relatively equal or synonymous with the phenothiazines in scope and intensity, differing only in frequency. Extrapyramidal syndromes are most common, with hematopoietic and cardiovascular problems next in order.

Allergic skin reactions, photosensitivity, and jaundice are minor and seldom reported. These agents, in conjunction with a potent analgesic, form the basis of the neuroleptanalgesia technique discussed further along in this chapter.

Phenothiazines

Although phenothiazine derivatives exhibit antihistaminic, antipruritic, and analgesic properties, their value in dental practice is primarily as tranquilizing agents and secondarily as antiemetics.

The tranquilizing action of the majority of the phenothiazines is similar, varying somewhat in depth and length of action. Chlorpromazine enjoys the widest latitude of use and is fairly representative of the remainder of the group.

Any classification of phenothiazines must, by the nature and complexity of the groups, be weak and arbitrary, blurred and imprecise.

There are roughly 30 separate derivatives of phenothiazine available — their only real differences being structural and quantitative, not qualitative. No more than five pheno-compounds are needed to completely cover the pharmacologic spectrum of this series.

The other derivatives, each with its share of confirmed disciples, present slight deviations in structure and action but some important differences in clinical application. But because of the escalating number of these derivatives and the extensive claims made for each, Table 5–3, attempting to differentiate and classify similar drugs in this category, is presented.

Originally conceived by Dr. Martin Gold in 1966, this table has been modified with additions and deletions by the author to fit current concepts.[24]

TABLE 5–3 PHENOTHIAZINE TRANQUILIZERS

I. PIPERAZINES

Prochlorperazine (Compazine)	Fluphenazine (Permitil, Prolixin)
Thiethylperazine (Torecan)	Acetophenazine (Tindal)
Trifluoperazine (Stelazine)	Carphenazine (Proketazine)
Thiopropazate (Dartal)	Butaperazine (Repoise)
Perphenazine (Trilafon)	Thioperazine (Vontil)

TOXICITIES:
Frequent: Parkinson's syndrome; akathisia; dystonic reactions; anticholinergic effects
Occasional: photosensitivity reaction; inhibition of ejaculation
Rare: cholestatic jaundice; blood dyscrasia; lenticular pigmentation; postural hypotension; allergic skin reactions; ECG abnormalities (usually without cardiac injury)

II. PROMAZINES

Promazine (Sparine)
Chlorpromazine (Thorazine)
Triflupromazine (Vesprin)
Methoxypromazine (Tentone)

TOXICITIES:
Frequent: oversedation; anticholinergic effects; postural hypotension
Occasional: pigmentary retinopathy; Parkinson's syndrome; akathisia; dystonic reactions; inhibition of ejaculation; photosensitivity reaction
Rare: cholestatic jaundice; blood dyscrasia

III. PIPERIDINES (ALIPHATIC)

Pipamazine (Mornidine)	Piperacetazine (Quide)
Propiomazine (Largon)	Thioridazine (Mellaril)
Mepazine (Palatal)	

TOXICITIES:
Frequent: oversedation; postural hypotension; anticholinergic effects
Occasional: cholestatic jaundice; Parkinson's syndrome; akathisia; dystonic reactions; inhibition of ejaculation; blood dyscrasia; photosensitivity reaction; allergic skin reactions
rare: lenticular pigmentation; ECG abnormalities (usually without cardiac injury)

IV. PHENOTHIAZINE (ANTIHISTAMINE)

Phenothiazine	Promethazine (Phenergan)
Diethazine (Diparcol)	Trimeprazine (Temaril)
Profenamine (Parsidol)	Methdilazine (Tecaryl)
Pyrathiazine (Pyrrolazote)	

It shows that potency (with toxicity usually paralleling) is determined by the type of side-chain addition. These additives categorize the analogs in synonymous groups and provide a method of relating and predicting their deviation from the parent drug, chlorpromazine.

These analogs are grouped and presented in Table 5–3 in a descending order of strength and effectiveness as tranquilizers, other actions being relative. Prominent specific toxicities as reported by The Medical Letter will be listed with each group. Unusual properties of individual members will be cited in succeeding paragraphs.

Although completely capable of tranquilizing, antiemetic and other actions, the fourth group in the table projects stronger antihistamine and antipruritic powers than most members of the family. Other things being relative or equal, such attributes should be known and should influence one's selection of a drug for a specific condition or illness.

Probably the least dangerous, but certainly the most dramatic, of all side effects of toxicities of the major tranquilizers (rauwolfias excepted) are the extrapyramidal syndromes—akathisia and dystonia. Bizarre is the only word to describe them.

Akathisia, characterized by inability to keep still, an irresistible urge to be in motion, and fright, is a prominent extrapyramidal tract symptom which appears frequently. The dystonic syndrome, involving tics, hypertonicity, or spasm of the muscles of the face, tongue, and neck with correspondingly bizarre facial expressions, and oculogyric syndrome (a contraction of the superior rectus muscles of the eye temporarily blinding the patient—only the white portion is visible to the observer) can and does occur in up to 10 per cent of patients on extended phenothiazine therapy. These rhythmical, intermittent muscle twitchings may be accompanied by anxiety and sweating. These toxic states — akathesia and dystonia — although not overly dangerous and ordinarily well controlled by anti-parkinsonian drugs, are disagreeable and very often frightening to the patient and his relatives and friends. However, tardive dyskinesia, which features vermiculation of the tongue muscles along with other symptoms heretofore described, is a lingering syndrome which some clinicians have declared a permanent disability.

MODERATE TRANQUILIZERS

Many categorizations are assailable — this one is no exception. Imitating the colors in a Madras print, the tranquilizers overlay and intermingle their intensities and toxicities to the extent that any designation is arbitrary and malleable. Mostly for the sake of clarity and comparison are the diazepines labeled moderate in action.

Since the publication of the second edition, the benzodiazepines have proliferated in numbers and swamped the sedative, anxiolytic, or neuroleptic muscle relaxant class in quantity by a vast margin. Diazepam (Valium) is the number one prescription item in our nation at this writing, and justly so when employed judiciously!

Chlordiazepoxide (Librium) exhibits both sedative and hypnotic effects on the CNS and has a selective action on the thalamus and hypothalamus which is thought to be the mechanism explaining its ability to suppress our anxious and aggressive tendencies. Librium in addition reduces cholinergic and adrenergic activity in the peripheral nervous system, thereby tending to lower blood pressure and tension. Diazepam (Valium) differs in that it has less effect on the CNS; nor is it a peripheral suppressor. Valium's primary targets seem to be the thalamus and hypothalamus, which should enhance its anti-anxiety effect while diminishing comcomitant CNS depression. Oxazepam (Serax) simulates diazepam in all its attributes, but seemingly has less anti-convulsant power.

Librium and Valium have demonstrated excellent anticonvulsant properties. In tests each exhibited strength enough to block strychnine-induced convulsions in animals, a feat not duplicated by chlorpromazine or reserpine, both reputed to be heavyweights in this field. Diazepines are premier agents for mild or moderate anxiety states, either parenterally or by mouth. They are occasionally used to reduce blood pressure in mild hypertension and show promise as a part of the multi-pronged efforts in rehabilitation of alcholics and addicts.

Flurazepam (Dalmane) is mainly proposed or prescribed for its hypnotic effects and is increasingly replacing other hypnotics because the results are as good with apparently less hazard of severe toxic effects. Although dependency and habituation are feasible (more psychological than physiological), considering the range and potency of the diazepines, their toxicity level is comfortably low.

The rapidity of onset and duration of action in this class of drugs is, of course, determined by metabolic degradation and the potency of the metabolites produced therein.

Rapid onset in approximate scale or order:
Diazepam (Valium) 2.5 — 10 mg T.I.D.
Oxazepam (Serax) 10 to 30 mg T.I.D.
Chlorazepate (Tranzene) 7.5 to 15 mg T.I.D.
Clonazepam (Clonopin) 0.5 to 6 mg T.I.D.
Chlordiazepoxide (Librium) 5 to 25 mg T.I.D.
Triazolam (Halcion); not used in U.S.

Slower onset:
Flurazepam (Dalmane) 15 to 30 mg H.S.
Prazepam (Vestran)

These are known to be slower in onset of clinical effects and therefore usually longer acting. These data should be considered arbitrary and based on rather sketchy observations, but this assumption has virtually confined their employment as hypnotics only. Newer analogs—medrazepam (Nobrium), nitrazepam (Mogadon) and fluctrazepam—either are in the testing stage or are unavailable in the U.S. at this writing.

. Lorazepam (Ativan) is very similar to oxazepam, but its narrow dosage range, 3 to 4 mg (5 mg or more incites a high incidence of side effects), has so far limited its use to premedication for general or neuroleptic anesthesia. In this area it produces significant antegrade amnesia (lack of recall) and a higher degree of somnolence than Valium, Serax, or Librium. This would seem to nullify its value in outpatient therapy.

Review of the literatures continues to confirm safety of Valium et al. One attempted suicide recovered completely after a 1500 mg oral dose.[54]

Even though a cardiac or cardiorespiratory arrest was attributed to diazepam in a recent Journal of Orthopedic Surgery article (Aug. 1977), subsequent investigation and interpretation of the event has cast doubt on its authenticity; four other drugs were involved, which is certainly a mitigating factor in the case described.

In several studies Valium was found to produce significant amnesia only with dosage of 10 mg or more while sedation and anxiety relief were present at as little as 2.5 mg dosage.

Morphine, Demerol, and other drugs that are known to delay gastric emptying, and atropine (with its anticholinergic effect on gastric motility), decrease uptake of oral diazepam and becloud its efficacy.

Although the manufacturer advises against water, normal saline, or 5 per cent dextrose as diluents, this advice is based on the remote possibility of a thrombus formation from a precipitate formed with these mixtures. This precipitate is fine enough to pass through ordinary filter paper, and it requires a severe stretch of the imagination to believe that this precipitate poses a danger to the patient. The author has personal knowledge of routine injection into a port of a high flow IV infusion with normal saline and 5 per cent D/W without complications of any kind! However, to be medicolegally secure, it is wiser to use a 5 to 10 cc syringe and aspirate blood as a dilutent for the 1,2, or 3 cc (5 mg per cc) dosage range you may select.

The pH of Valium (6.8) and the propyleneglycol vehicle will occasionally cause burning pain and subsequent, usually transitory, thickening at or proximal to the injection site (especially true in small veins), undesirable side effects of IV administration even when mixed with blood. While not morbid, this factor may elicit patient complaints postoperatively.

Libman and others have stated that Valium combined with local anesthesia is the safest and most effective neuroleptic for outpatient dental practice.[32]

In conclusion, most Medical Letter consultants believe that Librium, now available in the generic (chlordiazepoxide) form, may compare in efficacy with any other of the listed benzodiazepines. This is an important factor to a cost-conscious public when savings of 50 per cent or more are involved without sacrificing therapeutic value.

The contraindications for benzodiazepine therapy are:
Known allergies
Pregnancy
Acute narrow angle glaucoma
Untreated wide angle glaucoma
Certain depressed or suicidal syndromes or psychotic psychoses
Infants
Shock
Cautionary indications include:
Kidney disease
Acute or severe cardiovascular disease and severe respiratory disease
Gross obesity (improves appetite)
C.N.S. depressants and stimulants, including alcohol

Diphenylmethanes (Tranquilizers)

Lauded by many, dismissed as relatively weak and ineffective by others, the diphenylmethane derivatives are placed in the moderate category more for their breadth of action and potential than for their exhibited strength.

These drugs are structurally similar, but frequently pharmacologically different. They are related to various anticholinergics, antihistamines, antiemetics, narcotics, and even muscle relaxants, which have the diphenylmethane structure. Most are somewhat weak CNS depressants with multiple side effects more similar in nature to the major than to the minor tranquilizers.

Because of its immense popularity with dental and medical doctors, hydroxyzine (Atarax, Vistaril) will be exemplified as representative of its group.

Rapid-acting and mild, hydroxyzine exhibits sedative and tranquilizing powers along with antihistaminic properties. It has been suggested that hydroxyzine may arrest ventricular arrhythmias. One of its more popular applications in dentistry was in the field of psychosedation. Alone or in polypharmacal combinations (Demerol, scopolamine, etc.) for IV injection, it was the leading agent until 1970, when reports of vascular irritation and pathosis led to recommendation for discontinuing IV usages. Nevertheless, this is a veteran drug of proved usefulness and remarkably low direct toxicity with a possible exception in pregnancy, in which it has been shown that hydroxyzine has definite teratogenetic effects on some animal fetuses. Enough data to establish safety for human use are not yet available.

Because the differences among the diphenylmethane tranquilizers are insignificant, the others are listed below, without comment.

Benactyzine (Suavitil)
Pipethanate (Sycotrol)
Captodiamine (Suvren)
Pipradrol (Meratran)
Azacyclonol (Frenquel)
Buclizine (Softran)

MINOR TRANQUILIZERS

Carbamides, Ureides, and Higher Alcohols

Although the major tranquilizers affect not only behavior but also the autonomic nervous system, the minor agents, carbamides, ureides, and higher alcohols, are sedative in nature, anticonvulsant, and reduce skeletal muscle tone without significant autonomic effects.

Within this subgroup these agents differ from the phenothiazines, the diphenylmethanes, and rauwolfia in significant ways: (1) there are a variety of chemical structures involved; (2) they are not ganglionic blocking, adrenolytic, antihistaminic, antiserotonin, or antiemetic and they do not exhibit analgesia; (3) they are relatively nontoxic and resemble their close relations, the barbiturates; and (4) generally, they are not considered antihypertensive in clinical dosage.

These drugs exhibit three fundamental pharmacologic properties: (1) CNS depression, (2) muscle relaxation, and (3) anticonvulsant action.

The muscle relaxant group resembles the tranquilizers in most respects and exhibits the same basic pharmacologic properties, with heavy emphasis on muscle relaxant activity. Many of the muscle relaxants have been withdrawn from the market because of toxicity.

Meprobamate exhibits all the main characteristics of its group with approximately equal force and will serve as the prototype.

Miltown and Equanil are interneuronal blockers: central muscle relaxants with attendant sedative, tranquilizing (taming effect), and anticonvulsant properites. These eminently desirable requisites, combined with low toxicity and lack of depression, have made meprobamate an extremely popular and useful product.

Despite the glowing reputation and apparent safety, habituation and addiction (invariably involving patients taking massive doses over an extended period) are not unknown among the members of this supposedly minor, rather innocuous chemical group. However, neither affliction is particularly difficult to break, and withdrawal symptoms are mild and without sequelae when the patient is gradually weaned from the drug. Nonetheless, sudden withdrawal after addiction may result in toxic symptoms of a severe nature — tics, convulsions, and other irritative exacerbations of the CNS.

The Mephenesin and Substituted Propanediol Derivatives

I. *Tranquilizers (primarily):*

Meprobamate (Miltown, Equanil)
Mebutamate (Capla)
Emylcamate (Striatran)
Hydroxyphenamate (Listica)
Promoxolane (Dimethylane)

Oxanamide (Quiactin)
Phenaglycodol (Ultran)
Mephenoxalone (Trepidone)
Amphenidone (Dornwal)

II. *Muscle relaxants (primarily):*

Mephenesin
Meprobamate (Miltown, Equanil)
Carisoprodol (Soma, Rela)
Chlorzoxazone (Paraflex)
Methocarbamol (Robaxin)

Styramate (Sinaxar)
Phenyramidol (Analexin)
Chlormezanone (Trancopal)
Metaxalone (Skelaxin)
Zoxazolamine (Flexin) (discontinued)

III. *Nonbarbiturate CNS depressants (sedatives):*

Methaqualone (Quaalude)
Ethinamate (Valmid)
Ethchlorvynol (Placidyl)
Methylparafynol (Dormison)
Methyprylon (Nodular)

Glutethimide (Doriden)
Carbromal (Adalin)
Ectylurea (Nostyn)
Thalidomide (Kevadon) (discontinued)

Methaqualone has become a leading drug in the abuse category.

Tranquilizers Which Are Stimulants

Since most of us are members of the anxiety cult with its overt fears, we tend to forget the depressed citizens with their covert fears. A tranquil state can be approached from opposite directions — a depressor, to calm an agitated patient, or a stimulant, to elevate the mood of a morose one.

The MAOI's are prime examples — stimulants of the CNS to resolve psychotic depressant states. Reams of papers and articles have established both the need for and the efficacy of the MAOI's.

The amine oxidase inhibitors:

Phenelzine (Nardil)
Isocarboxazid (Marplan)
Pargyline (Eutonyl)
Etryptamine (Monase)

Nialamide (Niamid)
Tranylcypromine (Parnate) (discontinued)
Ipronizaine (Marsilid) (discontinued)
Pheniprazine (Catron) (discontinued)

Introduced innocuously as antidepressants, the MAO inhibitors have surfaced as controversial. A rather heterogenous group of drugs, they share one common trait: the ability to block oxidative deamination of naturally occurring amines. MAO's have prolonged and cumulative effects — two to three weeks after discontinuance.

Now the caution light is blinking and in two cases the red light is on. The width and intensity of toxic manifestations and potentiation associated with coemployment of the inhibitors with other common drugs (and foods) are stunning. Aged cheese, beer, wine, and certain heavy breads which harbor excessive amounts of tyramine are forbidden. Severe hypertension, convulsions, narcosis, and death are all lurking just around the corner for the unwary therapist or the unwarned patient.

Because of the increased activity and exploration of depression states, and the pressing need for less dangerous control agents, the dibenzazepines soon surfaced and became a factor.

Dibenzazepine derivatives (tricyclic).
Imipramine (Tofranil)   Trimipramine (Surmontil)
Amitryptyline (Elavil)   Protriptyline (Vivactil)
Desipramine (Pertofrane)   Doxepin (Sinequan)
Nortriptyline (Aventyl)

Effective, somewhat milder, easier to control, and lacking the extreme potentiating power of oxidase inhibitors, these agents resemble the phenothinazines in depth and range of toxicity. Anticholinergic effects and hypotension (antagonizes guanethidine) are frequent; parkinsonian activity with extrapyramidal features, mild seizures, cholestatic jaundice, and agranulocytopenia have been seen, along with drowsiness and allergic rash. Other negative aspects include a long latent period (often two to four weeks) and necessity for close, even daily, observation of the patient.

Before leaving the hypno-tranquilizers, several other agents with CNS and peripheral depressant and stimulatory action deserve mention:

CNS Depressants

Trimethobenzamide (Tigan) is widely known for its antiemetic properties. It has a unique chemical structure, is not a true phenothiazine, and should not be substituted in place of one. Most agents to control nausea are ineffective or at least controversial. Tigan seems to be as good as the best and less toxic than most.

Phencyclidine (Sernylan), like ketamine, is a dissociative anesthetic type drug producing a pseudocataleptic state with high analgesia and as such is employed in veterinary medicine. Although analogs may prove useful in the future, P.C.P., at present, is too toxic for human use. However, as one would expect, the cultists discovered it had hallucinogenic powers and now it is a leading drug of abuse, known in street parlance as "Angel Dust," "crystals," etc. The terrifying aspect is that it is simple and inexpensive to manufacture, thereby extremely difficult to control and it may be ingested, snorted, smoked, or injected with results of equal intensity. Symptoms are blank stare, bizarre behavior, confusion, ataxia, stupor or even combative, spasmodic episodes and unusual physical strength.

It is always dangerous to the physiology and often lethal in larger doses.[20]

Thioxanthenes

Chlorprothixene (Taractan) and thiothixene (Navane) are thioxanthenes whose conglomerate properties are so similar to the phenothiazines that it would seem needless to use them as substitutes until more knowledge is available.

CNS Stimulants

Data regarding bemegride, ethamivan, doxapram, and methylphenidate appear under the section on stimulants.

HISTAMINES AND ANTIHISTAMINES

A pyramiding group of drugs which block the effects of histamine at various receptor sites are referred to as antihistamines. They are useful not only in allergic diseases, but also for prophylaxis in motion sickness and as light sedatives, tranquilizers, and antiemetics. Their wide range of action and low toxicity have catapulted these agents into a prominent place in the dental armamentarium.

Antihistamines prevent or minimize the physiological effects of histamine. Theoretically there are three ways in which a drug might do this. First, by physiological antagonism of histamine (Adrenalin is an example of a drug many of whose actions are directly the opposite of those of histamine). Second, the drug might destroy histamine. Substances which do this are formaldehyde, nitrates, and an enzyme, diamine oxidase, known as histaminase. With the exception of histaminase, none of these other substances has therapeutic value as an antihistamine. Third, drugs may compete with histamine at its sites of action in the body, a phenomenon known as "competitive antagonism." The latter is the way all the currently prescribed antihistamines are believed to act. It is thought that these drugs, because their chemical structure resembles that of histamine, are accepted by the histamine receptors in the effector cells, thereby blocking out histamine. The evidence that histamine is implicated in the pathogenesis of many of the allergic diseases is inferred rather than proved, and it is therefore not altogether surprising that therapy with antihistamine drugs is not uniformly successful. The best results are obtained in acute urticaria and seasonal hay fever. In both these conditions the great majority of sufferers obtain a high degree of relief from the proper use of antihistamine drugs. In perennial vasomotor rhinitis, chronic urticaria, angioneurotic edema, and allergic skin reactions due to various allergens, including drugs, the results of treatment with antihistamines are of symptomatic value only; they do not shorten the course of the disease. In acute anaphylactic type reactions the drug of choice is Adrenalin. Antihistamines are of secondary value. In the field of allergic diseases the most disappointing result has been the failure of antihistamine drugs to benefit the vast majority of patients with bronchial asthma. The allergic basis of asthmatic attacks is undoubted; antihistamines are, however, seldom of value for either the prevention or the treatment of the acute asthmatic attack.

Often the choice of an antihistamine drug involves the consideration of the multitude of other effects it may have upon the patient besides that effect which is desired. Clearly it is undesirable to use an antihistamine which causes sleepiness for the treatment of hay fever in those citizens who must drive or perform precision tasks while taking the drug. On the other hand, sedation is a valuable attribute in a drug for the treatment of an acute urticarial reaction in a patient who is confined to bed.

Diphenhydramine (Benadryl) and tripelennamine (Pyribenzamine) have definite blocking and anesthetic effects on peripheral nerves and may be substituted for procaine, lidocaine, etc., in patients who are allergic or hypersensitive to these drugs. They are employed in the same relative dosage, i.e., 2 to 3 cc USP.

The antihistamines can be placed arbitrarily into six groups. This classification is based mainly on their relationship to the aminoethyl side chain of histamine and has value in that it provides a method of cataloguing agents which differ just enough to offer a selection to meet individual patient variations and to focus on specific needs.

1. *Ethylurediamine series.* This large group of general purpose antihistamines contains some very familiar proprietary names, including Neoantergen, Pyribenzamine, Histadyl, Anahist, and Antistine.

2. *Aminoalkylether series.* This group is strongly sedative almost to the hypnotic stage, and many have been used in nonprescription sleeping potions. Benadryl and Decapryn are the well-known members.

3. *Alkylamine series.* This group contains some of the newer and more potent antihistaminics which as a rule have a wider range of action and produce less drowsiness and sedation than the others. Chlor-Trimeton, Dimetane, Pyronil, and Forhistal are prominent names in this series.

4. *Individual or other series.* This group, represented primarily by Thephorin and Periactin, shows no clear relationship to the aminoethyl side chain, but its members are effective antihistamines, especially against serotonins. Many pharmacologists believe a fifth, or phenothiazine, classification is necessary in the grouping of histamine H receptor antagonists. Many of the phenothiazines act as antihistamines, the foremost example of which is promethazine (Phenergan). Others are trimeprazine (Temaril) and profenamine (Parsidol).

A new and exciting class of antihistamine drugs, the histamine H_2 receptor antagonists, are looming as important and effective in various areas of therapy. They inhibit gastric acid secretions stimulated by histamine released in the allergic phenomena.

Cimetidine (Tagamet) is the first to be released. Surprisingly, it also blocks secretion normally induced by insulin, foods, or vagal reflex; therefore it not only is classed with the antihistamines but also is a gastrointestinal drug for therapy in all duodenal and peptic ulcers and other conditions associated with gastric acid. It appears, *from the limited data available* at this writing, to be very effective and low in toxicity.

Another group of antihistamines, used primarily as anti-motion sickness agents, is listed separately. The vestibular apparatus is the site of motion sickness, and depression of this area by these agents relieves the symptoms of vertigo and nausea and also controls Meniere's syndrome. This depressant action is not solely antihistaminic, because many good antihistamines are ineffective; nor is it purely antiemetic, because chlorpromazine, a good antiemetic, is not a good anti-motion sickness agent. Dramamine, Marezine, and Bonine are able representatives in this class.

Side effects, although usually minor, may be unexpected and aggravating. Inability to concentrate, dizziness, and disturbances of coordination are fairly common. Dryness of the mouth, pharynx, and bronchial mucosa with an irritating dry cough may occur. Often unwanted gastrointestinal effects occur, surprisingly in view of the antiemetic effect of many antihistamines. Occasionally a vasovagal effect with syncopal attacks may occur, and rarely other bizarre reactions such as delirium, narcolepsy, fever, and dermatitis have been noted. Topical application is of questionable value, and may cause hypersensitivity.

It is wise to remember that antihistamines are more potent in preventing the actions of histamine than in reversing these actions once they develop. Antihistamines are synergistic with depressant drugs and as a rule cause drowsiness.

In comparison with other effective drugs, the toxic features of most antihistamines are remarkably benign. However, recent animal studies have revealed drug-induced fetal abnormalities following high dosages of hydroxyzine, meclizine, and buclizine. Clinical data in human beings are inadequate to establish safety in gestation, except for chlorphenaramine and diphenhydramine.

GENERAL ANESTHETIC AGENTS

General anesthesia is seldom used in the average dental office, but sedation, produced by the inhalation of anesthetic gases through special apparatus, is common enough to deserve mention. Nitrous oxide and occasionally trichlorethylene are the agents of choice. Greater than average care and skill are demanded of individuals contemplating or employing such a procedure. No other area of dental practice is fraught with more hazards. Recording the number of presedation precautions or steps necessary for safe administration of these agents and the side effects or number of toxic manifestations which may be encountered subsequent to their use is beyond the scope of this chapter. However, the basic properties of these drugs should be noted.

Nitrous oxide is inexorably linked with early dentistry, and still retains a lofty place in our favor. "Analgesia machines" invariably employ nitrous oxide as the chief agent. This gas, in combination with 30 per cent or more of oxygen, will produce good-to-excellent sedation with little if any direct toxic effects. But the hallucinations and struggling which can occur with improper administration may produce excitement and exertion which could be harmful to patients in a precarious state of health, or which could result in physical injury.

Recent reports have revealed an intensification of the hallucinatory effect when nitrous oxide sedation is employed on marijuana users. Although some are more placid, the usual response is heightened euphoria and exaggerated physical movements during administration, and prolonged after-effects. Consistent marijuana smokers require an increased percentage of nitrous oxide in the sedative mixture, leading to increased CNS initiation and increased difficulty of management, resulting in a generally ineffective and disruptive session in which little may be accomplished.

Trilene is one of the most potent analgesics in use today. It can be one of the most dangerous. Cardiac arrhythmias regularly appear, even with small concentrations, and cases of cardiac arrest have been reported during the analgesic state. Arrest can occur following sudden increase in concentration, even in the conscious patient. It is deceptively easy to administer and pleasant, and can be used alone or in conjunction with nitrous oxide and oxygen. Tachypnea is also an undesirable effect. A rebreather cannister containing either Ca or $MgOH_2$ must not be used anywhere in the anesthesia circuit. Phosgene, a lethal gas (used in WWI), is formed by mixing trichlorethylene and soda lime ($CaOH_2$). Trilene is not recommended.

The foregoing information may all be historical in nature, because at this writing, the FDA has proposed a ban on all uses of trichlorethylene because tests (1977) at the National Cancer Institute revealed liver cancer in mice after exposure to it.

FDA Proposes Ban on Trichlorethylene (Official Government Release)

The Food and Drug Administration has proposed a ban on the chemical trichlorethylene (TCE), in foods, drugs, and cosmetics. The substance has been shown to cause liver cancer in mice, according to tests performed by the National Cancer Institute. Trichlorethylene was once widely used to remove caffeine from coffee.

Trichlorethylene, under the name of Trilene, in the past was used quite commonly as a general anesthetic for dental surgery. In recent years its popularity has decreased owing to the use of newer, less-toxic agents.

Fluroxene (Fluoromar) should be listed because it enjoyed a flair of popularity, which then quietly expired. It resembles ethyl ether, but is less flammable, not as potent, and more toxic.

In fact, *Fluothane, Penthrane* and *Ethrane* are the only acceptable potent, nonexplosive, inhalation agents which are relatively safe for general anesthesia. *Ethyl ether* and *cyclopropane* are not only potent but highly flammable, and should be administered only by experienced personnel using proper equipment in a grounded room. *Chloroform* and *ethyl chloride*, while nonflammable, are cardiotoxic agents with a narrow margin of safety even in the best of circumstances. Their general use has been sharply curtailed.

Halothane (Fluothane) has replaced most of the other inhalation anesthetics because of its potency, nonexplosive nature, and lack of toxicity, even though some cases of hepatic damage have been reported.

Methoxyflurane (Penthrane) has been promoted largely for its analgesic properties. Disposable inhalers controlled by the patient are available to secure a high plane of analgesia for minimal procedures. Induction is slower; otherwise it approximates halothane in most respects.

Abbott Laboratories issued a warning about Penthrane late in 1970, concerning the increased incidence of renal tubular dysfunction, sometimes with a fatal termination. Long, deep anesthetics on obese or aged patients are mostly implicated, but of particular interest to clinicians is that *concurrent use of methoxyflurane on a patient who is taking tetracyclines may result in death from kidney failure.*

Enflurane (Ethrane) is another fluorinated hydrocarbon which is enjoying increasing use. It is very similar to halothane and methoxyflurane. Induction is fairly rapid and not unpleasant! Enflurane causes little nausea and vomiting, is chemically stable, and has minimal after effects. Like halothane it enhances the effect of non-depolarizing muscle relaxants.

Propanidid (Epontol) is an IV agent resembling ultra-short-acting barbiturates in induction and maintenance techniques. Its significant difference is a temporary stimulatory rather than depressive effect on respiration and blood pressure. Although widely used in Europe and Canada, it is little known in the U.S. Epontol may be substituted for barbiturates in patients with porphyria. It has been combined with methohexital, but the therapeutic value of the resultant mixture is highly questionable.

The ultra-short IV barbiturates (Pentothal and Brevital) are similar to the other barbiturates in action and toxicity except for their incredible speed in producing a state of unconsciousness and almost as rapid detoxification under normal physiologic conditions.

Neuroleptanalgesia Anesthesia

Neuroleptanalgesia is an anesthetic technique using a neuroleptic (major tranquilizer) and a narcotic analgesic in conjunction with inhalation anesthesia for induction and maintenance.

Innovar combines a potent major tranquilizer (droperidol) with a potent narcotic analgesic (fentanyl) to achieve the anesthetic state with or without premedication. Used by some anesthetists at 1 cc per 20 lbs and others at 1 cc per 50 lbs of body weight, Innovar provides the induction and basic control with nitrous oxide–oxygen as the supplemental agent. The technique is to give two-thirds of the total measured dose in one bolus, a muscle relaxant, intubation, then maintenance with 2:1 N_2O–O_2 and small increments of the remaining drug.

Toxic effects are the usual ones expected with CNS depression, plus a unique one: thoracic rigidity. Compliance of the lungs is reduced, and ventilation becomes a problem. This rigidity usually occurs with large doses and is susceptible to muscle relaxants; nevertheless, it is an annoying complication.

The main advantage is *professed* to be increased safety for poor risk patients in that profound analgesia and sedation are obtained without serious impairment of vital centers or function. However, Innovar has been condemned by Medical Letter as an unacceptable drug, not only because of its side effects but also because it is a potent compound with a fixed dose ratio which in this enlightened era of pharmacodynamics is not only frowned upon but subject to critical scrutiny from all angles.

It is possible to obtain a neuroleptic state without rigidity by judicious combinations of droperidol and fentanyl and other potent tranquilizers and analgesics. However, this is a jungle for the initiate or novice. Serious hypotension and respiratory depression along with other CNS problems often must be dealt with in this area of practice. The dental practitioner should be familiar with antagonists and analeptics, such as naloxone and physostigmine, and doxapram, and the selective employment of the proper vasopressors and/or analeptics in patients under MAO and trycyclic therapy, the restrictions involved with use of alpha (phenotolamine [Regitine]) and beta (propranalol [Inderal]) blockers, and other facts such as *possible epinephrine reversal with phenothiazines and occasionally with butyrophenones*. This information should be as familiar to you as is the use of O_2. Lack of knowledge concerning the alleviation and control of CNS vagaries with the proper agents and techniques should preclude ventures into this hazardous area of dental practice.

Disassociative Anesthesia

Disassociative anesthesia is another new technique defined as disassociation with profound analgesia in the presence of superficial sleep.

Ketamine HCl is the forerunner of what hopefully will be a new and exciting category of anesthetic agents. By definition it is not a true anesthetic. Its action is characterized by a peculiar state of unconsciousness in which sensory input is not blocked at the spinal or brain stem levels but afferent impulses received are interrupted in the association area of the cortex.

Outwardly the patient appears to be in a trance and unaware of painful stimuli; his eyes remain open, but he is oblivious to his surroundings.

The dosage is calculated by body weight and is injected *slowly* IV as a bolus, 1 mg per lb. Subsequent increments are at reduced strength (0.5 mg per lb). When excessive movements of the head or extremities occur (usually after 10 minutes) the injection of 0.5 mg per pound is repeated at these intervals until the surgery is completed.

The IM dose, which is especially useful for "hard-to-manage" children, is given in one quick "pop," 5 mg per lb. If additional anesthetic is needed, the strength is reduced to 2.5 mg per lb and repeated in 20 to 30 minutes.

Arbitrary limits for the number of repeated doses may be set at 15 for IV and five for IM.

There are several striking advantages evident in a ketamine anesthetic. The airway is not a major problem, because muscle tone and pharyngeal and laryngeal reflexes are largely unaffected. Cardiovascular and respiratory function are seldom impaired, and the CNS is not depressed significantly.

There is also a reverse and darker side of the coin. Sudden and drastic rise in blood pressure has been a factor often enough to curtail ketamine's use in hypertensive or arteriosclerotic patients. Mental complications are emerging in approximately 15 per cent of adult patients and are also prevalent in children. Delirium nightmares, hallucinations, and even schizoid reactions are seen during the recovery period. Although many are the result of improper handling, early aural, visual, or tactile stimulation must be avoided or kept minimal; the reactions are so strong and in some cases so persistent (for months) that ketamine's use should be restricted to specific cases until these psychic alterations can be eliminated or controlled. Valium has been used (with questionable success) by many investigators as a premedicant designed to reduce and/or negate these shattering psychic phenomena. At this time its value as a control remains controversial. Physostigmine will control most toxic phenomena.

The foregoing general anesthetic agents are included with brief comments only to maintain continuity and not with the intention of suggesting their use in any practice. Some — ether and cyclopropane — are too hazardous for office use; others — chloroform and ethyl chloride — are too hazardous for any use except in dire emergencies when other agents are unavailable. Fluothane and the IV barbiturates are potent drugs safe only in the hands of dentists properly trained in intratracheal anesthetic and resuscitative techniques.

LOCAL ANALGESIC AGENTS

The majority of local analgesics are esters of aromatic acids which usually contain an amino group and aliphatic amino alcohols. Ortho-amino, para-amino, meta-aminobenzoic acid, and benzoic acid esters are the predominant compounds. These ester types are primarily hydrolyzed in the plasma or in the liver by esterases. The aniline compounds, lidocaine (Xylocaine), propiticaine (Citanest) and mepivacaine (Carbocaine) compose the only other major local analgesic formulas suitable for injection. These drugs are not hydrolyzed in the plasma or liver, but depend on urinary excretion and redistribution into nonsensitive tissues for their detoxification.

The general aim in the synthesis of new anesthetic compounds is to produce more potent drugs with decreased systemic and local toxicity. In most cases, toxicity tends to rise as potency increases. If, however, the structural change responsible for the increased potency also increases the hydrolysis rate, then the toxicity of the new compound may be decreased. A good example of such a compound is 2-chloroprocaine (Nesacaine), which although twice as potent as procaine, is, because of its five times more rapid hydrolysis rate, less toxic. Since the temporary inhibition of conduction is the purpose of a local analgesic, diffusibility or the penetration of nerve sheaths in sufficient concentrations is a foremost consideration in determining its effectiveness.

Toxicity is a relative value. One local analgesic may initiate more frequent, even more severe episodes than another, but still not be as dangerous or lethal; for example, lidocaine is supposedly twice as toxic as procaine, but is not etiologic in nearly as many fatal or anaphylactic seizures.

Toxicity from overdose, yielding a blood level of the drug high enough to affect the vital centers, is caused either by intravascular injection, too large a volume, too concentrated a solution (percentage), or injecting rapidly into vascular areas.

A sparsely known fact of inestimable importance is that topical anesthetics are more rapidly absorbed from mucous membranes than from any other tissues. Blood level curves are similar to those following IV injection and grossly higher than subcutaneous or intramuscular infiltration. Vasopressors will not prevent or even retard absorption of the topical anesthetic, whether applied by swab or spray or gargle. Contrary to expectations, vasopressors offer no protection against sudden high levels.

The first symptoms of toxicity of the ester types are those of cerebral cortical stimulation characterized by talkativeness, restlessness, apprehension, excitement, and possibly convulsions. However, lidocaine and mepivacaine are different, causing cortical depression, lethargy, drowsiness, and sleep. If the toxic response is moderate to severe, medullary stimulation follows the cerebral cortical phase. Then, increased blood pressure, pulse rate, and respirations are evident. Nausea and vomiting also may occur. The final phase is medullary depression whose severity is directly proportional to the amount or degree of the previous stimulation. Blood pressure drops, pulse may become slow and thready, and respiration weakens or ceases. In almost all cases, death following a toxic overdose of a local analgesic drug is the result of respiratory depression or apnea.

While a great deal has been written concerning allergic reactions to local analgesic drugs, *true allergy is uncommon*. It has been extimated that only about 1 per cent of all reactions occurring during local analgesia are allergic in origin. However, when anaphylaxis strikes, manifested by sudden violent loss of vasomotor tonus (i.e., blood pressure and pulse), it is the most terrifying and hazardous reaction possible. Despite prompt and accurate treatment, even heroic measures, a fatal termination may be unavoidable.

Since it is a fact that some patients are allergic to local analgesics and that these allergies can be dangerous, it is also a fact that a patient who is allergic to any one drug usually will be allergic to every other drug of closely related chemical structure. Therefore, the local analgesics grouped according to their chemical structures are listed for edification and guidance in substituting one agent for another when allergy is suspected or confirmed.

    I. Benzoic acid esters
       Piperocaine (Metycaine)
       Meprylcaine (Orocaine)
       Kincaine (Kincaine)
    II. Para-aminobenzoic acid esters
       Procaine (Novocaine)
       Tetracaine (Pontocaine)
       Butethamine (Monocaine)
       Propoxycaine (Ravocaine)
       2-Chloroprocaine (Nesacaine)
       Procaine and Butethamine (Duocaine)
   III. Meta-aminobenzoic acid esters
       Metabutethamine (Unacaine)
       Primacaine (Primacaine)
   IV. Para-ethroxybenzoic acid esters
       Diethoxin (Intracaine)
    V. Cyclohexylamino-2 propylbenzoate
       Hexylcaine (Cyclaine)
   VI. Anilide or Amide
       Bupivacaine (Marcaine)
       Etidocaine (Duranest)
       Lidocaine (Xylocaine)
       Mepivacaine (Carbocaine)
       Propiticaine (Citanest)
       Quanticaine (Tarracine)

A new anilide derivative, bupivacaine (Marcaine) is a potent and long-acting local analgesic with good tissue penetrating properties and low incidence of side effects. Surprisingly, when compared with lidocaine, bupivacaine is superior in all areas: lower toxicity in equipotent doses, greater potency, quicker onset, longer duration (2 to 4 times), latent pain-free period after return to normal sensation in many patients, *and no requirement of a vasoconstrictor for consistent profoundness.*

It is contraindicated in children and retarded patients because of the possibility of lip chewing or self-mutilation.

Etidocaine (Duranest) is another amide or anilide derivative which is so similar in every respect to bupivacaine that a repetitive dissertation on its properties is not needed. A preference between the two brands may be determined after a lengthier trial but at this time none can be found in the literature.[18, 28, 41]

Until now, tetracaine held the longevity record, but duration is not a prime factor in most dental procedures, whereas toxicity is! Since tetracaine is also the most lethal of local analgesics, it has not been a favorite for office-type practice despite its proved worth.

As a general rule, the potency of a local analgesic depends solely on its chemical structure, while the duration, although markedly influenced by the molecular configuration, can also be altered by the addition of a vasoconstrictor drug. This additive has an important and sometimes vitally necessary function when one remembers that all the local analgesic agents in use in dentistry today, with the possible exception of Xylocaine, Carbocaine, and Monocaine, are vasodilators and, as such, are rapidly absorbed into the systemic circulation, thereby increasing the possibility of toxic overdose and decreasing local potency and duration.

The addition of beta-receptor blocking agents such as propranolol HCl to local anesthetic agents, in order to minimize or counteract undesirable cardiovascular and CNS symptoms, has been tested without significantly favorable results.

VASOPRESSORS OR VASOCONSTRICTORS

Despite the controversies that continue to swirl around the use, non-use, and abuse of the vasoconstrictor drugs, they are an integral part of most of the local analgesic solutions used in dentistry. Of the five sympathomimetic drugs commonly present as vasoconstrictors in dental analgesic solutions, all provide satisfactory results, with epinephrine being the most efficient, followed in order by Levophed, Cobefrin, Neo-Cobefrin, and Neo-Synephrine.

The importance of the sympathomimetic agents cannot be overstressed, particularly when it is considered that, because of their vasodilatory effect which increases with an increase in strength, very few if any of the local analgesics would produce satisfactory anesthesia for dental procedures without the addition of a vasopressor drug. Yet it is unlikely that there exists a dental practitioner in this country who has not received a note from the physician of a patient with cardiovascular disease, admonishing against the use of an anesthetic containing an adrenergic agent. Again, who will deny that the anxiety and stress created by painful dental treatment may provoke an ungovernable and unmeasurable release of endogenous epinephrine into this same patient's vascular system? It is the considered and published opinion of most cardiologists and internists that vasopressors should be used with local analgesics in treating patients with cardiovascular disease. Rather than increasing the hazard, it enhances the safety and comfort of dental procedures for these simple and sufficient reasons: (1) an increase in depth with the attendant psychic and physiologic benefits; (2) prevention of too rapid or too quantitative absorption of a potentially toxic and/or lethal drug (local analgesic) into the circulation; (3) reduction of bacteremia by decreasing circulation in the area of septic surgery; (4) reduction of hemorrhage in hypertensive patients; and (5) reduction of local tissue damage inherent with repeated injections and large quantities of irritating solutions. Provided proper precautions are observed (instrumentation and technique), the use of epinephrine within prescribed limits is considered safe for most cardiac patients. Knowledge of the anatomy, selection of the proper site before injection, good technique, and aspiration ordinarily will create a satisfactory plane of anesthesia even with minimal amounts of weaker analgesic solutions. Since the goal of chemotherapy is to achieve optimum therapeutic results with minimum alterations of normal physiology, one can hardly quibble when a majority of internists and anesthesiologists agree that 1 per cent solutions containing 1:200,000 parts epinephrine will provide a sufficient degree of anesthesia for most dental operations when properly employed. The reader is referred to Chapters 2 and 15 for further discussions of epinephrine.

Another cogent factor, often blithely ignored or disregarded, is that compounds containing racemic epinephrine, used in packing gingival areas to facilitate impression-taking of teeth prepared for restorative dentistry, can be extremely dangerous. The rapid absorption of large quantities of epinephrine through the abraded tissues of the gingiva and adjacent capillary plexuses may precipitate a profound cardiovascular reaction or crisis. One need only remember the swift and potent response to nitroglycerin when placed on the normal mucosa of the sublingual area to appreciate the amplified effect possible when other strong drugs are applied to lacerated and bleeding tissues in the same area.

Undoubtedly many untoward systemic reactions are attributed to the local analgesic drugs when the constrictors are the real offenders. The symptoms arising from toxic overdose of a vasopressor are mainly palpitation, tachycardia, hypertension, and headache, which differ from the signs of CNS stimulation and/or depression synonymous with local analgesic toxicity.

True allergic manifestations from vasoconstrictor drugs are extremely rare or do not exist. Many authorities state that any direct reactions attributable to the vasopressor drugs are due to overdose or idiosyncrasy and may be limited to those four mentioned above. All other complications which may ensue, other than occasional tissue slough from ischemia at the site of injection, should be blamed on other sources or agents.

ANTIBIOTICS

Most discussions on antibiotics and their usage end in impasse: there are few phases of medicine which provoke more passionate commitments and denouncements — more heat and less light.

Many enthusiastic practitioners will defend overusage on the grounds of beneficial secondary effects, such as lowered incidence of rheumatic fever because of prophylactic penicillin in pediatric nasopharyngeal infections.

Others will condemn this practice on the basis of a growing resistance of bacteria engendered by promiscuous application of these drugs, and the pyramiding number of allergic and toxic reactions appearing in the literature. This chapter is of course concerned with the latter.

There are several types of antibiotic toxicity: anaphylaxis — shock or acute cardiovascular collapse; simple allergy — edema, hives, rashes, etc.; auditory — damage to eighth cranial nerve and cochlea; hematopoietic — marrow damage and aplastic anemia; renal and hepatic — tubular (kidney) damage and necrosis of the liver; superinfection — disruption of normal bacterial flora, degenerative intestinal mucosa changes, fungus overgrowth, or chronic or persistent diarrhea.

The condemnation of piggy-back antibiotic combinations, alluded to in the first edition because of their questionable value and inherent dangers, has intensified to the point that their manufacture and distribution have ceased (with a few exceptions) and the shotgun concept has been virtually discarded. Antibiotics should be used as a rifle rather than a scattergun because they have an amazing degree of specificity. Accurate evaluation is virtually impossible with such conglomerate packaging.

The use of antibiotics in dental practice is not and should not be confined only to infections in and about the oral cavity. It is difficult for most of us to envision the potential danger and the very real chance of tragic consequences from relatively simple dental procedures performed on a patient with a history of cardiac damage. In individuals with rheumatic or congenital heart disease, bacteria present in the blood may lodge on damaged heart valves or other parts of the endocardium because of the roughened cauliflower-like surface of the scar tissue there. Concentration of bacteria or bacteremia, even though transitory, constitutes a measurable threat of bacterial endocarditis — a potential crippling or even fatal infection which often does not respond to massive doses of antibiotics.

It is well established that transitory bacteremia does result from tooth extraction, oral surgical procedures, manipulation of periodontal tissues, and removal of tonsils and adenoids.

In patients with cardiopathies it is recommended that antibiotics be used routinely in conjunction with the aforementioned procedures to decrease the likelihood that bacterial endocarditis will occur.

The purpose of antibiotic therapy is, of course, a prophylactic weapon to prevent bacteremia or reduce the magnitude or duration should it occur and to eradicate bacteria that may implant on heart valves before a vegetation is formed. Penicillin is the drug of choice. Although broad-spectrum antibiotics may decrease bacteremia, they cannot be relied upon to eradicate initial bacterial implants and for this reason they are not recommended. Erythromycin is always the second choice if an allergy to penicillin exists. Sulfonamides are completely unsatisfactory.

ROUTE OF ADMINISTRATION

The oral route of administration for dental infections involving the mucous membranes, skin, other soft tissues, and the sinuses is usually sufficient. Serious bone infections require parenteral IM injections for high effectiveness, while gross phlegmons (cellulitis, Ludwig's, etc.), which interfere with respiration or a patent airway, septicemia, and endocarditis are always treated with maximum IV doses.

The last infections mentioned are naturally of high morbidity, and the IV therapy is usually a combination of a penicillin and an aminoglycoside (i.e., carbenicillin and tobramycin, which together are potent in action and broad in spectrum), unless, of course, the patient is allergic or sensitive to one class or the other.

Regardless, potentially lethal infections of the oral maxillofacial complex require a consultation with an internist trained or specializing in antimicrobial therapy.

Classification according to molecular mechanism of action has an important part in the better understanding of the goals in antibiotic therapy.

I. Agents that alter structure and function of the cell wall (protein synthesis):
The penicillins
Cephalothin and analogues
Bacitracin
Vancomycin
Ristocetin
Cycloserine

II. Agents that restrict function of the cell membrane (penetrate cell wall and cytoplasm):
Nystatin
Amphotericin B
Polymyxin B
Tyrocidin
Gramicidin
Colistin

III. Agents that impair translation of genetic information (ribosome code, RNA, etc.) into protein synthesis:
The tetracyclines
Erythromycin, Oleandomycin, and TAO
Lincomycin and Clindamycin
Chloramphenicol
Neomycin
Streptomycin
Kanamycin
Gentamicin
Tobramycin

IV. Agents that impede replication of genetic information:
Nalidixic acid
Griseofulvin

Following is the list of the major and minor antibiotics in use at this time and the toxic effects which they may produce.

Penicillins

In many ways this drug is the most remarkable and effective weapon of modern medicine. Even with the extensive publicity given the newer "wonder drugs," penicillin remains the premier antibiotic. Were it not for its allergic potential, penicillin would be the safest and most useful agent of all. More research in the area of synthetic congeners may eliminate this danger.

Regardless of personal preference or safety reservations, penicillin is the standard by which most others are judged. Despite the knowledgeable air some therapists assume when the acquired resistance of bacteria to penicillin is discussed, there are, in fact, few significant data to support or structure this indictment. It still slaughters most streptococci and other gram-positive organisms with relative ease and impunity. However, penicillin-resistant staphylococci are a case apart.

Because of protein binding, acid sensitivity, and penicillinase problems, new analogs of penicillin have been evolved to solve or minimize the factors which render them weak or useless.

More data are certainly in order concerning the basic nature of antimicrobial agents, even though the majority of clinicians practicing today have been brought up in the antibiotic era. The penicillins act basically by interference with the biosynthesis of bacterial cell walls. Penicillin G, or benzylpenicillin, is the standard and exists in four therapeutic forms, aqueous, procaine, benzathine, and Oralpen. The *aqueous* form is given IV in million-plus unit doses and is effective for four to six hours, then must be repeated. Procaine is injected IM and lasts up to 24 hours. The procaine factor acts as an analgesic as well as a depot storage vehicle, therein slowing release of the penicillin. The usual dosage to maintain blood level is 600,000 to 1,000,000 units B.I.D. *Benzathine* is the long lasting (30 days) form permitting low dose (extended or continuous) for patients with rheumatic hearts and others who must have an effective blood level at all times in order to survive. The usual dose is 1.2 million units every 30 days. *Oralpen* is the ordinary Na or K form of penicillin G. These tablets must be used in high dosage forms, 1.5 million units or 1.5 to 2 gm, in order to provide adequate blood levels because exposure to gastric secretions destroys more than 50 per cent of the active drug.

Penicillin V, or phenoxymethyl penicillin, is the other form of the basic agent. Its primary virtue is the ability to resist degradation or destruction by gastric action to the point where 80 to 90 per cent of the oral dose remains effective.

Why, then, should penicillin V not be the drug of choice by the oral route? Scientifically it is, but economically it is not! Penicillin G is far less expensive than penicillin V, so even when two or three times as much is needed, it is still less costly. Physiologically, the amount makes little difference because penicillin is relatively nontoxic.

Methicillin is employed against penicillinase-producing staphylococcus. It is usually restricted to hospital use and must be given IV or IM. (Dosage 6–12 Grn/D IV.)

Carbenicillin (Carboxybenzylpenicillin) acts against the normal spectrum + penicillinase + gram negative bacilli (pseudomonas, proteus, and enterobacteria). It is frequently used in combination with gentamicin and tobramycin in potentially lethal infections. A great drawback in its employment is that bacteria develop resistance in a short time.

Cloxacillin and *dicloxacillin* are oral forms of synthetic or semisynthetic penicillins formulated to combat penicillinase-producing staphylococcus dosage: 250-500 mg Q.I.D.).

Oxacillin (Tegopen) and *Nafcillin* (Unipen), also in this group, are available in IM and IV formulation — 500 mg Q.I.D. Nafcillin (Unipen) yields better tissue levels in comparison. It is also mixed with aminoglycosides in therapy for highly morbid infections.

A good rule of thumb in suspected gram positive or staphylococcus infections is to start the patient on any one of these four agents before precise bacteriology is known, especially if the infection is a fulminating type!

Ampicillin (α-amino benzyl penicillin) and *amoxicillin* (same formula + H), which yield higher blood levels, are semisynthetic broad-spectrum penicillins which cover the penicillin G range plus many gram negative bacilli. However, they are ineffective against penicillinase-producing staphylococcus. The range includes *Escherichia coli, Proteus mirabilis, Salmonella, Shigella, Neisseria meningitides* and *Haemophilus influenzae.* Ampicillin is the drug of choice for influenza bacteria.

The ampicillins must be ingested at least 30 minutes before eating in order to prevent a decline or diminution of their effectiveness.

A majority of those colleagues who are really aware of all the vagaries and implications of penicillin therapy agree that the least expensive form of penicillin G if used in *large enough doses* will do the job as well as the more exotic and expensive relatives in its family. Penicillin should never be used topically, because ingestion through the skin, especially mucous membranes, greatly enhances the sensitivity effect. Toxic manifestation may be severe enough to be fatal (anaphylactoid shock and glottic edema) or mild enough merely to produce pruritus, rash, and hives. Toxic states with the severity of their symptoms somewhere between these extremes commonly occur. The signs may be immediate or may appear after a prolonged time, and their magnitude is variable and unpredictable.

Before we continue with other listings, a short dissertation on microbes will refresh your memory and aid substantially to your knowledgeable use of antibiotic compounds.

The five most common microorganisms found in odontogenic infections are, in order of frequency: *Streptococcus viridans, Neisseria catarrhalis, Staphylococcus albus* (DNase negative), *Staphylococcus aureus* (DNase positive), and anaerobic streptococci. These are all aerobic save the last and all are gram positive and therefore usually susceptible to the penicillins, the cephalosporins, erythromycin, and clindamycin.

Other common offenders are diphtheroids *Klebsiella, Hemophilus influenzae,* and occasionally *Proteus mirabilis,* H enterococci, *N. pharyngis,* and pneumococci. It would seem logical that most oral bacteria would be aerobic, but not so—over three fourths of mouth organisms extant are anaerobic. Since most cultures taken are only for aerobic tests, one can't help wonder if we are really aware of the true etiology in many head and neck infections. If moderate to *serious disease exists, it is wise to ask for and take anaerobic cultures with the special equipment needed.*

The most common anaerobics associated with oral and respiratory infections are *Bacteroides melaninogenicus,* fusobacteria (fusiform bacilli), and peptostreptococci. This group, along with others found in oral infection—*B. oralis, Clostridium* spp., and *Veillonella* spp.—are usually highly susceptible to penicillin G.

Cephalosporins

GROUP I

Cephalothin (Keflin), cephapirin (Cefadyl), and cephacetrile (Celospor) are all parenteral forms and are rapidly detoxified by the liver and excreted within 4 hours. This group is safe in most penicillin allergy cases. The IM dose is 500 mg every 8 hours, and the IV dose is 25 mg per kg every 3 to 6 hours. Higher or more frequent doses are mandatory in serious infections.

GROUP II

Cephaloridine (Loridine) and cefazolin (Kefzol, Ancef) are also parenteral forms but are long acting because of slow excretion and protein binding. They are considered best in meningitis, but are limited to a maximum dose of 4 gm per day because of their propensity for nephrotoxicity. Azotemia can be checked for with a Coombs' test.

GROUP III

Cephalexin (Keflex), cephaloglycin (Kafocin), and Cephadrine (Velosef, Anspor) are all oral forms with low protein binding and a high activity blood level. Kidney problems are minimal with unimpaired excretion.

As a group they are effective against penicillinase-producing staphylococci and are lower in allergic response.

In all serious infections where allergenicity is unknown and effectiveness against cell walls of gram positive or negative bacteria is needed, a cephalosporin is the drug of choice. They also will control *Staphylococcus epidermidis,* which is an increasingly morbid factor because it seems to have a predilection for metal. Heart valves, hip and other bone implants, and embedded mesh and wires are in jeopardy from this new manifestation in a formerly rather innocuous microbe.

All in all, the *broader spectrum* of the cephalosporins makes them more likely to *alter the normal microbial ecology of the host* and render him more susceptible to superinfections with resistant *Pseudomonas, E. coli,* and enterobacteria.

The Macrolides: Erythromycin (Ilosone, Erythrocin, E-mycin); Oleandomycin; TAO

Erythromycin operates best in the same bacterial spectrum (grampositive) as penicillin and as such is used as a penicillin substitute. Although not as effective, it is much safer. Hypersensitivity reactions and bacterial resistance are rarely encountered. Toxicity to erythromycin is almost negligible except for mild gastrointestinal irritation and diarrhea. Reports of allergy are scattered and inconclusive. The estolate salt has been linked with cholestatic jaundice. However, because of erythromycin's proven safety it is often prescribed as a placebo to the detriment of the efficacious ratio and its future value.

Erythromycin is bacteriostatic in normal doses but frequently moves into the bactericidal range when employed in large increments. The dosage is 1–2 gm or more per day.

A big drawback is its incompatibility with almost all IV medications, including catecholamines, vitamins, barbiturates, phenothiazines, phenytoin (Dilantin), lactobinate salts, succinate salts, and other antibiotics. It also influences many lab tests to give false readings (especially liver profile tests); this may be an important factor in total patient therapy.

Oleandomycin and Triacetyloleandomycin (TAO) fall in the same spectrum and category as erythromycin but are being phased out because they are less active and more toxic. They are limited to 10-day usage, with hepatic and GI problems (nausea, vomiting, and colitis) a not infrequent deleterious effect. Anaphylaxis has been reported which, along with the above, certainly removes oleandomycin and TAO from consideration in dental therapeutics.

Lincomycin (Lincocin); Clindamycin (Cleocin)

Isolated from the fungus *Streptomyces lincolnensis*, these antibiotics are usually bactericidal against gram-positive pathogens and effective to some degree against the remainder of the organisms in this class. No serious hypersensitivity reactions (angioneurotic edema, anaphylaxis, etc.) have been reported at this date, but gastrointestinal irritation (nausea, diarrhea, and cramps), colitis, and superinfection appear to be the major toxic manifestations. Lincomycin (parenteral), Lincocin, and clindamycin (oral) (Cleocin) inhibit protein synthesis (ribosomes and polypeptides). Because of their affinity or predilection for bone infections* and undoubted effectiveness against staphylococci, these drugs were accepted as heaven sent by most clinicians who daily deal with bacterial osteitis and occasional osteomyelitis. They are effective but not as potent as first hoped. Still, if you respect the limitations, they are second (at least on a par with erythromycin) to penicillin and the cephalosporins in pharyngitis, otitis media, dental infections (bone and soft tissue), septicemia, cellulitis, osteomyelitis[34a] and some thoracic infections. *They are not affected by probenecid but are antagonized by erythromycin, and the two should never be used together.* Protein binding is low, therefore they present a fairly high level of activity early. It is the preferred drug in anaerobic penicillin resistant (or allergy) infections,* especially *B. fragilis.* As mentioned, allergy is not a big factor and toxicity is mainly confined to the bowel but it must be stressed that its manifestations can be extremely serious (bleeding, ulceration, and slough). More than 300 cases of clindamycin-induced colitis, including 20 deaths, have been reported.[42] The dosage is 150 to 300 mg four times per day.

Tetracycline (Achromycin, Tetracyn, etc.), Chlortetracycline (Aureomycin), Oxytetracycline (Terramycin), Demethylchlortetracycline (Declomycin), Methacycline (Rondomycin), Doxycycline (Vibramycin), Rolitetracycline (Syntetrin, Velacycline), Minocycline (Minocin)

These are the major members of a large group of closely related antibiotics known for their broad spectrum of activity. Although this wide range is certainly a desirable factor, tetracyclines, unlike penicillin, which is bacteriolytic, are bacteriostatic and consequently are ordinarily neither as rapid nor as effective in overcoming severe infections. They are not first choice for any dental or pharyngeal infection, with the possible exception of *parotitis*

---

*Conjectured, but accepted by most.

(salivary adenitis). Minocin has a predilection for salivary glands (unfortunately it also has a high ratio of allergenicity), and *osteoradionecrosis* where Vibramycin has been effective. A recent study found tetracycline to be useless in the treatment of most periodontal diseases. Toxic effects are usually manifested by gastrointestinal symptoms of nausea, vomiting, and diarrhea, which can preclude the more serious alimentary mucous membrane degenerative changes resulting from superinfection. This change in resident bacterial flora offers the chance for monilial growth and persistent diarrhea. A relatively new and, from the dental standpoint, serious finding is that ingestion of tetracyclines by pregnant women may result in a faulty development and yellow discoloration of the dentition of the fetus in utero and in early childhood which persists throughout life. The platitude, shared by many in the past, that tetracyclines were rather innocuous and could be prescribed with alacrity as a placebo with an "I must do something positive for the patient; it can't hurt, and may help" attitude has been shattered. Fatal anaphylaxis is not an unknown entity.

Aminoglycosides

The aminoglycosides encompass a large group of antibiotics including old standbys and some of the newest "wonder" drugs.

Streptomycin, neomycin, kanamycin, gentamicin, tobramycin, paramycin and *amikacin* are now used in therapy, while sisomycin and lividomycin are expected to be released within a year's time.

Administration covers all routes, with kanamycin, paramycin, and neomycin available PO, and the others parenterally. Neomycin, of course, is effective topically. Amikacin is new and is the drug of choice to combat gram-negative bacteria which appear to resist the aminoglycosides.

Antibiotics of this class are synergistic and compatible with the penicillins, and exhibit bacteriostatic action in low doses and lytic action in high doses, especially against gram-negative bacilli. However, because of their extreme side effects, dental use should be limited (except for topical neomycin) to life threatening maxillofacial infections. Permanent damage to the auditory nerve, cochlear and vestibular labyrinthitis, and lethal nephrotoxicity are common with unrestricted or careless use of aminoglycosides.

Pre-therapeutic renal function tests are mandatory when extended usage is planned. Dosage is 3 mg per kg per day for 24 hours in lethal infections and 2 mg per kg per day thereafter. Aminoglycosides are more active in an alkaline atmosphere (8–60×) and less in high osmolality. Calcium ions (milk, etc.) may negate their action.

Spectinomycin (Trobicin)

This is very similar in all respects to the aminoglycosides, and, in addition, it builds up quick resistance. Its only use is for stubborn cases of gonorrhea where its effectiveness is determined by a definite and lethal affinity for the gonococci.

Chloramphenicol (Chloromycetin)

This drug exhibits a wide range of activity: gram-positive and gram-negative bacteria, rickettsias, typhoid, and some large viruses are susceptible to its action. It has a predilection for cerebrospinal fluid, and this and its broad spectrum make it valuable in bacterial meningitis. But the general usefulness of this potent agent is limited (except as a life-saving measure) because chloramphenicol has been found to produce blood dyscrasias and other gross degenerative changes. Although justification for the employment of Chloromycetin in any dental disease seems inconceivable, it should have a proper listing. Toxic effects are mainly concerned with marrow damage and resultant agranulocytosis or aplastic anemia, but newborn infants may be fatally poisoned by their failure to carry out the glucuronide conjugation necessary for metabolizing this agent. Temporary erythroid hypoplasia and gastrointestinal symptoms are other unwelcome side effects.

Carbomycin

Employed in the same situations and very similar to oleandomycin in action, this antibiotic precipitates minor gastrointestinal disorders, but dangerous toxicity has yet to be reported.

Novobiocin

Skin eruptions, jaundice-like discoloration of epithelium, possible liver damage, and blood dyscrasias are among the detrimental effects attributed to this antibiotic. These plus a narrow range of activity curtail its value.

Polymyxins

Reports of renal damage should provoke a hesitant attitude toward the general use of polymyxin B. It also causes postinjection pain.

The polymyxins A B C D E are all forms of this active group of antibiotics but only poly B and colistin (E) are in therapeutic use and then only topically, where they are bactericidal. Care is necessary because the toxic manifestations (nephrosis, peripheral neuropathy, and respiratory arrest) are severe.

Vancomycin

This is a dangerous nephrotoxic and ototoxic drug (resembling the aminoglycosides). Its use is restricted to treatment of coccal endocarditis and other morbid gram-positive coccal infections when the patient is allergic to all other appropriate antibiotics. Intermittent IV only with 1 gm every 12 hours.

Rifampin

Rifampin is an oral drug with great potential and low toxicity. It is effective against most gram-positive and gram-negative bacteria, some viruses, and *Mycobacterium tuberculosis*. Most experts in antimicrobial therapy feel its use should be limited to tuberculosis treatment, but it is effective in a broad spectrum, if needed.

Several of these listed antibiotics have little and often highly questionable application in dental infections, but are mentioned because of their popularity. Other new products, such as cycloserine, ristocetin, Coly-Mycin, nalidixic acid, fucidic acid, and viomycin, should also fall in this restricted category.

There are two other antibiotics whose primary value lies in topical application. They frequently appear in the form of lozenges, sprays, and creams in combination with many other agents. Despite their largely empirical employment, they do have therapeutic value. Bacitracin is effective on surface tissues against most of the gram-positive and some of the gram-negative cocci. It is not locally toxic or irritating.

Tyrothricin has a limited field of usefulness because its action is inhibited by the presence of gram-negative organisms, but it is bactericidal for streptococci and staphylococci in open wounds. This drug is remarkably low in sensitizing capacity to all tissues except the meninges. It is highly toxic when it is introduced accidentally or otherwise into the subarachnoid space. If such a possibility exists, the use of tyrothricin should be avoided.

Sulfonamides

Other agents used to control infections in the body are not true antibiotics, which by definition must be produced by living things, but synthetic compounds from the chemical laboratory. This chemotherapeutic group includes the sulfonamides, the antifungal drugs, the antiprotozoan drugs and the vermifuges. Only the first two classes are germane to dentistry and will be discussed.

Sulfadiazine is by consensus the most effective and least toxic of the sulfas, but sulfisoxazole (Gantrisin) and the triple sulfas are also widely and effectively employed, especially in urinary infections. Sulfas are highly bound in blood protein.

Sulfadimethoxine (Madribon) is another popular and potent product which has been accused of precipitating Stevens-Johnson syndrome (severe erythema multiforme with bulla formation) in a limited number of patients. Although rare, it is unfortunately a highly morbid disease.

In general, sulfonamides should be used guardedly and only after critical appraisal in patients with liver or renal damage, urinary obstructions, and blood dyscrasias. Skin rashes and angioneurotic edema do occur, but the major toxicity ordinarily encountered with the sulfas is crystalluria, which produces irritation of the kidneys and urinary tract and tubular obstruction. Adjuvant therapy with sodium bicarbonate will result in an alkaline urine, thus preventing crystal formation.

Fungicides and Fungistats

Three of the newer antifungal agents are widely, but not necessarily wisely, used in combination with the tetracyclines. Their effectiveness in short-term therapy is debatable.

Antifungal agents usually have a detergent-like effect on the fungal cell wall. In past years, a tetracycline-nystatin combination (Mysteclin F) was the antibiotic most commonly prescribed by the dental profession. No comment on the wisdom of this choice is necessary.

Amphotericin B is the best of the group for serious mycotic infection and is employed as an IV drip (50 mg every 6 hours). It is occasionally toxic to the kidneys and GI system, and can cause CNS depression with headache, fever, and chills.

Flucytosine is the safest of these agents and is the preferred choice for most mild to moderate cases. The dose is 500 mg four times a day by mouth.

Nystatin may be given orally or topically and is effective against *Candida* and *Monilia*, which is part of the normal flora. It is occasionally inactivated by gastric juice.

Griseofulvin is used primarily for dermatophytes (tinea) rather than systemic mycoses. It is taken orally for long periods, three to four weeks for skin infections and six to 12 months for nail infections. It acts by being deposited in the growing integument (keratin).

Nitrofurazone (Furacin)

A nitrofuran derivative, this agent is very effective against many organisms, both gram-negative and gram-positive, which are resistant to regular antibiotics and is bactericidal in a broad spectrum. It is applied topically in solution or ointment-like form. Continuous use for ten or more days often results in local tissue irritation and occasionally in generalized allergic skin reaction. In short term use, it is nontoxic, effective in blood or pus, and promotes healing. Furacin gauze is a favorite for packing infected antrums or covering wounds.

Other nitrofurans are nalidixic acid and methenamine.

Antiviral Agents

Like the Holy Grail, antiviral agents have been pursued assiduously but with little success, until recently, because viruses are intracellular and therefore difficult to eradicate without killing the cell itself. At present, there are 10 compounds under investigation.

The most recent and by far the most successful agent, *adenine arabinoside*, has quickened the pulse of the medical community. It has been employed successfully in 90 per cent of a group of patients with herpes encephalitis, which normally kills 70 per cent of its victims and leaves most survivors with serious neurological damage. At present, intensive studies are in progress to expand its horizons along with promising analogues of this "potential" miracle drug. Cytosine arabinoside appears effective in herpes genitalis. More data are needed and forthcoming.

Interferon is a long known antiviral factor produced by the tissue lymphocytes of the reticuloendothelial (immunological) system, but has a species specificity.

Rifampin, mentioned before, is primarily an antibacterial but has had some success against herpes and pox viruses.

Amantadine has been used with mixed (actually little) success against viral influenza.

Pyrimidine shows some activity in negating Herpes, while *Isatin* is, at present, investigational.

Anti-Protozoan Agents

Chloroquine, one of the few medications bound intracellularly rather than to blood protein, is active against malaria, amebiasis, trypanosomiasis, leishmaniasis, giardiasis, and toxoplasmosis. Fortunately the dental profession is not involved with these maladies and they are mentioned for clarification and academic interest only.

There are few areas of dental treatment in which more acumen is desirable and less is displayed than in the application of antibiotics.

Improper choice, employment of multiple or shotgun combinations, overuse of antifungal agents, reliance on highly toxic or potentially toxic agents when safer ones will suffice, inadequate and/or prolonged period of usage, and failure to secure identification and sensitivity tests from cultures are all errors of judgment common to most practices.

Thoughtful reflection on all the ramifications of antibiotic therapy and the setting of specific goals with specific weapons should replace the helter-skelter approach which presently relies on overblown claims and inadequate or inaccurate information as a substitute for cerebration.

Reproduced without change is a chart from *The Medical Letter,* listing toxicities (and their frequencies) of most of the major and minor antibiotics, fungicides, and fungistats.[56]

PRINCIPAL ADVERSE EFFECTS OF ANTIMICROBIAL DRUGS

Adverse effects of antimicrobial drugs can vary with dosage, duration of administration, concomitant therapy, age of the patient, and the state of the patient's renal and hepatic function. The principal adverse effects of antimicrobial agents are listed in the table on page 31 [of *Medical Letter*]. It is difficult to estimate the incidence of adverse effects from published reports alone; the frequencies indicated in the table are based on the experience of Medical Letter consultants as well. Major interactions of the drugs are also listed in the table.

ALLERGIC REACTIONS — Severe allergic reactions to antimicrobial agents are most likely to occur after parenteral administration. Penicillins frequently cause delayed allergic reactions such as drug fever, skin eruptions, and serum sickness; anaphylactic reactions are rare, especially with oral administration, and particularly in children. A person allergic to one penicillin should be considered allergic to all others. Ampicillin causes maculopapular rashes more frequently than other penicillins. Although the cephalosporins are often used in patients allergic to the penicillins, such patients may have allergic reactions to cephalosporins. Other antimicrobial drugs that are likely to cause allergic reactions are demeclocycline, flucytosine, nalidixic acid, novobiocin, the sulfonamides, and trimethoprim-sulfamethoxazole.

ADVERSE EFFECTS OF ORAL ADMINISTRATION — Oral antimicrobial drugs often cause gastrointestinal disturbances such as nausea, vomiting, and diarrhea. These effects are usually dose-related and may result from irritation, superinfection, or changes in flora; they can occur with parenteral as well as oral administration. Diarrhea is especially common with tetracyclines, ampicillin, lincomycin, clindamycin, or the cephalosporins. Clindamycin and lincomycin can cause severe diarrhea and pseudomembranous colitis; other antibiotics can also occasionally cause colitis. Serious systemic adverse effects sometimes result from the absorption of "nonabsorbable" antibiotics such as neomycin; the risk of such effects is greater in infants and in patients with renal failure, though they may occur in any patient with prolonged oral administration.

SUPERINFECTIONS — Antimicrobial agents administered by any route can predispose to superinfection in the gastrointestinal tract and other organs. Superinfection is most likely when large doses are taken repeatedly or when combinations of drugs are used; it is relatively frequent with the tetracyclines and other broad-spectrum drugs. Enterocolitis caused by Staphylococcus aureus and pneumonia and sepsis caused by staphylococci, gram-negative bacilli, or Candida are among the most serious superinfections. Stomatitis, glossitis, anal itching, and vulvovaginitis associated with oral administration of antimicrobials are often caused by fungi, particularly Candida species, though fungal cultures in patients with these symptoms may be negative.

RENAL DAMAGE AND RENAL INSUFFICIENCY — Many antimicrobial agents are excreted unchanged, mainly in the urine. Others are metabolized, and the metabolites, along with some unchanged drug, are excreted in the urine or through the biliary tract. Some antimicrobials excreted mainly by the kidneys can cause renal damage, leading to accumulation of the drug in the blood and further injury to the kidneys; these include bacitracin, neomycin, vancomycin, cephaloridine, trimethoprim-sulfamethoxazole, and the sulfonamides. Most patients with impaired renal function can tolerate the usual first dose of a drug excreted mainly by the kidneys; thereafter, to minimize the risk of toxicity, total daily dosage may be reduced by increasing the interval between doses or reducing the individual dose or both (F O'Grady, Br Med Bull, 27:142, 1971; WM Bennett et al, JAMA 230:1544, 1974). For specific dosage recommendations in renal insufficiency, see page 26 [of *Medical Letter*].

PREGNANCY — Although there is no firm evidence that any antimicrobial agent is teratogenic in humans, these drugs, like drugs generally, should be prescribed for pregnant women with special caution. Griseofulvin is embryotoxic and teratogenic in rats, and is contraindicated during pregnancy. Tetracyclines administered after the fourth month can produce staining and hypoplasia of the teeth in the newborn child. Parenterally administered tetracycline has caused severe liver damage in pregnant women. Sulfonamides given near term may contribute to the development of kernicterus in the newborn.

ADVERSE EFFECTS OF ANTIMICROBIAL DRUGS

°Relatively new drug; the possibility that other adverse effects will appear is greater than with older drugs.

AMANTADINE (Symmetrel)
  Frequent: livedo reticularis and ankle edema; insomnia; dizziness; lethargy
  Occasional: depression; psychosis; confusion; congestive heart failure; orthostatic hypotension; urinary retention; GI disturbance; rash; visual disturbance; increased seizures in epilepsy
  Rare: convulsions; leukopenia; neutropenia; eczematoid dermatitis; oculogyric episodes

(INTERACTION: Hallucinations, confusion, nightmares with anticholinergics)
AMINOSALICYLIC ACID (PAS)
  Frequent: GI disturbance
  Occasional: allergic reactions; liver damage; renal irritation; blood dyscrasias; thyroid enlargement; malabsorption syndrome
  Rare: acidosis; hypokalemia; encephalopathy; vasculitis
(INTERACTION: Increased toxicity with probenecid)

°*AMOXICILLIN*—see Penicillins

AMPHOTERICIN B (Fungizone)

Frequent: renal damage; hypokalemia; fever; thrombophlebitis at site of injection

Occasional: hypomagnesemia; normocytic, normochromic anemia

Rare: hemorrhagic gastroenteritis; blood dyscrasias; rash; blurred vision; peripheral neuropathy; convulsions; anaphylaxis; arrhythmias; acute liver failure

(INTERACTIONS: Concurrent use may increase toxicity of other nephrotoxic agents, curariform drugs, and digitalis glycosides)

AMPICILLIN — see Penicillins

AMPICILLIN-PROBENECID

(Polycillin-PRB; Probampacin; Trojacillin-Plus) (Probably same as for ampicillin, except that either component can cause rashes, which therefore are likely to be more frequent)

BACITRACIN

Frequent: renal damage; local pain with IM use; GI disturbance

Occasional: blood dyscrasias; rash

(INTERACTION: Concurrent use may increase toxicity of other nephrotoxic agents)

CAPREOMYCIN (Capastat)

Occasional: renal damage; eighth-nerve damage; hypokalemia

Rare: allergic reactions; neuromuscular blockade and apnea with large IV doses, reversed by neostigmine or calcium gluconate

(INTERACTIONS: Increased toxicity with other ototoxic or nephrotoxic agents)

CARBENICILLIN — see Penicillins

CEPHALOSPORINS (cefazolin [Ancef; Kefzol]; cephalexin [Keflex]; cephaloglycin [Kafocin]; cephaloridine [Loridine]; cephalothin [Keflin]; *cephapirin [Cefadyl]; *cephradine [Anspor; Velosef])

Frequent: thrombophlebitis with IV use; serum sickness-like reaction with prolonged parenteral administration

Occasional: allergic reactions, rarely anaphylactic; GI disturbance

Rare: hemolytic anemia; hepatic dysfunction; blood dyscrasias; renal damage (especially with cephaloridine)

(INTERACTIONS: Toxic renal damage may be potentiated by concurrent use of aminoglycosides, probenecid, or rapid-acting diuretics such as furosemide or ethacrynic acid)

CHLORAMPHENICOL (Chloromycetin; and others)

Occasional: blood dyscrasias, rarely aplastic anemia, possibly leukemia; gray syndrome in infants; GI disturbance

Rare: allergic and febrile reactions; peripheral neuropathy; optic neuritis and other CNS injury.

(INTERACTIONS: Antabuse-like symptoms with alcohol; increased anticoagulant effect with dicumarol; increased hypoglycemia with sulfonylureas; increased phenytoin toxicity)

CLINDAMYCIN (Cleocin)

Frequent: diarrhea; allergic reactions

Occasional: pseudomembranous colitis, sometimes fatal

Rare: blood dyscrasias

(INTERACTION: Neuromuscular blockade with curariform drugs)

*CLOFAZIMINE (Lamprene)

Frequent: red or red-purple skin pigmentation, gray-blue pigmentation of lesions, and urine discoloration with prolonged high dosage

Occasional: epigastric distress; diarrhea; headache

COLISTIMETHATE — see Polymyxins

CYCLOSERINE (Seromycin)

Frequent: confusion; coma

Occasional: peripheral neuropathy; liver damage; malabsorption syndrome; folate deficiency

Rare: seizures; psychosis

(INTERACTION: Increased convulsions with chronic alcohol abuse)

*DAPSONE (Avlosulfon)

Frequent: rash

Occasional: blood dyscrasias including hemolytic anemia; nephrotic syndrome; liver damage

DOXYCYCLINE — see Tetracyclines

ERYTHROMYCINS (Erythrocin; and others)

Occasional: stomatitis; GI disturbance; cholestatic hepatitis with erythromycin estolate in adults

Rare: allergic reactions; transient deafness

ETHAMBUTOL (Myambutol)

Occasional: optic neuritis; allergic reactions; GI disturbance; mental confusion; precipitation of acute gout

Rare: peripheral neuritis

ETHIONAMIDE (Trecator)
 Frequent: GI disturbance
 Occasional: liver damage; CNS disturbance including peripheral neuropathy; allergic reactions; gynecomastia
 Rare: hypothyroidism; optic neuritis
 (INTERACTION: May increase hypoglycemia with sulfonylureas)
FLUCYTOSINE (Ancobon)
 Frequent: GI disturbance; rash; hepatic dysfunction; blood dyscrasias, including pancytopenia
 Occasional: confusion; hallucinations
FURAZOLIDONE (Furoxone)
 Frequent: nausea; vomiting
 Occasional: allergic reactions, including pulmonary infiltration; headache; orthostatic hypotension; hypoglycemia; polyneuritis
 Rare: hemolytic anemia in G–6PD deficiency and infants less than one month
 (INTERACTIONS: Antabuse-like reaction with alcohol; possible hypertensive crises with other monoamine oxidase inhibitors, tyramine-containing foods or beverages, sympathomimetic amines such as phenylephrine, ephedrine, and amphetamines, and with levodopa; hyperpyrexia and convulsions with tricyclic antidepressants; hyperprexia, hypertension, or hypotension and coma with meperidine)
GENTAMICIN (Garamycin)
 Occasional: vestibular damage; renal damage; rash
 Rare: auditory damage; neuromuscular blockade and apnea, reversible with calcium or neostigmine
 (INTERACTIONS: Increased nephrotoxicity with cephalosporins, polymyxins; ototoxicity with ethacrynic acid; neuromuscular blockade with curariform drugs)
GRISEOFULVIN (Fulvicin-U/F; and others)
 Occasional: GI disturbance; allergic and photosensitivity reactions
 Rare: proteinuria; blood dyscrasias; mental confusion; paresthesias
 (INTERACTION: Decreased anticoagulant effect with warfarin)
*HYDROXYSTILBAMIDINE (Hydroxystilbamidine isethionate)
 Frequent: hypotension; vomiting; renal damage
 Occasional: liver damage; neuropathies

ISONIAZID
 Occasional: peripheral neuropathy; glossitis and GI disturbance; liver damage, particularly in patients more than 35 years old; allergic reactions; fever
 Rare: blood dyscrasias; psychosis; optic neuritis; hyperglycemia; folate and B_6 deficiency; pellagra-like rash; keratitis; lupus erythematosus-like syndrome
 (INTERACTIONS: Psychotic episodes, ataxia with disulfiram (Antabuse); enhances toxicity of phenytoin; increased incidence of hepatitis with alcohol; diminished isoniazid effect in some patients with chronic alcohol abuse)
KANAMYCIN (Kantrex)
 Occasional: eighth-nerve damage affecting mainly hearing that may be irreversible and may not be detected until after therapy has been stopped (most likely with renal impairment); renal damage
 Rare: rash; fever; peripheral neuritis; parenteral or intraperitoneal administration may produce neuromuscular blockade and apnea, not reversed by neostigmine
 (INTERACTIONS: Increased nephrotoxicity with cephalosporins, polymyxins; ototoxicity with other ototoxic drugs, ethacrynic acid, furosemide, or other rapid-acting diuretics; neuromuscular blockade with curariform drugs)
LINCOMYCIN (Lincocin)
 Frequent: diarrhea, sometimes progressing to severe pseudomembranous colitis
 Occasional: allergic reactions, rarely anaphylactic
 Rare: blood dyscrasias; hypotension with rapid IV injection
 (INTERACTION: Neuromuscular blockade with curariform drugs)
METHENAMINE MANDELATE (Mandelamine; and others) and METHENAMINE
HIPPURATE (Hiprex; Urex)
 Occasional: GI disturbance; dysuria; allergic reactions
*METHISAZONE (Marboran)
 Frequent: severe vomiting; nausea; anorexia
 Occasional: diarrhea; transient fluid retention; allergic reactions
 Rare: hyperbilirubinemia
 (INTERACTION: Increased adverse effects with alcohol)

MINOCYCLINE — see Tetracyclines

NALIDIXIC ACID (NegGram)

Frequent: GI disturbance; rash; visual disturbance

Occasional: CNS disturbance; acute intracranial hypertension in young children; photosensitivity reactions, sometimes persistent; convulsions

Rare: cholestatic jaundice; blood dyscrasias; arthralgia or arthritis

(INTERACTION: Increased effect of oral anticoagulants)

NEOMYCIN

Occasional: eighth-nerve and renal damage, same as with kanamycin but hearing loss may be more frequent and severe and may occur with oral, intraarticular, or topical use; GI disturbance; malabsorption with oral use; contact dermatitis with topical use

Rare: neuromuscular blockade and apnea that may be reversed by intravenous neostigmine or calcium gluconate

(INTERACTIONS: Increased nephrotoxicity with other nephrotoxic drugs; increased ototoxicity with ethacrynic acid and other ototoxic drugs; neuromuscular blockage with curariform drugs)

NITROFURANTOIN (Furadantin; and others)

Frequent: GI disturbance

Occasional: allergic reactions, including pulmonary infiltration and a lupus-erythematosus syndrome; blood dyscrasias; hemolytic anemia; peripheral neuropathy, sometimes severe

Rare: cholestatic jaundice

NOVOBIOCIN (Albamycin)

Frequent: cholestatic jaundice; allergic reactions; GI disturbance; neonatal hyperbilirubinemia

Occasional: severe blood dyscrasias

NYSTATIN (Mycostatin; Nilstat)

Occasional: allergic reactions; GI disturbance

OXOLINIC ACID (Utibid)

Frequent: CNS disturbance; nausea

Occasional: GI disturbance; anorexia; pruritus

Rare: allergic reactions; blood dyscrasias; photophobia

(INTERACTION: May increase effect of oral anticoagulants)

PENICILLINS (amoxicillin [Amoxil, Larotid, Polymox]; ampicillin [Polycillin; and others]; carbenicillin [Geocillin, Geopen, Pyopen]; cloxacillin [Tegopen]; dicloxacillin [Dynapen, Pathocil, Veracillin]; hetacillin [Versapen]; methicillin [Celbenin, Staphcillin]; nafcillin [Unipen]; oxacillin [Bactocill, Prostaphlin]; penicillin G, penicillin V, phenethicillin [Maxipen, Syncillin])

Frequent: allergic reactions, rarely anaphylactic; rash (more common with ampicillin than with other penicillins); diarrhea (most common with ampicillin)

Occasional: hemolytic anemia

Rare: muscle irritability and seizures, usually after high doses in patients with impaired renal function; renal damage; hyperkalemia and arrhythmias with IV potassium penicillin G given rapidly; bleeding diathesis; granulocytopenia or agranulocytosis with semisynthetic penicillins; pseudomembranous colitis with ampicillin; hepatic damage with semi-synthetic penicillins; abnormal behavior and neurological reactions with high doses of procaine penicillin G; hypokalemic alkalosis and/or sodium overload with high doses of carbenicillin; platelet dysfunction with carbenicillin

POLYMYXINS (colistimethate [ColyMycin]; polymyxin B [Aerosporin, Polymyxin B])

Occasional: renal damage; peripheral neuropathy; thrombophlebitis at IV injection site with polymyxin B

Rare: allergic reactions; neuromuscular blockade and apnea with parenteral administration, not reversed by neostigmine but may be by IV calcium chloride

(INTERACTIONS: Increased nephrotoxicity with aminoglycosides; neuromuscular blockade with curariform drugs)

PYRAZINAMIDE (Pyrazinamide)

Occasional: liver damage; hyperuricemia; GI disturbance

Rare: photosensitivity reactions

RIFAMPIN (Rifadin; Rimactane)

Occasional: liver damage; GI disturbance; allergic reactions

Rare: flu-like syndrome, sometimes

with thrombocytopenia, hemolytic anemia, and renal failure, particularly with intermittent therapy (INTERACTIONS: Decreased effect of oral anticoagulants; decreased effect of oral contraceptives; toxicity enhanced by probenecid)

*RIFAMPIN-ISONIAZID (Rifamate; Rimactazid) — see individual drugs (Although both drugs are hepatotoxic, it appears that hepatotoxicity is no greater than with isoniazid alone)

SPECTINOMYCIN (Trobicin)
Occasional: urticaria; dizziness; nausea; chills and fever; insomnia

STREPTOMYCIN
Frequent: eighth-nerve damage (mainly vestibular), sometimes permanent; paresthesias; rash; fever
Occasional: pruritus; anaphylaxis; renal damage
Rare: blood dyscrasias; neuromuscular blockade and apnea with parenteral administration, usually reversed by neostigmine; optic neuritis; hepatic necrosis; myocarditis
(INTERACTIONS: Increased nephrotoxicity with cephaloridine, cephalothin, polymyxins; ototoxicity with ethacrynic acid; neuromuscular blockade with curariform drugs)

SULFONAMIDES
Frequent: allergic reactions (rash, photosensitivity and drug fever)
Occasional: kernicterus in newborn; renal damage; liver damage; Stevens-Johnson syndrome (particularly with long-acting sulfonamides); hemolytic anemia; other blood dyscrasias; vasculitis
(INTERACTIONS [long/acting]: Increased effect of oral anticoagulants; increased hypoglycemia with sulfonylureas)

TETRACYCLINES (chlortetracycline [Aureomycin]; demeclocycline [Declomycin]; doxycycline [Vibramycin; and others]; methacycline [Rondomycin]; minocycline [Minocin; Vectrin]; oxytetracycline [Terramycin; and others]; tetracycline hydrochloride [Achromycin; and others])
Frequent: GI disturbance; bone lesions and staining and deformity of teeth in children up to 12 years old, and in the newborn when given to pregnant women after the fourth month of pregnancy

Occasional: malabsorption; enterocolitis; photosensitivity reactions (most frequent with demeclocycline); vestibular reactions with minocycline; increased azotemia with renal insufficiency (except doxycycline); parenteral doses may cause serious liver damage, especially in pregnant women and patients with renal disease receiving 1 gram or more daily
Rare: allergic reactions; blood dyscrasias; increased intracranial pressure in infants; fixed-drug eruptions; diabetes insipidus with demeclocycline
(INTERACTIONS: Nephrotoxicity with methoxyflurane; decreased tetracycline effects with oral antacids, iron; decreased doxycycline effects with barbiturates, carbamazepine)

*TOBRAMYCIN (Nebcin)
(Probably same as with gentamicin)

TRIMETHOPRIMSULFAMETHOXAZOLE (Bactrim; Septra) (Same as sulfonamides, but possibly higher incidence of hematologic reactions and renal damage)

TROLEANDOMYCIN (Cyclamycin; TAO)
Occasional: stomatitis; GI disturbance; cholestatic jaundice
Rare: allergic reactions

VANCOMYCIN (Vancocin)
Frequent: thrombophlebitis; chills, fever
Occasional: renal damage; eighth-nerve damage (mainly hearing) especially with large or continued doses (more than 10 days), in presence of renal damage, and in the elderly
Rare: peripheral neuropathy; urticaria
(INTERACTION: Increased toxicity with other ototoxic or nephrotoxic agents)

VIOMYCIN (Viocin; Viomycin)
Frequent: eighth-nerve damage (vestibular and hearing) with large or continued doses (more than 10 days) or in presence of renal damage
Occasional: rash; renal damage; electrolyte disturbances
(INTERACTIONS: Increased toxicity with other ototoxic and nephrotoxic agents; neuromuscular blockade with curariform drugs)

ANTICHOLINERGIC DRUGS (BELLADONNA ALKALOIDS, ETC.)

Atropine and scopolamine are the most important of the parasympatholytic group, which includes hyoscyamine and the synthetics Tral, Banthine, and Pro-Banthine. They enjoy wide use in medicine for treating a varied and long list of maladies, including cardiopathies, parkinsonism, gastric dysfunction, intestinal spasm, and mydriasis. They are antidotal in combating excessive actions of some other drugs, including the respiratory depression of morphine and the barbiturates.

In dental practice, atropine, a CNS excitant, is employed as an antisialagogue in conjunction with local analgesics and to diminish secretions in the nasopharynx and the bronchial tree, which reduces the hazard of aspiration in the unconscious anesthetized patient. Scopolamine, a CNS depressant, has stronger antisecretory properties and in addition produces drowsiness, euphoria, and amnesia. Comparison would seem to place scopolamine above atropine in desirable qualities, and this would be true if it were not for the paradoxical effects — excitement, hallucinations, and delirium — often seen after scopolamine administration.

Serious toxicity to either drug is seldom experienced, even though the symptoms of poisoning with agents of this group are very violent. Dysphagia, great thirst, visual disturbance, flushing of face, neck, and chest, rise in temperature, tachycardia, and delirious excitement followed by giddiness and stupor are recorded. Despite this formidable array of toxic effects, most victims recover without sequelae. Atropine and scopolamine usually are contraindicated for use in patients with glaucoma because of their mydriatic and cycloplegic actions. Increase in the intraocular pressure may lead to rupture or damage of the eyeball. Atropine causes tachycardia by blocking vagal inhibitory action on the heart, and this is undesirable in some cardiac conditions. These drugs are always prescribed with caution to geriatric patients, for in their age bracket appear most of the ailments which restrict the use of the belladonna alkaloids.

Cholinergic Drugs (Pilocarpine, etc.)

The parasympathomimetic or cholinergic agents, methacholine, carbachol, and bethanechol, are potent drugs whose medical uses are restricted to conditions which demand rather drastic treatment, such as postoperative urinary retention, ileus, and delayed gastric emptying after vagotomy.

Pilocarpine, probably the weakest member of this group, is sometimes used in dentistry as a sialagogue. It very effectively combats the dry mouth experienced by many patients who are taking ganglionic blocking agents (veriloid, apresoline) for the treatment of hypertension. Besides xerostomia, which often prohibits denture wearing and drastically interferes with mastication and deglutition, other distressing complaints are constipation, dryness of the eyes, and difficulty in micturition. Pilocarpine overcomes all these symptoms and may be given orally. Its toxic manifestations are essentially the opposite of the ganglionic blockers, and include sweating, lacrimation, salivation, urinary urgency, and incipient pulmonary edema. Consultation with the patient's physician is desirable when the dental doctor considers this treatment for any "dry-mouth" patient.

STIMULANTS AND ANALEPTICS

Amphetamine (Benzedrine)

This drug and its family, including dextroamphetamine (Dexedrine) and methamphetamine (Desoxyn and Methedrine [speed]), probably are the most improperly used products in the entire formulary. To improve the mood or relieve the outward manifestations of depression in mildly disturbed patients is their primary mission. Occasionally they are indicated to temporarily curb the appetite (anorexia) in some obese patients or to induce wakefulness in others. They also have some value as a respiratory stimulant in barbiturate poisoning. But gross misuse and the toxic ramifications thereof have caused the beneficial effects of the amphetamines to be accepted with diminishing fervor when their potential for harm is considered.

Toxicity to large or continued dosages is rapid and severe. Symptoms include insomnia, hallucinations, mania, hyperpyrexia, and convulsions, which if persistent and unrelieved may lead to death. Subtle or less dramatic toxic manifestations are the loss of sound judgment (which in auto and truck drivers has precipitated many fatal accidents) and interference with reasoning ability and intelligence. This interference can delude a person on "pep-pills" ("uppers") into believing that all is well in life when in reality it is not. The possible tragic consequences of such an attitude can well be imagined. The last but not least danger is that amphetamines are habituating, and the number of addicts is large, growing, and widespread throughout the country.

Diphenylmethanes

These cerebral or psychic stimulants, although related to amphetamine, are much milder in function with greatly reduced toxicity. Meratran and Ritalin are known in dental practice and may be employed with less hazard than most other stimulants. Hyperexcitability, some irritability, and insomnia are the undesirable but not usually dangerous toxic effects which may appear in some patients.

Often mentioned or suggested as an antidote for barbiturate or other drug depression states, Ritalin is slow and so mild as to be relatively tepid for real analeptic action. However, it is also mild in toxicity rating and may be expedient as a mood elevator.

Diphenylhydantoin (Dilantin Sodium)

This agent is the best of a large group of anticonvulsants prescribed to control epilepsy and other similar disorders. It may also be used occasionally in cardiac patients to control arrhythmias. Since this convulsive dysfunction is fairly common, a dental article should find a niche, however small, for information concerning Dilantin and similar drugs used in grand mal patients. Surprisingly, these anticonvulsant agents do not ordinarily becloud the mind or depress cortical activity, but all exhibit some toxic reactions in the CNS at normal dose levels, and excessive doses yield incapacitation with frightening symptoms. Ataxia, blurred vision, nystagmus, hyperreflexia, lethargy, and coma, along with mental aberrations, degenerative epithelial changes, visceral dysfunction, and blood dyscrasias, are the general toxic manifestations which may arise subject to excessive or prolonged ingestion of Dilantin. There are fortunately no apparent incompatibilities with other agents which could precipitate an acute crisis in a dental office, although an increase in CNS excitation originating from apprehension to the forthcoming procedure could trigger a seizure. Another toxic factor important from the dental standpoint is the frequent, often gross and obstructive hyperplasia of the alveolar gingival tissues found in patients on long-term Dilantin therapy.

Caffeine

Belonging to the xanthine group, caffeine is certainly the world's premier stimulant, and the safest, too! Appearing naturally in coffee, tea, and cocoa, it is also available in tablet and injectable form with sodium benzoate. Regardless of the method of assimilation, it stimulates all parts of the CNS to produce alertness, wakefulness, and talkativeness. Other effects, which may or may not be desirable, depending on the patient, are increase in respiration and diuresis. Toxicity is seldom a problem, but restlessness, irritability, and insomnia can be dangerous in some patients.

Hydrazines

The hydrazines or monoamine oxidase inhibitors often are listed with the stimulants but have wide ranging effects in other areas. Isocarboxazid (Marplan) is the only popular, relatively nontoxic drug in this group at this time. It has little, if any, use in dentistry. (See Tranquilizer section.)

Bemegride (Megimide)

Bemegride was introduced as an antagonist of the barbiturates, via competitive inhibition, but this virtue has yet to be proved. Present evidence indicates that it stimulates respiration and other neural functions by mechanisms similar to older analeptics, but is milder and less toxic. As with most CNS stimulants, overdose yields convulsions.

Ethamivan (Emivan)

Touted mainly as a stimulant useful in hypoventilatory states associated with chronic pulmonary disease, Emivan may be employed for general respiratory stimulation when such an agent is called for. Although this drug has a good margin of safety, it is a convulsant in large doses.

Doxapram (Dopram)

This agent is a promising respiratory stimulant of low toxicity. It is unique in that the dose required for respiratory stimulation is below that necessary to evoke excessive cerebral cortical activity.

PSYCHOTOMIMETICS

Damned by the majority on definition alone — psychoto (deep, far-reaching, prolonged mental disorders), mimetic (to mimic or simulate) — these black sheep in the drug family are unfortunately popular enough to demand attention. They require space in this text on the strength of the unpredictable nature of the interactions possible when patients experimenting with these potent agents are given common dental prescriptions. To avoid unpleasant, frightening, or possibly violent incidents, it is wise to postpone treatment of any kind for those who are known or suspected "users" of (1) lysergic acid diethylamide, (2) cannabis, (3) mescaline, or (4) psilocybin.

Lysergic Acid Diethylamide

LSD is a synthetic and the most potent hallucinogen. Its only legitimate use has been in experimental psychiatry. It is thought to obtain its profound effects from an antagonistic action on serotonin and the direct effect of an unusual amine.

Toxicities are broad and not well established, but persistent psychoses and chromosomal damage are evident in chronic users.

Cannabis

Marijuana has become a household word. The mountains of publicity it has garlanded have not been adverse enough to suit this author. The bevy of entertainers and some highly placed members of the academic world who dismiss its harmfulness, condone it, or jest about its illegal use have brought a modicum of respectability to this prostitute of the drug family.

Its alleged psychological benefits must be weighed against its acknowledged destruction or disruption of the will to excel or even to compete in our society, and against mounting evidence of insidious pathosis.

In the frantic search by its advocates for virtues to legitimize its use, only one positive aspect has presented. Tetrahydrocannabinol, the active chemical ingredient, has, in some cases, successfully counteracted the nausea caused by antimetabolites and other chemotherapeutic agents used in therapy for malignant tumors.

Mescaline (Peyote)

Mescaline is obtained from the mescal cactus. The dried buttons when ingested produce a stuporous state accompanied by brilliant visual hallucinations.

Toxicity is thought to be low, but little is known at this time owing to lack of data.

Psilocybin (Mexican Mushrooms)

Psilocybin resembles LSD, but seems much milder in all respects.

HORMONES (NATURAL)

Hormones are substances secreted by the ductless glands which regulate most body processes. The natural hormones have a multitude of effects, many of which at this time are not well understood.

Hypothyroidism (myxedema), hypoinsulinism (diabetes), and hypopituitarism (dwarfism) are examples of diseases which result from inadequate production of hormones by the thyroid, pancreas and pituitary glands. In other conditions, the endocrine glands, although normal, do not secrete enough hormone to meet the extra demands the body makes in its efforts to overcome severe stresses. An example is the use of norepinephrine and epinephrine in the alleviation or reversal of shock.

One may well question the necessity or desirability of including these exotic drugs in a dental treatise. It should be unnecessary to remind the reader that an inordinate number of patients who present for dental treatment may be on thyroxin for weight loss, estrogens for menopausal disorders, progesterones for menstrual and associated disorders, and oxytocin (posterior pituitary extract) in pregnancy complications.

Patients with Addison's disease may need supplemental vasopressor therapy. Asthmatics may require control with these same agents. Such patients must be carefully evaluated before stressful dental procedures are attempted; otherwise, toxic conditions may be precipitated which are exceedingly difficult to control or reverse. These include gastrointestinal distress and cramps, uterine bleeding, tachycardia, retention of electrolytes and water, and skin disturbances.

HORMONES (SYNTHETIC)

The cortisone derivatives are used extensively in many therapeutic situations. At present they are for the most part synthetic in origin, diverse, often obscure in action, transitory rather than curative in nature, and *potent*! These agents are capable of producing dramatic temporary improvement, but rarely permanent relief, from many afflictions.

One fundamental action of cortisone is its ability to suppress the inflammatory and immunologic responses of the body. This requisite is the basis of most of the clinical applications of cortisone and related drugs. Its use in therapy for various dermatoses, arthritis and allied collagen diseases, and allergic manifestations is particularly widespread. Anti-inflammatory and antiallergic actions of corticosteroids include reduction of the exudation of leukocytes and plasma constituents, maintenance of cell membrane integrity, inhibition of lysozyme release from granulocytes, other modes of phagocytosis inhibition, and stabilization of intracellular lysosomal membranes. Glucocorticoids inhibit amino-acid transport into muscle and reduce new protein synthesis. Cortisol, the natural hormone secreted by the adrenal cortex, is required for liver gluconeogenesis utilizing amino acids. All the corticosteroids tend to cause hypokalemia by increasing urinary losses of potassium. Effects of glucocorticoids on the central nervous system and on blood cells are notable and sometimes deleterious.

On the question or category of allergy, now is the proper time to place the corticosteroids in correct perspective for the step-by-step treatment of an-

ORAL GLUCOCORTICOIDS

Drug	Anti-inflam-matory Potency	Mineralocorti-coid Potency	Equivalent Doses
Cortisone	0.8	0.8	25 mg
Cortone (Merck)			
Cortisone Acetate (Upjohn)			
Hydrocortisone	1.0	1.0	20 mg
Cortef (Upjohn)			
Hydrocortone (Merck)			
Prednisolone	4.0	0.8	5 mg
Delta-Cortef (Upjohn)			
Fernisolone (Ferndale)			
Prednicen (Central)			
Prednis (USV)			
Sterane (Pfizer)			
Prednisone	4.0	0.8	5 mg
Delta-Dome (Dome)			
Deltasone (Upjohn)			
Fernisone (Ferndale)			
Keysone (Hyrex-Key)			
Lisacort (Fellows-Testagar)			
Meticorten (Schering)			
Orasone (Rowell)			
Paracort (Parke, Davis)			
Pred-5 (Saron)			
Servisone (Lederle)			
Sterapred (Mayrand)			
Meprednisone	4.0	0	4 mg
Betapar (Parke, Davis)			
Methylprednisolone	5.0	0	4 mg
Medrol (Upjohn)			
Triamcinolone	5.0	0	4 mg
Aristocort (Lederle)			
Kenacort (Squibb)			
Paramethasone	10.0	0	2 mg
Haldrone (Lilly)			
Stemex (Syntex)			
Fluprednisolone	15.0	0	1.5 mg
Alphadrol (Upjohn)			
Dexamethasone	25.0	0	0.75 mg
Decadron (Merck)			
Deronil (Schering)			
Dexameth (USV)			
Dexone (Rowell)			
Gammacorten (Ciba)			
Hexadrol (Organon)			
Betamethasone	25.0	0	0.6 mg
Celestone (Schering)			

aphylaxis and other emergency situations. Contrary to many articles and popular opinion, steroids are too slow-acting to be life-saving in acute episodes, and are the last drugs administered in emergency procedures. Although essential in combating immunologic reactions and regaining homeostasis, they are virtually ineffective in those first precious moments of crisis. Deviation from this concept could cost a life.

Even discounting the multitude of patients ingesting steroid preparations as a regimen for the control of inflammatory symptoms, the escalating number of dental nostrums featuring hormones is sufficient reason for the clinician to be acutely aware of the potency of these agents.

The list of natural and synthetic steroids is vast, but the actions and the toxicity of virtually all closely approximate those of cortisone.

Mineralocorticoids

Used in adrenocortical insufficiency states (Addison's disease, etc.) and salt losing adrenogenital syndrome, deoxycorticosterone acetate (DOCA) is the only pure mineralocorticoid, with fluorocortisone (Florinef) not far behind.

They are employed in close conjunction with glucocorticoids, glucose, fluid and electrolyte control, and antibiotics (in case of infection) in order to retain hormonal and physiologic balance in the patient. The general principles of corticosteroid therapy are as follows:

1. Use only for an established diagnosis and when less harmful therapies have failed.
2. Use the smallest therapeutically effective dose.
3. Use alternate-day therapy whenever possible.
4. Teach patients about the need for higher steroid doses during stress. Procedures for cessation of therapy are recommended.

TOXICITY

Cortisone and other steroids can and do mask the objective and subjective symptoms of serious infections until they become unmanageable — conceivably to the point of extremis. Because of toxic influence on the CNS, steroids may initiate psychotic behavior in patients with a basic predisposition in this direction. Cortisone-induced disturbances in metabolism and electrolyte balance may produce osteoporosis in bone and lead to pathologic fractures.

In the presence of diseases in which body defenses are essential, such as tuberculosis and peptic ulcer, cortisone and other steroids are contraindicated. Simulated Cushing's syndrome (recognized by the following symptoms: moon face, acne, facial hirsutism, edema, weakness, and depression) often appears in patients during a course of hormone therapy. Fortunately, this syndrome is reversible and the signs disappear when treatment is discontinued.

Prolonged cortisone ingestion usually results in adrenal atrophy which may persist for six months *or longer* after the drug is discontinued. This factor is of prime importance when general anesthetics are indicated for dental treatment. A crisis during the anesthetic period may precipitate a state of acute adrenocorticotropic insufficiency with a fatal termination.

VITAMINS

Seemingly innocuous and out of place in a chapter on toxicity, this group of drugs may qualify as the most used, most abused, and least understood of all the common therapeutic agents. Although relatively simple organic compounds which are essential nutrients required for normal metabolism, some vitamins are highly toxic in large and extended doses. This attribute is especially true of A and D and to some extent the other fat-soluble vitamins because they can be stored in the body. In contrast, the water-soluble vitamins, B complex and C, are rapidly excreted and exhibit minimal, if any, harmful effects.

Vitamin A

The fat-soluble lipochromes, alpha, beta, and gamma carotene and cryptoxanthin, occur naturally in plants and animal tissues and are converted into vitamin A in the intestinal mucosa and liver.

Vitamin A has a marked antikeratinizing effect on epithelial tissue and has been suggested for use in oral troches to treat leukoplakia. The therapy period is long, two to six months, but results appear to be promising, and no toxicity has been reported. However, the small number of patients involved in this particular research project precludes acceptance of the value of vitamin A for this specific application until more data are available.

Dosage above the normal may be required in steatorrhea, hepatic disease, or intestinal inflammation, but overdosage in the healthy patient produces hypervitaminosis, which is characterized by anorexia, irritability, pruritus, alopecia, cracked lips, hepatomegaly, and periosteal thickening.

Vitamin D

This fat-soluble vitamin occurs naturally in plant and animal tissues, usually in the form of a precursor, ergosterol or 7-dehydrocholesterol. These precursors are converted to the active form by ultraviolet light.

Large doses often yield severe toxic disturbances by increasing the renal excretion of phosphorus and the intestinal absorption of calcium, thereby upsetting the normal Ca-P balance in the body. This results in the mobilization of calcium from osseous structures, causing rarefaction and soft spots in the bone and calcification in the muscles and kidneys. This metastatic calcification in vital organs is a dangerous and sometimes irreversible condition.

Vitamin E

Another fat-soluble vitamin occurring naturally as alpha-tocopherol in plant and animal tissues, vitamin E has been linked to the fertility factor in animals. Despite the fact that lack of E results in germinal atrophy and defective development in some animals, its performance in humans is indefinite and equivocal.

There is no available evidence that overdosage can or does produce toxic effects.

Vitamin K

This liquid-soluble vitamin occurs naturally as naphthoquinines in plant and animal tissues, and is synthesized as menadione and phytonadione salts, which are water soluble. These analogs are known commercially as Hykinone, Synkayvite, and Mephyton. Since vitamin K promotes the formation of prothrombin in the liver, its use is mainly in blood coagulant therapy when hypoprothrombinemia is a factor and in negating or controlling coumarin effects in patients with vascular disease.

It is directly toxic to premature infants, producing jaundice and fatal kernicterus in large doses, and indirectly toxic when it interferes with controlled anticoagulant therapy in adult patients.

B Complex Vitamins

This group of water-soluble vitamins includes thiamine, niacrin, riboflavin, pyridoxine, pantothenic acid, and biotin. Except for pantothenic acid and biotin, these are important agents in the maintenance of oral health. Further description is superfluous here, other than the citing of harmful effects.

The toxicity of the B vitamins is nil, even in extreme overdoses, but thiamine occasionally elicits an allergic response of low magnitude, and in large doses a ganglionic-blocking action with resultant hypotension is possible. Niacin may produce a transient vasodilatation causing flushed or hyperemic areas on the skin.

Vitamin C

This water-soluble vitamin (ascorbic acid) occurs naturally in plant and animal tissues and has been synthesized since 1932. Probably the single most important vitamin in the maintenance of oral soft tissue health, vitamin C cannot be stored by the body and should be ingested daily.

Serious toxic reactions have never been reported from ascorbic acid, regardless of the state of the patient's health or the size of the dose. Dr. Pauling's well publicized theories on the role of Vitamin C in the prevention of common colds are at this date still in doubt. An intensive and extensive study by a team from the University of Pittsburgh (1976–77) has negated most of Pauling's theory. Another problem, reported in J.A.M.A. 237 (8):768, 1977, concerns the increase in urinary oxalate which can and does lead to the formation of uroliths (urinary tract stones). The possibility of oxalate stones is always a consideration in users of excessive amounts (approximately 1 gm or more daily) of Vitamin C.

Fluorine-Vitamin Compounds

These compounds are becoming extremely popular as a safe, simple method for ingestion of fluorides in areas where natural water content of fluorine is nonexistent or insufficient to help control dental caries. At this printing, toxic effects, local or systemic, have not emerged or been reported.

ENZYMES

Enzymes are relatively new but assiduously promoted by many manufacturers, and as a result are increasingly employed in the practice of dentistry.

Hyaluronidase, streptokinase-streptodornase, papase, trypsin and chymotrypsin are the important enzymes and enjoy the widest use. Although they may seem quite innocuous by nature and physiologic in action, it should be remembered that because some are derived in most part from animal tissue and bacteria, they are capable of producing foreign-protein anaphylaxis. They also may be instrumental in the spread of infection by breaking down natural body defenses. Persistent, unexplained hyperpyrexia is a new phenomenon associated with long-term enzyme therapy. Leukocytosis is assumed to be an etiologic factor in this temporary and reversible condition. One must struggle to make a good case for their use in dental practice.

ANTACIDS

This classification of drugs should be mentioned because of the gross quantities consumed by the general public to allay ulcer pain and to relieve functional indigestion. These drugs fall into two main groups: the inorganic alkaline salts and the insoluble buffered salts.

The inorganic alkaline salts are represented by $NaHCO_3$, $CaCO_3$, and MgO, only one of which is toxic enough to cause concern. Sodium bicarbonate, while effective and rapid in action, produces rebound acidity and, with overuse, alkalosis.

The insoluble buffered salts are commonly called gels: aluminum hydroxide (Amphogel), aluminum phosphate (Phosphaljel), and mixtures of magnesium hydroxide (Maalox) are the well known products in this category. Their toxic potential is very low, thereby casting them in the favored role for long-term antacid therapy.

VACCINES

The use of vaccines, while in the embryonic stage, is becoming a useful modality in dental medicine.

Herpes simplex virus causes some of the most aggravating and painful lesions known to man. Autogenous vaccines and vaccinia (smallpox) vaccine are often employed in the treatment of herpetic infections, and the results have been encouraging. Tetanus antitoxin and/or toxoid should be a part of the rationale of therapy for puncture wounds of the face and oral cavity or when severe trauma causes gross contamination of this area by dirt and debris. But, as is the case with all foreign protein substances, injection may elicit a toxic response.

All the signs and symptoms of severe histamine poisonings, cutaneous flushing, dizziness, nausea, fainting, tachycardia, vascular hypotension, and asthma, may occur from the injection of these sera or vaccines. In addition, urticaria is a frequent complaint. The delayed reaction, five to seven days later, features joint and muscle pain.

GERMICIDES, DISINFECTANTS, AND ANTISEPTICS

Germicides which kill bacteria, disinfectants which either kill or render organisms inert, and antiseptics which prevent further growth are all employed, sometimes ignorantly, in dental offices to reduce the pathogen population on equipment, instruments, and living tissues. The very nature and purpose of this group of drugs ensures their toxicity, in varying degrees, to all viable cells. Many of these agents — phenol, mercurials, boric acid, and iodine — are highly poisonous and cause severe local or general symptoms when applied to the skin or when they are ingested by other routes, whereas Zephiran, pHisoHex and peroxide usually are quite benign in normal situations.

Phenol

Phenol or carbolic acid and related phenolic compounds should merit consideration in any discussion of drug toxicity. Creosote, eugenol, guaiacol, thymol, resorcinol, "Campho-Phenique," and other mixtures of phenolic compounds are often subjected to vigorous and indiscriminate use in dentistry with apparently little thought being given to the possible consequences of such use. Usually, phenol et al. have a self-limiting penetration when applied topically, but deep placement in the bone or soft tissues (e.g., root canal therapy, drains, and bone packing for deep seated infections) may result in serious toxicity. An early symptom of mild systemic poisoning is dark-colored urine. Moderate poisoning may produce delirium, then convulsions, collapse, and unconsciousness. With severe systemic toxicity, there is cerebral edema, cardiac dilatation, degeneration of the kidneys, and necrosis of the liver. Ordinarily, fatal or severe poisoning results only from oral ingestion of fairly large amounts, and local application produces little more than surface tissue necrosis. However, there are cases on record where the application of small amounts to the epithelium have resulted in some or all of the gross toxic manifestations listed above.

Organic Mercurial Compounds

Three of the oldest and best known antiseptics are in this class — Metaphen, Merthiolate, and Mercurochrome. Despite their popularity, these drugs are at best only bacteriostatic, and their real worth has long been suspect and the subject of much controversy. Then, too, mercury causes toxic effects in many people, and in severe cases can be grossly destructive to both soft tissue and bone. Therefore, in patients who are sensitive to mercury, the use of these compounds should be avoided.

Iodine

The USP tincture and other iodine preparations are ordinarily rapid and efficient in disinfecting tissues. However, iodine, especially the alcoholic (and some aqueous) solutions, frequently causes acute pain and irritation when applied to abraded areas. Inflammatory changes at the wound edges interfere with healing and may produce adhesions or other cicatricial changes.

Iodophors

These are aqueous complexes of iodine usually combined with a detergent (povidone, etc.) to produce potent surgical scrubs (Betadine, Septodyne, Prepodyne, etc.) of low irritation to the skin and high activity against both gram-positive and gram-negative bacteria.

Alcohol (Isopropyl and Ethyl)

Seventy per cent is the most effective strength but is quickly vaporized and is drying to human tissues. It is an acceptable temporary antiseptic agent only for its activity against gram-positive and gram-negative bacteria.

Chlorhexidine

Hibiclens is a new preparation which promises to be the most effective yet. It covers the same range as the iodines but is quicker and longer lasting in action. In a recent study, it was significantly more effective than other preparations and there was no irritation.

Chlorhexidine resembles the iodophors in activity against gram-negative and gram-positive bacteria but has the added advantage of cumulative or persistent action in the skin, while the iodophors dry the integument!

Boric Acid

This old standby drug, despite its prevalent use, is vigorously condemned as worthless from a therapeutic standpoint by many of our leading pharmacologists. Boric acid may be absorbed from mucous membranes and denuded areas, and, because it is neither irritating nor painful to the tissues, many people consider it to be innocuous and apply the powder or solution in gross quantities. Nothing could be further from the truth, because boric acid is one of the most toxic of all the drugs in use today. In reviewing the literature, the Goldblooms (1953) found 55 per cent mortality in 109 cases of boric acid poisoning. The usual toxic symptoms are vomiting, diarrhea, rash and desquamation of the skin, hypothermia, hematuria, and signs of meningeal irritation. Regression may end at any of these stages, but unless the trend is reversed, circulatory collapse ensues, leading to a fatal termination.

Hydrogen Peroxide

This familiar nostrum in the pure form, and as the active agent in Sodium Perborate and other proprietary compounds, is found in most dental offices. It oxidizes organic matter and loosens debris and pus by effervescence during the release of nascent oxygen. It is claimed to be highly germicidal, but the action is fleeting or transient.

Toxicity is not a real problem, but extended use of this drug often results in a rebound effect which aggravates rather than relieves the tissue symptoms.

Benzalkonium Chloride (Zephiran)

This was once the best and at the same time the least toxic of all the cold sterilizing agents. It has detergent, keratolytic, and emulsifying actions; therefore, soap is unnecessary prior to its application to instruments or tissues. In fact, soap film will negate or reduce Zephiran's disinfectant power.

Toxicity is negligible when this drug is properly used. Its major drawback is its ineffectiveness against some gram-negative bacilli, especially *Pseudomonas aeruginosa* (common in hospitals and offices) and tubercle bacilli.

Hexachlorophene (pHisoHex)

This drug is used primarily in detergent soaps or creams for preparation of a surgical area and as a preoperative scrub agent for the surgeon's hands. It is active mainly against gram-positive organisms. Some toothpastes now contain this agent. Dermatoses have been noted subsequent to its use, but these are thought to be largely the fault of the detergent.

Silver Salts

Silver nitrate and Argyrol are venerable bacteriostatic agents which have largely been replaced by newer, better, and less toxic drugs.

TOOTHPASTES AND MOUTHWASHES

Before this chapter is ended, a brief comment on toothpastes and mouthwashes is in order.

Since practically all of these compounds contain a detergent and a flavoring agent, they are capable of generating sensitivity reactions in some patients. Detergents such as sodium lauryl sulfate, whether in toothpaste or soap, frequently are guilty of producing persistent and occasionally disabling skin eruptions and other allergic manifestations. Cinnamic aldehyde and methyl salicylate are two common flavoring agents which frequently cause gingivitis, glossopyrosis, and similar symptoms throughout the oral cavity.

While we may expect such reactions from products which contain antibiotics or strong astringents, these two lesser known factors frequently are ignored but will be etiologic for the above complaints in many patients.

Finally, in what is probably one of the most fraudulent and certainly one of the most objectionable areas of television and magazine advertising, a light is shining. In an order dated September 1970, the FDA finally zeroed in on mouthwash commercials. Ten leading brands were ordered to furnish real proof of germicidal power and banishment of halitosis or to cease their outlandish claims. The alternative was a government suit and banishment from the shelves. Hopefully most clinicians are aware that the average mouthwash is clinically worthless and that its promoters deal in the realm of fantasy![54]

SUMMARY

It is assumed that any practitioner who prescribes or administers a certain drug or compound to a patient knows the normal dosage of that agent; therefore the purpose of this chapter is not to list dosages, but to increase the doctor's awareness of the gross and the subtle toxic manifestations which may erupt with catastrophic suddenness or emerge slyly after long-term therapy.

The maze of new compounds and their questionable worth in some cases has been emphasized, along with the fact that an understanding of the pharmacology of all prescribed drugs is mandatory for the successful prophylaxis of drug intoxication. Mention has been made of the site and duration of action, relative strength, potentiation, metabolism and excretion, antagonism, and chemical structure as factors which determine the toxic potential or effects of a great number of drugs individually and in compatible compounds. Disease states which alter the effects of drugs and physiologic conditions which require dosage variant from the normal have been cited and discussed along with the advisability of a cautious approach in the administration of any drug to patients who are on delicate to strict regimens of chemotherapy.

A significant clue to the formidable nature of the problem of drug toxicology and its complexities is that while great progress has been made in recognizing and treating toxic responses to known chemical agents, there is emerging a brand new class of iatrogenic or "physician-made" drug diseases complete with appropriate and different signs, symptoms, and responses. Also, because of this, increasing scientific attention is being focused on the subject of teratology. Studies of teratogenicity are demonstrating that a fairly impressive number of drugs, when administered to laboratory animals (generally at doses substantially exceeding the comparable human dose), produce malformations among the offspring.

These phenomena no doubt lend substance and some respectability to that old adage, "The cure is sometimes worse than the disease."

The following material has been reproduced (with permission) from Medical Letter, Vol. 17, No. 5 (Issue 421), February 28, 1975.

ADVERSE INTERACTIONS OF DRUGS*

This article brings up to date material last reviewed in The Medical Letter in Volume 15, p. 77, 1973.

Two or more drugs administered at the same time or in close sequence may act independently, interact to increase or diminish the intended effect of one or both of the drugs, or may cause a new unexpected reaction.

---

*Extensive reviews of confirmed or suspected interactions between drugs are provided in P. D. Hansten, *Drug Interactions*, Philadelphia: Lea & Febiger, 2nd ed., 1973; American Pharmaceutical Association, *Evaluations of Drug Interactions*, 1973, Suppl. 1974.

DETECTION OF INTERACTIONS — The following table represents many reports and a consensus of views of many consultants; it lists only major interactions that have been observed clinically and is offered as a guide that may help to prevent unwanted interactions. Because of the risks of interactions, physicians should prescribe as few drugs as possible for concurrent use. Patients should also be asked routinely what prescriptions or over-the-counter medications they have been taking.

MECHANISMS OF INTERACTIONS — Many interactions result from changes in the metabolism of drugs caused by inhibition or induction of hepatic microsomal enzyme activity, changes in the binding of drugs with plasma protein or tissue receptor sites, changes in the distribution of drugs to the active receptor site, or changes in excretion. Genetic differences can also affect drug metabolism and interactions, and an interaction may occur with high doses of some drugs but not with smaller doses.

INTERACTIONS OF ALCOHOL — Interactions of alcohol with other drugs vary from one individual to another, with the amount of alcohol consumed, and with the duration of use of large amounts of alcohol. Concurrent use of excessive and sometimes ordinary doses of central-nervous-system depressants and intoxicating or large amounts of alcohol can lead to coma and death. When a person drinks an intoxicating amount of alcohol, hepatic metabolism of many drugs may be inhibited, leading to increased therapeutic or toxic effects of the drugs (E. Rubin and C. S. Lieber, Science, 162:690, 1968). On the other hand, in some individuals who drink more than eight ounces of 80-proof whiskey or the equivalent daily for a prolonged period, hepatic metabolism of drugs may be enhanced, which will diminish the therapeutic effects of many drugs, including some of those enhanced by acute intoxication with alcohol (Medical Letter, Vol. 16, p. 91, 1974).

Adverse Interactions of Drugs

Interacting Drugs	Adverse Effect	Probable Mechanism
ALCOHOL, with:		
Antabuse (disulfiram)	Abdominal cramps, flushing, vomiting, psychotic episodes, confusion	Inhibits intermediary metabolism of alcohol
Anticoagulants, oral	Diminished anticoagulant effect with chronic alcohol abuse	Enhanced metabolism
	Enhanced anticoagulant effect with acute intoxication	Reduced metabolism
Anticonvulsants		
Phenytoin (Dilantin; and others)	Diminished anticonvulsant effect with chronic alcohol abuse	Enhanced metabolism
	Enhanced anticonvulsant effect with acute intoxication	Reduced metabolism
Antimicrobials		
Chloramphenicol (Chloromycetin; and others)	Minor Antabuse-like symptoms	Inhibits intermediary metabolism of alcohol
Isoniazid	Increased incidence of hepatitis	Not established
	Diminished isoniazid effect in some patients with chronic alcohol abuse	Enhanced metabolism
Quinacrine (Atabrine)	Minor Antabuse-like symptoms	Inhibits intermediary metabolism of alcohol
Hypoglycemics[1]		
Chlorpropamide (Diabinese)	Minor Antabuse-like symptoms	Inhibits intermediary metabolism of alcohol
Phenformin (DBI; Meltrol)	Lactic acidosis	Synergy
Tolbutamide (Orinase)	Diminished hypoglycemic effect with chronic alcohol abuse	Enhanced metabolism
	Enhanced hypoglycemic effect with ingestion of alcohol, particularly in fasting patients	Suppression of gluconeogenesis
	Minor Antabuse-like symptoms	Inhibits intermediary metabolism of alcohol

Adverse Interactions of Drugs (Continued)

Interacting Drugs	Adverse Effect	Probable Mechanism
MAO inhibitors[2] (With Chianti wine and some other alcoholic beverages)	Hypertensive crisis	Inhibit metabolism of tyramine, resulting in increased release of norepinephrine
Salicylates	Gastrointestinal bleeding	Additive
Sedatives and Hypnotics		
Barbiturates	Diminished sedative effect with chronic alcohol abuse	Enhanced metabolism
	Enhanced central-nervous-system depression with acute intoxication	Additive; reduced metabolism
Chloral hydrate (Noctec; and others)	Prolonged hypnotic effect	Mutual potentiation
Diazepam (Valium)	Enhanced central-nervous-system depression	Additive
Meprobamate (Miltown; and others)	Diminished sedative effect with chronic alcohol abuse	Enhanced metabolism
	Enhanced central-nervous-system depression with acute intoxication	Additive; reduced metabolism

ANTIBIOTIC, CHEMOTHERAPEUTIC, & ANTIPARASITIC AGENTS

Interacting Drugs	Adverse Effect	Probable Mechanism
Aminoglycoside antibiotics,[3] with:		
Cephaloridine (Loridine)	Nephrotoxicity	Not established
Cephalothin (Keflin)	Nephrotoxicity	Not established
Curariform drugs[4]	Neuromuscular blockade	Additive
Ethacrynic acid (Edecrin)	Ototoxicity	Additive
Polymyxins (Aerosporin; Coly-Mycin)	Nephrotoxicity	Additive
Aminosalicyl acid (PAS), with:		
Probenecid (Benemid)	Aminosalicylic acid toxicity	Inhibition of renal excretion
Amphotericin B (Fungizone), with:		
Curariform drugs[4]	Increased curariform effects	Hypokalemia
Digitalis drugs	Increased digitalis toxicity	Hypokalemia
Cephaloridine (Loridine), with:		
Aminoglycoside antibiotics[3]	Nephrotoxicity	Not established
Ethacrynic acid (Edecrin)	Nephrotoxicity	Additive
Furosemide (Lasix)	Nephrotoxicity	Additive
Probenecid (Benemid)	Increased cephaloridine toxicity	Inhibition of renal excretion
Cephalothin (Keflin), with:		
Aminoglycoside antibiotics[3]	Nephrotoxicity	Not established
Chloramphenicol (Chloromycetin; and others), with:		
Alcohol	Minor Antabuse-like symptoms	Inhibits intermediary metabolism of alcohol
Anticoagulants, oral	Increased anticoagulant effect with dicumarol	Inhibition of microsomal enzymes
Hypoglycemics[1]	Increased sulfonylurea hypoglycemia	Inhibition of microsomal enzymes
Phenytoin (Dilantin; and others)	Increased phenytoin toxicity	Inhibition of microsomal enzymes
Griseofulvin (Fulvicin-U/F; and others), with:		
Anticoagulants, oral	Decreased anticoagulant effect with warfarin	Induction of microsomal enzymes
Isoniazid, with:		
Alcohol	Increased incidence of hepatitis	Not established
	Diminished isoniazid effect in some patients with chronic alcohol abuse	Enhanced metabolism

Adverse Interactions of Drugs *(Continued)*

Interacting Drugs	Adverse Effect	Probable Mechanism
Aluminum antacids	Decreased isoniazid effect	Inhibition of isoniazid absorption
Antabuse (disulfiram)	Psychotic episodes, ataxia	Alteration of catecholamine metabolism
Phenytoin (Dilantin; and others)	Increased phenytoin toxicity	Inhibition of microsomal enzymes
Lincomycin (Lincocin), with:		
Kaolin-pectin (Kaopectate)	Decreased lincomycin effect	Inhibition of lincomycin absorption
Nalidixic acid (NegGram), with:		
Anticoagulants, oral	Increased anticoagulant effect	Displacement from binding sites
Polymyxins (Aerosporin; Coly-Mycin), with:		
Aminoglycoside antibiotics[3]	Nephrotoxicity	Additive
Curariform drugs[4]	Neuromuscular blockade	Additive
Quinacrine (Atabrine), with:		
Alcohol	Minor Antabuse-like symptoms	Inhibits intermediary metabolism of alcohol

ANTIBIOTIC, CHEMOTHERAPEUTIC, & ANTIPARASITIC AGENTS

Interacting Drugs	Adverse Effect	Probable Mechanism
Rifampin (Rifadin, Rimactane), with:		
Anticoagulants, oral	Decreased anticoagulant effect	Induction of microsomal enzymes
Contraceptives, oral	Diminished contraceptive effect	Increased estrogen metabolism
Probenecid (Benemid)	Increased rifampin toxicity	Decreased hepatic uptake of rifampin
Sulfonamides, long-acting, with:		
Anticoagulants, oral	Increased anticoagulant effect	Displacement from binding sites
Hypoglycemics[1]	Increased sulfonylurea hypoglycemia	Not established
Tetracyclines, with:		
Antacids, oral	Decreased effect of tetracyclines	Inhibition of tetracycline absorption
Barbiturates	Decreased doxycycline (Vibramycin) effect	Induction of microsomal enzymes
Carbamazepine (Tegretol)	Decreased doxycycline (Vibramycin) effect	Induction of microsomal enzymes
Iron, oral	Decreased effect of tetracyclines	Inhibition of tetracycline absorption
Methoxyflurane (Penthrane)	Nephrotoxicity	Not established

ANTICOAGULANTS, ORAL, with:

Interacting Drugs	Adverse Effect	Probable Mechanism
Alcohol	Diminished anticoagulant effect with chronic alcohol abuse	Enhanced metabolism
	Enhanced anticoagulant effect with acute intoxication	Reduced metabolism
Allopurinol (Zyloprim)	Increased anticoagulant effect	Inhibition of microsomal enzymes
Anabolic and androgenic steroids	Increased anticoagulant effect	Not established
Barbiturates	Decreased anticoagulant effect	Induction of microsomal enzymes
Chloral hydrate (Noctec; and others)	Increased anticoagulant effect	Displacement from binding sites
Chloramphenicol (Chloromycetin; and others)	Increased anticoagulant effect with dicumarol	Inhibition of microsomal enzymes
Cholestyramine (Questran)	Decreased anticoagulant effect	Decreased absorption
Clofibrate (Atromid-S)	Increased anticoagulant effect	Displacement from binding sites
Contraceptives, oral	Decreased anticoagulant effect	Increase in activity of some clotting factors
Dextrothyroxine (Choloxin)	Increased anticoagulant effect	Not established
Disulfiram (Antabuse)	Increased anticoagulant effect	Inhibition of microsomal enzymes
Glutethimide (Doriden)	Decreased anticoagulant effect	Induction of microsomal enzymes
Griseofulvin (Fulvicin-U/F; and others)	Decreased anticoagulant effect with warfarin	Induction of microsomal enzymes
Hypoglycemics[1]	Increased sulfonylurea hypoglycemia with dicumarol	Inhibition of microsomal enzymes

Adverse Interactions of Drugs (Continued)

Interacting Drugs	Adverse Effect	Probable Mechanism
Nalidixic acid (NegGram)	Increased anticoagulant effect	Displacement from binding sites
Phenylbutazone (Butazolidin; Azolid) and oxyphenbutazone (Tandearil; Oxalid)	Increased anticoagulant effect	Displacement from binding sites
Phenytoin (Dilantin; and others)	Increased phenytoin toxicity with dicumarol	Inhibition of microsomal enzymes
Rifampin (Rifadin; Rimactane)	Decreased anticoagulant effect	Induction of microsomal enzymes
Salicylates	Increased anticoagulant effect	Reduction of plasma prothrombin
Sulfonamides, long-acting	Increased anticoagulant effect	Displacement from binding sites
Thyroid hormones	Increased anticoagulant effect	Increased clotting factor catabolism

ANTIDEPRESSANTS, TRICYCLIC,[5] with:

Barbiturates	Decreased antidepressant effect	Induction of microsomal enzymes
Guanethidine (Ismelin)	Decreased antihypertensive effect	Blockade of uptake at target site
MAO inhibitors[2]	Hyperpyrexia, convulsions	Not established
Sympathomimetic amines[6]	Hypertensive crisis	Inhibition of norepinephrine uptake by neuron

ANTIHYPERTENSIVE DRUGS, with:

Anesthetics, general	Hypotension	Usually additive
Antidepressants, tricyclic[5]	Decreased antihypertensive effect of guanethidine	Blockade of uptake at target site
Hypoglycemics[1]	Increased hypoglycemia with guanethidine	Not established
Phenothiazines	Hypotension	Blockade of dopamine; additive
Sympathomimetic amines[6]	Decreased hypotensive effect	Inhibition of norepinephrine uptake by neuron

BARBITURATES, with:

Alcohol	Diminished sedative effect with chronic alcohol abuse	Enhanced metabolism
	Enhanced central-nervous-system depression with acute intoxication	Additive; reduced metabolism
Anticoagulants, oral	Decreased anticoagulant effect	Induction of microsomal enzymes
Antidepressants, tricyclic[5]	Decreased antidepressant activity	Induction of microsomal enzymes
Corticosteroids	Decreased steroid effect	Induction of microsomal enzymes
Tetracyclines	Decreased doxycycline (Vibramycin) effect	Induction of microsomal enzymes

CONTRACEPTIVES, ORAL, with:

Anticoagulants, oral	Decreased anticoagulant effect	Increase in activity of some clotting factors
Rifampin (Rifadin; Rimactane)	Diminished contraceptive effect	Increased estrogen metabolism

CURARIFORM DRUGS,[4] with:

Aminoglycoside antibiotics[3] and polymyxins (administered parenterally)	Neuromuscular blockade	Additive
Amphotericin B (Fungizone)	Increased curariform effects	Hypokalemia
Diuretics (causing potassium loss)	Increased curariform effects	Hypokalemia
Narcotic analgesics	Increased respiratory depression	Additive
Quinidine	Increased curariform effects	Additive

DIGITALIS DRUGS, with:

Amphotericin B (Fungizone)	Increased digitalis toxicity	Hypokalemia
Cholestyramine (Questran)	Decreased digitoxin effect	Binding in intestine
Diuretics (causing potassium loss)	Increased digitalis toxicity	Hypokalemia
Sympathomimetic amines[6]	Enhanced tendency to cardiac arrhythmias	Additive effect on pacemaker

Adverse Interactions of Drugs *(Continued)*

Interacting Drugs	Adverse Effect	Probable Mechanism
DIURETICS		
Ethacrynic acid (Edecrin), with:		
Cephaloridine (Loridine)	Nephrotoxicity	Additive
Furosemide (Lasix), with:		
Cephaloridine (Loridine)	Nephrotoxicity	Additive
Potassium-losing diuretics, with:		
Corticosteroids	Enhanced potassium loss	Additive
Curariform drugs[4]	Increased curariform effects	Hypokalemia
Digitalis drugs	Increased digitalis toxicity	Hypokalemia
Spironolactone (Aldactone), with:		
Potassium salts	Hyperkalemia	Additive
Salicylates	Decreased natriuresis	Not established
Triamterene (Dyrenium), with:		
Potassium salts	Hyperkalemia	Additive
HYPOGLYCEMICS,[1] with:		
Alcohol, see ALCOHOL		
Anabolic steroids	Increased hypoglycemia	Not established
Chloramphenicol (Chloromycetin; and others)	Increased sulfonylurea hypoglycemia	Inhibition of microsomal enzymes
Dicumarol	Increased sulfonylurea hypoglycemia	Inhibition of microsomal enzymes
Guanethidine (Ismelin)	Increased hypoglycemia	Not established
MAO inhibitors[2]	Increased hypoglycemia	Not established
Phenylbutazone (Butazolidin; Azolid) and oxyphenbutazone (Tandearil; Oxalid)	Increased sulfonylurea hypoglycemia	Inhibition of microsomal enzymes
Propranolol (Inderal)	Increased hypoglycemia	Not established
Salicylates	Increased hypoglycemia	Displacement from binding; additive
Sulfaphenazole and possibly other long-acting sulfonamides	Increased sulfonylurea hypoglycemia	Not established
LEVODOPA (Dopar; and others), with:		
MAO inhibitors[2]	Hypertensive crisis	Increase in storage and release of dopamine, norepinephrine, or both
Phenothiazines	Decreased antiparkinson effect	Inhibition of dopamine uptake
Pyridoxine	Decreased antiparkinson effect	Enhancement of decarboxylation of levadopa at periphery
MAO INHIBITORS,[2] with:		
Alcohol (Chianti wine and some other alcoholic beverages)	Hypertensive crisis	Inhibit metabolism of tyramine, resulting in increased release of norepinephrine
Antidepressants, tricyclic[5]	Hyperpyrexia, convulsions	Not established
Hypoglycemics[1]	Increased hypoglycemia	Not established
Levodopa (Dopar; and others)	Hypertensive crisis	Increase in storage and release of dopamine, norepinephrine, or both
Meperidine (Demerol; and others)	Hypertension; or hypotension and coma	Not established
Sympathomimetic amines[6]	Hypertensive crisis	Increase in storage and release of norepinephrine
Tyramine in foods[7]	Hypertensive crisis	Inhibit metabolism of tyramine, resulting in increased release of norepinephrine

Adverse Interactions of Drugs (Continued)

Interacting Drugs	Adverse Effect	Probable Mechanism
SALICYLATES, with:		
Anticoagulants, oral	Increased anticoagulant effect	Reduction of plasma prothrombin
Hypoglycemics[1]	Increased hypoglycemia	Displacement from binding; additive
Methotrexate	Increased effect and toxicity of methotrexate	Displacement from binding sites
Probenecid (Benemid)	Decreased uricosuric effect	Not established
Spironolactone (Aldactone)	Decreased natriuresis	Not established
SYMPATHOMIMETIC AMINES,[6] with:		
Antidepressants, tricyclic[5]	Hypertensive crisis	Inhibition of norepinephrine uptake by neuron
Antihypertensive drugs	Decreased hypotensive effect	Inhibition of norepinephrine uptake by neuron
Cyclopropane and halogen-ated hydrocarbon anesthetics	Cardiac arrhythmias	Not established
Digitalis drugs	Enhanced tendency to cardiac arrhythmias	Additive effect on pacemaker
MAO inhibitors[2, 8]	Hypertensive crisis	Increase in storage and release of norepinephrine
THYROID HORMONES, with:		
Anticoagulants, oral	Increased anticoagulant effect	Increased clotting factor catabolism
Cholestyramine (Questran)	Decreased absorption of thyroid	Binding of hormone in intestine
MISCELLANEOUS DRUGS		
Allopurinol, with:		
Anticoagulants, oral	Increased anticoagulant effect	Inhibition of microsomal enzymes
Azathioprine (Imuran)	Azathioprine toxicity	Inhibition of azathioprine metabolism
Cyclophosphamide (Cytoxan)	Cyclophosphamide toxicity	Inhibition of cyclophosphamide metabolism
Mercaptopurine (6-MP)	Mercaptopurine toxicity	Inhibition of mercaptopurine metabolism
Cholestyramine (Questran), with:		
Anticoagulants, oral	Decreased anticoagulant effect	Decreased absorption
Digitalis drugs	Decreased digitoxin effect	Binding in intestine
Thyroid hormones	Decreased absorption of thyroid	Binding of hormone in intestine
Methotrexate, with:		
Salicylates	Increased effect and toxicity of methotrexate	Displacement from binding sites
Neostigmine, parenteral (Prostigmin), with:		
Quinidine	Decreased neostigmine effect	Anticholinergic effect of quinidine
Phenytoin (Dilantin; and others), with:		
Alcohol	Diminished anticonvulsant effect with chronic alcohol abuse	Enhanced metabolism
	Enhanced anticonvulsant effect with acute intoxication	Reduced metabolism
Chloramphenicol (Chloro-mycetin; and others)	Phenytoin toxicity	Inhibition of microsomal enzymes
Dicumarol	Phenytoin toxicity	Inhibition of microsomal enzymes
Isoniazid	Phenytoin toxicity	Inhibition of microsomal enzymes
Probenecid (Benemid), with:		
Aminosalicylic acid (PAS)	Aminosalicylic acid toxicity	Inhibition of renal excretion
Cephaloridine (Loridine)	Increased cephaloridine toxicity	Inhibition of renal excretion
Rifampin (Rifadin; Rimactane)	Increased rifampin toxicity	Decreased hepatic uptake
Salicylates	Decreased uricosuric effect	Not established

Footnotes—Adverse Interactions of Drugs

1. Hypoglycemics include insulin, phenformin (DBI; Meltrol), and the sulfonylureas (acetohexamide [Dymelor]; chlorpropamide [Diabinese]; tolazamide [Tolinase]; tolbutamide [Orinase]). Any drug with marked stimulant effect on the sympathetic nervous system can potentiate insulin release and consequently the action of sulfonylureas.
2. MAO inhibitors include furazolidone (Furoxone), isocarboxazid (Marplan), pargyline (Eutonyl), phenelzine (Nardil), and tranylcypromine (Parnate).
3. Aminoglycoside antibiotics include gentamicin (Garamycin), kanamycin (Kantrex), neomycin and streptomycin.
4. Curariform drugs include d-tubocurarine, gallamine, and succinylcholine.
5. Tricyclic antidepressants include amitriptyline (Elavil), desipramine (Norpramin; Pertofrane), doxepin (Sinequan), imipramine (Tofranil; Presamine), nortriptyline (Aventyl), and protriptyline (Vivactil).
6. Sympathomimetic amines include amphetamines, ephedrine, epinephrine (Adrenalin), isoproterenol (Isuprel), methylphenidate (Ritalin), norepinephrine (Levophed), phenylephrine (Sudafed; and others), and many appetite-depressing drugs; also amines in many over-the-counter cough, cold, and sinus remedies, including nasal decongestants.
7. Foods containing tyramine include aged cheeses, Chianti wines, beer, sherry, pickled herring, yeast extracts, chicken liver, chocolate, broad beans, sour cream, canned figs, raisins, and soy sauce.
8. Of the sympathomimetic amines (footnote 6), the most dangerous in patients on MAO inhibitors would be amphetamines, ephedrine, phenylephrine, and phenylpropanolamine.

Partial List of Trade Names

Acenocoumarol—(see Anticoagulants)
Aerosporin—Polymyxin
Aldactone—Spironolactone
Anisindione—(see Anticoagulants)
Antabuse—Disulfiram
Aspirin—(see Salicylates)
Atabrine—Quinacrine
Atromid-S—Clofibrate
Azolid—Phenylbutazone
Benemid—Probenecid
Bishydroxycoumarin—(see Anticoagulants)
Butazolidin—Phenylbutazone
Chloromycetin—Chloramphenicol
Choloxin—Dextrothyroxine
Colistin—(see Polymyxins)
Coly-Mycin—(see Polymyxins)
Coumadin—(see Anticoagulants)
Cytoxan—Cyclophosphamide
Danilone—(see Anticoagulants)
DBI—Phenformin
Demerol—Meperidine
Diabinese—Chlorpropamide
Dicumarol—(see Anticoagulants)
Dilantin—Phenytoin
Diphenylhydantoin—(see Phenytoin)
Dopar—Levodopa
Doriden—Glutethimide
Dyrenium—Triameterene
Edecrin—Ethacrynic acid
Fulvicin-U/F—Griseofulvin
Fungizone—Amphotericin B
Grifulvin—Griseofulvin

Hedulin—(see Anticoagulants)
Imuran—Azathioprine
Inderal—Propranolol
Ismelin—Guanethidine
Keflin—Cephalothin
Lasix—Furosemide
Lincocin—Lincomycin
Loridine—Cephaloridine
Meltrol—Phenformin
Miltown—Meprobamate
Miradon—(see Anticoagulants)
NegGram—Nalidixic acid
Noctec — Chloral hydrate
Orinase—Tolbutamide
Oxalid—(see Phenylbutazone)
Oxyphenbutazone—(see Phenylbutazone)
Panwarfin—(see Anticoagulants)
PAS — Aminosalicylic acid
Penthrane—Methoxyflurane
Phenindione—(see Anticoagulants)
Prostigmin—Neostigmine
Questran—Cholestyramine
Rifadin—Rifampin
Rimactane—Rifampin
Sintrom—(see Anticoagulants)
6-MP—Mercaptopurine
Tandearil—(see Phenylbutazone)
Tegretol—Carbamazepine
Valium—Diazepam
Vibramycin—Doxycycline
Warfarin—(see Anticoagulants)
Zyloprim—Allopurinol

REFERENCES

1. Adriani, J.: The Chemistry and Physics of Anesthesia. 2nd ed., Springfield Ill., Charles C Thomas, 1970.
2. Adriani, J.: The Pharmacology of Anesthetic Drugs: A Syllabus for Students and Clinicians. 5th ed., Springfield, Ill., Charles C Thomas, 1970.

3. Adriani, J.: Techniques and Procedures of Anesthesia. 3rd ed., Springfield, Ill., Charles C Thomas, 1969.
4. Adriani, J.: Fundamentals of General Anesthesia for Students and Practitioners of Dentistry. Springfield, Ill., Charles C Thomas, 1958.
5. Adriani, J.: Selection of Anesthesia: The Physiologic and Pharmacologic Basis. Springfield, Ill., Charles C Thomas, 1955.
6. Artusio, J. F., and Mazzia, V. P. B.: Practical Anesthesiology. St Louis, C. V. Mosby, 1962.
7. Beckman H.: Pharmacology — The Nature, Action, and Use of Drugs. 2nd ed., Philadelphia, W. B. Saunders Co., 1961.
8. Brady, E. S.: A Calculated Risk. Alumni Review, University of Southern California, November, 1964.
9. Birch, A. A., and Tolmie, J. D.: Anesthesia for the Uninterested. Baltimore, University Park Press, 1976.
10. Brechner, Verne L.: Pathological and Pharmacological Consideration in Anesthesiology. The Proceedings of the Twelfth Biennial Western Conference on Anesthesiology. U. of Utah Press, 1972.
11. Burton, A. C.: Physiology and Biophysics of the Circulation. 2nd ed., Chicago, Year Book Medical Publishers, 1972.
12. Catron, D. C.: The Anesthesiologist's Handbook. 2nd ed., Baltimore, University Park Press, 1976.
13. Chas. Pfizer & Co., Inc.: Package inserts, May 1966.
14. Cohen, D. D., and Dillon, J. B.: Anesthesia for Outpatient Surgery. Springfield, Ill., Charles C Thomas, 1970.
15. Cutting, W. C.: Handbook of Pharmacology. 2nd ed. New York, Appleton-Century-Crofts, 1964.
16. DeJong, R. H.: Physiology and Pharmacology of Local Anesthesia. Springfield, Ill., Charles C Thomas, 1970.
17. Dornette, W. H. L.: Anatomy for the Anesthesiologist: A Stereoscopic Atlas '63.
18. Drug Bulletin — L.A.C.–U.S.C. Medical Center, L. A., California, 8/10/77.
19. Drugs in Breast Milk. The Medical Letter. Vol. 16, No. 6, March, 1974.
20. Eastman, J. W., and Cohen, S. N.: Hypertensive crisis and death associated with phencyclidine poisoning. J.A.M.A., 231:1270–1271, 1975.
21. Farr, R. S.: Denver National Jewish Hospital, Denver, Colorado, 1970.
22. Fragen, R. J., and Caldwell, N.: Lorazepam premedication: Lack of recall and relief of anxiety. Anesth. Analg. (Cleve.) 55(6):792, 1976.
23. Garb, S., and Crim, B. J.: Pharmacology and Patient Care. New York, Springer Publishing Co., 1962.
24. Gold, M. I.: Tranquilizers and anesthesia. J.A.D.S.A., April, 1967.
25. Goth, A.: Medical Pharmacology, 5th ed., St. Louis, C. V. Mosby Co., 1970.
26. Greenfield, W.: Anesthesia progress. J.A.D.S.A., 23 (4): July-Aug, 1976.
27. Handbook of Non-Prescription Drugs, 1969 edition.
28. Hunter, A. R., and Bush, G. H.: General Anesthesia for Dental Surgery. Springfield, Ill., Charles C Thomas, 1971.
29. LaDu, B. H.: New York University School of Medicine.
30. Laskin, J. L., Wallace, W. R., and DeLeo, B.: Use of bupivacaine hydrochloride in oral surgery — a clinical study. J. Ortho. Surg., 35:25, 1977.
31. Lee, J. A.: A Symposium of Anesthesia. Chicago, Year Book Medical Publishers, 1973.
32. Libman, R. H.: Anesth. Prog., Sept-Oct, 1976.
33. Lorhan, P. H.: Anesthesia for the Aged. Springfield, Ill., Charles C Thomas, 1971.
34. McCarthy, F.: Emergencies in Dental Practice. 2nd ed., Philadelphia. W. B. Saunders Co., 1972.
35. Medical Letter: Vol. 15 (23), Issue 387, November 9, 1973.
36. Medical Letter: Vol 17 (5), Issue 421, February 28, 1975.
37. Monheim, L. M.: General Anesthesia in Dental Practice. St. Louis, C. V. Mosby Co., 1960.
38. Monheim, L. M.: Local Anesthesia and Plain Control in Dental Practice. 2nd ed. St. Louis, C. V. Mosby Co., 1961.
39. Mulay, D. N., and Urbach, F.: Local therapy of oral leukoplakia with vitamin A. A.M.A. Arch. Dermat., 78:637, 1958.
40. National Prescription Audit, 12th ed. Philadelphia. Lea and Febiger, 1972.
41. Ngai, S. H., and Papper, E. M.: Metabolic Effects of Anesthesia. Springfield, Ill., Charles C Thomas, 1962.
42. Olson, R. E., Morello, J. A., and Kreff, E. D.: Antibiotic treatment of oral anaerobic infections. J. Ortho. Surg., 33;. Aug. 1975.
43. Parke-Davis & Co.: Package inserts.
44. Powell, W. F.: Comprehensive Background for Anesthesiology. Springfield, Ill., Charles C Thomas, 1966.
45. Pricco, D. E.: J. Ortho. Surg., 35:129, 1977.

46. Pryor, W. J., and Bush, D.C.T.: A Manual of Anesthetic Techniques. 4th ed., Chicago, Year Book Medical Publishers, 1973.
47. Saidman, J., and Moya, F.: Complications of Anesthesia. Springfield, Ill., Charles C Thomas, 1970.
48. Salter, F. J.: University of Michigan Hospital Pharmacy Letter for Physicians, Vol. 5, No. 1. Jan., 1970.
49. Schwartz, H., Ngai, S. H., and Papper, E. M.: Manual of Anesthesiology for Residents and Medical Students. 2nd ed., Springfield, Charles C Thomas, 1962.
50. Shore, M. F.: Drugs can be dangerous during pregnancy and lactation. Can. Pharm. J., Dec., 1970. Reprinted by Upjohn Co.
51. Smith, J. W.: Manual of Medical Therapeutics, 19th ed. Boston, Little, Brown and Co., 1969.
52. Smith, R. H.: Pathological Physiology for the Anesthesiologist. Springfield, Ill., Charles C Thomas, 1966.
53. Sohn, D. M.: Valium. Anesth. Prog., May-June, 1975.
54. Steiner, R. B., and Thompson, R. D.: Oral Surgery and Anesthesia. Philadelphia, W. B. Saunders Co., 1977.
55. Stephen, C. R., Ahlgren, E. W., and Bennett, E.: Elements of Pediatric Anesthesia. 2nd ed., Springfield, Ill., Charles C Thomas, 1970.
56. The Medical Letter on Drugs and Therapeutics. New York, Drug and Therapeutic Information, Inc., 1970.
57. Thienes, C. H., and Haley, T. J.: Clinical Toxicology. 4th ed., Philadelphia, Lea & Febiger, 1969.
58. Vereby, K., Volavka, J., Mulé, S. J., et al.: Naltrexone: disposition, metabolism, and effects after acute and chronic dosing. Clin. Pharmacol. Ther. 20:315–328, 1976.
59. Walton, J. G., and Thompson, J. W.: Pharmacology for the Dental Practitioner. British D. J., Vol. 127, 1969.
60. Wynn, R. L., and Kohn, M. W.: The Pharmacology of Intravenous Sedation. Am. Soc. Ortho. Surg. 1976
61. Young, J. A.: The Medical Messiahs. Princeton, Princeton University Press, 1967.

Introduction to Psychosedation

The balance of Part 1, Prevention of Serious Medical Emergencies, is composed of five chapters which review control of the dental pain/anxiety complex. The background of pain, anxiety, and stress is examined, with special reference to the medically compromised patient, then is presented the art and science of human behavior, which utilizes non-drug methods for producing sedation in the anxious patient (iatrosedation), followed by the three routes for effective pharmacosedation: oral, inhalation, and intravenous. The intramuscular route is of questionable value and will not be reviewed.

The record of pain/anxiety control in the dental office is far superior to the still medieval practices one finds in the average medical office. Great advances have been made in dental psychosedation in the past 20 years, with special reference to the vastly increased use of inhalation sedation (nitrous oxide/oxygen). Much remains to be done, however, in increasing predoctoral and postdoctoral training in *all* sedation modalities. Comprehensive dental care cannot be offered if comprehensive pain/anxiety control is lacking. Nearly half of the general population seeks only emergency dental care because of apprehension. Regional anesthesia alone is not sufficient for a large percentage of patients.

Although the subject of anxiety control may appear to be inappropriate in a book on emergencies in dental practice, apprehension plays a major role in the production of life-threatening emergencies, and thus anxiety must be effectively treated if we are to significantly decrease the incidence of serious morbidity and mortality in the dental office. The reader is invited to review the chapter *Sudden Death* for sobering facts on the influence of stress in sudden death. Adequate pain/anxiety control is second only to a proper pretreatment physical evaluation in the prevention of serious medical emergencies. I expect the health practitioner to be held morally and legally responsible for complications resulting from his or her failure to adequately control anxiety in the high-risk patient.

Psychosedation by the oral route is within the capabilities of all experienced dental practitioners. Both the inhalation and the intravenous routes require adequate undergraduate or postgraduate training and experience. The chapter on the intravenous route includes deep sedation and ultralight general anesthesia techniques for the sake of completeness. The practitioner without adequate general anesthesia training should utilize light sedation only, during which the patient is conscious with intact protective reflexes, including the ability to maintain an airway, and is capable of rational response to question or command.

Remarkable advances are being made in control of the dental pain/anxiety complex. They are included here as a concise, single reference source.

6

PSYCHOSEDATION

Part 1:   The Nature and Control of Pain,
          Anxiety, and Stress

JOHN M. GREGG

INTRODUCTION

If the clinician is to provide dental health care with a minimum of harm to patients' psyche and physiology, four primary negative factors must be confronted: *pain, anxiety, stress* and pre-existing *disease* (Figure 6–1). These factors exist to some degree in all patients. They differ only in intensity, manner of expression, and significance to a particular patient. Counterbalancing these negative factors are a variety of states that can be induced therapeutically; these include *analgesia, hypnosis, hyporeflexia, amnesia, tranquilization* and *dissociation*. The specific approaches to be used in therapy and the degree of success obtained will depend on how well the clinician understands the basic mechanisms of both the negative and the counterbalancing factors.

PAIN

Because of major scientific breakthroughs in the past 15 years, the anatomy and physiology of pain are much clearer, and a more precise definition of pain is now possible. Pain is defined as a human response to a poten-

This research was supported in part by NIH research agent number DE 02668 and from the National Institute of Dental Research and by NIH grant number RR 05333 from The Division of Research Facilities and Resources.

Figure 6-1 Counterbalancing negative and positive factors in the control of pain, anxiety, and stress.

tially tissue damaging (noxious) stimulus that involves dual aspects of sensory perception and suffering. Noxious stimuli release a variety of chemical substances which appear capable of initiating the pain response; most notable are histamine, bradykinin, prostaglandin EG, and substance P.* These chemicals activate a specific class of peripheral nerve fibers called *nociceptors,* which are of the A delta and C fiber class. The primary nociceptors are small, 2 to 5 μ in diameter, with thin or no myelination, and enter the central nervous system to synapse on specific secondary nociceptor cells. In the case of the head and neck, the nociceptors distribute primarily to the subnucleus caudalis region of the spinal nucleus of cranial nerve V, where two kinds of physiologic activity occur that have great bearing on the nature of facial pain as we know it.

The first event is that the primary nociceptors appear to activate two different populations of centrally projecting cells, which may account for the biphasic nature of pain sensation. The so-called "first pain" is rapid, stinging, and precise in quality as compared to the delayed, duller, and more diffuse "second pain." A second major event occurring in the subnucleus caudalis region is the neuromodulation or "gating effect" that results in *pain thresholds.*

Two levels of pain threshold are generally recognized; a pain *perception threshold,* defined as the lowest level of noxious stimulation which is perceived as being painful, and a higher pain *tolerance,* or reaction, *threshold,* which is the lowest level of noxious stimulation that cannot be tolerated and that produces attempts at protective reflex withdrawal. The perception threshold has been found to be rather constant and similar between individuals across cultures, and it does not change markedly when analgesic drugs are given in controlled settings. In contrast, the pain tolerance

---

*Whether noxious chemicals can be released as a response to an internal stimulus such as anxiety, thereby initiating a pain response, is still an important question of scientific debate, as will be seen in the next section, on anxiety.

threshold is markedly influenced by a wide range of centrally acting drugs that are classified as analgesics.

Changes in pain tolerance thresholds from analgesic drugs have been correlated with suppression of activity in the secondary nociceptors of the pars reticularis of the subnucleus caudalis, but it has been learned that the threshold changes in these cells are actually due to neurochemical events that occur at higher levels. Clusters of neurons, known collectively as *opiate receptors,* are found in many areas of the anterior brainstem, especially the limbic forebrain, the hypothalamus, and the reticular gray matter of the midbrain, which appear to be a source of nerve fibers that descend to synapse on the threshold nociceptors in regions such as the trigeminal subnucleus caudalis. The opiate receptors are so named because they are selectively activated by exogenous opiate analgesics and inactivated when narcotic antagonists are given. They are especially rich in 5-hydroxytryptamine and dopamine, two substances which have been implicated not only in analgesia and pain threshold determination but also in key psychiatric states such as certain forms of depression and sleep disorders.

Among the best studied and perhaps most important of the opiate receptors are those found in the periaqueductal gray (PAG) region of the midbrain. The PAG region, in addition to responding to exogenous opiates, is believed to respond to two different endogenous sources of stimulation, one neural and one hormonal. First, projections to PAG are known to arise in limbic paleocortical centers, especially the median forebrain bundle. The limbic projections to PAG opiate receptors are important because they appear to be a major anatomic basis for the link between human emotions and pain. The limbic structures appear to be sources of such functions as aggression-rage reactions, euphoria, memory and learning functions, and certain aspects of anxiety.

In addition to these neural influences from limbic regions, the PAG opiate receptors are also influenced by recently discovered peptide hormones called endorphins ("endogenous morphine-like substances"). The endorphins appear to originate as small portions of a larger 91 amino acid peptide hormone known collectively as beta-lipoprotein, which appears to be synthesized in the hypothalamus from the same precursors that make up adrenocorticotropic hormone (ACTH), and, like ACTH, are secreted into the blood by the anterior pituitary gland as a response to sustained trauma or stimulation of the central nervous system.

Once in the blood, beta-lipoprotein breaks up into a number of biologically active subparticles, including B-endorphin, which finds its way to the opiate receptor cells through the cerebrospinal fluid. The endorphins appear capable of inducing profound analgesia which, as with exogenous opiates, is brought on slowly over a matter of 15 to 20 minutes and is also reversed by the narcotic antagonists. Therefore, an endogenous neurohormonal system seems to exist in the brainstem to provide a basis for natural changes in pain tolerance thresholds and appears useful to the individual under conditions that are threatening and potentially painful. However, it is apparent that the positive and protective benefits of this system can be markedly altered and overridden by functions of the limbic cortex which collectively we call *anxiety.*

ANXIETY

Anxiety can be defined as an unpleasant feeling of apprehension or impending danger that occurs in the presence of a threat of pain which is out of proportion to the actual threat and which produces an exaggerated emotional response. Anxiety produces meaningless frenzy, rigid or distorted expressions, and often a withdrawal and shutting off of useful activity which may lead to a state of near sensory and motor paralysis. Fear, in contrast, is an appropriate defensive reaction, a sharpening of the senses, and a readiness to respond to a real environmental danger.

Pain and anxiety are known to be interconnected human experiences. As anxiety increases, so does the likelihood of the patient interpreting stimuli as pain. High anxiety trait personalities have been shown to be more pain responsive. Anxiety differences between groups of people may also explain the ethnic differences in responsiveness to pain. Jews and Italians, for example, have been shown to be more reactive to clinical pain than "old Americans," and women have rather consistently been more reactive than men. Patients who are fatigued, debilitated, and depressed tend to respond to threats with a higher degree of undifferentiated anxiety and are correspondingly more "pain reactive."

From a developmental standpoint, the startle pattern of the infant is the precursor to both the fear and anxiety experiences. The socialization of the child and the establishment of a culture can be seen as a product of the individual or society being able to differentiate between real and imagined threats (fear versus anxiety). In conquering anxiety, the mature and effective neocortex is able to inhibit or tone down the intensity of anxiety and simultaneously control rage reactions. The importance of the cortical control has even been seen in experimental decorticate animals where emotional excitement has led to uncontrolled rage leading to death. Similar loss of cortical control may explain voodoo deaths in which anxiety persists without physical release.

It is apparent that the level of uncontrolled anxiety is transferred to the physiologic upheaval that we know as the stress response. Studies have shown that urinary metabolites of epinephrine and plasma norepinephrine are significantly higher in dental patients with phobias than in control dental patients. In order to understand the full significance of uncontrolled anxiety, a review of the *stress response* is necessary.

THE STRESS RESPONSE

When stimulated by pain or anxiety, a series of physiologic responses occur which make up the stress response. They encompass protective skeletal muscle reflexes, the autonomic nervous system responses, and endocrine responses (Table 6–1). Acute stress responses in skeletal muscles include withdrawal actions such as head turning, grimacing, vocalization, raising of the hands, heightening of muscle spindle activity, and dilation of intramuscular blood vessels in preparation for "fight or flight." The autonomic acute stress response is predominantly sympathetic, with elevated heart rate, increased ventilation, dilation of pupils, decreased and mucoid

TABLE 6-1 ADAPTIVE AND MALADAPTIVE STRESS RESPONSES

Adaptive (Acute) (Sympathetic Dominant)	Maladaptive (Acute) (Parasympathetic Dominant)	Maladaptive (Chronic) (Psychophysiologic Disorder)
Increased heart rate	Decreased heart rate	Neurodermatitis
Increased blood pressure	Decreased blood pressure	Peptic ulcer
Increased ventilation	Decreased ventilation	Ulcerative colitis
Decreased gut motility	Increased gut motility	Bronchial asthma
Decreased salivation	Increased salivation	Raynaud's disease
Decreased sweating	Increased sweating	Dysmenorrhea
Increased skeletal muscle tone	Decreased skeletal muscle tone	Hypertension
Peripheral vasoconstriction	Peripheral vasodilatation	Hyperthyroidism
Pupillary dilation	Pupillary constriction	Rheumatoid arthritis
Urinary retention	Urinary release	Migraine
Increased blood sugar	Decreased CO_2 sensitivity	Paroxysmal tachycardia
Dysphoria, alertness	Agitation, confusion	Herpetic stomatitis
		Myofibrositis syndrome

salivation, and a generalized peripheral cutaneous vasoconstriction (Table 6-1). Norepinephrine released by the adrenal medulla increases the rate and force of myocardial contractions. The acute endocrine stress responses are primarily due to release of ACTH and probably endorphin precursors from the pituitary gland. Secondary steroid secretion by the adrenal cortex releases glycogen from the liver as an energy substrate.

These classic physiologic responses to a fearful situation, it can be seen, prepare the individual very well for "fight or flight," for combat or rage reactions. As such, the responses are adaptive. If, however, the stress is overwhelming and the individual is restrained in some way from physical outlet of the stress response, as is the usual case in fear producing dental-surgical settings, then maladaptive stress responses occur.

Two main types of maladaptive stress responses occur, acute responses such as syncope and chronic responses such as psychosomatic disease. During unresolved acute pain or anxiety, the maladaptive stress response tends to be a rapid switch from sympathetic organ readiness to parasympathetic dominance. The pulse rate slows markedly to below normal as the vagus nerve predominates. Respirations become shallow, choppy, and rapid. A cold sweat, profuse serous salivation, and nausea are experienced as a result of increasing gut peristalsis. Great proportions of circulating blood are pooled in the greatly dilated venous splanchnic beds, and cardiac return from the appendages is slowed because of the flaccidity of the venules and the skeletal muscles (Table 6-1). The final result is inadequate perfusion of the brain with oxygen and glycogen, and the patient finally faints.

The other type of maladaptive stress response is chronic and, as Hans Selye has pointed out in his classic work on the "general adaptation syndrome," may result in many forms of secondary somatic disease. Even though modern medical science has defined the major infectious vectors, autoimmune responses, and traumatic causes for many diseases, the majority of disease conditions of the modern civilized world are known to be either direct results of or markedly influenced by maladaptation to stress.

The list of psychosomatic syndromes is well known (Table 6–1): hypertension, asthma, dermatitis and mucositis, obesity, peptic ulcer, cardiac murmur, hyperglycemia in diabetes, myofibrositis and muscle spasm syndromes, herpetic outbreaks and susceptibility to infections. It is ironic that when people become ill in somatic ways, anxiety tends to disappear; and as anxiety-stress responses and neurotic behavior become more overt, the organic disease becomes less severe.

It can be seen, therefore, that maladaptive stress responses to unresolved pain and anxiety situations such as stressful dental care may lead to both acute maladaptations, such as syncope, and chronic psychosomatic disease conditions. When maladaptive stress occurs in young, basically healthy people, it results in further emotional upset, interference with the delivery of dental-surgical care, and transient psychosomatic inconveniences. When seen in older, higher medical risk patients, however, uncontrolled pain and anxiety, and maladaptive stress responses are the calling cards of major medical emergency.

HIGH RISK PATIENTS AND STRESS

Uncontrolled pain, anxiety, and stress response is most devastating when coupled with certain pre-existing disease states. Four categories of patients present special problems: those with cardiovascular, pulmonary, endocrine and psychiatric disease.

Cardiovascular. The courses of both hypertension and atherosclerotic disease of coronary and cerebral vessels are directly influenced by stress.

Although the causes of coronary artery disease and its dramatic endpoint, the myocardial infarction, are multifactorial, protracted stress response in the "Type A" personality is a clear prime factor in the long term disease course. In the acute situation, stress from pain and emotional upset are the most common precipitators of angina pectoris. As endogenous stores of epinephrine and norepinephrine reach the heart, its rate and force of contractions increase, placing greater demands for oxygen delivery on the coronary vessels. The patient whose coronary vessels have become relatively rigid from atherosclerosis and whose collateral perfusion of muscle is atrophic cannot adapt to these increased stress demands, and ischemic myocardial cell death results. The best treatment, of course, is prevention, both in the long term disease course and most clearly in the acute stressful dental operatory. If heart attack does occur, the level of pain and anxiety continues to be a prime determinant of outcome. In the patient who has survived a myocardial infarction, stress control becomes even more important. The post-MI patient often manifests arrhythmias due to myocardial fibrosis, and dental manipulations such as extraction are known to precipitate arrhythmias greater than 40 per cent of the time even among non-cardiac patients.

Patients whose atherosclerotic disease has also involved cervical and cerebral vessels are prone to transient cerebral ischemia (TCI), manifested as brief periods of disorientation or weakness due to partial occlusion of the vessels. If the occlusion is prolonged, typically because of venous emboli, then neuronal infarction (CVA) will occur. A not uncommon victim of such embolization is the atherosclerotic patient whose legs have been elevated and immobilized in a dental chair and whose blood flow past potential venous emboli is suddenly increased by pain or emotional upset.

Hypertension also has a multifactorial basis, involving renal, suprarenal, and, most often, underlying vascular disease. Central nervous system factors involving the release of neurogenic amines and ACTH as part of the chronic stress response are also felt to play a key role, particularly in idiopathic forms (essential hypertension). Although the hemorrhagic CVA is seen less frequently (15 per cent) as the cause of death than cerebral infarction in the general population, it is the most likely form to be seen in the dental office. Acute elevations of blood pressure appear to be the major predisposing factor in acute hemorrhagic CVA, and the risk has been estimated as increasing by 30 per cent for every 10 mm Hg elevation of systolic pressure above 160.

Pulmonary. The control of stress is also important for the well-being of patients with certain types of pulmonary disease. Bronchial asthma is usually classified in two different forms: allergenic (extrinsic Type I) and non-allergenic (intrinsic). The allergenic form is almost always begun by antigens that trigger the release of chemical mediators such as histamine, bradykinin, and slow reacting substance of anaphylaxis (SRS-A) from the bronchial mast cells. The non-allergenic form is usually provoked by non-allergenic pollutants and physical and emotional stress. Both forms of asthma result clinically in episodes of wheezing and progressive expiratory dyspnea. In all cases, uncontrolled anxiety can play an important role. In some patients, particularly children and phobic adults, it is a primary trigger for an attack, and removal of the source of anxiety (such as a dreaded dental operation) may dramatically reverse symptoms. In most patients the degree of anxiety will largely determine the extent of the attack once it has begun.

Similarly, the patient who is experiencing acute pulmonary edema must receive adequate stress and pain control. This condition presents with clinical symptoms of dyspnea, increased respiratory rate, nocturia, orthopnea, and, late in the disease course, paroxysmal nocturnal dyspnea. The predisposition is usually to left heart failure, a more common entity than right ventricular failure. Acute crisis may be precipitated by stress in the dental chair, and patients will show signs of cough and suffocating dyspnea, pallor, sweating, increased diastolic blood pressure and eventually cyanosis.

Endocrine. Another high risk category of patients includes those with endocrinopathy, especially those who are brittle diabetics, who have adrenal insufficiency, or who have thyroid dysfunction. Although symptomatic hyperglycemia in the diabetic is a gradually developing and usually non-life-threatening problem, if untreated it will progress to acidosis and coma. Hyperglycemia is often precipitated by upsets in secondary disease states, by dehydration, and by fever of some duration, not an uncommon set of circumstances for a patient with a dental abscess. The patient presents with a flushed, hot, and dry face, rapid pulse, low blood pressure, and hyperventilation.

In contrast, hypoglycemia is a much more rapidly evolving emergency problem. The diabetic patient who has not eaten and is under stress will have rapid consumption of available glucose. As blood glucose falls below the critical 50 mg per 100 ml, signs of brain dysfunction appear, with confusion, yawning, and lethargy along with nausea and hunger. As blood glucose continues to drop, the patient enters a phase of increased sympathetic activity in which there are sweating, tachycardia, and increased anxiety just prior to loss of consciousness. It is important that the signs of CNS dysfunction not be misinterpreted as a purely psychogenic-based syncope, and especially critical that depressant drugs, including local analgesics, not be administered to the patient who is in impending hypoglycemic or hyperglycemic shock.

An ordinary endocrine response to stress involves the release of ACTH from the pituitary gland and the consequent release of a number of glucocorticoid hormones by the adrenal cortex. The glucocorticoids, primarily cortisol, aid in the adaptation to stress by increasing metabolic rate, increasing sodium retention, and making small blood vessels more responsive to the pressor effects of norepinephrine. If glucocorticoids are insufficient, the stress response becomes a downhill course of depleted extracellular fluid, hyperkalemia, and eventually death due to peripheral vascular collapse and ventricular asystole.

Adrenal cortical insufficiency may exist as a primary disease (Addison's disease) or much more commonly as adrenal atrophy secondary to the administration of exogenous steroids. There is, of course, wide use of steroids in the treatment of allergic-inflammatory states, often over long periods of time. There is also evidence that adrenal hypofunction can continue as long as two years after drugs have been stopped. Patients with Addison's disease and secondary insufficiency can often tolerate ordinary day-to-day stresses but may not be able to respond to maladaptive crises in the dental office. Acute adrenal crisis must be prevented by providing increased exogenous cortisols to meet anticipated stresses and by reducing stress.

Patients with thyroid gland dysfunction are also a higher risk population. Hypothyroidism, producing the syndrome of myxedema, is a rather common disorder, which, if recognized, is easily treated with exogenous thyroxin. Myxedematous patients are at higher risk for two general reasons. First, they have a high incidence of cardiovascular disease due to cardiac enlargement. Second, the myxedematous patient is extremely sensitive to the actions of sedatives such as barbiturates, narcotics, and minor tranquilizers. The potential for drug overdose at ordinarily safe dose levels is quite high. This is because thyroid hormone is the basic determinant of basal metabolic rate (BMR) and because the capacity of liver cells to detoxify sedative agents is reduced in the hypothyroid condition.

Complications may also arise among patients with hyperthyroidism. Because of the elevation in BMR, these patients are prone to cardiac irritability, and conditions such as angina pectoris may be exacerbated. For this reason they should not be given a vagal blocking agent such as atropine, and vasopressor agents contained within local analgesic solutions should be used with extreme caution to avoid an uncontrollable sympathetic response. Although the exact cause of hyperthyroid disease is not known, it occurs mostly in areas where there are iodine deficiencies in water and food, and it is often first manifested in patients during periods of intense physical and emotional stress. As an added source of difficulty, mild hyperthyroidism may closely resemble acute anxiety states, but would not be expected to respond as well to psychosedation.

Psychiatric. Patients with psychiatric disorders are higher risk patients for two general reasons; first, uncontrolled anxiety and stress responses directly exacerbate this disease, and second, they are often being treated with drugs with considerable side effects and interactions. Certain subgroups of psychiatric patients present special problems, particularly psychotics, hysterics, and depressives. Psychotic patients are readily identified because of their extreme behavioral and thought dysfunction. The challenges in achieving behavioral control are usually obvious. The heightened risk is in large part related to the fact that many psychotic patients are debilitated secondary to nutritional and endocrine deficits and also that the drug regimes used to manage these states are often complex and variable in their side effects. Many of the psychotropic drugs such as the phenothiazines and the butyrophenones have marked effects on peripheral vasomotor reflexes, making the patients prone to orthostatic hypotension. These effects may be potentiated by psychosedative drugs likely to be used in controlling pain and anxiety.

Hysteria is seen as a non-adaptive physical response to an anxiety producing situation. Examples include non-organic hemiparesis, hysteric blindness, immobility of body parts including the jaws, chest pains, and hyperventilation. These patients are difficult diagnostic problems, and experience has shown that a good history and preventive pain and anxiety control are the best treatment.

The most common psychiatric syndrome that will present risk problems to the dental practitioner is depression. Actually a spectrum of related disorders, depression is characterized by vegetative disorders of sleep, appetite, bowel and sex functions, and mood disorder producing despair, apathy, and acute lowering of intellectual performance. Often the depression may be masked in a physical complaint or coupled with a compulsive personality with manic episodes. These patients are high risks because their physiologic responses to stress and to psychosedative drugs are so unpredictable and variable from day to day.

A depressive patient suffering anxiety in the dental chair may respond very nicely to sedation with intravenous diazepam during the stress period, only to suffer a marked deepening of the depression *for days* postoperatively. The drugs used to treat depression may also increase the risk of management. Many patients use anxiolytic agents such as alcohol, minor tranquilizers, and barbiturates, often in an uncontrolled, self-titrated manner. Each of these drug classes, when combined with usual psychosedative techniques may produce drug interaction, including risk of serious respiratory depression. Many other depressed patients are being treated with antidepressants. Two general classes of antidepressants are in use; the monoamine oxidase inhibitors (MAOI) and the tricyclics.

The MAO inhibitors have been implicated in severe hypertensive and hypotensive crises when patients have received intravascular injections of local analgesic with vasoconstrictors.

The MAO inhibitors have also been found to be incompatible with the narcotics and barbiturates as well as certain foods containing tyramine. The tricyclics, now more widely used in clinical psychiatry, have also recently been shown to have potential interaction with local analgesic vasopressors. More commonly, tricyclic therapy may be complicated by increased cardiac arrhythmias, and diaphoresis with fluid retention in appendages and abdomen. These patients are less able to adapt to physiologic stress and may develop more severe arrhythmia and hypotension as a result.

Drug Abuse. Patients who abuse drugs are especially high risks in the stressful dental care setting. Patients who abuse the classic sedative-hypnotic drugs, alcohol, barbiturates, and narcotics are often not good stress responders because they are debilitated and have neither psychic nor physical reserves. The alcoholic with hepatic cirrhosis may not have sufficient liver function to detoxify psychosedative agents that might be given. Ironically, because of the mechanisms of enzyme induction, and drug tolerance, many sedative-hypnotic drug abusers will require massive doses of usual psychosedatives before the desired behavioral relaxation is seen. Then as the excitement and euphoria passes, the patient often manifests a "rebound" physiologic *depression* of vital functions.

Many drug abusers, fearful of dental treatment, will "fortify" themselves before an appointment with their drug. In the case of alcohol, this practice is relatively easily detected and the clinician can avoid compounding problems by not attempting to operate on or sedate an intoxicated patient. The signs of intoxication by other drugs, particularly the hallucinogenic agents such as tetrahydrocannabinol (marijuana) and amphetamine, are more difficult to detect. These are drugs whose half-lives are very long, in the order of days, and which depot in body stores to be released in times of stress and excitement. Recent studies have shown clearly that the hallucinogens, *including the widespread cannabinols*, when combined with the stress of dental care, may precipitate marked elevations in anxiety, psychotic-like responses, increased likelihood of syncope, and potentially dangerous tachycardias.

CONTROLLING THE PAIN-ANXIETY-STRESS EXPERIENCE

More precise knowledge of the basic mechanisms of pain, anxiety, and stress response are leading to safer and more effective clinical controls. Pharmacotherapy is still the most widely used approach, and has been aided by the introduction of the benzodiazepines in the 60s with their excellent safety record, by the development of conscious neuroleptic approaches in the 70s, and by the establishment of comprehensive teaching guidelines for the use of nitrous oxide. There is new interest in the use of local analgesics, with the introduction of less toxic and less allergenic agents, the demonstration of the effectiveness of more dilute concentrations of vasoconstrictors, and the proven applications of longer duration agents such as bupivacaine and etidocaine.

Recently there has been an expanded application of non-pharmacologic techniques to the control of pain, anxiety, and stress. Behavioral approaches such as hypnosis, autogenic relaxation training, and biofeedback have been applied to the stressful dental setting. They are proving especially useful when combined with adjunctive psychosedative drugs. Physiologic ap-

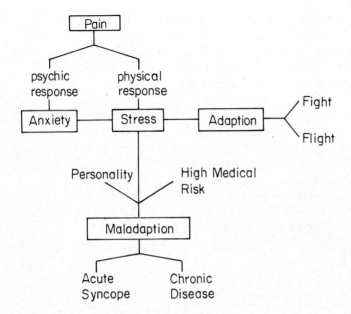

Figure 6-2 Interrelationships of pain, anxiety, and stress.

proaches to pain control have not found wide acceptance as yet. However, it has been demonstrasted that acupuncture stimulation and transcutaneous electrical neural stimulation can induce changes in the pain threshold that may be due to the activation of the opiate receptor system in the brain. Behavioral and physiologic methods for controlling pain, however, still represent the least developed of potential methods of patient control.

Whatever approach might be used, it is now clear that pain, anxiety and stress are not controlled through a single psychologic or physiologic process, as one would turn down the volume on a radio. Rather, they can be controlled by inducing a number of specific psychophysiologic states within the nervous system. Those primary control states are: *analgesia, hypnosis, hyporeflexia, amnesia, tranquilization,* and *dissociation* (Table 6–2).

Analgesia. For purposes of routine dental analgesia, care can be divided into two types: regional and systemic. Regional nerve block analgesia-

TABLE 6-2 CNS STATES THAT MODIFY PAIN, ANXIETY, AND STRESS RESPONSE

Analgesia	—a systemic raising of thresholds for pain perception or tolerance. "When it happened it didn't feel like pain"
Hypnosis	—an artificial induction of sleep processes. "I was too sleepy to be aware of pain"
Hyporeflexia	—decreased ability to respond to painful stimulation. "It hurt but I didn't react"
Amnesia	—interference with learning or recall. "It didn't happen"
Tranquilization	—a calming and dampening of anxiety. "It was happening but didn't scare me"
Dissociation	—a feeling of depersonalization; a detachment of the "self" from reality. "It was happening to someone, but it wasn't really me"

may be a preferred term for the effects of local anesthetic agents, since true anesthesia, the "absence of all sensation," is rarely achieved with nontoxic concentrations of local anesthetics. Systemic analgesia is a raising of thresholds for pain perception and, more often, pain tolerance. As we have seen in an earlier section, analgesic drugs activate descending opiate receptor systems, which arise in the anterior brainstem. In the trigeminal system morphine and nitrous oxide have been shown to suppress activity in the nociceptor cells of subnucleus caudalis, presumably through the descending opiate receptor mechanism. Unfortunately, virtually all current major analgesic drugs also have potentially dangerous actions in the anterior brainstem in addition to their opiate receptor actions. Specifically, the variable stimulation of reticular formation centers in midbrain, pons, and medulla may induce respiratory depression because of reduced responsiveness to lowered pCO_2 levels.

Hypnosis is a CNS state that has classically been sought as a means of reducing acute pain, anxiety and stress. It implies an artificial induction of a sleep process and appears to dull the awareness of pain stimuli and the drive to respond to them. Certain agents appear to exert their primary pain and anxiety control through hypnosis, notably the barbiturates, which at the same time have little or no analgesic action. In contrast, the potent analgesic-narcotic fentanyl has little hypnotic action, and nitrous oxide produces mild to moderate levels of both hypnosis and analgesia. The mechanism of drug induced hypnosis is tied to the diffuse "reticular activating" network in the core of the brainstem. The barbiturates are known to induce sleep by suppressing neural activity in this system. However, recent neuropharmacologic research has shown that unconsciousness may also be caused by stimulating certain reticular centers, inducing a seizure-like activity in which the rapid eye movement (REM) phase of sleep predominates. Neuroleptic drugs, the dissociative agent ketamine, and to some degree nitrous oxide appear to induce sleep through this active stimulation rather than through classic depression of reticular functions.

Hyporeflexia. Lowered responsiveness to stimuli is a potentially useful state for controlling the effects of pain and anxiety. It implies the suppression of unwanted aversive skeletal muscle reflexes and lowering of autonomic and endocrine stress responses. It is a state which aids the patient by preventing entry into the maladaptive stress phase, and helps the clinician because the patient is quiet and physiologically stable. Atropine and scopolamine induce hyporeflexia for activities of the parasympathetic system and particularly the vagus nerve. They prevent the maladaptive fear-induced vasovagal bradycardia and hypotension which lead to syncope. Certain of the narcotics, particularly when used in neuroleptic combinations with narcotics, markedly suppress skeletal muscle aversive reflexes, presumably through CNS mechanisms. Succinylcholine and curare produce skeletal muscle hyporeflexia when used in low doses and areflexia at higher therapeutic levels; they act not on the CNS but on the neuromuscular endplate. The suppression of skeletal muscle reflexes, although desirable to some degree in conscious sedation for the control of dysfunctions such as gagging and spasticity, is also a source of potential danger when protective functions such as cough and laryngeal reflexes are decreased.

Amnesia, or loss of memory for the pain-anxiety experience, has become a powerful tool in recent years. It has been shown that this state can be attained even though the patient is conscious and otherwise intellectually competent. Most effective sedation methods and some autosuggestion techniques attain some degree of amnesia. The benzodiazepine tranquilizers, particularly diazepam, have been shown to be very potent amnesics, capable of "erasing" up to 100 per cent of the memory of local analgesic injections and even very painful incisions at very small doses. Neuroleptic combinations such as fentanyl and droperidol are also very powerful amnesics, whereas nitrous oxide and the belladonna alkaloids, commonly used in sedative drug combinations such as in the Jorgensen technique, have a mild and variable amnesia potency. In all types of sedative amnesic drugs studied thus far, the amnesia is strictly anterograde, meaning the loss of memory for events which follow the administration of the drug. This is in direct contrast to the retrograde amnesia brought on by cranial concussion, in which physical injury to temporal cortex memory stores appears to occur. The mechanism of sedative-amnesia action appears to be an interference with the "consolidation" phase of learning in which a short-term memory trace is transferred, probably through protein synthesis mechanisms, to permanent memory storage. The primary amnesic effect, therefore, is on long-term memory, and there appears to be little interference with the patient's ability to recall events that happened seconds or a few minutes previously.

Tranquilization implies a psychic relaxation, diminished anxiety, and decreased concern for the painful event. The active induction of tranquility appears to involve centers in the limbic cortex which can be activated either chemically or neurally from higher neocortical pathways. The limbic system mediates the psychophysiologic events that we know as "emotion" and, through its direct feedback controls over the hypothalamic-pituitary and probably opiate receptor systems, it is a primary determinant of the pain response. Certain classes of drugs appear to be more specific for action in limbic centers, notably the "minor" tranquilizers such as benzodiazepines and the "major" tranquilizers such as the phenothiazines. Other drugs, such as nitrous oxide and the narcotics, may have tranquilizing effects also, but they appear to depend more on indirect influences from other cortical areas. Therefore, the euphoria seen with nitrous oxide and morphine may have a tranquilizing effect on the properly oriented patient, but may on occasion have a paradoxical dysphoric and non-tranquilizing effect if patients are not reassured.

Dissociation is a fascinating and poorly understood CNS state which may have profound effect on pain and anxiety. It is an active "depersonalization" or shifting of the individual out of his usual mental image of "self" and has been likened to a transient schizophrenia. In response to pain and anxiety, the patient is able to dissociate the events occurring in the body (pain) from the real self and therefore does not physically or emotionally react. This state is closely associated with hallucinogenic activity in the brain, and theorists have suggested that it represents a dominance of the primitive paleocortical brain and suppression of the conscious neocortex. Many common drugs can induce varying degrees of dissociation, as can certain mental and physical deprivation states. Starvation, sensory deprivation, self-induced trances, and extreme fear may precipitate dissociation. Alcohol, amphetamines, nitrous oxide, and belladonna alkaloids are mild and variable dissociators, dependent on dose. The major dissociative drugs currently available include LSD, cocaine, ketamine, and the cannabinols (marijuana). Experimentation with these potent dissociatives in the pain-anxiety setting has produced highly mixed and sometimes disturbing results. Nevertheless, it represents a promising futuristic approach to pain control.

GUIDELINES FOR PATIENT CARE

No single therapy currently available, whether it is behavioral, physiologic, or pharmacologic, can reliably produce the ideal blend of CNS states described above. Nevertheless, the clinician may orchestrate patient care by seeking the best combinations of effects for a given patient, at the same time adhering to a few general guidelines (Table 6–3):

Guideline 1. Be preventive in controlling pain and anxiety. Maladaptive stress responses, it has been seen, are the outcome of unresolved pain-anxiety conflict and are best treated preventively, especially in the high risk population.

Guideline 2. Use control techniques as positive reinforcement measures, not as methods of restraint. The backbone of proper pain and anxiety control is patient-clinician rapport and an enhancement of natural positive measures of psychophysiologic control. Drugs which act on the nervous system do not replace the need for patient communication, suggestion, and reinforcement of positive (adaptive) behavior. It has been observed many times, for example, that most centrally acting drugs, particularly narcotics and the hallucinogens, can produce either euphoria or dysphoria, depending on the nature of the environment and the suggestions given to the patient. Nor does good patient relaxation or the use of analgesic drugs eliminate the need for regional nerve block analgesia and atraumatic tissue handling.

Guideline 3. Depend most heavily on preoperative assessment of physical and emotional status to determine correct pain and anxiety control methods. It is important to select patients properly, to know when a more severe behavioral problem or a higher physical risk exists. Once the operation has begun, continuous monitoring of psychic and physiologic responses will warn of impending problems.

TABLE 6–3 GUIDELINES FOR MANAGING PAIN, ANXIETY AND STRESS

1. Be *preventive* in controlling pain and anxiety.
2. Use control techniques as *adjuncts for positive reinforcement*, not as methods of restraint.
3. Emphasize preoperative assessment and intraoperative monitoring of patient physical and emotional status.
4. *Adapt* and *select* control techniques that fit the patient's needs rather than fitting patients to preferred techniques.
5. Use *"titration"* pharmacosedation techniques rather than predetermined dose schedules.

Guideline 4. Adapt and select control techniques that fit the patient's needs. This is opposed to the use of a single control approach for all patient problems. Error is commonly made, for example, in attempting to control moderate to severe behavorial problems with nitrous oxide sedation techniques alone, an approach that often leads to ineffective control or unsafe levels of anesthetic use.

Guideline 5. Use *titration* pharmacosedation techniques rather than predetermined dose schedules. Although usually effective dose ranges and toxic doses should be known, psychosedative drugs should be added slowly until objective and subjective levels of relaxation and psychophysiologic control are attained. *If predetermined boluses of drug are used, there is risk of inadequate depth of sedation or overdose due to the marked variation in patient responsiveness to CNS agents.*

REFERENCES

1. Alderman, E. L.: Analgesics in the acute phase of myocardial infarction. J.A.M.A., 229:12, 1974.
2. Berger, H.: Hypoglycemia: A perspective. Postgrad. Med., 57:81, 1975.
3. Campbell, R. L., Gregg, J. M., et al.: Vasovagal response during oral surgery. J. Oral Surg., 34:698, 1976.
4. Cannon, W. B.: Bodily Changes in Pain, Hunger, Fear and Rage. 2nd ed., New York, Appleton-Century-Crofts, 1927.
5. Cannon, W. B.: "Voodoo" death. Amer. Anthrop., 44:169, 1942.
6. Edmonson, H. D., Roscoe, B., and Vickers, M. D.: Biochemical evidence of anxiety in dental patients. Brit. Med. J., 4:7, 1972.
7. Epstein, S. E., et al.: Angina pectoris: Pathophysiology, evaluation, and treatment. Ann. Intern. Med., 75:263, 1971.
8. Felig, P.: Pathophysiology of diabetes mellitus. Med. Clin. North Am., 55:821, 1971.
9. Flod, N. E., Franz, M. L., and Galant, S. P.: Recent advances in bronchial asthma. Am. J. Dis. Child., 130:890, 1976.
10. Friedberg, C. K.: Syncope, pathological physiology, differential diagnosis and treatment. Mod. Concepts Cardiovasc. Dis., 40:55, 1971.
11. Gregg, J. M., Functional anatomy of facial pain, In Alling, C., and Mahon, P. (eds.): Textbook of Facial Pain. Philadelphia, Lea and Febiger, 1977, pp. 25–44.
12. Gregg, J., Small, E., et al.: Emotional response to intravenous delta 9-tetrahydrocannabinol during oral surgery. J. Oral Surg., 34:301, 1976.
13. Gregg, J. M., Ryan, D. E., and Levin, K. J.: The amnesic actions of diazepam. J. Oral Surg., 32:651, 1974.
14. Grindal, A. B., and Toole, J. R.: Headache and transient ischemic attacks. Stroke, 5:603, 1974.
15. Hughes, J., Smith, T. W., Kosterlitz, H. W., et al.: Identification of two related pentopeptides from the brain with potent opiate agonist activity. Nature, 258:577, 1975.
16. Kannel, W. B., and Feinleib, M.: Natural history of angina pectoris in the Framingham study: Prognosis and survival. Am. J. Cardiol., 29:154, 1972.
17. Locksley, H. B.: Hemorrhagic strokes: Principle causes, natural history, and treatment. Med. Clin. North Am., 52:1193, 1968.
18. Malamed, S. F.: Handbook of Medical Emergencies in the Dental Office. Saint Louis, The C. V. Mosby Co., 1978.
19. May, R.: The Meaning of Anxiety. New York, W. W. Norton, 1977.
20. Mayer, D. J., and Price, D. D.: Central nervous system mechanisms of analgesia. Pain, 2:379, 1976.
21. Menendez, C. E., and Rivlin, R. S.: Throtoxic crises and myxedema coma. Med. Clin. North Am., 57:1463, 1973.
22. Messing, R. B., and Lytle, L. D.: Serotonin-containing neurons: their possible role in pain and analgesia. Pain, 4:1, 1977.
23. Price, D. D., and Dubner, R.: Neurons that subserve the sensory-discriminative aspects of pain. Pain, 3:307, 1977.
24. Schachter, J.: Pain, fear and anger in hypertensives and normotensives. Psychosom. Med., 19:17, 1957.

25. Selye, H.: The Stress of Life. New York, McGraw-Hill, 1976.
26. Snulyan, H., Gilber, R., and Eich, R. H.: Pulmonary effects of heart failure. Surg. Clin. North Am., 54:1077, 1974.
27. Snyder, S. H.: Opiate receptors and internal opiates. Sci. Am., 236:44, 1977.
28. Staples, A. F.: Cardiopulmonary crisis in the dental office. Dent. Clin. North Am., 17:473, 1973.
29. Sternbach, R. A.: Pain Patients: Traits and Treatment. New York, Academic Press, 1974.
30. Streeten, D. H. P.: Corticosteroid therapy. I. Pharmacological properties and principles of corticosteroid use, J.A.M.A., 232:944, 1975.
31. Streeten, D. H. P.: Corticosteroid therapy. II. Complications and therapeutic indications. J.A.M.A., 232:1046, 1975.
32. Wepman, B. J.: Psychological components of pain perception. Dent. Clin. North Am., 22:101, 1978.
33. Woodrow, K. M., et al.: Pain tolerance: differences according to age, sex, and race. Soc. Psychosom. Med., 34:548–556, 1972.

7

PSYCHOSEDATION

Part 2: Iatrosedation

NATHAN FRIEDMAN

INTRODUCTION

Fear of dentistry is a worldwide health problem of considerable significance. In the United States it is estimated that 20 to 40 million people
avoid the dental practitioner because of fear. For these people, fear is a
more destructive lesion than caries or periodontal disease, since it is the
major obstacle to their seeking dental health care.

Avoidance of usual preventive dental care frequently results in extensive pathology. Consequently, such patients are eventually driven to the
doctor by some crisis-like situation: either pain, swelling, acute infection,
or the last-ditch need to have a badly destroyed dentition treated. However, the doctor cannot "get to" the teeth until the barrier of fear is removed
in some way. Attempting to ignore the wall of fear usually leads to great
frustration and stress for the doctor and a higher fear level for the patient.

A recent survey of dental practitioners indicates that 57 per cent of
those responding considered the "difficult patient" to be the most stressful
single factor in their practices.[8] It is clear that for both the doctor and pa-

tient, fear must be viewed as a signficant syndrome requiring treatment. In a sense, each time the clinician is faced with a fearful patient, he or she is dealing with an emergency: not a dental emergency, but the emergency of fear. For the patient, facing the practitioner triggers an acute mobilization of fear. For the doctor, facing the fearful patient may create considerable stress, a sense of inadequacy, and frustration unless he or she is equipped to deal with the problem expertly.

The clinician has a variety of ways to help the fearful patient. The use of drugs is the traditional modality. The techniques of inhalation and intravenous and oral sedation have been taught for years in dental schools and, postdoctorally, through continuing education channels. The techniques are well structured and the goals quite clear, and the doctors using these modalities are confident of their effectiveness. However, it must be recognized that pharmacosedation does not reduce or eliminate fear; it temporarily circumvents it. Its value lies primarily in making dental treatment approachable for the patient by diminishing awareness and producing a temporary state of tranquility.

Treatment of the fear syndrome requires a different technique, one by which the fear is eliminated or significantly reduced by means of a relearning process. The relearning process is the result of interactions designed for this purpose and initiated by the doctor.

Traditionally, sedation has been equated with the use of drugs to induce calmness. Although in a vague way it is conceded that the behavior of the doctor is helpful in calming the anxious patient, it is considered a haphazard, intuitive effort. The concept of fear treatment to be developed in the following pages is based on a system of simple behavioral techniques designed to accomplish the goal with maximum efficiency and minimum use of time. This system is iatrosedation.

TERMINOLOGY

Iatrosedation is defined as the act of making calm by the doctor's behavior. Behavior, in this sense, includes a broad spectrum of verbal and non-verbal communication (behavior). The word was formulated by the author through combining the prefix "iatro" (pertaining to the doctor) with sedation (the act of making calm).

Pharmacosedation is defined as the act of making calm with the use of drugs.

Psychosedation (as used in this book) refers to psychological calming, making the person calm. It is distinguished from organ sedation wherein some part of the body is calmed, such as cardiac sedation. Psychosedation, then, is the generic term for psychological calming and includes iatrosedation and pharmacosedation.

In treating the fearful patient, iatrosedation is primary and pharmacosedation is secondary. The fear is reduced to the lowest level possible with iatrosedation. If this level is not sufficiently low to permit the patient to cope with the dental experience, pharmacosedation is used supplementally. In most instances, however, iatrosedation alone will reduce the fear to a functional level.

COMPONENTS OF IATROSEDATIVE PROCESS

Iatrosedation has two components: (1) the iatrosedative interview and (2) the iatrosedative clinical encounter.

1. The Iatrosedative Interview

The first meeting of doctor and patient is an interview in the literal sense of the word; that is, it is a view between two people. If in the course of this interchange the patient indicates either verbally or nonverbally that he or she is anxious, the doctor responds by initiating an iatrosedative interview. The procedure is designed to identify the fear problem, make a diagnosis, and initiate treatment. The fear level will drop as the interview progresses so that a substantive decrease will be achieved at its completion. Usually, the interview does not complete the relearning process in which the fear is eliminated or maximally reduced. This occurs during the second phase of the iatrosedative process, the iatrosedative clinical encounters.

2. Iatrosedative Clinical Encounters

The first clinical encounter is crucial. This is the "firing line." The patient and doctor are going to face together what the patient perceives as dangerous. The doctor's behavioral technique must be structured to blend with his or her clinical techniques to provide the maximum feeling of safety for the patient. Often this first clinical interaction will result in a successful learning experience, eliminating the fear entirely; that is, dropping the level to what is considered within the normal anxiety range. If this does not occur, subsequent clinical encounters will continue to decrease the fear until the maximum effect of iatrosedation is achieved.

There are instances when the iatrosedative interview does not drop the fear level sufficiently and the patient requires some pharmacosedation to face the first clinical encounter. The choice of modality is worked out together, based on the patient's previous experiences and feelings about the use of drugs and the methods of administering them. Many people have anxieties about inhalation sedation because of imagined threat to breathing, some about intravenous sedation based on a feeling of loss of control, while others object to the use of drugs in any form.

DENTAL FEARS

Every doctor is familiar with the more obvious fears patients may have, for example:

1. *Fear of pain*
2. *Fear of the "drill"*
   There may be several components besides that of producing pain; for example, mutilation due to slipping, the sense of cutting, the noise, smell, or other.

3. *Fear of the "needle"*
   The most common fear is that of pain of injection. There are others, however, such as:
   a.   Fear of deep penetration
   b.   Fear of tissue injury
   c.   Fear of numbness, etc.
4. *Fear of surgery*
   Periodontal and oral surgery may be feared because of fantasies of mutilation, threat to body image, pain, or for other reasons.
5. *Fear of the loss of teeth*
   This partial list will suffice. However, other fears invariably are combined with the above obvious ones. Frequently these are more important fears which are not apparent to the patient or the doctor until they surface during the interview. These are fears that all people have normally but which are exaggerated when bound up with the dental fears listed above. They are:

1. Fear of the unknown
2. Fear of helplessness and dependency
3. Fear of body damage and body change
   Each of these heightened fears, when they exist, must be dealt with in the iatrosedative process. As we shall see, there are specific techniques designed to deal with these components of the problem.

HOW DENTAL FEARS ARE LEARNED

Basically, fear of the dental practitioner is learned. It can be learned in a variety of ways and is expressed in seemingly limitless kinds of experiences. However, irrespective of how the fear was learned and what the central focus is — be it pain, the "drill," or the "needle" — *the ultimately important element usually is the behavior of past doctors.* As a consequence, *the ultimately important element in defusing that fear will be the behavior of the present doctor* and the feelings generated in the patient as a consequence of such behavior.

Fear may be learned as a consequence of *direct* or *indirect* experiences. A direct experience is one in which the individual has suffered some traumatic incident or threat of trauma in a dental or medical therapeutic situation. Traumatic experiences not related to medicine or dentistry can spread to the dental situation if there is some triggering reminiscent occurrence.

An *indirect* experience is one in which the fear is learned vicariously. The most frequent vicarious source is the family; father, mother or sibling.[11] The child may learn to be fearful as a consequence of observing a parent's experience or hearing of it. The same would hold true for those of siblings or friends. Other vicarious experiences result from viewing motion pictures, television skits, and cartoons portraying painful or threatening dental scenes.

These experiences most frequently occur during childhood. The memories of the events and the feelings associated with them may persist throughout life unless relearning occurs. Fortunately, the ability to unlearn and relearn is resident in each individual.

THE CONDITIONING ASPECT OF DENTAL FEARS

Classical Conditioning

Heightened fear of the clinician and the dental experience may be viewed as a conditioned response in some instances, similar to the response found in pavlovian classical conditioning. A brief review of this paradigm is:

Pavlov offered food (unconditioned stimulus) to dogs and this resulted in salivation (unconditioned response). Pavlov then presented food to the same dogs, but simultaneously paired it with a bell tone (conditioned stimulus). After a critical number of pairings, the sound of the bell became a sufficient stimulus to produce salivation (conditioned response).

An example of a direct dental experience that can be likened to conditioning is as follows:

A child is taken to a dental practitioner. An aversive stimulus such as pain elicits a response of high fear. The pain may be caused by the "drill" or the "needle," but it is the doctor who is paired with the instrument that produces the pain. The doctor then may be considered a conditioned stimulus and the fear associated with the appearance or thought of the practitioner may be likened to a conditioned response.

Although the above example is likened to classical conditioning, an overlay of interrelated variables may be conceptualized. The histories of many patients reveal fear-learning patterns, leading to an assumption that more is involved than the simple pairing of the doctor with the pain or the instrument causing the pain. The behavior of the practitioner seems to be a powerful component of the traumatic experience. The normal fears of helplessness, dependency, and the unknown are markedly intensified and become, with the pain, a part of the conditioned response. Hence the doctor, as a conditioned stimulus, may trigger a conditioned response which includes all of those fears. Yet the fear will be labelled simply fear of pain.

A simple example of such conditioning is reflected in the behavior of a 45 year old male patient who visited the dental practitioner for an examination. He was extremely anxious and had been for two days prior to the visit. His history revealed that, when he was about five years of age, he was taken to a practitioner by his father to have a tooth extracted. He had a vivid memory of pain and of being pinned down by his father and the doctor. During the struggle the overwhelming experience of force, pain, injury, and total violation of trust and denial of any protection against frightening danger was imprinted on the child's brain. His father's behavior compounded that of the clinician's, and the conditioning was magnified in intensity. The fears of helplessness, dependency, and the unknown clearly are integrated with the painful experience.

One such traumatic event can result in a lifelong conditioned response of high anxiety unless relearning or counterconditioning takes place. Iatrosedation is designed to reduce or eliminate high anxiety through relearning (counterconditioning).

Generalization

Conditioning also results in generalization; that is, its effects spread from the original traumatic circumstances to situations which have similar elements — for example, medical experiences generalize to dental situations if similar cues are involved.

Childhood experiences with surgery such as tonsillectomies are a common source of fear learning that may be generalized to the dental scene. This is true not only in relation to mutilation or pain but to the experience with general or local analgesia.

Injections for immunization or for the administration of antibiotics or local analgesics to dress or suture traumatic wounds may be originating circumstances for the heightening of fear and anxiety. An example of generalization is as follows:

Joe B., a muscular, vigorous-looking man, 30 years of age, during the initial interview stated that he did not want local analgesia for any restorative procedure. When asked if there was some reason for this he said that he feared injections; that in the past he reacted to them with nausea and "palpitations," and would "turn white" even at the thought of a "shot." Pain was not a factor but in the course of the interview it became apparent that the *deep penetration of the needle*, as in a mandibular injection, seemed to have been a disturbing experience. Pursuing this cue precipitated an association with childhood experiences. Between the ages of seven and 10, Joe had suffered a number of accidental injuries, such as scalp wounds and deep cuts about the face and legs. Each time these emergencies arose he was rushed to the physician or hospital amid considerable anxiety and would have an injection to permit suturing, followed by an injection of an antibiotic. Consequently, *injections became associated with body injury, crisis, fear, and pain*, and a locked-in conditioned response developed. Each time Joe had to face an injection of any type, or in any area of the body, he would suffer acute anxiety. This was generalized to an intraoral injection for regional anesthesia. In an attempt to avoid this anxiety when having dental restorative procedures, he refused to have injections of local analgesics.

MODELLING

Another method of learning is through modelling.[1] This is an indirect or vicarious learning experience. Fears often arise in children because of their observations of traumatic experiences of parents, siblings, or friends, or hearing stories of these experiences. This kind of learning also may take place as a result of seeing traumatic dental scenes portrayed in television skits, motion pictures, or cartoons.

The parental scene is a common and powerful learning arena for fear, as evidenced by the following history. Here, the patient refuses injections for regional anesthesia just as Joe B. (above) did, but the fear is based on a modelling learning experience rather than a direct one.

A woman, 45 years of age, refused injections for dental treatment, stating that she feared them tremendously. When asked what there was about the injection that she feared, she responded that she didn't know. She had not had any traumatic experiences at the hands of dental or medical practitioners as a child or as an adult. Seemingly there was no reason for the fear. When questioned about blood tests she replied that she would not have them. When asked about immunization injections as a child she said that neither she nor her sister had them because her mother, a nurse, "didn't believe in them." The clinician interpreted this to indicate that a small child being told this by her mother (a nurse as well) would feel that "shots" were dangerous and must be avoided. His approach to the solution of the problem was to use this interpretation as the starting point.

In the above history, the fear was not linked with the behavior of a doctor or some other authoratative figure. This usually is not the case. In most instances the tales heard from others or scenes viewed on television will include the doctor's unsympathetic behavior linked with the traumatic event. A small child accepts these impressions as real and universal and, consequently, may face the *first* dental experience with fear.

A dental practitioner who is cognizant of the symptoms of fear can dispel this type of anxiety quite easily. If, on the other hand, he or she is unaware of or ignores the symptoms, a more powerful fear-learning experience will occur, precipitated by the doctor's inept behavior when trying to treat a frightened patient.

An example of modelling based on observation of events portrayed on the screen is as follows:

A 47 year old male stated, "I have a terrible fear of dentists." He characterized his mouth as a "disaster area," not having had treatment for a number of years. He stated that he tolerated pain well, that he has had pain all of his adult life since he was injured and disabled in service. "It's probably more the anticipation than the actual act that worries me. I tolerate pain fairly well." Learning to fear the dental practitioner started as a child because, as he stated, "It seems to be part of our social syndrome to be afraid of dentists. I remember I used to see movies — comedies, you know — the guy gets in there, 'this isn't going to hurt' and wow!...you know. It's supposed to be funny but it scares you and you're supposed to overcome that fear..." The story unfolded in a way that suggested that when he did go to the dental clinician he had high anticipatory anxiety, including a heightened fear of the unknown which he characterized as "...the strangeness of having a hand groping in there with sharp instruments and cutting away at things that normally are not cut upon . . ." Interrelated with the unknown was the potential body damage that the "strange hand" may create.

Knowledge of the learning paradigms is essential to the effective use of the technique of iatrosedation. Similarly, it is important to understand the significance to the patient of the doctor's behavior in all aspects of dental care. The significance of such behavior becomes even more consequential where anxiety is a dominant factor.

THE PATIENT'S PERCEPTION OF THE DOCTOR

Fearful patients require a specific type of behavior from doctors. Janis constructed a blueprint of such behavior based on his results obtained from a five year study of the psychological stress endured by patients preparing for and undergoing major and minor surgery, including operative dentistry.[7]

He explored, in great depth, the emotions, needs, and responses of these patients relative to the doctors who were caring for them. The behavior of the doctors was determined to have a powerful influence on the patient's fear and stress levels. What they needed from their doctors became apparent. To begin with, Janis concluded that the patient perceives his doctor in two important ways: (1) as a Danger Control Authority and (2) as a Protective Authority.

Surrounding the perception of the doctor in these roles were strong feelings and needs. Janis summarized them as follows:

The doctor controls what the patient perceives as threatening or dangerous and is the only one able to protect him from that danger. The patient facing a threatening situation becomes anxious and looks for emotional support. The Danger-Control Authority, able to protect him from that danger, becomes invested with strong emotional significance. His behavior and communications assume greater importance than would ordinarily be expected. The patient's ability to tolerate stress and learn to cope with his fear depends upon his being able to develop a sense of trust and maintain high confidence in the Protective Authority figure. In order to do this and develop a feeling of safety, there must be a "working through" before the patient is exposed to what he considers dangerous.

This "working through" is the iatrosedative interview, the first interaction between the fearful patient and the doctor. Skillfully performed from a base of knowledge, it ordinarily should not exceed five to 10 minutes. Janis' findings suggest two questions that must be answered in order to solve the problem. They are:

1. What does the patient perceive as threatening or dangerous?
2. What can the doctor do to make the patient feel safe, that he or she will be protected from the danger?

The answers to these questions are the heart of the iatrosedative process.

THE IATROSEDATIVE INTERVIEW

The iatrosedative interview has been fashioned after the traditional open-end interview.[3] It begins with an open-ended question such as, "Are you having any difficulties?" The question provides the patient maximum opportunity to reveal what is uppermost in his or her mind; it permits the patient to establish his or her priority of "difficulties." If the patient elects to begin with a statement about his sensitive teeth or bleeding gingiva or a need for examination because he suspects caries, the doctor responds to each particular cue. He will go on to get information about the problem or need until he is satisfied that he has all that is required to help make a diagnosis and treatment plan.

Most patients are not inordinately fearful and manage their anxieties well, in which case the iatrosedative interview is not needed. However, should the patient respond with any of the many statements of anxiety, such as, "I'm a coward about teeth," or "I'm the worst patient you'll ever have," or "I'm scared to death," the interview should be put on an iatrosedative course immediately.

Strategies of the Interview

Two strategies are involved: (1) a verbal, fact-finding, interpretive strategy, and (2) a nonverbal, empathic strategy.

The verbal fact-finding strategy is divided into two major categories: (1) gathering information and (2) giving information.

Gathering information has a Sherlock Holmes quality about it. The objective is to ferret out pertinent information quickly and concisely. The first question, as suggested from Janis' findings, the doctor (Danger Control Authority) must have answered is, "What is it that the patient perceives as threatening or dangerous?"

Once the patient's fear is determined, the second step is to determine how the fear was learned. Knowledge of the learning paradigms mentioned above can be helpful at this point. Again, this information can be elicited quickly and concisely in a matter of four or five minutes, or less. This is not meant to be an in-depth, prolonged inquiry.

Good information gathering requires an adroit questioning technique, the ability to listen and "hear" what is central in the patient's communication and to respond in a way that will facilitate the unfolding of the story.

After gathering information, the doctor switches to giving information. It is his turn to talk and the patient's turn to listen.

In *giving information*, the doctor (Protective Authority) answers Janis' second question, "What can the doctor do to make the patient feel safe, protected from danger?"

The gathered information is valueless unless it is sorted out and interpreted. It is then fed back to the patient in a way that will give him or her insight into the specifics of the fear, how it was learned and how it can be unlearned. The doctor then states his commitment as to how he will behave and what effect he expects his behavior to have on the patient's ability to relearn.

This verbal communication, coupled with empathic nonverbal communication, will initiate a feeling of trust. If the trust is maintained and subsequently deepened by the iatrosedative clinical encounters, the fear may be eliminated because fear is soluble in trust.

Model of the Iatrosedative Interview

A simple five step model of the above strategy is:

Gathering Information	1. Recognition of the anxiety
	2. Facilitation of the cues
	3. Ventilation by the patient ("talking it out")
Giving Information	1. Management of the information gathered
	2. Commitment by the doctor

The following is a brief explanation of each of these steps:

Recognition of the anxiety is a dual process. The doctor responds verbally to some expression of anxiety by the patient; that is, turns his attention to it. In addition, the nonverbal communication with which the words are transmitted tells the patient that he understands, empathizes, and wants to help him cope with the problem.

Facilitation of the cues is a technique of encouraging the patient to elaborate on the initial statement of anxiety and subsequent cues, a "tell me more" technique. This is the Sherlock Holmesian listening and exploration that will ferret out the critical information needed to identify the problem. This leads to:

Ventilation, which discharges some of the anxiety in the telling of the story, the nature of the fear, its origin and intensity. Most important, the behavior of the previous doctors (or other people involved) may be described.

Management of the information gathered is a "feedback" mechanism by which the patient who learned to be fearful can unlearn this fear and re-learn a different set of feelings and behavior. In the telling, the doctor's statements are supportive and suggestive. This leads to:

Commitment by the doctor to behave in a protective way, different from the previous doctor(s). Some statement of how the feared object or situation will be handled should be given at this time. It should be done with sufficient clarity and depth to elicit a response from the patient, verbally and nonverbally, that the anxiety level has dropped.

Technique of the Iatrosedative Interview

Although the verbal, fact-finding-interpretive aspect of the technique is discussed and exemplified below, I wish to emphasize that the separation of the verbal and nonverbal aspects is artificial. Obviously the verbal and nonverbal communications are, in reality, united and inseparable. However, looking at the techniques separately simplifies the presentation.

Once a patient responds to the opening question with a statement of anxiety or fear such as, "I'm petrified of dentists," a simple but precise tactical design should become operative. The doctor must progress from the general statement of fear to the determination of what the patient *specifically* fears. Eliminating or reducing the fear level is thereby made much easier; it is virtually impossible to make a commitment of behavior if the specific fear is unknown. Once the specific fear is known, the next step is to learn the circumstances of its origin. Graphically stated:

General Statement⟶Specific Fear⟶Origin of Fear

The most economical and expeditious technique for moving from the general to the specific to the origin is by the use of brief, highly specialized questions in responding to the patient's statements. We will label these questions as "what" questions and "can you tell me" questions.

These "on target" questions are succinct. The doctor at this stage of the interview does a minimum of talking and a maximum of listening and responding. (This will be reversed when the time comes for him or her to give information.)

Examples of these "what" and "can you tell me" questions can be illustrated briefly as follows:

Patient: "I'm petrified of dentists." (general statement)

Doctor: "*What* is it you are petrified about?"

Patient: "The drill."

Doctor: "*What* is it about the drill that bothers you?"

The patient may respond to this question by relating the specific aspect of the "drill," stating that it is the pain; that she had always had painful experiences. An appropriate response would be, "*Can you tell me more about it?*" The objective is to have the patient elaborate on the history of her experiences. Another such question is: "*Can you tell* me *what* happened?"

Example and Analysis of an Iatrosedative Interview

The doctor initiates an open-ended interview, unaware that the patient is fearful.

Doctor: "Are you having any difficulties?"

The usual open-ended question; the doctor knows nothing of the patient's feelings. This question permits the patient to establish his or her priority of "difficulties."

Patient: "Doctor, I'm terribly afraid of anything to do with my teeth."

With this general statement of fear, the doctor signals his recognition and acceptance of the problem by responding with the first of the "what" questions. This also sets him on course to determine the specific fear.

Doctor: "What is it that you are afraid of?"

The first of the basic "what" questions.

Patient: "I hate needles."

This is more specific but not specific enough. There are many reasons people fear injections, such as deep penetration, pain, sense of body damage, and others.

Doctor: "What is it about injections that bothers you?"

Another "what" question designed to pinpoint the specifics of the fear.

Patient: "It's the pain of the shot that bothers me."

This is the specific threat. Now the questions should be directed toward revealing the origin of the fear and the behavior of past doctors which may be responsible for this learning.

Doctor: "Have you had painful injections in the past?"

This is a precise question, repeating the word "pain" (painful) to get to the origin.

Patient: "Yes ... I have ... many times and I'm really afraid of them ..."

Sometimes the patient will continue the story, particularly if facilitation is shown by a nodding of the head. If not, then ——

Doctor: "Can you tell me what happened?"

Bringing the patient closer to the origin.

"As a child I had shots for fillings and the needle hurt a lot . . . they were awful.

This pairing of pain with injections may be traumatic enough to set up a conditioned response, but if the doctor's behavior is traumatic as well the threat increases.

"I cried and squirmed and they got angry which frightened me more. . . .

The sense of helplessness is magnified here, the danger is intensified by the doctor; he offers this little girl no protection — the distrust is compounded by his anger — in all creating a traumatic experience of considerable power.

"It got worse because sometimes the shots didn't take, but he drilled anyway — it was terrible!"

The fear of the unknown is added to the other fears — she did not know if she would have protection from pain or not — again compounded by the doctor's not caring.

At this point the strategy shifts from gathering information to giving information. The elements of the conditioning are painfully clear: the pain, the distress, the fear of helplessness and the unknown coupled with a non-protective, angry authority figure. The counterconditioning process begins with an empathic statement of support followed by your interpretation of the effects of the experience on the patient and an explanation of why you believe she can relearn. Suggestion is used in conjunction with a commitment of how you will behave when both of you face the first injection together. This commitment will state: (1) how you will behave, (2) what you will do, and (3) how you will do it.

Doctor: "I can understand why you would be afraid of injections. . . .

Support, respect and empathy

"It seems to me that you learned you couldn't trust that doctor to protect you from pain. You were depending on him but he didn't seem to want to help you. These feelings still exist within you and you are still feeling today the same terror and distress you felt as a child.

Interpretation and explanation of why she is still fearful years after the original events.

"But you can unlearn and learn a new set of feelings based on our relationship.

Suggestion and a promise of a new and different kind of relationship.

"Let me tell you how I think things will go. First, I am confident that I can give you an injection with very little, if any, pain. If there is some, it will not be enough to be upsetting.

Beginning of the commitment. This offer is based on the ability to give injections in that way. To promise what you cannot deliver would be disastrous.

"I will keep you informed at all times — .

This, to dispel the fear of the unknown.

"If you feel any concern or discomfort I will stop. I will not perform any treatment until you are ready and the area is numb.

To dispel fear of helplessness and dependency and to create some sense of control for her —as well as a sense of trust.

"I know from past experiences that you can learn not to be afraid."

Suggestion that she can learn not to be afraid is coupled with the assurance of the doctor's knowledge and expertise.

The "Third Ear" and the Interview

The above interview is a reconstruction of a relatively uncomplicated interchange. It seems simple, merely a matter of "common sense." However, it is technically highly structured, proceeding in an arrow-like projection straight to the target.

More complicated histories require additional skills. The ability to be effective will depend upon how well one "hears" what is being said. One may listen but not "hear." "Hearing" relates to the picking up of obscure cues; words and phrases that contain the clue to the fear being expressed, cues less obvious than "pain," "drill," and "needle." Hence they may go "unheard." Success will depend upon the doctor's knowledge of these cues and the development of his "third ear," which permits him to "hear" the subtle and less obvious statements of fear.

What follows is an example of an interview in which some obscure cues are put forth by the patient. She is not aware of their meaning, yet without knowing the significance of these cues, she is compelled to give them. The interview was performed by a relatively inexperienced third year predoctoral student as part of a course on iatrosedation. He did quite well up to a point, but his "third ear" was not developed sufficiently to enable him to pick up the more obscure cures.

Student: "Are you having any difficulties?"

Patient: "Yes, I have a tooth that has been aching and I need to have it fixed; but I can't take novocaine . . . and the whole idea makes me very nervous."

Student: "Is there some reason why you cannot have a local anesthetic?"

Patient: "My doctor said I am allergic to all of the 'caine' family and therefore I must have a general anesthetic to get my work done."

Student: "How did your doctor come to the conclusion that you are allergic? What happened?"

Patient: "Well, I had to have a tooth pulled that was in my palate, an eye tooth. The dentist gave me several shots and then left while it took effect. All of a sudden I couldn't breathe. It felt like something terribly heavy on me. My heart started palpitating, pounding, and I was choking and having a terrible problem. The dentist came back, was upset, and said that I had to have an EKG immediately . . . he wouldn't work on me, so I went to the doctor he called. There was nothing wrong with my heart . . . he said I can't take local anesthetics."

Student: "Have you had dental treatment since then? What did you do?"

Patient: "I had all my work done without a local, even the rebuilding of a tooth with spikes in it. I so dread it . . . it's worse than having a baby, which I also had without a local."

Student: "How did you feel when you did get injections?"

Patient: "There's a little tenseness, but not bad. The needle doesn't bother me, but I'm scared. I think most people are anxious, don't you? It has nothing to do with the dentist as a person. I don't know, there's just something about it . . . it's sort of a frightening experience; you don't know if you're going to choke or something. It's more a matter of being able to control the situation."

This interview had been videotaped as part of the course on iatrosedation. A teacher reviewed the tape with the student and pointed out that the patient had repeated a cue three times to which he had not responded. She had said, ". . . I couldn't breathe . . . I was choking . . . you don't know if you're going to choke or something, . . ." and then added, "It's more a matter of being able to control the situation."

Generally speaking, when a patient reacts to a dental situation with a sensation of not being able to breathe, or feeling like he or she is choking, the cue suggests some previous experience that was a threat to breathing. The student was advised to resume the interview with the patient, stating that during the review of the tape it was noticed that she mentioned having had difficulty with breathing and choking. He was to ask the patient if she ever had an experience that was a threat to her breathing. Her response was, "Yes, now that I think of it, when I was a young girl I almost drowned." So indeed, she had suffered the harrowing experience of suffocation, and the assumption can be made that any sensation which suggests interference with the airway may trigger the feeling of panic that accompanies suffocation. The suffocating experience was generalized to the dental scene.

The probable sequence of events was reconstructed in order to offer the patient an interpretation of the origin and cause of her fear. Working with such an interpretation is helpful to the patient in diminishing the fear and permits the doctor to plan for the clinical phase of the iatrosedative process.

The evidence was pieced together in the following manner:

The doctor had given several injections to produce palatal anesthesia. This undoubtedly extended to the soft palate producing numbness and a feeling of largeness that so many patients report with a posterior palatal injection. This feeling of intrusion on the airway triggered off a feeling of panic, resulting in the acute anxiety attack the doctor faced on his return to the operating room.

The student was advised to have the patient tested for tolerance to one of the local analgesics. Results of the testing indicated that she was not allergic. Armed with this information and the reconstruction of the past events, he proceeded to explain and interpret what he thought was the origin of her anxiety, suggesting that she could unlearn the feeling involved and learn a new way to respond to the situation. He suggested that by starting with treatment wherein no palatal anesthesia was involved she would undoubtedly tolerate it very well. This is indeed what happened. The treatment phase started with the use of infiltration injections for anesthesia. The patient tolerated this very well and the relearning process expanded as treatment continued, to the point in fact where palatal injections did not set off a high anxiety response.

Another indirect cue that must be "heard" and understood is the word "gag" or "gagger." Gagging frequently is a panic response, related to a feeling that some threat to breathing or swallowing is about to occur. This feeling has its roots in the past, similar to the cue discussed in the previous history, and is the result of an experience of actual or anticipated suffocation, a traumatic surgical experience involving the throat, or a choking incident.

In the following iatrosedative interview, this type of cue arises. The "what" questions are used to track down the specificity and origin of the fears but, in addition, the cues are facilitated by the use of *reflection*.

"Reflection" is a major method of facilitating cues. The work or phrase is reflected or repeated, either exactly as stated or in a similar form. This echoing or repeating of the patient's word or words acts as an invitation to continue talking about the subject. It is the most economical and productive facilitating tactic in the repertoire.

In the interchange that follows, the key words (cues) will be italicized, as will the reflective responses of the doctor. In addition, the "what" questions will be italicized.

Doctor: "Good morning, Mrs. Caswell. How are you?"

Mrs. C: "Good morning, Doctor. I'm fine, thank you."

Doctor: "Tell me, are you having any difficulties?"

Mrs. C: "Well, yes. I'm a terrible *coward* about anything to do with my teeth."

Doctor: "You are? In *what* way are you a *coward?*"

Mrs. C: "I'm *terrified*. I guess that sums it up. I really get very jittery."

Doctor: "Have you any idea *what* happened to *terrify* you?"

Mrs. C: "Yes, well, I . . . when I was a little girl I had very bad baby teeth I guess, and the dentist I went to was kind of *mean* . . . and also . . . I'm a *gagger* . . . those two things . . . when I was 18, I made about three appointments, showed up and then ran out."

Reflecting the words "coward" and "terrified" accomplished several objectives swiftly. The doctor communicated his recognition of the patient's fear and invited her to tell him more about it. Simultaneously, he moved from the general statement of fear toward the specific fear. The past doctor's behavior was stated in a general way ("he was mean"), and an indirect cue was sprung ("gagger"). The doctor then combined a "what" question with the reflected word "mean" to continue the facilitation.

Doctor: "In *what* way was he *mean?*"

Mrs. C: "I have a horrible memory of the nurse grabbing me and holding me while the doctor worked on me . . . and *not being able to get my breath.*"

The vivid image of the behaviors of the doctor and his assistant, though briefly stated, expresses the patient's feelings about that behavior. In addition, an important indirect clue is uncovered: the "not being able to get my breath." Gagging is the physical expression of panic; in this case, the panic associated with "not being able to get my breath." This is the specific fear. If the interviewing doctor did not "hear" the cues "not being able to get my breath" and "gagger," and if he did not know that there was an important relationship between them, he probably would have gone off on a time-consuming and unproductive tangent. Instead, he moved straight to the target of determining the origin.

Doctor: "Did you ever have an experience where you were *not able to get your breath?*"

Mrs. C: "That's a very interesting question, Doctor. I'll tell you why. When I was a child I had diphtheria. I remember fighting trying to get my breath, and the memory of a band of fire around my throat . . . and faces coming very close to me. I remember my breath, you know . . . they were trying to decide — the doctors — whether or not to give me a tracheotomy. My grandmother told me . . . they didn't . . . but I do remember all those faces — and even now, if anyone gets too close to my face I feel like my breath is being cut off. It's the memory of that fear and the distrust of my first dentist, . . ."

The specific fear apparently stems from this experience. It's generalized so that any doctor coming close in a therapeutic situation triggers the associated feeling of panic. This, presumably, is what occurred with her first dental practitioner. Using this as a basis for initiating a relearning process, reducing the anxiety and offering support, the doctor at this point switches from gathering information to giving information. He interprets and explains past events and suggests that change can occur.

Doctor: "Yes, the heads coming close to your face became associated in your *mind with the choking and the panic you felt when you were gasping* for air. When your first dental practitioner approached you, you panicked. He ignored this, had you held down and intensified your fear. This created distrust. Since then, you've invested all dental doctors with this distrust and fear. But this can be changed. What we have to cope with is the present."

Mrs. C: "You sound very psychologically oriented."

The doctor accepts this recognition of expertise and uses it to expand on his interpretation of suggestion, finally leading to commitment:

Doctor: "I am, and for a very important reason. What we have to deal with here, the dominant issue, is your fear, not the condition of your teeth. If I cannot assure you that I will take care of you as a person, then you'll run away from me in the same way you did from other dental doctors — and you'll not get what you want and need."

Mrs. C: "Yes, that's right . . . and as you pointed out, I would not really be reacting to the fear here — the reality of the situation — but rather to the earlier fear rooted in my childhood."

Doctor: "Exactly. Just as your mind can record and retain a vivid image of something that happened thirty years ago, so it has the capacity to relearn. And that's what we're going to talk about now. You are not that child, you do not have diphtheria, you are not going to choke. I will keep you informed in advance at all times of what I plan to do and what you may expect in the way of discomfort or lack of it. And I will ask for feedback from you as to how you feel about it. In short, you will have a great deal of control over the situation. I believe that my approaching you will not set off the panic button and we will be able to accomplish what you want. Just remember, I will keep in mind at all times how you feel."

Mrs. C: "All right. Thank you, Doctor; I do feel better now."

This statement by the patient implies that she feels less anxious. It remains for the clinical iatrosedative encounter to determine this and to continue the fear reduction process.

The concept of determining the specific fear, its origin, interpretation, explanation, suggestion, and commitment is a general one. It is used here in a particular manner. Each individual will use it in a way peculiar to himself. The principles are sound. The manner of implementing them is individualistic.

A common thread seems to weave through most histories of fearful patients. It is an unholy quartet of feelings consisting of: (1) the specific fear ("needle," "pain," "drill," etc.) invariably combined with (2) distrust, (3) an intensified fear of helplessness and dependency, and (4) an intensified fear of the unknown — a sense of being unsafe and unprotected from the perceived threat or danger.

The variations on this theme seem endless. The following history is quite typical. It is not as obscure as the last two, but more complicated than the report preceding them.

Doctor: "Good morning, Mrs. Brown."

Patient: "Good morning, Doctor."

Doctor: "Are you having difficulties?"

Open-ended question.

Patient: "Yes, my gums bleed and *I think I have pyorrhea.*"

Doctor: "You *think you have pyorrhea?*"

Facilitation by reflection.

Patient: "Yes, I've heard that bleeding gums is the beginning of pyorrhea and can cause teeth to loosen and they have to be pulled. And this makes me very *nervous.*"

It is best not to take for granted what "makes me very nervous" means, therefore facilitate the cue.

Doctor: "*What* is it that makes you *nervous?*"

The "what" question is combined with reflecting "makes me nervous."

Patient: "Well, the idea that I might lose my teeth and . . . the kind of treatment I might need."

The "what" question yields a new clue — closer to the specific fear we want to uncover.

Doctor: "*What* kind of treatment are you referring to?"

Patient: "Surgery — that some cutting might have to be done —"

This seems to be the dominant problem and more specific.

Doctor: "*What* is there about the surgery that disturbs you?"

The "what" is an attempt to learn the specific fear.

Patient: "The whole idea ... I was told to have my gall bladder removed three years ago and I refused to do it."

What is "the whole idea"? What is behind "the whole idea"?

Doctor: "Is there some reason why you feel this way about surgery?"

An "on target" question designed to uncover the specific fear or fears surrounding the surgery. It may elicit information of its origin as well.

Patient: "Yes, there is ... when I was about five or six years old I had my tonsils removed. Although I do not remember anything specific about it—I was not prepared for this—and the experience left me fearful."

The origin begins to unfold as does an important element of the fear—the unknown.

Patient: "When I was eight years old I went to an orthodontist who looked at my teeth but nothing was done. A few months later my mother said she was going to take me to a party the orthodontist was giving for all of his patients. I put on my party clothes and we went. When we arrived I was immediately grabbed, forced in the dental chair, held down and given gas. I was terrified ... when I came to, I found that I had wet myself and was crying bitterly."

Distrust of the mother (authority) based on deceit.
Distrust of the doctor, exaggerated fear of helplessness and dependency; and fear of the unknown probably are intensified.

Fear of surgery is not the total problem. This fear may be viewed as a vehicle carrying the powerful feelings of distrust, helplessness, and the unknown with it. For this reason the maxim "Fear is soluble in trust" seems credible.

The promises, therefore, made in the commitment are important, since they tend to initiate a feeling of trust and security with an attendant drop in the fear level. It remains for the iatrosedative encounter to fulfill the promises made and the hopes raised.

IATROSEDATIVE CLINICAL BEHAVIOR

The clinical encounter begins the moment you pick up an instrument, whether it be a mirror or a probe. An important commitment should be made at this time, to wit: the quality of your tactile behavior. How delicately or roughly you use your instrument tells the patient something of your involvement with him: your awareness, concern, and skill. The more threatening an instrument is, the more significant is your manner of wielding it and the more important are the verbal communications made in conjunction with its use. What you are about to do with it and what you anticipate the effects on the patient will be are two important happenings that should be shared with him or her. In short, you should communicate in a way that will prepare your patient for what is about to occur. Skill in the use of such preparatory communications is essential to iatro-sedation.

Preparatory Communications

Let us consider Preparatory Communications in relation to the "normal" patient first. The non-fearful patient is subject to normal anxiety, which is an anticipatory state of expecting threat or danger and preparing for it. We all tend to be apprehensive when dependent on another whose actions hold the threat of pain or body damage or both. We have no control and are helpless. The unknown is disturbing: that disquieting sense of not knowing what the other person is going to do, the threatening silence when the "needle" or other potentially painful or cutting instrument is picked up. All of these feelings are exaggerated when the person in control gives us no information with which to brace ourselves psychologically, no assurance that he is aware or concerned about us.

Preparatory communications are brief communications made to the patient prior to using an instrument or performing an action which could be perceived as threatening. The communication is intended to prepare the patient for what is about to happen or may be experienced, such as discomfort, pain, noise, or pressure. Such preparatory communications tend to dispel the fear of the unknown and the sense of helplessness through the simple act of foretelling. The patient receives an additional sense of control over his situation because he knows what to expect.

Control through knowing (cognitive control) tends to increase with the use of preparatory communications. When the Danger Control and Protective Authority shares his knowledge with the patient, it tends to reduce anxiety significantly. Egbert's studies clearly demonstrate this.

Egbert and his colleagues demonstrated the effects of preparatory communications on the anxiety level of patients scheduled for major surgery.[2] A number of clinical experiments were performed by his group of anesthesiologists to determine the effects of the doctor's behavior and communication on the anxiety level of surgical patients. One such study measured the effect of the anesthesiologist's preoperative visit with his patients in producing calmness versus the effect of pentobarbital for preanesthetic medication. They summarized their findings this way:

"Patients who had received a visit by an anesthetist before operation were not drowsy but were more likely to be calm on the day of operation. Patients receiving pentobarbital one hour before an operation became drowsy but it could not be shown that they became calm. If the purpose of preanesthetic medication is to allay anxiety, our data suggest that pentobarbital, causing drowsiness, does not achieve the desired result alone."

Their data also suggested that the psychological impact of the preoperative visit made the effects of the pentobarbital seem inconsequential. In their comment, Egbert et al. stated:

"At first sight it would seem surprising that an anesthetist, in a 5 to 10 minute interview, would be able to exert a psychologic effect demonstrable the following day. The patient's interest in knowing about anesthesia would not seem to be an adequate explanation. A better explanation is provided by Janis. He found that persons facing a frightening situation became anxious and looked for emotional support . . . an authority supposedly able to modify the dangers, becomes invested with strong emotional significance. The statements made by this authority assume greater importance than would ordinarily be expected."

Iatrosedation on the "Firing Line"

Mrs. X., the patient whose iatrosedative interview revealed she feared painful injections (p. 246) is now on the "firing line," the first clinical encounter in which the injection will be given.

Doctor: "How are you feeling this morning?"

Patient: "Fine, thank you. I'm a lot less nervous about the shot than I was before we talked, but I'm still somewhat nervous."

Doctor: "Well, I would expect that; but I think you will learn today to be a lot less nervous than you are now. As I told you, I am confident that I can give you an anesthetic with very little if any pain . . . should you feel anything I think it will be something you will be able to handle very well. I will keep you informed as we go along as to what you can expect. I will be responding to you . . . and between us I feel sure you will develop a new set of feelings. Okay?"

Patient: "Okay."

Doctor: "Is there anything else you would like to talk about?"

A combination of manual and communicative techniques are involved in order to carry out, as succinctly as possible, the promise of an atraumatic experience with this injection. Although we are using the injection as a model, this concept should be carried out in *all* aspects of clinical treatment. Each doctor must develop his own style of iatrosedative behavior.

THE MANUAL COMPONENT (INFILTRATION)

The syringe is prepared beforehand with a warm cartridge. It is kept out of sight behind the patient, to be passed over the shoulder below the line of vision. The objective of penetrating the tissue noiselessly and painlessly (or with the minimal amount of pain) is achieved by:

1. applying a topical anesthetic at the site of penetration (in this case the reflection of the alveolar mucosa);
2. making the mucosa as taut as possible by pulling the lip or cheek out without discomfort;
3. establishing a firm finger or hand rest to provide maximum stability and control of the syringe;
4. delicately penetrating the taut mucosa, the bevel toward the tissue, to the depth of the bevel (1 to 2 mm.) only;
5. very slowly injecting a drop or two of anesthetic. After a few moments,

penetrate 1 to 2 mm. and deposit a few more drops. Move slowly into an anesthetized area until the target area is reached.

This manual technique is combined with preparatory communication in the following manner:

Doctor: "I am going to put a surface anesthetic on your gum to numb it so that you will be more comfortable."

This is said as you approach with the topical. The mucosa is pulled taut with syringe poised to penetrate.

"I don't expect you to feel this."

The needle is inserted to the depth of the bevel, stopped, and a few drops injected.

"Do you feel it?"

If the patient indicates that he does not, the doctor answers:

"Good. I will be injecting very slowly . . . it may take longer than usual. I won't be using any more than the normal amount but it will be easier for you. Do you feel anything?"

If the patient indicates "No," reply:

"Good."

If the patient indicates in any way that he or she *does* feel something, it is wise to respond by saying, "I'm sorry, but I don't think you will feel anything from now on. I will be going very slowly." This is not said defensively, but merely to let the patient know you care.

These simple preparatory communications carry much more weight for the patient than one would suspect. An interpretation of what they may mean follows:

1. Using a topical anesthetic communicates the concern of the doctor and the wish to minimize pain.
2. "I don't expect you to feel this" states, I am about to inject and will do all I can to do it without pain.
3. "Did you feel it?" — I have already started injecting and I want to know how it is with you. This is a continuing involvement and I want feedback from you.
4. "Good" or "I'm sorry" — what you feel is important to me.
5. "I will be injecting slowly, no more than usual . . . etc." — I am keeping you informed, explaining in case you get upset because you may think I am using too much anesthetic, etc.

Communications of this kind should be used consistently with all operative procedures.

The above interpretation of the doctor's preparatory communications is based on feedback from patients with whom these kinds of interchanges have taken place. A patient who had stated that she was no longer fearful was asked why she felt this had occurred:

Doctor: "What is it that permitted you to overcome your fear?"

Patient: "Well, I think when you first saw me I had this tremendous fear built up because of my past experiences. I'd heard so many stories about the amount of pain I would suffer with your work . . . but I have to have it done . . . I've suffered so greatly with other dental work, surely I'll have mountains of pain with this . . . by the time I came to you and with my own frightening experiences . . . the thing that calmed me was your *ability to work psychologically* with me."

Expertise and recognition.

"First, *knowing* my tremendous fear. I had made just a couple of comments, you know, about one dentist and how I should have been here many years ago. . . .

"Hearing" and responding to critical cues during the interview.

"The method you used to *tranquilize me by words,* logically, something for me to accept within my fear, so strong that I automatically began to relate and listen to what you had to say instead of closing my mind; logically you approached me and tranquilized me. . . . I don't know how else to explain it.

Interpretation, explanation, suggestion and commitment.

"In other words, the very words that you used put me at ease enough to say, 'Listen, maybe he *is* telling the truth. . . .'" and I gained more confidence as you talked to me, *as you explained.*

Trust developing.

"I felt very confident; then when I came in for the surgery, I only had slight apprehension, yet I figured I might suffer the tortures of the damned . . . but I felt no pain whatsoever.

Iatrosedative interview dropped fear level, but was still higher than normal.

Doctor: "Well, you were very apprehensive, predicated on past experiences. You say the words that I used . . . what words?"

Patient: "You were willing to go out on a limb, knowing what you know, in *telling me what to expect* from what you were doing . . . you have a habit of *saying in advance* 'you may feel this, but it will not be very much if anything,' 'you will feel pressure but no pain.'

He made clinical preparatory iatrosedative communications so that she would know what sensations she may feel, thus minimizing the fear of helplessness and the unknown.

> "This in itself, when the surgery began, is the thing that puts your patients at east . . . because every time a dentist picks up an instrument, just like everybody else, they want to run away . . . because he sees you picking up all kinds of things . . . he *doesn't know what you are going to do* . . . and *it's the not knowing* that upsets the patient. . . ."

Knowing lessens the fear of the unknown.

Euphemistic Language

The term "euphemism", derived from the Greek *eu* (well) and phanai (to speak), originally meant "to use words of good omen." The definition of euphemism as we know it today is similar; it is the substitution of a mild or inoffensive expression for one that may offend or suggest something unpleasant. With respect to dentistry, the use of euphemisms is particularly indicated in place of fear-provoking or threatening words and technical terms.

The use of threatening and technical language is a frequent barrier to communication between doctors and patients. It either creates apprehension and confusion or intensifies them if they already exist. In order to prevent potential problems that can result from the use of emotionally charged language (with which dentistry is richly endowed) or technical jargon, the doctor must develop alternative methods of communicating potentially threatening information to patients.

Euphemistic language should be used with all patients. Since it tends to minimize anxiety, it is an integral part of iatrosedation. An example of its use may be seen in the communications used above for the atraumatic injection. Although these preparatory and explanatory communications are very brief and quite simple, thought has been given to substituting low threat words for threatening ones and non-technical words for technical ones. For example, few lay people know what a *topical* anesthetic is, hence it is referred to as a *surface* anesthetic. Instead of saying, "This won't *hurt*," the phrase used was, "I don't expect you to *feel* this." "I will be *injecting* slowly" is replaced with "I'll be *doing* it slowly" since some people may have disturbing imagery stimulated by the work "injecting," particularly if the injection is the primary fear problem.

These simple euphemistic substitutions are not earth-shaking. Most clinicians seem to be aware of the many threatening words and terms with which the dental vocabulary is laden: "drill," "needle," "shot," "cut," "clamp," etc. What is consequential is the decision to avoid these words, to replace them with euphemisms and to develop the constant, ongoing vigilance required to avoid falling into the trap of being verbally threatening.

When one considers the dilemma of describing, in non-threatening terms, a pulp tester and its use to an anxious patient, one realizes how euphemistically agile the doctor must be!

It is necessary to maintain the iatrosedative posture in all phases of involvement with your patient. Another communication principle for reducing threat in what might be a threatening situation is the use of a Preparatory Interview.

Preparatory Interview

The preparatory interview is a brief interview conducted with the patient prior to performing a treatment or diagnostic procedure for the first time with that patient which could be threatening to him. The objective is to learn two things:

1. Has the patient ever experienced this specific procedure before (e.g., endodontics, injection, periodontal probing, periodontal surgery)?
2. How does the patient feel about it?
    The general principle of knowing "how it is" with the patient before taking him into an area of potential threat seems irrefutably sensible and sensitive. Preparing to use potentially fearsome instruments or procedures with no knowledge of the person's experience with and feelings about them seems illogical.
    Let us assume that Mrs. X has successfully shed her fear of injections. However, in the course of continuing dental treatment it becomes apparent that endodontics is required. Following the examination the need for it had been discussed briefly. How should Mrs. X be approached? If the roentgenograms indicate that endodontics has been performed in the past, should you assume that no problem will be encountered, tell her of the need, and proceed to refer her to an endodontist or arrange an appointment to treat her? Or should you learn something of her feelings about having endodontic treatment? The obvious answer to an obvious question: yes.

Doctor: "Mrs X., if you recall I had mentioned that you would need to have root canal treatment. The X-rays indicate that you have had this kind of treatment. How did it go?"

Mrs. X: "Well (hesitantly), I really had a bad time with it."

Doctor: "A bad time?"

Mrs. X: "Yes, the tooth was very painful, it ached badly, and although the doctor gave me several shots, all of which scared me, when he took the nerve out I almost died, it hurt so much."

Doctor: "I can see that you did have a bad time of it and I can appreciate how you must feel about considering root canal treatment again. Fortunately, however, we have a different situation now. You see, when the tooth is very inflamed such as yours was last time, it is very difficult to get good anesthesia. This is not the case with the tooth now. As a matter of fact, no anesthesia is needed at all because . . ."

The remainder of the discussion need not be pursued here. The example is used to point out the wisdom of exploring potentially threatening procedures with the patient before starting treatment.

NONVERBAL EMPATHIC STRATEGY

It was stated that the iatrosedative interview technique is composed of two strategies:

1. a verbal fact-finding interpretive strategy
2. a nonverbal empathic strategy

It was further stated that these were separated for the purpose of discussion but the separation is artificial, since verbal and nonverbal communications are in reality inseparable.

The crucial function of nonverbal communication is the transmission of feelings.[9] The major feelings to be communicated to the fearful patient by the doctor are:

1. attentiveness and concern
2. acceptance of the patient and his problem
3. supportiveness
4. involvement with the intent to help

These feelings and nonverbal statements are created through the process of listening, "hearing" what you are listening to, then responding empathically.

Listening is the act of turning your attention to another person and permitting him to speak. "Hearing" is understanding what he is saying. Although these are nonverbal behaviors, they were discussed as part of the verbal fact-finding strategy because the "hearing" is a prerequisite for responding by facilitating the telling of the story, offering support and commitment. Reflecting and reacting to the patient's feelings and story by face, voice, and body is responding nonverbally to what one "hears."

The principal factor in listening is being attentive. This requires concentration, discipline, and the intentional use of your behavior. Attentiveness is communicated in two ways:

1. Through your physical presence (physical demeanor and posture)
2. Through your psychological presence ("hearing" the total communication of the patient, both verbal and nonverbal)

PHYSICAL ATTENDING SKILLS.

The skilled use of one's face, voice, and body will result in a posture of involvement. This is the medium that will communicate whether you really are or are not involved with your patient. The nonverbal signals you send out will either verify your words of concern and support or belie them.

Man's richest sign system is his head and face.[6] The voice and body have almost as much value as the face in the wordless communication system that plays such a powerful role in the creation of an empathic climate in which the doctor and patient will interact.

There are many components of nonverbal communication. Some of the significant ones considered here are:

1. Eye contact
2. Facial expressiveness
3. Vocal characteristics
4. Body orientation
5. Trunk lean
6. Proximity (distance)

Haase and Teffer carried out research on the nonverbal components of empathic communication.[4] The intent of the study was to explore the relative contribution of verbal and nonverbal behaviors to the communication of empathy. Their findings were:

1. A verbal message of medium empathetic value can be altered favorably by maintaining good eye contact, forward trunk lean, good body orientation, and good distance.
2. Conversely, high levels of verbal empathy can be reduced to unempathic messages when the communicator utters the message without eye contact, in a backward trunk lean, rotated away from the addressee, and from a far distance.

These findings add to the existing knowledge of the power of nonverbal communication, colloquially alluded to as "body language."

Eye Contact

Eye contact is a crucial key in the communication system. It is virtually impossible to create a sense of attentiveness and interest in a person if you are not looking at him. "Looking at him" means making eye contact.

This mutual looking tends to increase when the participants like each other and when they are involved in their interaction. It lessens when touchy subjects come up or unpleasantness develops between the interactants. A "noncollision course" is taken, a lowering of the eyes, a "dimming of the lights."

Good eye contact does not mean staring, or constant eye contact. This is very disconcerting. It should be varied. You should permit your eyes to drift to an object not too far away and then return to the patient. As in all nonverbal behaviors, this should be done naturally, in a relaxed, comfortable manner.

The eyes contribute to the facial expression in many ways. For example, in smiling, they can either lend warmth or put a chill on the smile. If when the mouth expresses a smile and there is no expression around the eyes, the smile tends to be "icy."

Facial Expressions

The face can be the best expression of emotions but it can also be a superb mask. However, it is the most difficult of our nonverbal behaviors to monitor. We are aware of what our eyes are doing, how our voice sounds, what movements we make, but the face is the one expressor from which we get no feedback. Hence, it is the most vulnerable area of our behavior. Many doctors avoid facial risks by wearing a noncommittal mask, a sort of professional "poker face." Generally, unless one has learned to pay attention to his nonverbal communications, he is almost totally ignorant of his facial behavior. Consequently he may be sending signals facially that he doesn't intend to, or may be inadequately expressing what he would prefer to say.

Facial expressiveness in skilled attending is used in two basic ways: (1) to send messages and (2) to respond appropriately to messages being received. When the doctor turns his attention to his patient at their first meeting, the facial signals most people would like to see are warmth, interest, and alert intention of being involved. Facial responsiveness should mirror the feelings of the patient to varying degrees; that is, concern should be reflected by concern and not by apathy, a faint smile, or exaggerated interest. The face is an instrument of wide range from broad to very subtle communications, some almost inperceptible. It is wise to remember the admonition, "Be careful what you say with your face when talking with your mouth."

Vocal Characteristics

The voice can be used like a musical instrument. It alters the meaning of words, either giving the lie to them or making them ring true. In our culture, we ascribe certain characteristics to voice sounds. The voice of authority generally is characterized as being low in pitch, resonant, and used with measured tempo. A fast, high-pitched, squeaky voice is associated with immaturity.

In attending, it is desirable to speak at an even tempo with moderate volume, at as low a pitch and with as much resonance as is consistent with your voice. There should be variations of these qualities to reflect and support the meaning of the words. Above all, one must be on guard to avoid mixed messages wherein the voice and the face are saying something different than the words. One of the commonest examples of a mixed message is that conveyed by the doctor who, hoping to assure the patient, says with disinterest in his voice and looking away, "Don't worry, everything will be all right."

One of the more penetrating studies performed to determine which message is dominant when two incongruent ones are sent was done by Mehrabian.[10] He set up situations in which the facial and vocal expressions were in conflict with the verbal messages. His conclusions indicate that in the communication of feelings, the words were responsible for only 7 per cent of the impact; the vocal expressions produced 38 per cent of the effect, and the facial expressions 55 per cent. Hence, if your face and voice do not match your words, you would best say nothing. On the other hand, the verbal promises of help and protection assume greater significance if supported by empathic nonverbal communication. In short, it is *how* something is said, not *what* is said, that builds or destroys relationships.

Body Orientation

Facing patients squarely tells them that you intend to pay attention. If you sit with your body rotated away from the patient, you are "turning away", thus creating an atmosphere of inattentiveness. This inattentive orientation is intensified if your position is at a 90 degree angle or less. In addition, such a position makes good eye contact difficult and strained.

If the interview is taking place in the dental treatment room, you should be in a position between 7 and 8 o'clock. Should you use your consultation room it would be preferable not to sit behind a desk. Two armchairs can be used in approximately the same position as above.

In my opinion, the interviews should take place in the treatment room. If the patient is fearful, the operatory may stimulate the expression of anxiety, in which case the issue is confronted. Sitting comfortably in a consultation room, which tends to be a more relaxed and social environment, provides little provocation to discuss one's fears.

Body Distance or Proximity

How close one sits in a situation such as we are discussing influences the communication. The degree of proximity engenders different feelings in different cultures. Hall[5] reports that most Americans tend to deal with space in the following way:

1. *Intimate Zone* — ranging from contact to 18 inches. This is the zone for handling secrets and whispered conferences.
2. *Casual–Personal Zone* — ranging from 1½ to 4 feet. This is the region for normal personal interaction.
3. *Social–Consultative Zone* — ranging from 4 to 12 feet. This is the area for handling impersonal business.
4. *Public Zone* — ranging from 12 feet to the limits of hearing. This is the region of the public speaker addressing an audience.

A distance between 3½ to 6 feet is appropriate when conducting the interview in the dental operatory. The distance will vary depending upon your comfort with the patient with whom you are interacting. The more your interest rises, the closer you will tend to be. As with eye contact, facial expression, and body orientation, there is the matter of a dynamic process; that is, you should not be fixed and rigid about any of these physical attendance components but maintain a moderate degree of fluidity.

Trunk Lean

A forward trunk lean is a powerful message of interest. Somehow it is difficult to be indifferent while leaning forward and listening to another person. The forward lean of the body is an eloquent statement of attentiveness. The reverse of this, leaning backward, and folding one's arms, is a statement of casual interest at best and nonattentiveness at worst.

The trunk lean is an effective facilitator. If a patient is speaking and pauses, merely leaning forward slightly will act as a request to "tell me more." Not only does it act as the body language of "tell me more," it also indicates interest and empathy.

Another of the many components of "body language" is tactile communication. During an interview, support, concern, and empathy can be conveyed by touching the forearm of the patient. This is the most acceptable and least intimate area of the body for tactile communication. Needless to say, in the clinical encounter tactile communication is constant. The delicacy or roughness of one's "touch" conveys a great deal of information to the patient about the doctor's "presence" and, more significantly, the doctor's awareness of the patient's presence.

SUMMARY

Fear is a major cause of avoidance of dental treatment for millions of people. Some of the common dental fears and how they originate are explored. What is presented here is a technique to treat fear with interpersonal skills utilizing simple behavioral principles. The goal is either to eliminate the fear or to reduce it to a level that permits the patient to cope successfully with the dental experience.

This technique has been termed "iatrosedation," and is defined as the act of making calm by the doctor's behavior. The two major categories of iatrosedation are:

1. the Iatrosedative Interview
2. the Iatrosedative Clinical Encounter

The iatrosedative interview is designed to initiate fear reduction through a relearning process. It is brief and economical, usually lasting no more than 10 minutes. The clinical encounter continues the process, thus dropping the fear level further. Examples of the clinical technique, including preparatory communications and other stress reducing communication principles complete the chapter.

REFERENCES

1. Bandura, A.: Principles of Behavior Modification. New York, Holt, Rinehart and Winston, 1969.
2. Egbert, L., Battit, G., Turndoff, H., and Beecher, H.: Value of the preoperative visit by an anesthetist, J.A.M.A., 195:553, 1963.
3. Enelow, A. J., and Wexler, M.: Psychiatry in the Practice of Medicine, Oxford, England, Oxford University Press, 1966.
4. Haase, R. F., and Tepper, D. T., Jr.: Nonverbal Components of Empathic Communication. J. Couns. Psychol., 19:417–424, 1972.
5. Hall, E. T.: Silent assumptions in social communication—disorders of communication. Res. Publ. Assoc. Res. Nerve. Ment. Dis., 42:41–55, 1964.
6. Harrison, R. P.: Beyond Words. New York, Prentice-Hall, Inc., 1974.
7. Janis, I. L.: Psychological Stress. New York, Wiley and Co., 1958.
8. Kahn, R. L., Cooper, C., and Mallenger, M.: Dentistry: What causes it to be a stressful profession, International Review of Applied Psychology, in press 1979.
9. Mehrabian, A.: Nonverbal Communication. Chicago, Aldine Press, 1972.
10. Mehrabian, A.: Silent Messages. Belmont, Cal., Wadsworth Publishing, 1971.
11. Shoben, E. J., Jr. and Borland, L.: An empirical study of the etiology of dental fears. J. Clin. Psychol. 10:171, 1954.

8

PSYCHOSEDATION

Part 3: Pharmacosedation — Oral Route

JOHN HAGEN
and STANLEY F. MALAMED

INTRODUCTION

The first two chapters of this psychosedation section reviewed the interrelationship of pain, anxiety, and stress, with particular reference to the medically compromised patient, and the non-drug technique of sedation called iatrosedation. Should iatrosedation prove to be ineffective in tranquilizing the anxious patient, drug therapy must be employed for sedation (pharmacosedation). This chapter will review sedative drugs which may be used by the oral route.

PREMEDICATION

In past years of inhalation general anesthesia by the irritating (and thus frightening) agent ether, the term *premedication* referred primarily to the use of drugs for sedation so that the patient was tranquil, nonanxious, and indifferent upon arrival in the operating room. A number of these drugs have the added effect of minimizing respiratory tract secretions and of intensifying the primary anesthetic agent.

The basic tenets of premedication have remained unchanged; however, the development of new drugs and techniques stresses the primary action of anxiety suppression, rather than supplementation of a general anesthetic agent. Ideally, in dentistry we wish to produce psychic depression and thereby reduce the patient's response to any untoward stimulus.

Although it is perfectly proper to use the term premedication for sedative drugs administered prior to dental therapy, the term pharmacosedation is now more widely used.

ORAL ROUTE VS INTRAMUSCULAR ROUTE

One of the problems associated with parenteral administration of drugs, with special reference to the intramuscular route, has been injection injury. The intramuscular route has generally been favored over the oral route because absorption is more rapid and is thought to be more predictable. However, administration by mouth is safer, as well as more convenient and economical. Studies have shown that, if food intake is restricted at the time the sedative drug is taken by mouth, gastrointestinal absorption is sufficient to make this route clinically practical. It is therefore felt that the intramuscular route offers no advantage over the oral route for sedation.

SELECTION OF THE PATIENT

Although every patient will experience some degree of anxiety before or during dental treatment, not all patients are candidates for pharmacosedation. In general, the selection process centers on those individuals who are incapable of controlling the extent of their reactions to an untoward psychic stimulus, and for whom iatrosedation is not effective.

The vast majority of our patients who require pharmacosedation include the hyperreactive adult and child, followed by the adult and child with mental or motor defects, the chronically infirm elderly patient who is able to withstand only nominal procedures, and the medically compromised patient. Examples of this last, very important group have been mentioned in Chapters 2 and 6, with special reference to patients with a history of congestive heart failure, myocardial infarction, angina pectoris, cerebrovascular accident, and arterial hypertension.

The iatrosedative interview (see Chapter 7) takes place as a matter of routine when the clinican performs the original physical evaluation. Having identified the patient requiring an iatrosedative consultation and clinical experience, the practitioner will then conclude whether drug therapy is additionally required, or this conclusion may be reached only after the initial clinical experience with iatrosedation proves to be unsatisfactory.

An anxiety evaluation questionnaire completed by the patient at the same time the medical history is completed has been suggested by Corah[5]. This patient, however, will be accurately identified during the doctor/patient interview, and the simple question "Do you have any fears or concerns about dental care?" is probably more accurate than a special questionnaire.

During physical evaluation when the doctor reviews the medical history and elicits any indicated dialogue history, the patient is routinely inspected for physical signs that may indicate disease. At this time signs of unusual anxiety may be observed, such as sweaty palms and forehead, unnaturally rigid posture in the examination chair, eyes constantly observing the doctor and assistant as if anticipating an attack, unusually rapid response to questions, and protective movements of the head or arms during the oral examination. Late recognition of anxiety may occur during an unsatisfactory clinical experience.

FACTORS MODIFYING DRUG ACTION

If a large number of individuals are administered the same dose of a drug there will be noted an extremely wide variation in the drug's clinical effectiveness. At one extreme will be a number of patients (approximately 15 per cent) who will exhibit unusually intense clinical signs and symptoms, while at the other extreme will be another group (again 15 per cent) who at this same dose will exhibit few if any of the desired clinical effects of the drug (that is, if previously anxious, they will remain so). The remaining 70 per cent will demonstrate varying degrees of acceptable clinical activity ranging from mild anxiety reduction to excellent clinical effectiveness. This individuality in response to drug therapy is called biologic variability. Most oral medications are available in three dosage forms, making it somewhat easier for the prescribing doctor to accommodate for individual variability in responsiveness.

Many other factors act to modify the clinical effectiveness of drugs. While all routes of drug administration are affected by these factors, it is the oral route which illustrates the greatest clinical variability. Among the factors acting to alter the manner in which a drug affects a patient are: age, weight (or body surface area), sex, physical status of the patient, *presence of other substances in the stomach*, presence of anxiety or stress, expectations of the patient, and degree of confidence in the administrator of the drug.

Because of these factors, which apply to all drugs, and because of biologic variability in reactivity to drugs, the administration of individualized doses via the oral route is very difficult. A major factor which prevents this individualization of drug dose is the latent period exhibited by orally administered drugs. For most oral drugs a period of at least 30 minutes must pass before a clinically effective blood level is achieved, and approximately 60 minutes for maximal clinical effectiveness to occur. It is therefore not possible to titrate drugs via the oral route. Titration represents the ability to administer small increments of a drug to a patient until the desired clinical action is achieved. This permits the drug administrator to achieve more profound levels of sedation with a greater degree of safety. Two techniques of pharmacosedation — inhalation and intravenous sedation — permit titration and are therefore used for *intraoperative* sedation at the desired levels. Sedation produced by the oral route is both preoperative and intraoperative.

ADVANTAGES AND DISADVANTAGES OF THE ORAL ROUTE

Oral administration is the most frequently used method of pharmacosedation in dental practice. It does possess several advantages over other techniques of sedation. These include ease of administration, almost universal acceptability, low cost, lower incidence of adverse reactions and, in most cases, decreased severity of those that do occur. The oral route does not require the use of additional equipment such as syringes and needles, nor does it require advanced education to be used safely.

On the negative side, however, we must include a reliance on patient compliance with prescribing orders, the prolonged latent period, the unreliable absorption of the drug into the circulatory system, the inability to titrate, and the inability to readily lighten or deepen the level of sedation.

Rational Use of the Oral Route

When all of the preceding factors are considered, it becomes obvious that the drug administrator does not maintain complete control over the ultimate clinical action of orally administered drugs as compared to the inhalation and intravenous routes. Because of this lack of control, the doctor must carefully weigh the potential risk versus the benefit to be gained from the oral route.

For tranquilization during dental treatment very light levels of sedation may prove to be inadequate for the degree of anxiety present. More profound levels of sedation may on occasion be sought via this route; however, the clinician should always keep in mind the lack of control maintained over drug action and the wide range of individual variability to a given drug dose. Drugs with a high therapeutic index (lethal $dose_{50}$/effective $dose_{50}$) can be used more readily for profound sedation than those with lower therapeutic indices. Minor complications such as oversedation or lack of cooperation and more serious side-effects such as respiratory depression and loss of consciousness are always possible consequences of drug administration. To minimize their occurrence, the drug administrator (or prescriber) must have a thorough knowledge of the pharmacological actions of the drug being administered as well as its adverse reactions. This person must also be capable of promptly recognizing and managing any adverse reactions that may develop.

Should more profound levels of sedation be desirable, other techniques of pharmacosedation which are more controllable (that is, where titration and reversal of sedation are possible), can be used in place of sedation by mouth. Both inhalation sedation and intravenous sedation are to be preferred in this situation, provided the clinician is well trained in their safe use.

What, then, represents a rational use for oral sedation in dental practice? From the standpoint of safety it is important that the drug administrator never seek to achieve levels of sedation beyond which he or she is comfortable and capable of recognizing and managing any undesirable side effects which may develop. In addition, the quality of dental therapy should never be compromised because of the use of pharmacosedation. For these reasons, a rational use of oral sedation would include the achieving of very light levels of sedation only. More profound sedative levels should be reserved for more controllable techniques or when indicated via the oral route by a doctor who through prior experience or training can adequately manage any adverse reactions that might develop.

There are two areas in which lighter levels of sedation are desirable. The first and most common use is for the reduction of anxiety in the hours immediately preceding a dental appointment. The goal of drug therapy in this instance is to reduce anxiety so that the patient will, in fact, appear for the appointment. After the patient is in the dental office, other techniques can be employed for the increased anxiety levels noted during actual treatment. An important consideration in the use of oral sedation for this purpose is the necessity for the doctor to advise the patient not to drive a motor vehicle to the dental office and to be accompanied by an adult if the drug has been taken at home. For medicolegal reasons the doctor should also enter this instruction on the chart.

A second important use of the oral route is for the reduction of anxiety in patients who are so apprehensive about their upcoming dental therapy that they are unable to sleep the night before the appointment. Oral sedation is used in this situation to allay apprehension, thus permitting the patient to sleep comfortably, therefore arriving at the office well rested and better able to tolerate the stresses of therapy.

THE DRUGS

A large number of oral drugs are available for use in the management of anxiety. The major categories include the sedative-hypnotics and the antianxiety agents, including the benzodiazepines. Other drugs such as antihistamines, narcotics, and carbamates, and ethyl alcohol are also used for oral sedation. The more commonly used oral drugs will be reviewed.

Ethyl Alcohol

Patients have long used self-administered alcohol as a sedative prior to dental treatment; however, prescription by the dental practitioner has not become popular. Alcohol has, in the past, been used for sedation in dentistry. Niels Bjorn Jorgensen, considered to be the father of sedation in American dentistry, first used alcohol for sedation in 1923. He originally prescribed 4 ounces of medicinal alcohol, later changing to aromatic elixir USP, which became known as Jorgensen's elixir.[17]

McCarthy and Hayden[23] have reviewed the history of alcohol and have presented a protocol for its use as a sedative in dentistry. The following is a brief review of their recommendations.

The practitioner is legally liable for any injury which results from improper medication, be the drug diazepam, pentobarbital, or alcohol. For this reason the use of all drugs including alcohol should be approached with a high degree of caution and concern for the patient's safety. While the use of alcohol is not contraindicated in pediatric dentistry, special precautions and care are necessary. The dosage forms to be described will therefore refer to the adult patient who is legally able to drink alcohol.

In discussing the advantages and disadvantages of this technique with respect to informed consent, the authors recommend use of the term "medicinal alcohol". Eighty proof (40 per cent) distilled neutral spirits are used, flavored if desired or administered in a pleasant vehicle such as fruit or vegetable juice. To avoid possible gastritis, the dose of alcohol should be diluted two times, for example 2 ounces of vehicle to 1 ounce of alcohol. The patient should not have consumed any alcohol within the past 12 hours, with a maximum consumption of 6 ounces of distilled spirits or equivalent during the past 24 hours. Other CNS-depressant drugs (sedative-hypnotics, narcotics, antianxiety agents, N_2O-O_2) ought not be employed along with alcohol to avoid possible undesirable drug reactions, unless the practitioner is thoroughly experienced in sedation/anesthesia and in basic life support.

The patient should eat a light, high carbohydrate meal (cereal and milk) three hours prior to dental therapy. An empty stomach should like-wise be ensured prior to the ingestion of other sedative drugs. Approximately 20 minutes before therapy is to start the alcohol is administered in the dental office. Duration of clinical sedation is approximately 60 minutes, although a degree of sedation will persist for an additional 10 to 20 minutes. In most instances the patient may be dismissed about 80 minutes after the medication is administered. The patient may be permitted to drive a car from the office, if the doctor considers the patient fully recovered from the drug effects. This represents a significant advantage over other forms of oral or parenteral sedation.

Dosage schedules are presented in Table 8–1. The higher dosage forms are used at subsequent visits if the initial dosages were inadequate. When the higher forms are used, it is recommended that the patient be retained in the dental office for 140 minutes from the time of administration before being dismissed.

The patient is advised to abstain from further alcohol or other CNS-depressants for a minimum of three hours after discharge. A light, high carbohydrate meal is suggested after dismissal.

Alcohol is contraindicated as a sedative in persons who have no social experience with the drug, are intolerant of it, have an aversion to alcohol for either religious or personal reasons, have a history of hypoglycemic reactions associated with alcohol, diabetes mellitus or malnutrition, hysteria, liver disease, or a past or present history of alcoholism. In addition, its use is to be avoided in persons taking medications whose actions could be additive or synergistic. Included are: barbiturates, antianxiety agents, monoamine oxidase inhibitors, and chloral hydrate. With respect to other diseases, the same precautions and principles of medical consultation apply as for any other sedative agent.

TABLE 8–1   RECOMMENDED DOSES OF ETHYL ALCOHOL

Weight in Pounds	First Appointment	Subsequent Appointments*
100	30 ml (1 oz)	45 ml (1½ oz)
140	30 ml (1 oz)	60 ml (2 oz)
180	60 ml (2 oz)	90 ml (3 oz)
220	60 ml (2 oz)	90 ml (3 oz)

*Increased dosage forms should be used only if first appointment doses prove inadequate.

When employed in proper dosage and with proper instructions, alcohol is an effective sedative for the relief of *mild* anxiety in dentistry. It possesses virtually no side effects when used as recommended; it is rapidly metabolized; and virtually all patients may be permitted to leave the dental office unescorted. Its antianxiety effect is equivalent to that of oral diazepam or pentobarbital; however, the unwanted effects of the latter drugs (depression, headache) are rarely encountered.

The Barbiturates

The barbiturates represented the first of the truly effective antianxiety drugs which were, and still are, widely prescribed. Pharmacologically the barbiturates are generalized central nervous system depressants, producing depression of the limbic system, cerebral cortex, and reticular activating system at therapeutic dose levels.[25] These actions produce a reduction in the anxiety level, decreased mental acuity, and a state of drowsiness. At high dosage levels, depression of the medulla is noted with barbiturates, leading to respiratory and possibly cardiovascular depression. The barbiturates are classified as sedative-hypnotic drugs which at differing dosage levels produce relaxation (sedation) or induce drowsiness (hypnosis). Barbiturates are usually categorized by their duration of action after an average oral dose. Table 8–2 lists the more commonly employed barbiturates, and their usual oral dosages. The long-acting barbiturates (16 to 24 hours) and intermediate-acting (6 to 8 hours) produce clinical levels of sedation for too long a period of time for the usual dental appointment. The long-acting barbiturates are commonly employed as anticonvulsants, while the intermediate-acting barbiturates are employed as "sleeping pills" in specific types of insomnia.

The short-acting barbiturates, most notably pentobarbital and secobarbital, with an average clinical duration of action of 3 to 4 hours, are better suited for use in dentistry. Most of the ultrashort-acting barbiturates are used intravenously for the rapid induction of general anesthesia. The two most notable examples of ultrashort-acting barbiturates are thiopental sodium (Pentothal) and methohexital sodium (Brevital). There is one ultrashort-acting barbiturate which is available in oral form as a sedative-hypnotic, hexobarbital. Its clinical applications will be discussed.

The disadvantages of the barbiturates are numerous. In fact, in the past

TABLE 8–2 AVAILABILITY OF ORAL BARBITURATES

Generic	Proprietary	Availability	Usual Sedative Dose*
Hexobarbital	Presed, Sombulex	250 mg	250 to 500 mg
Pentobarbital	Nembutal	30, 50, 100 mg	100 mg
Secobarbital	Seconal	30, 50, 100 mg	100 mg

*Dosage forms indicated are those for a normal, healthy 70 kg patient. It is suggested that the package insert or a textbook of pharmacology be consulted prior to drug administration.

decade since the introduction of other, more effective and pharmacologically specific antianxiety agents, the use of barbiturates has declined. This laudable trend should continue as more evidence accumulates regarding the adverse properties of the barbiturates.[6] Important properties of these drugs include dose-related respiratory depression, the potential for habituation and addiction, the development of tolerance, and drug interactions. Of especial importance is the action of barbiturates and the coumadin anticoagulants. Barbiturates inhibit the actions of these important drugs.[8, 12, 19] In addition, the barbiturates are the most frequently implicated drugs in suicide attempts.[9]

Another important consideration in the use of these drugs in dentistry is the fact that they lack the ability to obtund pain without inducing a concurrent decrease in the level of consciousness.[4] In sedative doses the barbiturates actually produce an increase in the patients response to painful stimulation.

Of the dozen or so barbiturates used clinically, only three are of significant value in dental practice and even then only in isolated instances. The intravenous agents, intermediate-acting agents, and long-acting agents have little place in dental practice for preoperative sedation. The three agents of potential value are: pentobarbital, secobarbital, and hexobarbital.

Pentobarbital (Nembutal) is a short-acting barbiturate with a half-life of 21 to 42 hours. Clinical effectiveness (onset of action) develops within 20 to 25 minutes on an empty stomach, with a duration of action of from 3 to 4 hours. The therapeutic index (lethal dose$_{50}$/effective dose$_{50}$) of pentobarbital is relatively high, which is uncommon among the barbiturates. For this reason, pentobarbital is preferred over most other members in this category for sedation in dental practice. Pentobarbital is available in 30, 50, and 100 mg capsules. The average adult dose for preoperative sedation is 50 to 100 mg administered one hour prior to dental therapy.

Secobarbital (Seconal), another short-acting barbiturate, has a half-life of 20 to 28 hours. Its clinical onset and duration of action are similar to that of pentobarbital; however, the therapeutic index of secobarbital is lower than that of pentobarbital with an attendant increased risk of undesirable effects and overdose. It is available in 30, 50, and 100 mg capsules. Usual adult dose is 100 mg taken one hour prior to dental therapy.

Hexobarbital (Presed, Sombulex) is an ultrashort-acting barbiturate available in oral dosage form. Its clinical onset develops rapidly, generally within 15 to 30 minutes. Hexobarbital is also metabolized rapidly and excreted from the circulatory system within 4 to 5 hours. The usual duration of clinical effectiveness with hexobarbital is from 60 to 90 minutes. Hexobarbital is available in 250 mg tablets and is normally administered 30 minutes prior to dental therapy in a dosage of 250 to 500 mg. In our clinical practice hexobarbital is reserved for those patients requiring additional sedation upon arrival in the dental office, but who are unable to receive other techniques of pharmacosedation (inhalation or intravenous).

USES OF BARBITURATES

The short-acting barbiturates, pentobarbital and secobarbital, are used for preoperative anxiety control, and on occasion for more profound intraoperative sedation. The latter use of these agents is not recommended unless the doctor is capable of recognizing and managing any adverse effects which might develop from their administration. Oversedation, manifested as uncooperativeness or respiratory depression, is the most commonly observed clinical sign. These agents may be employed where other, more effective antianxiety agents (i.e., benzodiazepines) are unavailable or have proven ineffective.

Effective sedation with barbiturates results in drowsiness. The patient must be accompanied by an adult and must not operate a motor vehicle or dangerous machinery for the balance of the calendar day.

The ultrashort-acting barbiturate hexobarbital is commonly administered to the patient within the dental office to achieve rapid-onset sedation when other techniques for sedation are unavailable. The drug is administered 30 minutes prior to the scheduled appointment. The same precautions regarding a companion, driving, and dangerous machinery apply.

BENZODIAZEPINES

The first benzodiazepine was synthesized in the late 1950's and marketed in 1960.[10] The agent was chlordiazepoxide, and it represented a significant step forward in the pharmacological management of anxiety. At present six benzodiazepine derivatives are available in the United States. Five are antianxiety agents and one is classified as a sedative-hypnotic. These agents, availability, and usual adult doses are listed in Table 8–3.

All of the benzodiazepines possess antianxiety, anticonvulsant, and skeletal muscle-relaxing properties. Oral forms are well absorbed from the gastrointestinal tract; however, unlike most other drugs, chlordiazepoxide and diazepam are absorbed more slowly and less reliably following intramuscular rather than oral administration,[2, 6, 7, 18] therefore, these two agents should be administered orally whenever possible.[14]

Pharmacologically, the benzodiazepines produce a depression of subcorti-

TABLE 8–3 AVAILABILITY OF ORAL BENZODIAZEPINES

Generic	Proprietary	Availability	Usual Dose*
Chlordiazepoxide	Librium	5, 10, 25 mg	10–25 mg
Chlorazepate	Tranxene,	3.75, 7.5, 15 mg	7.5–15 mg
	Azene	3.25, 6.5, 13 mg	6.5–13 mg
Diazepam	Valium	2, 5, 10 mg	5–10 mg
Flurazepam	Dalmane	15, 30 mg	30 mg
Lorazepam	Ativan	1, 2 mg	2–4 mg
Oxazepam	Serax	10, 15, 30 mg	15–30 mg

*Dosage forms indicated are those for a normal, healthy 70 kg patient. It is suggested that the package insert or a textbook of pharmacology be consulted prior to drug administration.

cal levels of the CNS. While their precise mode of action is unknown, it is thought that their anxioloytic actions are due to their depressant activity on the limbic system. A major advantage of the benzodiazepines is their high therapeutic indices. It is this factor which has led to the benzodiazepines becoming so frequently prescribed.

The benzodiazepines undergo biotransformation in the liver and are excreted in the urine. When administered orally the clinical duration of action is approximately three to four hours. There is, however, significant variation in the onset of action of several of these drugs. Chlordiazepoxide blood levels rise slowly following oral administration, reaching a maximum approximately 4 hours following administration;[26] diazepam reaches maximal blood levels in 2 hours;[28] however, 90 per cent of the maximal blood levels develops within one hour. Diazepam, therefore, is usually administered one hour prior to the scheduled dental appointment. As with other CNS depressant drugs, patients receiving diazepam must be cautioned that they should be accompanied by an adult and not operate a motor vehicle or other dangerous machines after taking these drugs. Oxazepam has a rapid onset of action (60 minutes maximal blood level) and a shorter duration of clinical effectiveness. The benzodiazepines have been reported to possess weak anticholinergic properties, therefore their use is contraindicated in patients with narrow-angle glaucoma.

Chlordiazepoxide

Chlordiazepoxide, the first of the benzodiazepines employed clinically, is an effective antianxiety agent when employed orally. Its use in densitry, however, has never approached that of diazepam. One important factor is its relatively slow onset of action. Maximal blood levels following oral administration are not achieved for up to four hours.[26] This makes the use of this agent for anxiety reduction in the preappointment period less attractive than a drug with a more rapid onset. Chlordiazepoxide is more practical when taken as an antianxiety agent the evening prior to dental therapy. The longer onset of action will be of negligible importance at this time. A significant advantage of chlordiazepoxide is its availability in generic forms, which has led to a decrease in its cost. Its equal effectiveness as an antianxiety agent (ignoring its prolonged onset) and its lower cost make chlordiazepoxide a drug to be considered when antianxiety drugs are selected.

Chlordiazepoxide is available in 5, 10, and 25 mg capsules. The usual adult dose for preoperative or night-time anxiety reduction is 25 mg one to two hours before the appointment or at bedtime.

Diazepam

Diazepam is the most commonly prescribed drug in the world.[28] Introduced in 1963, it is presently available under the proprietary name of Valium. Diazepam is effective as an antianxiety, anticonvulsant, and skeletal-muscle-relaxing drug. It may be administered orally or parenterally. Intramuscular administration is not recommended unless other routes of administration are not practical because of the erratic and inconsistent absorption of diazepam from muscle.[18] Indeed, when equivalent doses of diazepam are administered via the oral and intramuscular routes, a higher degree of clinical effectiveness develops with the oral dosage form.[23] Intravenous administration of diazepam has become a highly popular technique for conscious-patient sedation. It is discussed fully in Chapter 10.

Following oral administration, maximal blood levels are achieved in approximately two hours. Approximately 90 per cent of this maximal level is achieved within one hour, so that the agent may be administered 60 minutes prior to the scheduled appointment with satisfactory results. Patients must be cautioned that they should not operate motor vehicles or other dangerous machinery, and that they should be accompanied by an adult after receiving oral diazepam. Diazepam is available in 2, 5 and 10 mg tablets. The average adult dosage for preoperative anxiety reduction is 10 mg taken one hour prior to the scheduled appointment.

Flurazepam

Flurazepam is a benzodiazepine which is employed as a sedative-hypnotic for the induction and maintenance of sleep.[21] It is preferred to the barbiturates for a variety of reasons,[22] among which are a vastly superior therapeutic index, a significantly lower incidence of adverse reactions, a minimal potential for successful suicide attempts, and a lack of drug dependence, habituation, addiction, and tolerance. More realistically, when used as a hypnotic the evening before dental therapy, it induces a state of drowsiness, with a much lower incidence of "hangover" (lethargy, drowsiness, headache, and ataxia) the morning after its ingestion than is observed following barbiturate administration.[13]

Flurazepam, available in 15 and 30 mg capsules, is usually administered in the 30 mg form one hour prior to bedtime. The 15 mg form is reserved for younger and older patients, or debilitated persons. Flurazepam may be administered 60 minutes prior to the dental appointment when moderate to profound sedation is desired; however, more controllable techniques are to be preferred.

Other Benzodiazepines

Several other benzodiazepine derivatives are available for clinical use in the United States. These agents, chlorazepate, oxazepam, and lorazepam are effective antianxiety agents when prescribed in appropriate dosage form. They do not possess any advantage over the previously described drugs. They may be used in dentistry to achieve anxiety reduction in the immediate preoperative period for mild levels of anxiety. Drug package inserts or a textbook of pharmacology should be consulted prior to employing these agents.

The benzodiazepines have become the drugs of choice for the management of anxiety in the preoperative period in dentistry. The most compelling factor in their favor is their relative safety when compared to the barbiturates.

THE ANTIHISTAMINES

A side effect of most antihistamines is their ability to produce a degree of central nervous system depression (sedation).[29] One antihistamine, hydroxyzine, has been used in dentistry primarily because of this property. Hydroxyzine possesses sedative, antihistaminic, antiemetic, antispasmodic, and anticholinergic properties. Its primary use has been as a preoperative sedative in pediatric dentistry.[20]

Oral forms of hydroxyzine are well absorbed from the GI tract, clinical effects being noted within 15 to 30 minutes. Maximal effect develops in two hours, with a duration of action of three to four hours. Unwanted side effects are rarely observed following oral administration, drowsiness, and drying of the mouth being reported most frequently.[1] Fatal overdose has never been reported.

Hydroxyzine is available in two forms: the hydrochloride (Atarax), which is available in 10, 25, 50 and 100 mg tablets, as a syrup (10 mg per 5 ml), and as the pamoate (Vistaril), available as 25, 50 and 100 mg capsules and as a suspension (25 mg per 5 ml).

Hydroxyzine is indicated for timid, highly anxious or "high strung" children.[22] Its greatest effectiveness appears to be in preschool or younger school-age children. The liquid form of Atarax is more pleasant tasting to most patients than is Vistaril. Because of its relative safety, hydroxyzine may be used effectively with other techniques such as inhalation sedation or parenteral sedation, provided that reduced dosages of the other agents are employed and that careful monitoring of the patient is maintained.

CARBAMATES

Meprobamate (Miltown, Equanil) is an example of this class of drugs. It is useful in the management of anxiety and tension; however, it has also been demonstrated to be less effective than the benzodiazepines.[27]

Meprobamate is well absorbed following oral administration, however maximal blood levels do not develop for three hours. The drug has a half-life of 11 hours.[16] Respiratory depression and hypotension may develop with overdosage. Tolerance and physical dependence may develop with meprobamate, and successful suicide attempts have been reported.[11] Drowsiness and ataxia are the most frequently reported adverse side effects. Other side effects include nausea and vomiting, slurred speech, and headache. Both proprietary forms are available in 200 and 400 mg doses. Administered two hours before therapy, the 400 mg dosage form is the most frequently employed in the healthy adult.

NARCOTICS

Narcotics are classified as strong analgesics. Their primary function is the relief of pain of a moderate to severe nature. In addition, these agents will mildly alter a patient's psychological response to pain and will suppress anxiety and apprehension. Many of these agents are employed parenterally as preanesthetic medications because of their sedative, antianxiety, and analgesic properties. However, to achieve antianxiety effects, narcotics should not be administered via the oral route, absorption is not as consistent as with parenteral administration, and the incidence of unwanted side effects is considerably greater (postural hypotension, nausea, and vomiting). Oral narcotics should be reserved for the relief of pain when milder analgesics prove to be inadequate.

CONCLUSIONS

Pharmacosedation by the oral route is a moderately successful method of relieving mild apprehension. Because of the inherent difficulties attendant in achieving precise levels of sedation, it is recommended that only light levels of sedation be sought.

A great number of drugs are presently available for the relief of anxiety. In general, these agents fall into a limited number of drug groups: antianxiety agents, barbiturates, and antihistamines. Ethyl alcohol is also an effective mild antianxiety agent in dentistry. While all drugs may be safely employed by the knowledgeable, well trained dental doctor, the prudent doctor will limit his or her prescribing habits to a limited number of agents with which he or she is quite familiar. From a practical point, however, the benzodiazepines have virtually supplanted the barbiturates as the drugs of choice for anxiety reduction in dentistry. Although many benzodiazepines are available, diazepam and chlordiazepoxide are most frequently employed for mild anxiety, while flurazepam, classified as a sedative-hypnotic, is useful for more intense anxiety; it is taken the evening before dental therapy, or occasionally on the day of therapy.

Other drug groups should be considered for use whenever the benzodiazepines are contraindicated or ineffective, and when other more controllable techniques of conscious-patient sedation are unavailable.

In all situations, regardless of the drug to be employed, the practitioner must be fully aware of the pharmacologic properties of the drug, as well as its potential adverse reactions, and must be capable of managing these reactions. When used properly and cautiously, the administration of drugs for anxiety reduction can lead to a dramatic decrease in the incidence of anxiety-induced complications in dental practice.

REFERENCES

1. Bailenson G.: The Relaxed Patient: A Manual of Sedative Techniques. Philadelphia, J. B. Lippincott, 1972.
2. Baird, E. S., and Hailey, D. M.: Plasma levels of diazepam and its major metabolite following intramuscular administration. Br. J. Anaesth., 45:546, 1973.
3. Barraclough, B. M. Are there safer hypnotics than barbiturates? Lancet, 1:57, 1974.
4. Bennett, C. R. Conscious sedation in dental practice. Saint Louis, C. V. Mosby, 1974.
5. Corah, N.: Development of a dental anxiety scale. J. Dent. Res., 48:596, 1969.
6. Gamble, J. A. S.: Blood diazepam levels: Preliminary results. Br. J. Anaesth., 45:926, 1973.
7. Gamble, J. A. S.: Plasma levels of diazepam. Br. J. Anaesth., 45:1085, 1973.
8. Greenblatt, D. J., and Miller, R. R.: Rational use of psychotropic drugs. I. Hypnotics. J. Maine Med. Assoc., 65:192, 1974.
9. Greenblatt, D. J., and Shader, R. I.: Acute poisoning with psychotropic drugs. In Shader, R. I., and DiMascio, A. D. Psychotropic Drug Side Effects: Clinical and Therapeutic Perspectives. Baltimore, Williams & Wilkins Co., 1970.

10. Greenblatt, D. J., and Shader, R. I.: Benzodiazepines in Clinical Practice. New York, Raven Press, 1974.
11. Greenblatt, D. J., and Shader, R. I.: Meprobamate: A study of irrational drug use. Am. J. Psychiatry, 127:1297, 1971.
12. Greenblatt, D. J., and Shader, R. I.: The clinical choice of sedative-hypnotics. Ann. Intern. Med., 77:91, 1972.
13. Greenblatt, D. J., Shader, R. I., and Koch-Weser, J.: Flurazepam hydrochloride, a review. Clin. Pharmacol. Ther. 83:237, 1975.
14. Greenblatt, D. J., Shader, R. I., and Koch-Weser, J.: Slow absorption of intramuscular chlordiazepoxide. New Engl. J. Med., 291:1116, 1974.
15. Haider, I., and Oswald, I.: Effects of amylobarbitone and nitrazepam on the electrodermogram and other features of sleep. Br. J. Psychiatry, 178:519, 1971.
16. Hollister, L. E., and Levy, G.: Kinetics of meprobamate elimination in humans. Chemotherapia, 9:20, 1964.
17. Jorgensen, N. B. Pain control. In Royer R. W. (ed.): Current Therapy in Dentistry. Saint Louis, C. V. Mosby, 1970, Vol 4.
18. Kaplan, S. A., Jack, M. L., Alexander, K., et al.: Pharmacokinetic profile of diazepam in man following single intravenous and oral and chronic oral administrations. J. Pharm. Sci., 62:1789, 1973.
19. Koch-Weser, J., and Sellers, E. M. Drug interactions with coumarin anticoagulants. New Engl. J. Med., 285:487, 1971.
20. Kopel, H. M.: Hydroxyzine. In Wright G. Z.: Behavior Management in Dentistry for Children. Philadelphia, W. B. Saunders, 1975.
21. Kopel, H. M.: The clinical use of hydroxyzine as a preoperative sedative: An investigative double blind study with apprehensive children. Anesth. Prog., 18:127, 1971.
22. McCarthy, F. M., and Hayden, J., Jr.: Ethyl alcohol by the oral route as a sedative in dentistry. J.A.D.A., 96:282, 1978.
23. McCaughey, W., and Dundee, J. W.: Comparison of the sedative effects of diazepam given by the oral and intramuscular routes. Br. J. Anaesth. (Abstr.), 44:901, 1972.
24. Morgan, H., Scott, D. F., and Joyce, C. R. B.: The effects of four hypnotic drugs and placebo on normal subjects sleeping and dreaming at home. Br. J. Psychiatry, 177:649, 1970.
25. Pallasch, T. J.: Clinical Drug Therapy in Dental Practice. Philadelphia, Lea and Febiger, 1973.
26. Smyth, D., and Pennington, G. W.: Determination and excretion of chlordiazepoxide ("Librium") in human plasma and urine. Arch. Int. Pharmacodynam., 145:154, 1963.
27. Sterlin, C., Ban, T. A., and Jarrold, L.: The place of doxepin among the anxiolytic-sedative drugs. Curr. Ther. Res., 14:195, 1972.
28. Stolley, P. D., Becker, M. H., McEvilla, J. D., et al.: Drug prescribing and use in an American community. Ann Intern. Med., 76:537, 1972.
29. Tempero, K. F., and Hunninghake, D. B.: Antihistamines. Postgrad. Med., 48:149, 1970.

9 | PSYCHOSEDATION

Part 4: Pharmacosedation – Inhalation Route

NORMAN TRIEGER

and

SEYMOUR CARR

INTRODUCTION

Psychosedation with nitrous oxide and oxygen offers an approved approach to patient management in dental treatment. Properly administered, it can serve as an important adjunct to the control of anxiety in the conscious patient. This is accomplished by the effects created in the central nervous system by the inhalation of controlled amounts of nitrous oxide and oxygen, and by its potent effect as a placebo. Research has demonstrated that it diminishes sensitivity to noxious stimuli in the conscious and responsive patient even in the absence of true analgesia. It does not, however, substitute for local analgesia when the anticipated procedure is a painful one, or the need for a full general anesthetic when an unconscious patient is required.

PAIN CONTROL CONCEPT

Developing such a concept of pain control enables one to properly place nitrous oxide-oxygen sedation within a broad schema (Fig. 9–1)

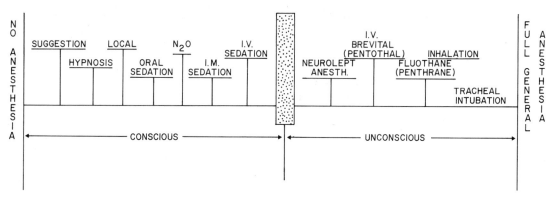

Figure 9–1   Schema of the spectrum of pain control in dentistry.

which ranges from no anesthesia through the several modalities, such as suggestion, hypnosis, acupuncture, local analgesia, oral sedation, nitrous oxide sedation, intramuscular and intravenous sedation. All of these are widely practiced and are effective methods of control of pain and anxiety in the dental office for the conscious patient. A significant barrier must then be recognized which separates the conscious from the unconscious patient. A conscious patient is defined as "one with intact protective reflexes, including the ability to maintain an airway, and is capable of rational responses to questions or commands." The schema may be continued with the use of more potent intravenous agents, such as Brevital and Pentothal, and inhalation agents, such as Fluothane, Ethrane and Penthrane, to reach the end point of full general anesthesia with tracheal intubation as is generally practiced in hospitals.

Frequently, combinations of these methods are employed to achieve optimal conditions for the rendering of dental treatment. Such combinations — for example, inhalation plus intravenous sedation administrered concurrently — may obscure the usual responses for each modality alone and lead to greater hazard. Caution dictates an approach based on even more controlled titration of agents and the ability and equipment to render appropriate emergency care. The utilization of *both* the inhalation and intravenous routes should be limited to the clinican who is trained and experienced in all anesthesia/sedation modalities and in basic life support.

Nitrous oxide-oxygen psychosedation may be used in dentistry for a variety of procedures: to aid in radiographic surveys, prophylaxis, and impression taking, to effectively reduce gagging, and to provide a more cooperative patient. Suture removal, changing dressings and packs, wire and splint removal, and cementation of crowns may be carried out more comfortably with the patient sedated with nitrous oxide-oxygen. Operative dentistry and crown and bridge and nonsurgical periodontics can be done with the aid of nitrous oxide-oxygen, though it is important to use local analgesia as an adjunct when the operation is anticipated to be a painful one. Extractions and periodontal surgery would generally require adjunctive local analgesia.

The rhetorical question may be asked, "If sedation is the desired end result, why not use many of the psychosedative drugs available, by either the oral, intramuscular, or intravenous route?"

The answer must be that none of the other modalities (with the exception of alcohol) obviate the need for a responsible person to accompany the patient or permit the patient to follow his normal routine shortly after a psychosedation session. In none of the others do we have an agent that produces onset of signs within 45 to 90 seconds, nor can the level of sedation be controlled and altered as rapidly as with nitrous oxide-oxygen.

Again it is worthwhile mentioning that in none of the other techniques do we have a return to normal as rapidly (120 to 180 seconds) as at the conclusion of nitrous oxide-oxygen psychosedation.

SAFETY

The record of safety experienced in the use of nitrous oxide-oxygen for conscious patients, in the manner to be detailed below, is remarkable. No serious complications have been reported in the performance of many millions of such cases in the past few years. Ruben,[35] in a Danish dental study in 1966, cited the administration of over 3,000,000 sedations without mishap. Important consideration must be given to the concentration of oxygen in this technique. *Psychosedation can be achieved and adequate oxygenation assured if the concentration of oxygen is never lower than 25 per cent or 2.5 liters per minute flow. Adequate sedation will generally be achieved without oxygen delivery below 50 percent.*

Nitrous oxide depresses bone marrow and peripheral white blood cell counts after prolonged use; that is, more than 48 hours of continuous use. However, its administration as a sedative agent in the manner in which it is generally used has failed to demonstrate any toxic effect. Jaffe, in a recent searching paper, reviewed the literature and concluded that, "Nitrous oxide used properly is still the least toxic of all anesthetic agents."[25]

Recently there has appeared in the medical and dental literature a number of reports indicating potential health hazards to dental practitioners and other operatory personnel. These potential health hazards are thought to be associated with prolonged exposure to atmospheric pollutants arising from the use of gaseous anesthetic agents.

Perhaps the earliest reference to the toxic effects of anesthetic agents was by Lassen et al.[29] in 1956. They reported agranulocytosis arising in patients exposed to continuous sedation with 60 per cent N_2O for three days.

One of the very early studies done in regard to operating room personnel and their prolonged exposure to atmospheric pollutants was by Vaisman[41] in 1967. He was led to undertake the study by what seemed to him a disproportionate number of headaches and spontaneous abortions occurring in people who worked in the operating suites of his hospital in Russia.

In 1968 Fink and Kenny[22] reported on the teratogenic effects on experimental animals related to the toxicity of anesthetics. In 1973 Corbett and Ball[19] studied embryotoxicity in experimental animals.

These early studies then directed greater attention to the hazards operating room personnel faced from chronic exposure to anesthetic room pollutants. In 1971 Cohen et al.[16] did a study which found increased abortion rates in operating room personnel.

Most definitive was a large scale study done in 1972 of the effects of trace anesthetic agents on the health of 40,044 operating room personnel. This study, sponsored by the American Society of Anesthesiology and the National Institute of Occupational Safety and Health, produced statistics that indicated operating room personnel produce a 25 per cent higher rate of birth defects, 50 per cent more spontaneous abortions and twice as much liver disease as other personnel in the hospital who do not work in the operating suites.

Further studies indicated that room pollution in dental offices[17] where nitrous oxide was being used as a sedation agent or in oral surgery offices[42] where it was being used as an adjunct to ambulatory anesthetic procedures had even higher pollution rates varying from 130 to 9000 PPM, when approximately 50 to 100 PPM is considered maximum for safety.

This increased pollution ratio was thought to be due to:

1. The semi-closed system in use.
2. The smaller size of dental operatories.
3. Exhaling gases from the patient's open mouth.
4. The inefficient machines, with their increased number of leaks, sometimes used in dental offices.

In a sincere effort to protect the personnel employed in hospital operating rooms and dental offices there has begun a movement toward developing significant restrictive legislation. Some of the discussed legislative measures possibly necessary for the operating room are being made equally stringent for the dental office.

However, the personnel in the dental office are not being exposed to the multiplicity of agents found in the operating room. Pollutants such as ethylene oxide, Fluothane, and Ethrane are not routinely used in the dental office. In addition, the periods of exposure in the dental office are considerably less than in the operating room, averaging no more than 90 minutes per day as compared to the operating room, where exposure is chronic.

As frequently happens with controversial issues, the pendulum has now begun to swing in the opposite direction. Questions are being raised concerning some of the animal studies and their unproven effects in man. Subsequent studies in regard to observed health hazards to operating room personnel have not verified earlier findings. Critical reviews of previously published data regarding spontaneous abortions in operating room personnel have not agreed with prior conclusions.

Scaramella, et al.[36] made several excellent observations that speak for moderation in modifications and restrictions that might be placed on the dental office by legislation in regards to scavenging devices. They found that the problems of pollution affecting performance, initially considered significant, have been challenged. They also noted that time-weighted samples taken over the day would produce less than 10 parts per million in the dental operatories. Gas flow in an eight hour day occurs only for approximately one to two hours. It is recommended that levels of less than 50 parts per million be sought.

In the absence of further evidence to the contrary, we strongly favor these measures:

1. Good nitrous oxide–oxygen hygiene
2. Good mask fit
3. Elimination of machine leaks

This might make it possible to reduce pollutant levels over an eight hour period to within less than 50 parts per million without resort to additional devices.

We agree that atmospheric pollution is undesirable and must be eliminated but, in view of the fact that its bad effects have not been conclusively proven, restrictive legislation should be avoided at this time. This does not mean that the authors are trying to discourage the use of scavenging devices, several types of which will be described in the section on equipment. We feel that the method of control of pollution in the dental office should at this time be determined by the individual practitioner, who may choose to use scavenging devices or passive techniques.

REVIEW OF CARDIOPULMONARY PHYSIOLOGY

Nunn and Freeman[32] have presented an important concept of "available oxygen" — the amount of oxygen available for tissue perfusion. This is related to cardiac output; to the arterial oxygen saturation; to the hemoglobin concentration (and a constant of 1.34 ml per gram which indicates the amount of oxygen that can combine with each gram of hemoglobin when fully saturated). This consideration of tissue perfusion by oxygen is a key one. We, at present, have no direct way to measure cardiac output, short of the experimental laboratory. Instead, we use other indirect measurements, such as the blood pressure, pulse rate, and the patient's color and responsiveness as indications that tissue perfusion is adequate.

This concept of available oxygen for the tissue is of further significance when one realizes that the determinants of available oxygen are not simply added together to achieve the resultant available tissue oxygen, but in fact are *multiples* of one another.

For example, a patient with a normal cardiac output, whose myocardial pump is in good condition, can respond to stresses of illness or surgery or anxiety by rapidly increasing output. A patient free of pulmonary disease can maintain adequate oxygen saturation of his blood, which the heart pumps to it. If this same patient had a hemoglobin which was lower than the normal 12 to 18 gm, he would still be able to manage satisfactorily in undergoing anesthesia. If, however, we have an elderly patient who has sustained some previous myocardial damage and also has compromised pulmonary function because of emphysema or airway obstruction and is also moderately anemic, then the product of these three parameters may produce a severe impediment to adequate oxygenation of tissues.

Cardiac output is diminished by all anesthetic agents or depressant drugs. Congestive heart failure, aortic and mitral stenosis, hemorrhage, and constrictive pericarditis also decrease the output of the ventricles. A decrease in venomotor tone, dependent pooling, or dilatation of the venous bed leads to a decrease in venous return and consequently a drop in cardiac output.

The position of the patient is also an important consideration. Elevation of the legs, as is customarily practiced in the new contour dental chairs, will diminish the likelihood of blood pooling in the lower extremities. Patients with cardiopulmonary disease generally have the greatest lung compliance in the sitting position. A combination of legs up and the head and thorax at a 30-degree angle is often practiced and may overcome some of the problems of patient positioning.

Induction of anesthesia is dependent upon (1) the partial pressure of the gas, (2) its solubility (i.e., rate of uptake by blood and then by tissues), and (3) its potency. In consideration of the pulmonary factor, a primary point is the rate of ventilation which determines the early uptake. Thus, breath holding would certainly delay the onset of the anesthetic effect and rapid deep breathing would tend to increase the rate of uptake. Transfer of the gas from the pulmonary alveoli to the blood is dependent upon its rate of diffusion. Diffusion is a function of (1) its solubility, (2) the rate of pulmonary blood flow (i.e., cardiac output), and (3) the tension of the gas in the arterial and venous blood. Further, the blood-to-tissue transfer is dependent upon the following: (1) Solubility of the gas in the tissues. With nitrous oxide, blood and tissue solubility, except for fat, are almost the same (nitrous oxide is relatively insoluble when compared to other inhalation anesthetics). (2) The rate of blood flow for perfusion of the tissues is another important determinant. In this regard, the brain's blood supply is many times greater than that of the fat areas of the body, and, hence, an effect is noted on the central nervous system very rapidly. (3) The tension of the anesthetic gas will also determine the exchange from blood to tissue and its saturation. Graphically, the induction of anesthesia may be pictured as a series of swinging doors at the several exchange points. The introduction of the gas into the lungs meets the alveolar barrier before entering the venous circulation. Once carried by the blood, it is pumped out by the heart where it encounters the barrier to the tissues.

NITROUS OXIDE INDUCTION

The initial absorption of nitrous oxide is extremely rapid. Approximately 1000 ml at a normal respiratory minute volume is taken up within the first minute. At the end of ten minutes, it drops to 350 ml and drops further to 200 ml in 30 minutes, and to only 100 ml in 100 minutes. Studies by Eger et al.[20] show that breathing 100 per cent nitrous oxide will require only one minute to reach 80 per cent alveolar concentration! At 1 per cent nitrous oxide, it takes four to five minutes to reach 80 per cent inspired concentration (Fig. 9–2).

It is readily demonstrable that it generally takes approximately 40 seconds of breathing nitrous oxide for patients to experience sensory changes such as tingling, feeling "high," feeling warmth, and other changes in perception. Hustead and Eastwood[9] have demonstrated, in the use of nitrous oxide for obstetrics, that when pain is present, during labor, only 30 per cent of patients reported decrease in pain with the administration of nitrous oxide-oxygen sedation. This percentage increased significantly when labor pains were of short duration, patients apparently having confidence that the

Figure 9-2 Graph illustrating the uptake of nitrous oxide.

gas helped to relieve their discomfort. N_2O is rapidly transmitted to the fetus across the placenta, but does not influence uterine contraction.[30] *This strongly suggests an important placebo effect acting in the control of pain.*

Patient variability, in response to nitrous oxide, is very great. Each patient must provide his own titration. There can be no arbitrary or predetermined levels, because we are dealing with individuals who vary tremendously in their response to the percentage of nitrous oxide.

RECOVERY FROM NITROUS OXIDE

The elimination of nitrous oxide follows a reverse pattern of uptake. A large volume is removed initially. This high initial outpouring of nitrous oxide may produce hypoxia (diffusion anoxia) on recovery by displacing oxygen. Though this is not usually found with nitrous oxide-oxygen sedation, following general anesthesia there is a tendency toward hypoventilation on recovery, as carbon dioxide is blown off and the respiratory rate falls. This diffusion hypoxia is most apparent during the first five to ten minutes in recovery. Oxygen administration at the end of each procedure is advisable.

CHARACTERISTICS OF NITROUS OXIDE

Nitrous oxide gas, which is prepared by heating ammonium nitrate, is compressed and liquefied in blue cylinders at a pressure of 800 pounds per square inch. It is stable and does not react with soda lime, which is often used to absorb carbon dioxide during anesthesia. It will support combustion, but will not explode or burn. No chemical reaction occurs in inhalation. It is eliminated by the lungs, skin, sweat, urine, and intestinal gas. It is a sweet-tasting gas and not unpleasant to inhale. More recently, it was shown that nitrous oxide's "analgesia" resembles opiate actions.[14] These effects can be blocked by the administration of narcotic antagonists such as naloxone. Nitrous oxide may function by causing the release of endogenous endorphins in the central nervous system. The release of such newly identified peptides with narcotic effects may account for the euphoric effects attributed to nitrous oxide as well as the increased pain tolerance and also the extended post-administration feeling of relaxation and lassitude. Subsequently, these findings were refuted.[38a]

With nitrous oxide inhalation psychosedation, all modalities of sensation may be affected, depending upon the concentration of gas administered. Acuity of hearing, sight, touch and pain, memory, concentration, and calculation are affected. Electroencephalographic changes are minimal. Cerebellar functions are affected and produce incoordination and psychomotor deficits, ataxia, and nystagmus. Nitrous oxide has a pronounced effect on the sensorium at subanesthetic levels. Changes in heart rate, cardiac output, blood pressure, or central venous pressure are generally insignificant except when approaching the excitement stage of anesthesia. At subanesthetic concentrations, blood pressure and pulse rate show a gradual and moderate decline which may well be a reflection of the sedation achieved. Myocardial depression by nitrous oxide has also been demonstrated.[21, 33] But it has also been successfully used as an analgesic adjunct in acute myocardial infarction where it produced considerable relief of mild pain. These decreases in heart rate and blood pressure tend to persist into the recovery period even after the patient's sensorimotor changes have been restored to normal. This may account for the postsedation feeling of being very relaxed. At higher concentrations, nitrous oxide has been found to produce signs of sympathetic activation with increases in cardiovascular parameters.[38] Venodilatation of the skin vessels occurs during nitrous oxide administration, and this may facilitate venipuncture. A diaphoresis or sweating often occurs with nitrous oxide induction. Belladonna alkaloids may help control this phenomenon.

CONTRAINDICATIONS

There are few contraindications to the use of nitrous oxide-oxygen sedation. There are, however, significant contraindications related to *any* elective treatment given to certain patients with significant health problems. Patients with congestive heart failure who are *decompensated* should not receive any elective dental treatment, as they are ASA Class IV at the moment, although medical treatment may elevate such a patient to Class III or even Class II status. See Chapter 2 for the ASA physical status classification. The rendering of emergency care to relieve pain and infection may become necessary. Similarly, patients who have sustained a myocardial infarction within the past six months should have all elective treatment deferred. Patients with advanced pulmonary disease, such as emphysema, are also poor candidates for anesthesia. However, these patients, as well as those with congestive heart failure and recent myocardial infarction, may benefit by the administration of oxygen during the performance of essential dental therapy. This often serves to provide an enriched oxygen atmosphere and aids to decrease anxiety and provide better tissue perfusion. You are reminded never to deliver more than a 30 per cent oxygen concentration to a patient with advanced pulmonary emphysema (rest dyspnea, ASA Class IV) (see Chapter 2).

Nasal obstruction, upper respiratory infections, and allergic rhinitis may be considered important contraindications for nitrous oxide-oxygen sedation. We are dependent upon the nasal airway, whether the mask or cannula is used. Patients who have significant nasal obstruction will not be able to benefit from this technique.

Patients with severe anemia may benefit from the adjunctive administration of high levels of oxygen, but should not be made to undergo anesthesia or other treatment which further depresses the oxygen-carrying capacity of the blood or cardiac function.

Patients receiving monamine oxidase inhibitors (such as Nardil, Marplan, Niamid, Parnate, Eutonyl, Octomal, Cavodil, Drazine, Marsilid, Parstelin, Perefenil, and Tersavid), generally prescribed for their emotional antidepressive effects, and those receiving cortisone or related steroid medications are particularly susceptible to hazards associated with stress and anesthesia.

One of the most significant contraindications to the use of nitrous oxide-oxygen psychosedation is emotional instability. Because this method causes some distortion of normal perception, it would be unwise to involve schizoid patients or drug addicts. It is undoubtedly far better when dealing with patients who are emotionally disturbed to maintain their tenuous contact with the reality of the treatment situation.

LIABILITY INSURANCE

Although the controlled administration of nitrous oxide-oxygen for psychosedation has been free of serious complications, some insurance underwriters have insisted that it be classified along with general anesthesia. There have been a few instances when this attitude has resulted in an increase in premium for malpractice insurance in specific areas in this country. This increase has been relatively small. More recently this increase in premium has been reduced by the insurance companies secondary to their favorable experience with the use of nitrous oxide-oxygen sedation. Offsetting this small increase in overhead cost, the doctor will be able to render more service to more relaxed patients. A specific charge is often made for the "anesthesia" as a specific service. A number of dental insurance programs provide a fee for sedation and anesthesia services.

PRETREATMENT EVALUATION OF THE PATIENT

The patient's medical history should precede the clinical examination. The reader is referred to Chapter 2, Physical Evaluation, for further detailed discussion of pretreatment considerations.

ROLE OF THE AUXILIARY PERSONNEL

It is important that all persons (secretaries, assistants, laboratory technicians, hygienists) employed in the office be made aware of the proper office demeanor when a patient is undergoing nitrous oxide-oxygen sedation. The office should have a quiet relaxed atmosphere prior to and throughout the psychosedation procedure. It is necessary to avoid loud noises or other distractions, such as excessive talking, in the presence of the patient. Remember that the patient under the influence of nitrous oxide-oxygen is *conscious*. Statements made within hearing of the patient may be distorted and misinterpreted.

The duties of the assistant can be accomplished with greater empathy and more efficiency if the assistant has experienced nitrous oxide-oxygen sedation. It is our belief that all personnel involved with patients having this procedure should experience the sensations produced by nitrous oxide, under supervision.

The duties of the dental assistant in regard to the preparation of the patient for nitrous oxide-oxygen sedation begin with her explanation to the patient about the steps that are about to be taken. Having experienced this method of sedation, she can describe to the patient the sensations he is about to experience. At this point, it is well to avoid unrealistic promises. Also, avoid use of the expression, "Don't worry." This is an impossible command to comply with and often suggests to the patient that perhaps there is something to be concerned about.

The assistant then adjusts the nasal hood or cannula to assure comfort during the psychosedation session. Under the doctor's direction, she regulates the flow of gases.

The procedure has been explained to familiarize the patient with what is about to happen, and the sensations of warmth and tingling he or she will experience are described. The nose mask or nasal cannula is adjusted comfortably, and the flow of 5 to 8 liters of oxygen per minute is continued for one minute.

At this point, the bag should be checked to avoid underinflation or overdistention. The liter flow per minute is determined by our estimate of the patient's tidal flow, based on the size and metabolic rate of the individual (Fig. 9–3). A brief review of the following information may be in order at this point.

Average tidal air... 500 ml
Complemental (including tidal)..................... 3000 ml
Supplemental (reserve)............................... 1000 ml
Vital capacity .... 4000 ml

Following the oxygenation period, begin nitrous oxide flow at 1 liter per minute and decrease oxygen at 1 liter per minute, pausing 30 to 45 seconds at each stop until the "baseline" area is achieved. When baseline is achieved for the patient with the 7.5 liter per minute flow, our flowmeter might then look like Figure 9–4.

To determine the actual percentages of gases flowing, the calculations are quite simple. A flow of 3 liters per minute of nitrous oxide and 4.5 liters

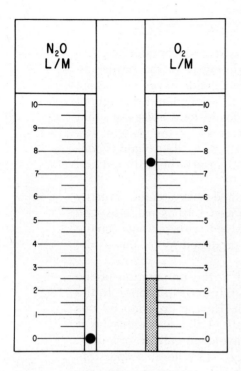

Figure 9–3 Flowmeters. Oxygen is set first to determine adequacy of total flow.

per minute of oxygen composes a total flow of 7.5 liters per minute, of which 40 per cent is nitrous oxide and 60 per cent is oxygen.

Generally, 50 per cent nitrous oxide or less will be effective in carrying the patient to the level of psychosedation desired. The alveolar concentration of nitrous oxide is a function of *time* as well as administered concen-

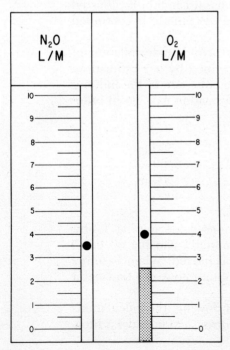

Figure 9–4 Flowmeters. Achieving baseline for psychosedation; individualizing is important.

tration of the gas. At lesser concentrations of nitrous oxide, psychosedation will be achieved in a few more minutes. Never give less than 2.5 liters (25 per cent) of oxygen.

Inevitably the question arises, "How do I know when baseline is achieved?" Remember that we are dealing with a *conscious* patient. We ask the patient, "Do you feel as if you're floating?" Are you dreaming?" Are you comfortable?" The patient may respond with hesitation. If the patient is questioned about the hesitation, the reply usually is something like, "I heard you, but it was too much trouble to answer." At this point, the patient's eyes are generally closed and he speaks with difficulty. The respira-

PSYCHOSEDATION LEVEL

DESIRED MAINTENANCE LEVEL

ULTRALIGHT ANESTHESIA LEVEL

UNDESIRABLE LEVEL

NORMAL PUPIL   CONSTRICTION CAUSED BY LIGHT   DILATED PUPIL

NORMAL PUPIL WITH VOLUNTARY MOVEMENT   DILATED PUPIL WITH INVOLUNTARY MOVEMENT

RELAXED   RESTLESS AND AGITATED

RELAXED AND COOPERATIVE   INAPPROPRIATE MOVEMENT

Figure 9–5 Signs that are a guide to the maintenance or baseline stage.

Illustration continued on following page.

PSYCHOSEDATION LEVEL

DESIRED MAINTENANCE LEVEL

ULTRALIGHT ANESTHESIA LEVEL

UNDESIRABLE LEVEL

NORMAL, SMOOTH BREATHING

SLOW, DEEP OR SHALLOW BREATHING

BLOOD PRESSURE INITIALLY UP
THEN DECREASES 8−10 mm/Hg

BLOOD PRESSURE INCREASING
WITH EXCITEMENT PHASE

PULSE RATE INITIALLY UP
THEN DECREASES WITH SEDATION

PULSE RATE INCREASING WITH EXCITEMENT

CONSCIOUS, RESPONSIVE BUT SEDATED,
NOT TRUE ANALGESIA

HYPER−REACTIVE, LOSS OF CONSCIOUSNESS,
ANALGESIA

Figure 9–5 *Continued.*

tions are normal and there is no holding of breath or grunting. If the patient should slip into deep sedation or ultralight anesthesia, there can be superficial slow breathing which is often irregular with prolonged inspirations, phonation, and grunting.

Other signs (Fig. 9–5) which help us know that we are maintaining our patient in the proper stage are the facial expressions of the conscious individual as compared to the facial expressions representing pain or semiconsciousness. The patient's eyes in the proper stage are also an aid, with

normal pupils which contract normally to light. There is no rolling of eyeballs. If the patient sinks too deeply, the pupils may become dilated and
contract actively to light, and the eyeballs roam. The pulse rate and blood
pressure are not definitive aids in determining the level of sedation.

Referring to Figure 9–6, it is our aim to maintain each patient at the
proper sedative level (barred zone). If the patient should approach the excitement or ultralight anesthesia level, he or she can be returned to baseline by decreasing the nitrous oxide and increasing the oxygen flow.

For patients who are to have a great deal of dental therapy performed,
it is useful to teach them to lighten the sedation by breathing through their
mouths or, if discomfort is experienced, to take deep breaths through the
nose to increase the concentration of nitrous oxide being delivered.

At the completion of the dental procedures, the nitrous oxide is turned
off and the oxygen flow is increased to the original 5- to 8-liter flow per
minute. The oxygen should be continued for approximately 2 to 4 minutes
until the effects of the sedation have disappeared.

Allow the patient to remain in the chair until he feels normal. The
patient should never be dismissed if he is still feeling sluggish.

SUBJECTIVE REACTIONS

All persons involved in caring for the sedated patient should experience nitrous oxide-oxygen sedation at all levels under close supervision.
Only when they have personally experienced it can they appreciate the
patient's feelings, reactions, and needs.

The early subjective symptoms, which are sometimes but not always
present, include tingling sensations in the toes, the fingertips, the tip of the

PRE-ANALGESIC STAGE	CONSCIOUS, ORIENTED, ANXIOUS
ANALGESIA-AMNESIA STAGE (DESIRED STAGE)	CONSCIOUS, RELAXED, FLOATING, WARMTH, LESSENED ANXIETY, EUPHORIA
"PRE"-EXCITEMENT and ULTRA-LIGHT ANESTHESIA STAGE	NON-ORIENTED, RESTLESS, HYPERRESPONSIVE TO STIMULI
SURGICAL ANESTHESIA PLANES 1 2 3 RESPIRATORY HAZARD	UNCONSCIOUSNESS (NITROUS OXIDE LACKS POTENCY TO ANESTHETIZE PATIENTS INTO SURGICAL PLANES OF ANESTHESIA)

Figure 9–6 Schematic of the level of the desired stage in relationship to the
planes of anesthesia.

tongue, or the lips. These feelings can be readily determined by direct questioning, because we are dealing with a conscious patient. If the patient cannot respond to our questions, this is a signal to us that he has sunk below the level of sedation. The operator should immediately decrease the liter flow of nitrous oxide and increase the oxygen by a corresponding amount.

Another useful sign of the patient's level is based on his ability to maintain his mouth in the open position. For this reason we do not recommend the use of a mouth prop, which is used routinely for patients who are undergoing a general anesthetic. The sedated patient who is being maintained at the proper level can keep his mouth open in a relaxed manner. If the mouth slowly begins to close, this indicates to the operator that the nitrous oxide flow should be slightly decreased, with a corresponding increase in the oxygen flow. Remember to maintain the total liter flow initially decided as the proper amount (tidal flow) for this patient, without underinflation or overdistention of the bag.

Another subjective symptom the patient may experience is a warm wave which sweeps over his entire body after the initial tingling sensations. He may experience a feeling of lethargy and relaxation. An occasional patient experiences a humming or vibratory sensation throughout his body, somewhat like a finely tuned motor softly purring. Patients at the ideal plane for operating often experience a floating sensation. At this point, we have established our baseline and this is where we want to maintain the patient. This is the ideal time to inject a local analgesic. The patient is conscious and responsive to the needle prick, but will care less about the discomfort produced.

OBJECTIVE REACTIONS

Minor alterations of blood pressure, pulse rate, and respirations are noted in patients undergoing nitrous oxide-oxygen sedation. These changes are best illustrated by use of Figures 9–7, 9–8, and 9–9. Incoordination does

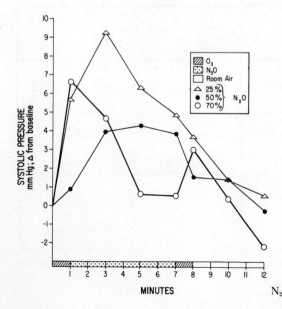

Figure 9–7 Influence of various concentrations of N₂O on the systolic blood pressure.

Figure 9–8 Influence of various concentrations of N_2O on the pulse rate.

become evident under inhalation sedation when the patient is requested to perform some specific activity.

A self-administered, simple line-drawing test was used to evaluate psychomotor function while patients were under the influence of nitrous oxide-oxygen.

The validity of this test has been previously verified in other studies on drug effects. Patients were asked to connect a series of dots on the test to complete the outline of the figure. A baseline drawing is taken prior to the influence of any agent. The test is then repeated at suitable intervals to determine decrement in performance, as well as recovery to the patient's own baseline. Figure 9–10 demonstrates a composite of several tests administered to the same patient undergoing sedation at a constant percentage of nitrous oxide and oxygen.

Figure 9–9 Influence of various concentrations of N_2O on the pulse pressure.

Figure 9–10   Series of tests by the same subject, showing impairment of psychomotor performance caused by drug effect, and recovery.

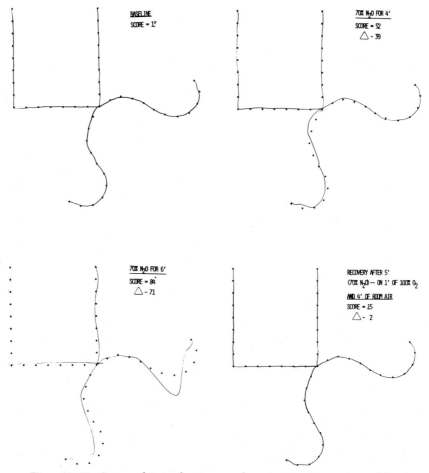

Figure 9–11   Series of tests showing psychomotor impairment in a subject receiving 70 per cent nitrous oxide.

Figure 9–12 Table showing objective data evaluated by statistical analysis.

Figure 9–11 shows a similar series of drawings under a higher concentration of nitrous oxide. In almost all cases studied, return to normal baseline occurs within 2 to 4 minutes after cessation of the nitrous oxide. This test can be numerically scored to yield objective data which can be evaluated by statistical analysis (Fig. 9–12).

In this same study, electrical stimulation of the lower lip was used to determine threshold reactions to a noxious stimulus. Although no correlation in this experimental set-up can be made to clinical pain situations, our results showed an "analgesic" effect attributable largely to placebo influence and less so to the nitrous oxide-oxygen administration (Fig. 9–13).

Such testing may help in the preanesthetic evaluation of patients. This test is a modification of the Bender-Motor Gestalt Test, which has been used extensively to measure psychomotor performance in brain-damaged children.[2]

Figure 9–13 The influence of N_2O on response to electric stimulation of the lower lip.

SAFETY EQUIPMENT

This section, devoted to the discussion of the nitrous oxide-oxygen psychosedation equipment, has been deliberately titled *safety equipment*. Those of us involved in research and teaching in this area have made an effort to convey to the manufacturers our ideas on details of construction and operating features which will enhance the safety of the patient. Manufacturers of the psychosedation apparatus have in turn been most cooperative in their efforts to comply with our recommendations. It is our hope that they will soon recognize the need to discontinue the use of the term "analgesia" in naming their machines. We recommend that the machine be called an inhalation sedation unit. This change would help emphasize that we are not attempting to reach a level of analgesia but rather to provide an adjunct to control of anxiety in the conscious patient.

The information on equipment necessary to treat a patient under nitrous oxide-oxygen psychosedation will be presented in two parts. In the first part we consider adjunctive aids and in the second part the actual components of the inhalation sedation unit.

It is understood that all the equipment and supplies necessary to perform the planned dental procedures be immediately available so that the maximal amount of therapy can be produced during the sedation period. The operating team will, of necessity, be well trained, coordinated, and efficient. The office should have available a sphygmomanometer, a stethoscope, a thermometer, a dental chair that can go into a fully reclining position, and aspirating equipment capable of sucking up at least ½ pint of liquid in 10 seconds.

The inhalation sedation unit is a compact continuous flow machine used for administering gases under controlled conditions. It is composed of first storage cylinders for the compressed gases, either remote in a separate storage area or attached to the machine with the portable cylinders by double yokes.

In regard to these yokes there is an interesting safety feature incorporated into them. There are two pins on the valve surface of the yoke, and there are two holes (Fig. 9–14) drilled in the corresponding surface of the valve on the cylinders. Each type of gas has its own combination of pins and holes. This Pin Index Safety System (P.I.S.S.) makes it impossible for the incorrect cylinder of gas to be connected to a yoke that is pin indexed for another type of gas.

While discussing safety features, it is necessary to mention that most machines, but not all, have a fail-safe system with or without an audible alarm. The fail-safe refers to the feature of the nitrous oxide being cut off immediately, should the oxygen in the supply line fall to less than 50 P.S.I. (pounds per square inch).

The gases go from these cylinders through regulators to the flowmeters which control the volume of the gases administered to the patient. These controlled volumes first pass through a reservoir bag from which they are guided to the mask or cannula on the patient by breathing tubes.

We state unequivocally that the unit should be a continuous flow type. Our own experience, as well as studies by McCarthy and Shuken[31] and Allen and others,[13] has convinced us that the demand flow unit is not as efficient and in

Figure 9–14 Note the difference in space between the two holes on the valve surface of the N₂O cylinder and the O₂ cylinder.

Figure 9–15 Continuous flow inhalation sedation unit of the portable cylinder type. (Courtesy of Dentatron Corporation.)

some cases is unsafe, whereas the continuous flow unit is efficient, safe, and ideal for this technique. The relative accuracy of the continuous flow unit is an acknowledged fact.

The reader will recall that the gases on a continuous flow machine move continually at the rates set on the flowmeters and are not related to the patient's respirations. The demand flow machine, also called an on-demand or intermittent flow machine, does not flow continually at a set rate. The dial is set at a given percentage for the proportions of the two gases, and the output responds and varies with the patient's respiratory needs.

Continuous flow inhalation sedation units can be of the portable cylinder type (Fig. 9–15) or part of a permanent installation system. Those units which are part of an installed system can be wall mounted (Fig. 9–16), stand mounted (Fig. 9–17), or cabinet mounted. This flexibility permits greater convenience in introducing an inhalation sedation unit into the office.

Cylinders

Cylinders come in a variety of sizes, designated A, B, D, E, F, G, H, M, and H H. These cylinders are made of ⅜-inch thick steel and are used to transport and store gases.

Figure 9–16 Wall-mounted permanent installation inhalation sedation unit. (Courtesy of Dentatron Corporation.)

Figure 9-17 Stand-mounted, portable, permanent installation inhalation sedation unit. (Courtesy of N. C. G. Division of Chemetron Corporation.)

Interstate Commerce Commission regulations state that any gas with a pressure exceeding 25 lbs per square inch at 25° C is classified as a compressed gas. The cylinders containing these gases must be subjected to test by interior hydrostatic pressure at least once every five years. The Commission requires that the cylinder be marked with the date of the test. These markings are located at the shoulder of the cylinder.

In addition, the American Hospital Association, in cooperation with the American Society of Anesthesiologists and the medical gas industry, has adopted a uniform color code to be used on all gases supplied in standard cylinders:

Oxygen .... green
Nitrous oxide.................... light blue
Nitrogen .... gray bottom, orange shoulder
Carbon dioxide.................. gray
Cyclopropane .... orange
Helium .... brown
Ethylene.......................... red

Figure 9–18 Multiple piping outlet. (Courtesy of N. C. G. Division of Chemetron Corporation.)

In regard to the ownership of cylinders, sizes A, B, D, and E must be owned by the individual. Cylinder sizes M, G, H, and H H may be owned by the individual, but it is considered economically more feasible to have them supplied by the medical gas supply company.

The medical gas industry makes a demurrage charge of from 6 to 10 cents per day on all cylinders (not doctor-owned) that are retained in the office for more than 30 days.

The most frequently used of the smaller cylinders are the E cylinders which attach directly to the machine. An E cylinder of oxygen contains approximately 625 liters. It can cost from 8 to 20 dollars, depending on distance from the supplier, number of suppliers in the area, and other variable factors. The E cylinder of nitrous oxide contains approximately 1600 liters. Cost can vary from 12 to 25 dollars.

The H cylinder of oxygen and the G cylinder of nitrous oxide are the most frequently used of the larger cylinders and are usually placed in a central storage area. The gases are brought to the piping outlets (Fig. 9–18) from the cylinder storage area through pressure hoses or copper tubing after first passing through a regulator (Fig. 9–19).

Figure 9–19 Regulators with attached pressure gauges for cylinder pressure and line pressure. (Courtesy of Littell's Oxygen, Inc.)

The regulator is actually a reducing valve which reduces the stored pressures of the gas in the cylinder to a safe and usable level. The nitrous oxide has a cylinder pressure of 750 lbs per square inch, and the oxygen has a cylinder pressure of 2400 lbs per square inch when full. These pressures are reduced by the regulator to an average of 50 to 60 lbs per square inch in the carrying line.

In regard to the cylinder pressures of the nitrous oxide and oxygen, there is a difference in the way the gauges will reflect the depletion of the cylinders. Nitrous oxide is present in the cylinder as a liquefied compressed gas and vapor in equilibrium. As long as liquid remains in the cylinder, the gauge shows a cylinder pressure of approximately 750 lbs per square inch. It is only after the liquid is almost depleted that the pressure begins to drop in relation to the gas outflow. This characteristic makes for an abrupt change from a full cylinder at 750 lbs to an empty cylinder. This characteristic also suggests the need for more than one cylinder of each gas connected to the manifold so that an additional source of the gas is immediately available.

Oxygen is a nonliquefied compressed gas, and consequently there is a direct correlation between the pressure recorded on the gauge and the state of depletion of the cylinder.

The cost of the larger cylinders that are usually not doctor-owned can also vary tremendously, depending on the user's geographical location. An H cylinder of oxygen which contains approximately 5300 liters can cost from 12 to 25 dollars. A G cylinder of nitrous oxide which contains approximately 13,800 liters can vary in cost from 46 to 100 dollars.

Piped gas models from a central supply of large G and H tanks are initially a more expensive installation. They require an initial piping installation, including pressure regulators and gauges, manifold, copper tubing, and wall outlets.

The small cylinder portable models using E size medical gas cylinders require no piping installation.

However, the use of the more economical G and H size medical gas cylinders soon offsets the initial expenses.

The comparative cost of gases on the West Coast, based on size of cylinders, is shown in the accompanying table.

| | E Size Cylinders | | G and H Size Cylinders | |
	Capacity	Cost	Capacity	Cost
Oxygen	625 liters	$8.00	5300 liters	$12.00
Nitrous oxide	1600 liters	$12.00	13,800 liters	$46.00

It is necessary to make several suggestions on the handling and storage of cylinders.

1. Full cylinders should be stored in the vertical position.

2. Cylinders should be stored in a place of even temperature, particularly avoiding heat.

3. Consideration should be given to the fact that cylinders should be closed each evening. Storage in a place where access is difficult should be avoided.

4. Cylinders should be handled with care, particularly to avoid dropping.

5. The use of grease, oil, or other lubricants on the cylinder valve should be avoided.

A final word in regard to the purity of the gases that are put into these cylinders: It is imperative that these gases be prepared, purified, and filtered according to standards set by the FDA. This can only be assured through the purchase of the gases from a reputable medical gas supplier.

Instances have been cited in the literature[11, 18] of cylinders being contaminated with nitrous dioxide. In Great Britain it was discovered that one supplier had distributed 65 cylinders so contaminated. On administration of this contaminated gas, nitric acid was formed with resultant dire consequences to the patients.

Regulators and Pressure Gauges

The pressure gauge (Fig. 9–19), which is an adjacent part of the regulator, indicates the pressure of the gas within the cylinder. In rare instances the glass face of the pressure gauge has shattered when the gas was turned on. The staff person performing this function should avert his or her eyes at the time.

The regulator, as previously mentioned, is a reducing valve which reduces the stored pressures within the cylinder to a safe and usable level. The approximately 2400 lbs per square inch pressure in the oxygen cylinder and the approximately 750 lbs per square inch in the nitrous oxide cylinder are reduced by the regulator to 50 to 60 lbs per square inch. This gas reduced in pressure goes from the regulator to the manifold.

Manifolds

Manifolds can operate automatically, switching from an emptying cylinder to the next full cylinder in the bank. Manifolds can also have an electric audible alarm and signal light which notifies the office staff which cylinder is depleted. From these manifolds the gas goes through copper tubing to wall outlets.

In regard to the tubing that brings the gases from the cylinders to the wall outlets, it is important to ascertain, by testing the gases prior to use, that the plumbing has been done correctly. There have been instances of transposition of the tubing from the oxygen cylinder to the nitrous oxide outlet and vice versa. Patient fatalities have occurred.

Wall Outlets

These outlets are supplied by a number of manufacturers. It is important that they too incorporate certain desirable features. They should be quick connectors. They also should have the safety feature of differently spaced and shaped connecting ends (Fig. 9–18). These connectors are coded to fit the proper outlet. From these quick-coupling coded wall connectors should run high pressure, color-coded hoses to the inhalation sedation unit. The inlets on

Figure 9–20 Front view of flowmeters. Note the oxygen flush bar readily available. (Courtesy of the Foregger Company.)

the machine are fabricated under the Diameter Index Safety System (D.I.S.S.), which provides threaded connections of a specific diameter to match only a similar diametered connector on the specific hose, for each gas. The gas which reaches the machine goes first to the flowmeters.

Flowmeters

The flowmeters (Fig. 9–20) record the flow of liters per minute for each of the gases on a readily visible scale graduated in liters. Flowmeters operate simply. A ball of given proper diameter is placed within a tapered, transparent tube, and it will rise and fall, depending on the quantity of gas forced into the tube.

Oxygen Flush

The pushbutton direct oxygen flush (Fig. 9–20) bypasses the regular flowmeters, providing a minimal flow of 30 liters per minute of oxygen into the mask. This is for use in an emergency to fill the bag or whenever a sudden increase in oxygen is desirable.

Reservoir (Rebreathing) Bags

These are available in a variety of sizes from 1 to 8 liters. The 3- and 5-liter sizes are most commonly used.

It is essential that the unit have a reservoir bag for several reasons. In the technique we advocate, observation of the bag gives the operator an accurate guide to the patient's tidal flow. It is particularly important that the inhalation sedation unit have a bag in the breathing circle for certain emergencies. This bag can be used to provide positive pressure oxygen by squeezing the bag to assist respirations.

Bags can be obtained in either rubber or plastic. The rubber deteriorates more rapidly than the plastic, particularly in large cities where atmospheric pollutants are high.

Breathing Tubes

The purpose of these tubes is to transport the gases from the inhalation sedation unit to the mask or cannula on the patient.

Tubes can be made of either corrugated rubber or plastic in a variety of lengths. A selection of connectors should be available to efficiently change to different attachments.

Breathing Masks and Cannulas

Either a nasal mask (Fig. 9–21) or a cannula (Fig. 9–22) may be used to deliver the gases from the breathing tube to the patient. It is our belief that the

Figure 9–21 Nasal mask of single hose variety.

Figure 9–22   Nasal cannula.

nasal mask with a functioning expiratory valve is much more efficient and desirable to the procedure than the cannula.

The cannula has the disadvantage of being wasteful. Because of the discrepancy in size between the nares and the cannula tube, a good deal of the gases is dissipated into ambient air. In addition, some patients complain of the irritating and drying effect on the nasal mucosa created with the cannula. Lastly, the use of the cannula does not permit the reservoir bag to function, an omission we consider detrimental to the technique we endorse. There are, of course, some patients whose previous anesthetic experiences with a mask were unpleasant, and this could preclude the use of a mask, making the use of the cannula a necessity. In addition, there may be a number of patients whose anatomy in the upper anterior region would make dental procedures in that area difficult while using a mask.

A final word in regard to nasal masks, to decry the use of an air dilution valve. A study by Hamilton and Eastwood[24] has shown that a 15-gauge needle inserted into a full face mask will allow up to 60 per cent dilution of the inspired gases with room air. Surely the presence of an open air dilution valve would even further dilute the inhaled gases, making an accurate determination of the concentration of inhaled gases impossible. Allen[12] stated the matter perfectly when discussing the effort some manufacturers make to grade the resistance on expiratory valves. "If, therefore, such sensitivity of expiratory valves is attempted, it seems fatuous to have an air valve on the nasal mask to allow air dilution of the inspired gases."

A full face mask (Fig. 9–23) has no place in the nitrous oxide sedation technique but should be available in case of an emergency in which it becomes necessary to provide positive pressure oxygen by squeezing the bag to assist respirations. The nasal mask is easily removed from the breathing tube and the full face mask substituted via the appropriate connector.

Figure 9–23 Full face mask has no place in the nitrous oxide psychosedation technique. The full face mask should be available to utilize the inhalation sedation unit as a resuscitator in case of an emergency.

In regard to the use of 100 per cent oxygen on a patient in distress who continues to deteriorate, it should be a cardinal rule that the use of the machine should be discontinued at least temporarily. Discontinuance gives the operator a chance to observe if the patient improves on room air. If the patient should improve after discontinuance of the 100 per cent oxygen from the machine, it would certainly indicate a malfunction of the machine, a rare but possible occurrence.

Finally, the previously alluded to scavenger devices must be mentioned. This is a relatively new area of development and we feel sure that the definitive scavenging system has not been attained. We will briefly discuss the three basic systems now being used in many variations. We are aware that systems other than the ones described are available and perhaps favored on a regional basis.

The modified Allen T circuit (Fig. 9–24) has a proximal expiratory valve and can be utilized with a passive evacuation system. It is easy to maintain and the "D" and "E" models have a satisfactory profile, being able to maintain satisfactory levels (<30 ppm). The system's disadvantages are related to difficulty in obtaining a good mask fit and necessity for modification if the unit is to be used for resuscitation.

The Brown system (Fig. 9–25) effectively maintains levels of less than 30 ppm but, unlike the Allen T system, requires a suction connection. This can lead to problems with sterilization of the equipment. The mask is bulky with a high profile.

The Circle system (Fig. 9–26) does a satisfactory job of scavenging but is a complicated circuit. The general practitioner of dentistry is usually not trained

Fresh
Expired
Mixed

Figure 9-24   Modified Allen T circuit. (Courtesy Dr. G. D. Allen.)

in the use of this system. It has low flows and is more difficult to maintain. In addition, this system requires periodic replenishment of the soda lime.

We would like to remind practitioners that a good deal can be done to reduce pollution in the dental office by observing good nitrous oxide–oxygen hygiene. This would include the following:

1. Correction of faulty equipment such as:
    a. leaky wall connectors
    b. deformed compression fittings
    c. loose high pressure hoses
    d. loose, defective or missing gaskets or seals
    e. loose slip joints or threaded connectors
    f. loose flowmeter tubes
    g. worn out bags and breathing hoses

Figure 9-25   Brown system.

SCAVENGING VALVE   EXPIRED GAS

SODA LIME

FRESH GAS

(check valves) = ▽

Figure 9–26 Circle system (Courtesy Dr. G. D. Allen.)

2. Correction of the physical plant, such as:
    a. air conditioning system that does not recirculate the air
    b. proper location of vents
    c. weather-stripping the operatory doors

3. Correction of personnel habits by:
    a. minimizing traffic through the operatories
    b. not engaging the patient in unnecessary conversation

Safety Measures

It should be office policy to consider the inhalation sedation unit as equipment not to be used for other than professional purposes. Inhalation of nitrous oxide is not indicated as fun and games for the office staff.

In addition, the habit practiced in some offices of a morning "whiff" of the gases to be sure they are flowing properly is to be discouraged. Nitrous oxide is not addictive, but it can be habit forming. Under no circumstances should it be self-administered.

Maintenance

The inhalation sedation unit should be checked when indicated for malfunctions, particularly regarding the accuracy of the flowmeters and the function of the fail-safe mechanism. This service is provided by medical gas supply companies.

Recommendations for Greater Safety

The desirable features which we feel should be available on all units to enhance the safety and effectiveness of the inhalation sedation equipment are as follows:

1. All gauges and meters should be in full view.

2. Standardization of the flowmeter scales to conform to medical anesthesia machine practice.

3. Flowmeters calibrated for nitrous oxide and oxygen, with positive control valves controlling the flow. Each complete revolution of the control knob should result in a 1-liter increase or decrease in the flow.

4. Flowmeters should be protected and covered with a safety shield.

5. We strongly recommend that a system be established whereby turning on of either the nitrous oxide or the oxygen will immediately cause the oxygen flow to jump to 2.5 liters flow per minute of oxygen. This would ensure the patient's always having at least 2.5 liters of oxygen per minute, the minimum of oxygen desirable for patient safety.

6. A fail-safe that discontinues the deliverance of nitrous oxide whenever the outflow of oxygen from the machine drops below 2.5 liters per minute is mandatory. It is also desirable for this fail-safe to activate an audible alarm, calling the operator's attention to the fact that the gas flow has been discontinued and corrective action must be taken immediately.

7. The pushbutton oxygen flush should be readily accessible and easily visible on the front of the inhalation sedation unit.

8. All units should have a bag holder tee with a 2- to 5-liter bag incorporated into the line. The reservoir bag should be easily observed by all members of the team.

9. The machines should be compact and well made and should incorporate all the previously listed safety features, such as P.I.S.S. and D.I.S.S. systems. The machine should be built to take long hours of use without need for frequent repairs.

Complications

Expectoration.   Patients should be discouraged from expectorating. This can be helped by making liberal use of the aspirator. If it is absolutely necessary for the patient to expectorate, the assistant should place her hand on the patient's forehead to guide him and prevent him from bumping his head on the cuspidor when bending over.

Nausea.   This condition is rare with nitrous oxide sedation, though it may occur with patients who have consumed a heavy meal prior to their dental appointment or have been carried too deeply into the pre-excitement stage. Although we do not usually advise abstinence from food prior to a sedation appointment, it may be necessary to do so with these patients. Some patients who are prone to develop motion sickness may also be more prone to develop nausea.

Vomiting.   If vomiting occurs, the gas must be discontinued. The nasal mask is removed and the patient tipped forward to allow facilitation of emesis.

Perspiration.   Usually perspiration can be disregarded unless it is accompanied by pallor and other evidence of cardiovascular distress, such as decrease in blood pressure and increase in pulse rate.

Behavior Problems.   Patients who become too deeply anesthetized may develop dissociation, with emotionally disturbing dreams and psychic distortions and reactions. We must be on guard for this type of untoward reaction and prevent the patient from reaching this stage. Some patients with prior adverse reactions to general and even spinal anesthesia may develop intense anxieties while undergoing the sensory change of nitrous oxide sedation. It is often best to discontinue the administration, allow the patient to discuss the recall of experience, and then, if agreeable, suggest a subsequent opportunity to try it again in the near future. Reassure the patient that he can stop the procedure if this severe anxiety returns by signaling and by taking some deep breaths through his mouth. Some patients may resent the threat of feeling "out of control" when they begin to experience subjective tingling, floating, or numbness. These patients are usually very rigid, "up-tight" people. Nevertheless, their wishes should be honored and they should be given time and opportunity to learn how to control their nitrous oxide sedation.

The advantages of rapid onset of sedation and rapid recovery may well be voided by the administration of other drugs orally, intramuscularly, or intravenously. Also, it may confuse the anticipated reactions by the patient. It is best to use nitrous oxide-oxygen sedation with adjunctive local analgesia only. Not all patients are appropriate candidates for nitrous oxide sedation. Some will require a complete general anesthetic, whereas others are cooperative patients with only local analgesia and the application of iatrosedative principles. Each patient must be uniquely evaluated and managed.

It has been recommended that oxygen and a means to efficiently administer it to patients are integral parts of any dental practitioner's armamentarium. The presence of an inhalation sedation machine in the office satisfies this requirement. It can be helpful as an adjunct in the management of many conditions.

Although emergencies are extremely rare with nitrous oxide-oxygen sedation the authors feel that members of the dental profession must be prepared for any emergency which can occur in the dental office.

Airway Obstruction.   Obstruction of the airway through whatever cause demands immediate attention. In this technique of nitrous oxide-oxygen sedation, one is dealing with a *conscious* patient who responds rapidly to an intrusion threatening his airway. The operator must exercise care in the use of high-speed instrumentation and its copious water flow, with the aid of a high-volume suction in addition to the watchful eyes of the operator and assistant. The airway may be aspirated with tonsil tip suction to evacuate any large quantity of fluid. Additionally, there are a few maneuvers which will very quickly assist in re-establishing a good airway. The simplest of these is to elevate the patient's chin and to hyperextend the neck or pull the mandible forward. The operator may also place his forefingers behind the angles of the jaw and push the mandible forward, which will free the airway by simultaneously pulling the tongue and tissues of the floor of the mouth out of the oropharynx. See Chapter 11 on basic life support.

In the unconscious patient, this simple maneuver will often result in a deep inspiration and the patient's return to consciousness. If respirations are depressed, oxygen should be administered via the nasal mask. The additional attachment of a face mask may be helpful to assist depressed respiration. The use of endotracheal tubes and laryngoscope requires significant training in anesthesiology and is well beyond the scope of those not trained in general anesthetic techniques.

OTHER INHALATION AGENTS

Methoxyflurane (Penthrane) has shown promise for the production of both psychosedation and true analgesia by the inhalation route. However, mounting evidence of renal damage virtually eliminates Penthrane from consideration for office use.

At the present time, no inhalation agent other than nitrous oxide-oxygen is recommended for sedation.

SUMMARY

Nitrous oxide-oxygen sedation, properly administered to the *conscious* child or adult, provides an important adjunctive aid to the management of the dental patient. It helps establish enhanced rapport by decreasing anxiety while promoting a more tranquil and often euphoric mood. *It cannot substitute for local analgesia when painful procedures are undertaken.*

A minimum concentration of no less than 25 per cent oxygen (generally 2.5 liters per minute) will ensure adequate oxygenation of the patient. Generally, less than 50 per cent nitrous oxide will suffice to achieve adequate sedation of your patient. Numerous studies have verified the safety of this technique. Our aim is to maintain a conscious and responsive patient free of the hazards of hypoxia and excitement. The desired level of relaxation and sedation is also attainable at much higher levels of oxygenation.

Each patient serves as his own determinant of the most appropriate concentration of nitrous oxide and oxygen. A stepwise procedure has been presented to facilitate each individual's titration to achieve a baseline of sedation.

Inhalation sedation, properly administered, requires additional education and experience. We urge the clinician to seek further knowledge through university postgraduate extension programs. We commend those dental schools now providing the requisite education to their undergraduates in the safe and effective management of the dental patient with inhalation techniques of psychosedation.

REFERENCES

Books:
1. Adriani, J.: Appraisal of Current Concepts in Anesthesiology. St. Louis, C. V. Mosby Co., 1969.
2. Bender, L.: A Visual Motor Gestalt Test and Its Clinical Use. New York, American Orthopsychiatric Association, 1938.
3. Bennett, C. R.: Monheim's General Anesthesia in Dental Practice. St. Louis, C. V. Mosby Co., 1974.
4. Dripps, R. D., Eckenhoff, J. E., and Vandam, L. D.: Introduction to Anesthesia: The Principles of Safe Practice. Philadelphia, W. B. Saunders Co., 1964.
5. Green, C. D.: *In* Eastwood, D. W. (ed.): Nitrous Oxide. Philadelphia, F. A. Davis Co., 1964.
6. Jorgensen, N. B., and Hayden, J., Jr.: Premedication, Local and General Anesthesia in Dentistry. Philadelphia, Lea & Febiger, 1967.
7. Langa, H.: Relative Analgesia in Dental Practice — Inhalation Analgesia and Sedation with Nitrous Oxide. 2nd ed., Philadelphia, W. B. Saunders Co., 1976.
8. Papper, E. M., and Kitz, R. J.: Uptake and Distribution of Anesthesic Agents. New York, McGraw-Hill Book Co., 1963.

9. Hustead, R. F., and Eastwood, D. W. (eds.): Clinical Anesthesia; Nitrous Oxide. Philadelphia, F. A. Davis Co., 1964.
10. Trieger, N.: Pain Control. Chicago, Quintessence Pub. Co., 1975.

Periodicals:
11. Albright, R., L., and Bakett, J. A.: Poisonous effects of the impurities of nitrous oxide. J. Oral Surg., 26:643, 1968.
12. Allen, G. D.: The enigma of air dilution. Anes. Progress, 17:53, 1970.
13. Allen, G. D., Gehrig, J. D., and Tolas, A. G.: An evaluation of demand-flow anesthetic machines in dental practice. J.A.D.A., 78:91, 1969.
14. Berkowitz, B. A., Ngai, S. H., and Finch, A. D.: Nitrous oxide "analgesia": Resemblance to opiate action. Science, 194:967–968, 1976.
15. Cohen, E.: Symposium: Analgesia in dental practice — some aspects of operative dentistry under analgesia. New York Dent. J., 32:209, 1966.
16. Cohen, E. N., Belville, J. W., and Brown, B. W.: Anesthesia, pregnancy and miscarriage: A study of operating room nurses and anesthetists. Anesthesiology, 35:343–347, 1971.
17. Cohen, E. N., Brown, B. W., Bruce, D. L., et al.: A survey of anesthetic health hazards among dentists: J.A.D.A., 90:1291, June 1975.
18. Contaminated cylinders of nitrous oxide. Brit. Med. J., September 1966, p. 658.
19. Corbett, T. H., Ball, G. L.: Respiratory excretion of halothane after clinical and occupational exposure. Anesthesiology, 39:342–345, Sept. 1973.
20. Eger, E. L., II, Saidman, L. J., and Brandstater, B.: Minimal alveolar anesthetic concentration: A standard of anesthetic potency. Anesthesiology, 26:756, 1965.
21. Eisele, J. H., Reitan, J. A., Massumi, R. A., et al.: Myocardial performance and N_2O analgesia in coronary artery disease. Anesthesiology, 44(1):16–20, 1976.
22. Fink, B. R., Kenny, G. E.: Metabolic effects of volatile anesthetics in cell culture. Anesthesiology, 29:505–516, May-June 1968.
23. Glaser, P.: Use of nitrous oxide analgesia for the modern practitioner. J. La. Dent. Assoc., 25:6, 1967.
24. Hamilton, W. K., and Eastwood, D. W.: A study of denitrogenation with some inhalation anesthetic systems. Anesthesiology, 16:861, 1955.
25. Jaffe, M.: Nitrous oxide — hemopoietic toxin? Anes. Prog., 17:8, 1969.
26. Kappel, P. F.: Nitrous oxide-oxygen analgesia in general dental practice. Northwestern Dent. J., 46:269, 1967.
27. Kelner, G. M.: Symposium: Analgesia in dental practice — analgesia in pedodontic practice. New York Dent. J., 32:209, 1966.
28. Kurland, P. A.: A new technique for dental analgesia. Brit. Dent. J., 125:302, 1968.
29. Lassen, H. C. A., Henriksen, E., Neukirch, F., and Kristensen, H. S.: Treatment of tetanus: Severe bone marrow depression after prolonged nitrous oxide anesthesia. Lancet, XVI of vol. 1:527–530, 1956.
30. Marx, G. F., Joshi, C. W., and Orkin, L. R.: Placental transmission of nitrous oxide. Anesthesiology, 32:429, 1970.
31. McCarthy, F. M., and Shuken, R. A.: Appraisal of the demand flow anesthetic machine and review of the literature. J. Oral Surg., 27:624, 1969.
32. Nunn, J. F., and Freeman, J.: Problems of oxygenation and oxygen transport during hemorrhage. Anaesthesia, 19:206, 1964.
33. Price, H. L.: Myocardial depression by nitrous oxide and its reversal by Ca^{++}. Anesthesiology, 44:211–215, 1976.
34. Rothchild, H.: The physiological basis of analgesia. New York Dent. J., 32:163, 1966.
35. Ruben, H.: Nitrous oxide analgesia for dental patients. Acta Anaesth. Scand. (Suppl. 25) 419, 1966.
36. Scaramella, J., Allen, G. D., Adams, O., and Randall, F.: Nitrous oxide pollution levels in oral surgery offices. J. Oral Surg. (in press).
37. Senday, V. I.: The role of analgesia on oral reconstruction. New York Dent. J., 36:164, 1966.
38. Smith, H. T., Eger, E. D., Stoelting, R. K., Whayne, T. F., Cullen, D., and Kadis, L. B.: The cardiovascular and sympathomimetic responses to the addition of nitrous oxide to halothane in man. Anesthesiology, 32:410, 1970.
38a. Smith, R. A., Wilson, M., and Miller, K. W.: Naloxone has no effect on nitrous oxide anesthesia. Anesthesiology, 49:6–8, 1979.
39. Tekavec, M. M., Baum, J. J., and Chrisman, D.: Blood-oxygen levels during use of nitrous oxide-oxygen analgesia. Anes. Prog., 16:8, 1969.
40. Trieger, N.: Ambulatory anesthesia in management of patient with cardiopulmonary disease. Anes. Prog., 14:169, 1967.
41. Vaisman, A. I.: Working conditions in surgery and their effects on the health of anesthesiologists. EKSP, KHIR 12:44 May-June 1967.
42. Whitcher, C. E., Zimmerman, D. C., Tonn, E. M., and Piziali, R. L.: Control of occupational exposure to nitrous oxide in the dental operatory. J. Am. Dent. Assoc., 95:763–776, 1977.

10

PSYCHOSEDATION

Part 5:   Pharmacosedation — Intravenous Route

PETER A. FOREMAN

INTRODUCTION

Although great technical advances have been achieved in dentistry during recent years, the problems of pain and anxiety remain factors that must be overcome if these advances are to be enjoyed by all. Several authorities[1-3] consider that our public image has not changed; that a majority of patients still avoid dental treatment owing to apprehension, often preferring extraction while they are anesthetized to conservation while they are conscious; that state-operated health schemes such as that of the United Kingdom do not necessarily lead to substantial improvements in dental health; and that many dental practitioners are unaware of, or refuse to believe, the extent of the problem.

Until recent years, the problem of the fearful, apprehensive dental patient, like that of the mentally and physically handicapped, was partially solved by treatment under general anesthesia. However, this had obvious disadvantages, including the risk of anesthetic complications, particularly during long operations, as well as postanesthetic complications such as delayed recovery, nausea and vomiting, and succinylcholine pains — none of which endeared the method to the busy practitioner as a means of treating ambulatory dental patients. Moreover, the dangers of subjecting anxious high-risk patients to the emotional and physiological stresses of prolonged general anesthesia need no elaboration.

The inevitable result has been that over the years many patients have sought only emergency treatment for pain, eventually becoming edentulous through neglect of their teeth because of fear of dentistry. Obviously, what was needed was a means of bridging the gap between local analgesia and general anesthesia, so that dental treatment could be brought to nervous patients and others with the advantages but without the risks and disadvantages of general anesthesia.

In the past decade there has been growing interest in the use of intravenous psychosedation for dental procedures, particularly in restorative dentistry for highly apprehensive patients who, because of fear, might otherwise receive less than adequate care, and also for those patients whose time is valuable and who prefer treatments to be completed in the fewest possible visits. This interest has been largely stimulated by the introduction of the ultra-short-acting anesthetic methohexital sodium (Brevital sodium, Brietal sodium); the nonbarbiturate anesthetics propanidid (Epontol) and Althesin; tranquilizers, of which the most useful to date is diazepam (Valium); and the use of various drug combinations to produce sedation (Jorgensen technique) or basal narcosis on which small increments of methohexital are superimposed to deepen the level of sedation temporarily as required (Berns, Shane, Foreman).

Analgesia is usually improved by the administration of local or regional analgesic agents; inhalation supplements are sometimes used for this purpose.

It is, of course, vital to the success of any pharmacological technique that the doctor has taken the time to establish a good interpersonal relationship with his patient (see Chapter 7, Iatrosedation). Close doctor-patient rapport will improve patient cooperation, trust, and relaxation, as well as increasing suggestibility and placebo response. These factors *must* be considered if we are to achieve maximum therapeutic effects from drugs administered for sedation.

Several intravenous techniques in current use[4] will be briefly described in this chapter. Training in these techniques and their allied pharmacology, and experience under supervision, of course, are essential before such procedures are undertaken. Although patients readily accept intravenous methods, their use can only be justified if the safety factor equals or surpasses that of other techniques in general use. Also the standard of treatment attainable must at least equal that attainable through other methods. If these criteria cannot be met, there is no place for these techniques in dentistry. Experience to date, however, has shown that safety and a high standard of treatment can be achieved by skilled, conscientious dental practitioners who are trained in the proper use of the intravenous route. Since the publication of the American Dental Association Council on Dental Education's "Guidelines for the Teaching of Comprehensive Pain and Anxiety Control in Dentistry" in 1971,[52] a significant milestone, it is encouraging to see increasing numbers of dental schools introducing comprehensive patient management programs at both undergraduate[56] and continuing education levels.[41]

The intravenous route has several important advantages over other methods of drug administration:

1. It is accurate. Because the effect is seen quickly, dosage need never be arbitrary, and the administration of the drug can be carefully adjusted to suit the patient's requirements ("titration"). Thus the risk of overdosage is minimized, but at the same time the disadvantages of underdosage are avoided. Requirements vary widely between patients. For example, in the intravenous premedication technique (Jorgensen) the dose range of sodium pentobarbital may show individual variation between 30 and 300 mg. When such wide variation occurs, any attempt to individualize oral dosage would be useless.

2. The full effect of an intravenously administered drug is seen almost immediately — within a few minutes at the most.

3. The patient will not experience pain, providing that a meticulous technique of venipuncture is used. A sharp, sterile, fine-gauge disposable needle should be used, and a surface obtundent such as ethyl chloride may be applied to the site of injection.

4. The rate of recovery from an intravenously administered drug is much faster, after a peak effect that occurs within minutes of injection. The duration of after-effects is thus considerably reduced.

Disadvantages of the intravenous route include the possibility of such local complications as intra-arterial injection, extravascular injection, thrombophlebitis, and venous thrombosis. Systemic complications such as respiratory and circulatory depression may be caused by overdosage, or there may be allergic reactions, muscle tremors, and other effects caused by pharmacologic action of the drug. However, overdosage should never occur, as the proper use of the intravenous route allows much greater precision in assessing correct dosage. Systemic effects of the drug, of course, are not confined to its intravenous administration.

THE IDEAL PSYCHOSEDATIVE AGENT

1. Safety
   Low toxicity
   Wide therapeutic safety margin (ED_{100} vs LD_{50})
   Reliable, predictable actions
   Rapid, complete recovery following treatment
2. Selectivity
   Anxiolytic
   Retention of patient cooperation (verbal contact maintained)
   Amnesia for unpleasant procedures
   Muscle relaxant (especially muscles of mastication — long procedures)
   Analgesia (less important when supplemented with local analgesia)
3. Freedom from side effects
   Local, such as thrombophlebitis
   Systemic, such as respiratory and/or circulatory depression
4. Freedom from drug interactions
   For example, meperidine + MAO inhibitor (hypotension); diazepam + barbiturate (respiratory depression)

5. Simplicity of administration
6. High degree of patient acceptance
7. Higher quality of treatment possible than with other means

INTRAVENOUS TECHNIQUES IN CURRENT USE

During recent years, several techniques have found increasingly wide-spread use in dental practice. These include:

1. Intravenous diazepam sedation.[8-12]
2. Intravenous premedication (the Jorgensen technique).[13]
3. Intermittent methohexital sodium anesthesia.[14, 15]
4. Intermittent methohexital sodium sedation.[16-18]
5. Intermittent propanidid anesthesia and sedation.[19, 20]
6. Intermittent Althesin anesthesia and sedation.[21]

In addition, several modifications of these basic methods have been developed. These modifications consist of basal sedation upon which nitrous oxide sedation or small increments of methohexital are superimposed as required to cover unpleasant or painful procedures, or to extend the period of sedation. Meperidine hydrochloride or pentazocine lactate have also been used for this purpose.

7. Diazepam plus nitrous oxide sedation.
8. Diazepam plus meperidine hydrochloride or pentazocine lactate.[55]
9. Sodium secobarbital/meperidine hydrochloride plus methohexital supplementation.[7]
10. Hydroxyzine hydrochloride/alphaprodine hydrochloride plus methohexital supplementation.[64, 65]
11. Diazepam plus methohexital supplementation.[29]

Other techniques which have been investigated include neuroleptanal-gesia[63] and the use of dissociative drugs such as ketamine hydrochloride (Ketalar).[18] Unfortunately, a high incidence of undesirable side effects makes several of these drugs unsuitable for general use in the dental office.

There are problems of nomenclature, particularly in presentation to the patient, to whom an intravenous injection usually means "Pentothal" and general anesthesia. In fact the main objective with many of these methods is the avoidance of general anesthesia in its traditionally recognized sense, with total loss of consciousness and normal protective mechanisms. It is my practice to tell the patient that he will receive intravenous sedation, *not* general anesthesia; that he will feel very sleepy and totally relaxed throughout the procedure; that he will feel absolutely no pain nor will he be aware of the passage of time, owing to the actions of the drug; and that he will awaken feeling relaxed and refreshed.

I. BASIC TECHNIQUES

Intravenous Diazepam Sedation

One of the most promising drugs to appear in recent years for the treatment of dental patients is the short-acting tranquilizer diazepam (Valium).[16, 23, 30, 36, 59] In fact, diazepam comes closer to meeting the criteria for the ideal psychosedative agent than any other presently available. Given intravenously, it produces well-controlled sedation and relaxation for dental procedures of up to an hour's duration. Diazepam has a wide therapeutic safety margin *and has now become the drug of choice for the trained general dental practitioner, as well as for the introduction of dental students to intravenous sedation.* A useful degree of amnesia is produced by the drug, and its use is routinely combined with local analgesia.

Diazepam is a benzodiazepine tranquilizer, chemically and pharmacologically related to chlordiazepoxide (Librium), nitrazepam (Mogadon), flurazepam (Dalmane) and oxazepam (Serepax, Serax). It possesses powerful anxiolytic, sedative, amnesic, and muscular relaxant properties, exerting a major action on the limbic system, the area of the cortex concerned with emotional response to external stimuli.

Diazepam is used in premedication,[12, 26] in the management of mentally handicapped patients,[43] to alleviate muscle spasm in cerebral palsy[20, 49] and tetanus,[26] in psychiatry,[6] in cardioversion[50] as an anesthetic induction agent,[14] and as an anticonvulsant.[3] When it is given alone, even large doses have little effect on respiratory or cardiovascular function in normal healthy subjects beyond that which results from reduced demand in the tranquilized state. However, marked potentiation of central depressants such as barbiturates has been observed with diazepam[29, 36] This effect must be remembered if such combinations are used, as severe respiratory depression may result. Also, elderly patients may show a marked response to extremely small dosages to diazepam; e.g., 1–2 mg. This possibility must always be kept in mind, as profound respiratory depression and even apnea can occur with this group.

There is a latency of approximately 1 to 2 minutes in the onset of effects and a wide individual variation in response to diazepam when it is administered intravenously. Its duration of clinical action also varies, but in most cases 30 minutes or more of light sedation occur, a sufficient period for most short dental procedures; many patients will tolerate therapy that extends beyond this time.

An important point to remember when using diazepam intravenously is the possibility of recurrence of clinical symptoms 4 to 6 hours after administration.[4] This "rebound effect," which coincides with increased plasma levels of diazepam and its metabolite desmethyldiazepam, appears mainly to be due to the remobilization of unmetabolized diazepam from a storage site within the body, possibly the gall bladder or gut wall, and often follows the ingestion of food. Patients treated with intravenous diazepam sedation should therefore be warned of this possibility, along with the person accompanying them from the dental office. Although plasma rebound may be a disadvantage after morning appointments, where the patient becomes sleepy after lunch, it can, in fact, be an advantage following afternoon appointments. For example, a patient undergoing oral surgery at 2 PM is less likely to require post-surgical sedation that night, as a useful degree of sedation is likely to recur by about 7 or 8 PM following an evening meal.

For dental procedures in most healthy adults, the intravenous administration of 5 to 20 mg of diazepam at a maximum rate of 2.5 mg (0.5 ml of undiluted solution) per 30 seconds usually results in a relaxed, nonapprehensive patient, who is moderately sedated. Atropine sulfate (0.5 mg) is sometimes administered prior to the diazepam if an antisialogogue is required. Diazepam should not be diluted, or mixed with other drugs.

The supine position is advised, the manufacturers of diazepam recommending that the patient be kept supine for at least an hour after administration. When the desired degree of relaxation and sedation has been achieved, local analgesic injections are placed and the dental procedure commenced.

In my own experience, diazepam has proved a very useful drug, not only in the management of nervous patients but also for the control of severe gag reflexes.[16] It may also be commended as oral premedication before dental treatment, particularly in children,[28] as well as a safe nocturnal sedative, although nitrazepam or flurazepam may be more useful for the latter purpose, due to their more prolonged hypnotic action. See the chapter on *psychosedation, oral route*. I have also found oral diazepam useful in the management of severe intermittent and stress-related episodes of bruxism.

Jorgensen Technique

From 1946 until his death in 1974, that great pioneer of dental pain/anxiety control Niels B. Jorgensen of Loma Linda University used a combination of sodium pentobarbital (Nembutal sodium), meperidine* (Demerol), and scopolamine to produce a state of sedation, relaxation, and a degree of postoperative amnesia in apprehensive dental patients.[48] Sodium pentobarbital is injected slowly (10 mg per 30 seconds) until initial cortical symptoms are observed. These symptoms may take the form of slight dizziness, tiredness, and release of apprehension. An additional 10 to 15 per cent of the dose administered to this baseline level is then injected. The syringe is then exchanged for one containing a usually standardized mixture of 25 mg of meperidine hydrochloride and 0.4 mg of scopolamine hydrobromide. Because of the incompatibility of meperidine with barbiturates, blood is aspirated into the pentobarbital syringe before the meperidine/scopolamine mixture is injected, or, if an IV drip or infusion technique is being used, the IV line is flushed before administration of meperidine/scopolamine. Dosage of meperidine/scopolamine is reduced proportionately when less than 100 mg of pentobarbital produces initial cortical symptoms.

The combination of pentobarbital (for sedation), meperidine (for sedation, euphoria, and some analgesia), and scopolamine (for antisialosis and anterograde amnesia) usually results in a cooperative, relaxed, and sedated patient who will calmly accept up to three hours of concentrated restorative or surgical treatment under local analgesia without apparent discomfort, remaining conscious throughout and able to assist the operator when necessary. Monitoring studies[28] have demonstrated the safety of intravenous premedication, and that minimal impairment of cardiovascular and respiratory status occurs when the technique is used for light sedation.

With few exceptions, use of this technique results in greatly improved operating conditions (particularly when the patient is extremely nervous)

---

*Generic name pethidine hydrochloride outside U.S.

without the problems and responsibilities of general anesthesia. It is helpful for prolonged operations such as multiple quadrant restorative dentistry, crown and bridge therapy, periodontal surgery, and oral surgery for which the patient usually receives local analgesics.

Intravenous premedication, together with other methods outlined in this chapter, is complementary to four-handed dentistry and the use of the supine position. It is welcomed not only by the apprehensive, but also by patients who need extensive restorative treatment but who have limited time at their disposal, and who therefore prefer to complete their treatment in the fewest possible visits. The technique (together with intravenous diazepam) has been found a valuable introduction to intravenous procedures for both undergraduates and qualified practitioners, and has also proved useful in the treatment of some patients who have cerebral palsy.

Disadvantages include a relatively long recovery period, as well as a relatively long induction time (10 minutes or more), that reduce its usefulness for treatments requiring less than two hours.

Intermittent Methohexital Anesthesia

Methohexital sodium (Brevital sodium, Brietal sodium) is administered in controlled intermittent dosage via suitable apparatus[24, 68] to produce and maintain a state of very light anesthesia throughout the operative procedure; normal protective reflexes may be depressed with overdosage. When utilized primarily for oral surgery, rather than restorative dentistry, protective reflexes are more likely to be depressed by the larger dosage increments necessary. The technique consists of an initial induction dose — 40 to 60 mg for an adult woman, 60 to 100 mg for an adult man; maintenance doses of approximately half the induction dose are administered when the patient's response to stimuli indicates the need. Total time of anesthesia should, as a general rule, be restricted to 20 minutes, and total dosage to 200 mg. Cumulative effects have been observed with the use of higher dosages.

Atropine sulfate (0.6 mg) is often administered intravenously before induction if the dental procedure is going to take more than five minutes. This drug reduces salivary and mucous secretions (Fig. 10–1).

Intermittent Methohexital Sedation

Successive 10 to 20 mg increments of methohexital sodium are administered until the patient is deeply sedated but still able to hear and respond to the operator's instructions.[31, 32, 36] At this level the patient is totally amnesic, and the operative procedure may be commenced cautiously. Should response to painful stimulus occur, no further methohexital should be given. Instead, the injection of a short-acting local analgesic and the use of verbal suggestion and reassurance will usually provide good operating conditions. Sedation and amnesia are maintained by small increments of methohexital as required throughout the treatment. Protective reflexes remain intact.

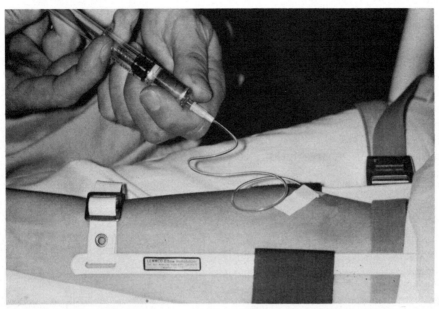

Figure 10–1 Administration of atropine sulfate via an IV infusion set, following which the remaining atropine is flushed from the infusion set with 5 per cent dextrose or normal saline, etc., before the administration of other drugs.

Discussion. Methohexital sodium has been found to have several important advantages over earlier ultra-short-acting intravenous barbiturates such as sodium thiopental, particularly in the treatment of dental patients who are ambulant. These advantages include shorter duration of action and faster clinical recovery, reduced cumulation, relative absence of local complications, amnesia, and stability in solution.[17, 38]

The very fast clinical recovery seen after low doses of methohexital sodium is due to rapid redistribution and metabolism[13, 67] of the drug.

Intermittent methohexital sodium anesthesia and sedation are more suited to short procedures of 20 minutes or less and should be used only in restorative and minor oral surgical procedures of short duration. If this limitation is observed, and if the patency of the airway is ensured at all times by effective mouth packing, intermittent methohexital anesthesia and sedation are safe and useful techniques. However, they should not be overextended. In my opinion, when airway control is a problem, the patient is better protected by endotracheal intubation for more prolonged and extensive surgical procedures such as complex multiple extractions, difficult removal of impacted teeth, and other major oral surgery. I believe that for most short routine dental procedures, methohexital need only be used to produce a state of relaxation, sedation, and amnesia, supplemented with local analgesia as necessary. In this way, the continued presence of the patient's protective mechanisms is guaranteed, and because of lower dosages, a more rapid and complete recovery occurs. Criticism of the "operator-anesthetist" is also invalid under these circumstances.[10, 11, 47]

Although the term "intravenous sedation" has been used to distinguish the state produced by low dosages of methohexital from the state of general anesthesia in which protective mechanisms do not function, methohexital sodium is in fact a potent anesthetic drug, and it could be used improperly.[33, 69] In the past, particularly with drugs such as sodium thiopental, complications caused by overdosage have arisen. Rather illogically, the drug, rather than its administrator, has been condemned. Methohexital sodium and other intravenous drugs should *never* be administered by anyone who has not had proper training and experience under supervision in the use of these drugs.[46, 53, 54]

Correctly used, both intermittent methohexital sodium anesthesia and sedation are safe and will seldom cause complications. A survey[58] of 445,386 administrations has revealed a 0.1 per cent incidence of nausea or vomiting, a 0.1 per cent incidence of laryngeal stridor or spasm, and a 0.2 per cent incidence of recovery prolonged beyond one hour.

Significant respiratory depression does not occur with the dosages recommended, although temporary respiratory disturbances may sometimes be observed during induction. Hiccups may also occur on occasion. In my own experience as well as that of others,[5, 42] such disturbances appear related to the speed with which the induction dose is injected, as well as to the concentration of the drug. For this reason, I prefer always to use a 1 per cent solution of methohexital. Muscular twitching, often combined with exaggerated response to even slight stimulus, may also be seen in some patients, particularly in children and adolescents. This is possibly due to idiosyncrasy to the methyl groups in the methohexital molecule. Such a reaction should not be confused with shivering, which may occur during cold weather if room temperature is low and the methodexital sodium solution is below body temperature. The problem of the highly resistant, restless type of patient who is not easily controlled by methohexital sodium alone may often be overcome by the prior intravenous administration of diazepam, which has valuable muscular relaxant, anxiolytic, and amnesic properties.[29, 36]

The most potentially serious complication of these and other intravenous techniques is probably that of vasodepressor syncope. An inexperienced administrator could conceivably confuse fainting in the upright position with the onset of sedation or anesthesia. The consequences could be disastrous.[8, 9] For this reason, it is desirable that all dental intravenous procedures be carried out with the patient supine.* This position is also complementary with the now standard operating technique of seated, four-handed dentistry (Fig. 10–2).

Intermittent Propanidid Anesthesia and Sedation

These techniques[15, 19] are similar to those of intermittent methohexital anesthesia and sedation, with the important advantage that the initial rapid recovery is due to detoxification of the drug rather than redistribution. Recovery from propanidid is therefore more complete at an earlier stage.

Exceptions: hiatus hernia, advanced pregnancy, gross obesity, acute bronchial asthma, and cardiac insufficiency with orthopnea. In these conditions, the patient should be treated in a semireclining position. Also, for all practical purposes the reclining position, utilizing a contour dental chair, is virtually equivalent to the supine position.[37]

Propanidid (Epontol) is also administered in intermittent dosage in the same way as methohexital sodium, except that a larger gauge needle must be used for injection because of the high viscosity of propanidid. Dilution is possible, but the weaker solution must be rapidly and continually administered to maintain anesthesia. The initial induction dose required to produce anesthesia usually ranges from 200 to 300 mg for an adult woman, and 300 to 500 mg for an adult man. As with methohexital sodium anesthesia, 25 to 50 per cent of the induction dose is injected when reaction to stimulus becomes apparent. For sedation, a similar administration technique to that used for intermittent methohexital sedation is employed, using smaller dosages.[19]

Intermittent propanidid anesthesia and sedation, like intermittent methohexital sodium anesthesia and sedation, are useful for short procedures when the duration is not expected to exceed 20 minutes. Propanidid may be regarded as the drug of choice for patients who are allergic to barbiturates and those who have a history of porphyria or severe liver dysfunction.

Unfortunately, in spite of the more rapid and complete recovery seen with propanidid, there appears to be less jaw relaxation and much less amnesia than with methohexital sodium; there is also an increased tendency to local vascular complications, hypotension and allergic reactions. However, it is a useful drug for short procedures, particularly when extremely rapid recovery is required. Propanidid is not presently available in the United States.

Intermittent Althesin Anesthesia and Sedation

These techniques[21] are again similar to intermittent methohexital anesthesia and sedation.

Althesin is a combination of two steriods, alphadolone and alphaxalone, and is therefore administered on a volume basis, instead of the usual weight of drug in milligrams basis employed for other techniques. The onset of anesthesia or sedation is much slower than with methohexital, and the initial dose and subsequent increments have a more prolonged effect, thus accurate judgment of when and how much to administer is more difficult. Overdosage effects, such as apnea, must therefore be expected on occasion. However, there is less accumulation than with methohexital when used intermittently for long appointments, and, like propanidid, recovery is more complete at an earlier stage. Unlike propanidid, postoperative thrombophlebitis is seldom a problem, and jaw relaxation is better, but hypotension, muscle twitching and allergic reactions have been reported. There is also less amnesia than with methohexital.

For anesthesia in adult patients, an induction dose of 0.05 ml per kg usually suffices (2.5 to 5.0 ml for adults weighing between 50 and 100 kg), with maintenance increments of approximately half the induction dosage as required. For sedation, up to 2.5 ml is injected very slowly, while closely observing the effect on sleepiness, slowing of speech, and response to commands — the aim being (as with other sedation techniques) to cause drowsiness while maintaining a cooperative and relaxed patient. Further increments of up to 0.5 ml are administered as required to maintain sedation.

Althesin and propanidid anesthesia and sedation have been included in this chapter for the sake of completeness, but this author strongly believes that their disadvantages generally outweigh their advantages, and that methohexital still remains the drug of choice in most situations.

II. MODIFICATIONS OF BASIC TECHNIQUES

Diazepam plus Nitrous Oxide Sedation

Although nitrous oxide sedation and intravenous diazepam sedation have become standard basic techniques for the general practitioner and in the teaching of undergraduate dental students, along with the Loma Linda (Jorgensen) technique for the more experienced, there are occasions when it is useful to extend or supplement the basic single drug techniques. For example, the clinical duration of action of diazepam when injected intravenously is usually 30 to 60 minutes, which may be insufficient time to complete some dental procedures.

Some operators advocate the administration of further, reduced increments of diazepam in order to prolong sedation after the effects of the initial induction dose have worn off. I do not favor this approach because of probable increases in recovery times due to diazepam's rebound effect.[8] In fact, where several increments have been used, it is not uncommon to see cases where the patient is unable to return to his normal duties for 1 to 2 days following treatment, a situation I regard as quite unacceptable.

While other modifications outlined in this section are useful in the hands of the doctor who is trained in anesthesiology, I believe the simplest and safest approach for the general practitioner who is experienced with both nitrous oxide sedation and intravenous diazepam sedation lies in a combination of these two techniques.

Nitrous oxide sedation alone is usually satisfactory for most patients who are moderately apprehensive. Unfortunately, where a high level of anxiety is present, it is often ineffective by itself. In such patients, a reduced induction dose of diazepam followed by nitrous oxide will often overcome this problem, as well as prolong the relatively short period of sedation provided by diazepam alone. Alternatively, where diazepam has been used but its clinical action has terminated, nitrous oxide may be introduced in order to prolong sedation without recourse to further increments of diazepam or other drugs which may compromise safety or prolong recovery.

It should be noted that diazepam will often markedly enhance the effects of nitrous oxide, and for this reason its administration should always precede that of the latter. In my experience, approximately one half to two thirds of the patient's normal requirements of nitrous oxide provides an acceptable depth of sedation when preceded by a minimal amount of diazepam; e.g., 5 to 10 mg for a healthy young adult. Higher dosages of diazepam followed by "normal" concentrations of nitrous oxide may lead to much deeper levels of sedation, or even to the production of general anesthesia. The use of both inhalation and intravenous techniques requires the doctor to be highly trained and experienced in all anesthesia/sedation areas and in basic life support. However, as long as the possibility of potentiation is borne in mind and nitrous oxide supplementation is approached with caution, this is an extremely useful technique.

Diazepam plus Meperidine or Pentazocine

With resistant patients, or in procedures requiring intraoperative or postoperative analgesia (e.g., oral surgery), analgesics such as meperidine (pethidine) hydrochloride (Demerol) or pentazocine hydrochloride (Talwin, Fortral) are sometimes used to supplement diazepam as well as to reinforce and prolong its sedative action. Fentanyl citrate (Sublimaze) has also been used for this purpose.

As with nitrous oxide, barbiturates, and other CNS-acting drugs, the depressant effects of the analgesics may be greatly enhanced by diazepam, and respiratory depression is an ever-present possibility which must be closely watched for. Even minimal supplements of meperidine, pentazocine, or fentanyl may result in profound respiratory depression in some patients, necessitating resuscitative procedures and the use of a narcotic antagonist such as naloxone hydrochloride (Narcan). It would thus appear advisable to restrict the use of such combinations to specific cases such as highly resistant patients or major surgical procedures where a simpler approach is ineffective.

I strongly believe that diazepam should always be the *first* drug administered, never subsequent to barbiturates, analgesics, or other CNS depressants, because of its profound potentiating effects. Injection following other drugs may result in severe respiratory and circulatory depression in some patients.

The technique I prefer is to administer diazepam as outlined earlier, followed by *slow* injection of up to 25 mg meperidine, up to 30 mg pentazocine, or up to 100 *micro*grams of fentanyl; with close attention to respiratory rate and depth throughout and following administration. Naloxone should be immediately at hand if required, along with resuscitative facilities.

Although useful in certain situations, techniques employing analgesic supplementation of diazepam are not without hazard and should only be used by the doctor who is trained in general anesthesia. Whatever the technique, the motto "the simpler it is, the safer it is" should be applied. It makes good sense to start with the simplest approach possible, e.g., intravenous diazepam alone, before the addition of other drugs which in many patients may be totally unnecessary and in fact may lead to undesirable or even serious complications.

Secobarbital/Meperidine/Methohexital

Joel Berns[7] has developed a technique in which basal narcosis is obtained with the slow intravenous administration of up to 50 mg of sodium secobarbital (Seconal sodium), followed by 25 to 50 mg of meperidine hydrochloride. Increments of methohexital sodium (20 mg) are then superimposed to deepen sedation temporarily to anesthesia for painful procedures such as extractions, local injections, and so forth. Advantages claimed include the ability to tailor sedation to the length of the procedure, so that the recovery period is shorter than that required by techniques such as intravenous premedication. Protective reflexes are depressed at anesthesia levels.

Hydroxyzine/Alphaprodine/Methohexital

In a similar method developed by Sylvan Shane,[64, 65] a tranquilizer, hydroxyzine hydrochloride* (Vistaril, Atarax), is used in combination with the analgesic alphaprodine hydrochloride (Nisentil) and atropine sulfate. Methohexital sodium is then used to deepen sedation temporarily as required. As with Berns' technique, local analgesia is an integral part of this procedure.

Diazepam/Methohexital

Experience with the foregoing techniques led to the conclusion[36] that there could be advantages in combining intravenous diazepam with intermittent methohexital sodium sedation. After the initial induction with 5 to 20 mg of diazepam, 5 to 10 mg increments of methodexital sodium are superimposed to cover unpleasant procedures; the periods of deepened sedation last up to five minutes. Local analgesia is again used routinely.

I have found this drug combination extremely useful,[29] particularly for procedures requiring 30 to 90 minutes' operating time. The opportunity to reduce the barbiturate dosage significantly is attractive; it is not unusual to find that 10 to 20 mg of diazepam and 50 to 100 mg of 1 per cent methohexital sodium (in 5 to 10 mg increments) are sufficient for procedures lasting more than an hour. Amnesia is greatly enhanced by the addition of methohexital, an important factor in the treatment of some patients who want to be "asleep" during the operative stage.[39] In fact, the anterograde amnesia which accompanies this drug combination is almost unbelievable, the patient remaining conscious and able to converse with the operator throughout treatment, yet remembering nothing of this later.

Care must be taken to use *small* increments of methohexital with this technique. Larger doses will lead to sedation levels approaching general anesthesia, resulting in loss of contact and patient cooperation during treatment and more prolonged recovery, as well as periodic depression of protective reflexes.

The diazepam/methohexital combination is often useful in the management of those patients who have previously been restless with methohexital alone. In many of these there is an improvement, probably because of

---

*Following reports of complications from inadvertent intra-arterial injection of hydroxyzine, the manufacturers (Pfizer) have recently withdrawn their recommendation for administration of hydroxyzine intravenously, and are now recommending that hydroxyzine be administered via the intramuscular route only. This technique is reported here for its historical interest.

the pharmacological properties of diazepam. Diazepam has also been used in combination with propanidid instead of methohexital, but although post-operative recovery is faster using propanidid, amnesia is less reliable, and deeper levels of sedation are required. Many variations of these intravenous sedation techniques have been promoted by various authors using different drugs to produce desired results, e.g., promethazine, scopolamine, fentanyl, etc. However, modifications combining the use of diazepam and nitrous oxide sedation, or diazepam and methohexital, have proved most satisfactory in my experience, as well as the safest and most reliable.

It should also be remembered that there is no panacea, and there will always be the exceptional patient who requires a different form of management such as full endotracheal anesthesia, which can also have its problems in the difficult, resistant patient.

Neuroleptanalgesia and Dissociative Anesthesia

In neuroleptanalgesia[63] extremely powerful narcotic analgesics, phenoperidine (Operidine) or fentanyl citrate (Sublimaze Citrate) are used in combination with droperidol (Droleptan), a major tranquilizer with anti-emetic properties, to produce a state of general analgesia without loss of consciousness. However, the analgesic drugs may produce severe respiratory depression and droperidol may lead to postoperative agitation or depression in psychologically disturbed patients. A useful substitute for droperidol has been found in hydroxyzine hydrochloride (Vistaril), which is also antiemetic but seldom causes psychological side effects. I have found that less than half the analgesic dosage recommended for hospital treatments is required for dental restorative procedures. Adverse respiratory effects are avoided by the lower dosage, but the technique cannot be recommended for general use in the dental office because of its potential dangers.

An interesting future possibility may be the use of short-acting dissociative drugs such as ketamine hydrochloride (Ketalar) which produce intense analgesia without adverse circulatory or respiratory side effects in most patients, although hypertension has been recorded in some[18] Its use appears contraindicated in psychologically disturbed patients who may experience unpleasant hallucinations during the recovery phase, and in hypertensives. Most workers with experience of ketamine agree that its main application is in the management of difficult children, and as an alternative to more sophisticated anesthetic and psychosedative techniques in remote communities where anesthesiology training and facilities are minimal.

Some of these latter methods may have side effects that make them generally unsuited to routine use in the dental office; they have been mentioned only for the reader's interest. It is my belief, however, that safe, short-acting drugs which will eliminate anxiety and provide sedation, amnesia, and possibly analgesia will be introduced during the next decade. The dental profession and dental practice could be profoundly affected. At present, diazepam sedation, intravenous premedication as described and taught by Jorgensen, and intermittent methohexital sodium sedation and anesthesia, together with the techniques that employ the supplementary use of nitrous oxide sedation or minimal increments of methohexital sodium, remain the only methods clinically proven by many administrations.

Although evidence has been produced[27] to show that the prolonged administration of certain psychosedative drug combinations to patients *seated upright in the dental chair* can result in decreased cardiac output, rate, and minute work, it must be noted that Bourne[8, 9] has repeatedly stressed that (with few exceptions) all patients treated with intravenous psychosedation or anesthesia should be kept supine throughout. It should also be noted that even more pronounced circulatory and other changes have been recorded during natural sleep,[60] which if recorded during sedation or anesthesia would undoubtedly cause great consternation. Obviously, in our present state of knowledge, not enough is known about normal physiological patterns for us to assume automatically that experimentally recorded variations during sedation or anesthesia necessarily indicate potential clinical hazard or even abnormal physiological behavior in any particular individual. Although the need for continued experimental and clinical research in anesthesiology cannot be overestimated, caution is indicated before making dogmatic assertions concerning any particular drug or technique, owing to the many factors involved.

In my experience, the techniques described in this chapter have proved clinically safe and acceptable, providing that there are no contraindications to their use, the patient is kept supine, the number of drugs used, the drug dosages, and the duration of administration are kept to a minimum, and the operating team is properly trained and experienced in the use of these techniques and in the management of the patient before, during, and after treatment.

PREVENTION OF COMPLICATIONS AND EMERGENCIES

No chapter on patient management and psychosedation can be considered complete without including a section on the prevention of dental office complications and emergencies. Although many, including this author, firmly believe that serious medical emergencies are, in fact, *less* likely to occur when anxious patients are properly sedated, it must also be recognized that the use of drugs may increase the risk in some situations. Fortunately, the great majority of emergencies can be prevented, provided certain basic rules are employed. It is the purpose of this section to emphasize the means of *prevention* of complications and emergencies when using intravenous sedation. For management of serious medical emergencies, see Part II of this book.

Patient Selection and Evaluation

In view of possible drug reactions and interactions, a comprehensive medical history is mandatory for all patients receiving dental treatment, whether by the methods described, full general anesthesia, local analgesia, or no medication at all. I personally prefer the use of a questionnaire which is completed and signed by the patient at the initial consultation. Reports of deliberately misleading medical histories (some of which have led to fatalities) and the withholding of important medical information by patients indicate the importance and possible medicolegal implications of a medical history which has been signed by the patient. Patients who are using drugs illegally are often reluctant to sign the medical history, and the doctor should always be alert to this possibility. Needless to say, any patient who refuses to sign should be refused treatment. A useful, brief but pertinent medical history is that published in the 1977–78 edition of Accepted Dental Therapeutics (see Fig. 2–1), and is available through the order department of the American Dental Association. Alternatively, a questionnaire designed to meet individual office requirements may be preferred.

The history must also be thoroughly discussed with the patient, with particular reference to past and recent serious illness, present treatment by medical practitioners, and previous as well as current drug therapy. If doubt exists, consultation with the patient's physician is essential. Whenever possible, high-risk patients should be hospitalized and not accepted for treatment in the dental office. All medical histories must be regularly revised at future appointments. See the chapter on *physical evaluation*.

Special attention must be paid to patients who may be, or may have been, receiving corticosteroid therapy, sleeping drugs, tranquilizers, and antidepressants, particularly monoamine oxidase inhibitors, for whom the use of meperidine hydrochloride is absolutely contraindicated. Meperidine dosage must be reduced in myxedema (hypothyroidism) and cardiovascular disease, in which its use may lead to hypotension. It should also be reduced for patients who are pregnant or who are taking oral contraceptives,

Figure 10–2 Treatment of patient under intravenous sedation. Note: patient supine; assistant supporting chin and operating high volume suction; oral prop and sponge flange pack with external ties; intermittent administration apparatus; wrist immobilized to prevent dislodgment of indwelling needle; pulse monitor lead attached to finger.

and in whom a reduced urinary excretion of meperidine and its metabolites may occur. Generally, I consider it inadvisable to carry out other than emergency treatment on a woman who is in the first trimester of pregnancy, and the use of tranquilosedative drugs should be avoided whenever possible, in accordance with current accepted medical practice. For further information on management in pregnancy, see Chapters 5 and 13.

Diazepam is rarely contraindicated, although it must be used with caution in patients taking barbiturates or narcotics, in whom synergistic effects may occur. Its use should also be avoided in patients with severe respiratory or liver disease, narrow-angle glaucoma, or psychiatric states such as depression. When administered intravenously, diazepam may produce thrombophlebitis, particularly in small veins, and patients must be warned of this possibility and to seek early treatment if necessary. The incidence of thrombophlebitis may be reduced by using large veins whenever possible, as well as a post-diazepam flush.[51]

Barbiturates should be used with caution, or avoided entirely in patients who have severe cardiovascular disease or respiratory and liver dysfunction, and are absolutely contraindicated in porphyria and dystrophia myotonica.

Belladonna derivatives such as atropine and scopolamine must be avoided in patients who have thyrotoxicosis, hypertension, or glaucoma; and scopolamine should not be administered to elderly patients or young children, because it may produce disorientation, depression, or excitation. (In general, dosages of most drugs considered in this chapter must be reduced in the elderly) See the chapter on *drugs*.

Local analgesics containing epinephrine and norepinephrine must be used with caution in patients who have thyrotoxicosis and severe cardiovascular disease, as well as in those who are taking monoamine oxidase inhibitors and tricyclic antidepressants, particularly the latter.[40] For such patients the use of an alternative such as prilocaine hydrochloride (Citanest hydrochloride) with felypressin (Octapressin) may be advisable. Many still consider that endogenous epinephrine production is more likely to produce adverse cardiac symptoms in apprehensive patients than the relatively small amounts contained in local analgesic solutions, providing that total dosage is small, and the patient is adequately sedated. Evidence,[1, 2] however, suggests that felypressin may be safer than epinephrine as a vasoconstrictor for local analgesics in patients with cardiovascular disease. The routine use of aspirating syringes and a slow rate of injection are of course essential in high risk patients. See the chapter on *complications from local analgesia*.

Pre-operative Patient Management

Having decided that pharmacosedation is indicated, it is important to present it in such a way that the patient will readily accept it. Those referred by other patients are usually less apprehensive, but some are afraid of anything outside their experience. It is essential that a strong doctor/patient relationship built on trust is established wherever possible *before* treatment is carried out. The patient's fears must be considered, and

---

INSTRUCTIONS PRECEDING INTRAVENOUS SEDATION

MEDICAL HISTORY: Any personal illness, weakness or allergy must be reported; also details of any drugs recently prescribed or being taken — especially sleeping drugs, tranquillizers or cortisone preparations.

PREPARATIONS: No food or drink must be taken within FOUR hours of the appointment time and the previous meal should be light and easily digestible.

No tight clothing should be worn, sleeves should be easily drawn up past the elbow. Dentures, spectacles or contact lenses to be removed — nurse will arrange safe keeping.

FOLLOWING SEDATION: The patient must be accompanied by a friend.

Any patient accepting a sedation appointment must specifically agree:—
   NOT to drive a vehicle or operate any machinery the same day;
   NOT to undertake any responsible business matters;
   NOT to drink any alcohol.

(Although there are normally no after-affects following this form of treatment, because of traffic regulations, etc., the above precautions must be strictly adhered to.)

Figure 10–3 Instructions printed on reverse side of appointment card.

reassurance provided at the consultation appointment. The procedure should be explained, without going into unnecessary detail, and any questions the patient may have, answered. Avoidance of complications, and the effectiveness of the sedation technique employed are directly related to the interpersonal relationship established before the treatment appointment. Where severe anxiety is present, oral sedation should be considered in order to ensure a sound rest the night before treatment. The safest and most useful drugs for this purpose at present are flurazepam (Dalmane) 15 to 30 mg, or nitrazepam (Mogadon)* 5 to 10 mg.

Pre-operative instructions must be stressed, and strictly adhered to by the patient. These can be incorporated in the appointment card (Fig. 10–3). They should include the restriction of food and drink for 4 to 6 hours pre-operatively, removal of dentures and contact lenses, attendance to toilet requirements, and arranging for a responsible escort following treatment. Patients must be warned against driving, operating machinery, undertaking important business matters, and drinking alcohol after treatment. Observance of these regulations must be checked before treatment is commenced.

Failure to follow instructions should result in cancellation of the appointment. If exceptions are made, such as in the case of diabetics and the fasting rule, it may be clearly pointed out to the patient that a specific exception is being made and why. Patients accepted for treatment who have not obeyed instructions will quickly tell others of such casual attitudes, and the risk of future complications and emergencies will increase

---

*Not available in the U.S.

accordingly. If rules are made, they must be kept, and those who break the rules must be refused treatment. It is surprising how quickly the word spreads among patients that "the doctor means what he says" (or doesn't mean what he says) and such cancellations are extremely rare in well-run practice.

Do not keep anxious patients waiting. Have everything in readiness so that when the patient arrives, he or she is taken immediately to the treatment area. If a mildly anxious patient is kept waiting, an active imagination may result in having to deal with a highly anxious patient in the operatory, thereby decreasing the effectiveness of the sedation technique, increasing drug requirements and thus the risk of complications.

Patient Care During Treatment

The supine position (or semireclining position in a contour dental chair with the head and feet at the same level) should be used routinely wherever psychosedation techniques are employed. This will greatly reduce the risk of syncope and its potentially serious sequelae. Use of this position is, of course, complementary with modern operating techniques.
There are, however, some disadvantages which must be considered:

1. The risk of foreign bodies entering the pharynx is increased; e.g., amalgam and tooth debris, calculus, reamers, burs, etc. Proper mouth packing or the use of rubber dam is essential for protection, along with effective use of suction by an alert dental assistant. Where oral sponge packs are used, they should be replaced frequently before they become saturated, and discarded when fraying occurs. Spare suction tips should be readily available in case of blockage.
2. The risk of gastric regurgitation is more likely in the supine position, although uncommon. Hiatus (esophageal) hernia predisposes toward this. It is therefore doubly important to stress preoperative fasting instructions in such patients. On the other hand, should regurgitation or vomiting occur, it is more easily managed than with a patient who is seated upright.
3. Women in advanced pregnancy are usually more comfortable in a semireclining than a supine position, where fainting may occur due to pressure from the fetus on the inferior vena cava, resulting in obstruction of venous return.

    Obese patients, acute asthmatics, patients with hiatus hernia, and those with cardiac insufficiency and orthopnea are also more comfortable in the semireclining position.
4. The risk of foreign bodies entering the patient's eyes is increased, and the use of a protective shield should be considered.

The doctor and his staff must be properly trained in the care of the unconscious patient, know how to position the patient correctly, and be capable of maintaining a patent airway during treatment. Although most of the techniques described in this chapter are *conscious* patient sedation techniques when correctly employed, incorrect use, overdosage, hypersensitivity, etc. may lead to deeper levels of sedation approaching general anesthesia. Even patients treated with light sedation can doze off, and their respiratory efficiency may be impaired if the airway is not properly cared for. During treatment, the assistant should support the patient's chin and watch respiratory movements. A common early warning sign of partial respiratory obstruction is snoring, a sign which should never be ignored.

It is possible that the so-called "sigh reflex," which is abolished during general anesthesia, may be depressed by some sedation techniques. Loss of this reflex may result in reduced alveolar exchange due to miliary atelectasis, leading to a progressive and insidious hypoxia. During anesthesia, this possibility is prevented by intermittent hyperinflation through squeezing the reservoir bag. It would thus seem a sensible precaution during sedation to instruct the patient to take two or three deep inspirations every 10 to 15 minutes.

The dental assistant should be trained to monitor the carotid pulse, eye signs, and patient's color, as well as respiration. An intelligent assistant can also be trained to record blood pressures. She should be observant, and report anything unusual such as respiratory disturbances, swallowing attempts, needle blockage, low nitrous oxide or oxygen pressures, etc. Particles of amalgam and tooth debris should be removed immediately with suction, and she should request "time out" from operating in order to remove debris from difficult to reach areas.

Postoperative Patient Management

Following treatment, patients should be slowly raised to the seated position for a short time before being asked to stand, to prevent postural hypotension. They should then be taken to the recovery area, supported if necessary, where they may be given coffee while waiting for a responsible escort to take them home. During this immediate postoperative period, they should be supervised by the office staff, who must also know not to give scalding coffee to a sleepy patient who may still have a numb lip due to local analgesia.

Postoperative instructions must be clearly established and agreed to before treatment (Fig. 10–3A). Patients should not be permitted to leave the

---

POSTOPERATIVE INSTRUCTIONS

INSTRUCTIONS TO PATIENT:
    You must NOT drive, or operate any machinery today.
    You must NOT undertake any responsible business matters today.
    You must NOT drink alcohol today.

INSTRUCTIONS TO PERSON ACCOMPANYING PATIENT:
    This patient has had dental treatment carried out painlessly with the aid of intravenous sedation. Occasionally, some of the sedative drugs used may produce drowsiness for several hours, particularly after long appointments.

    You are therefore requested to:
    1. See the patient safely home, and arrange for responsible supervision the remainder of the day.
    2. See that the patient obeys the above instructions.

Figure 10–3–A

office unaccompanied, short procedures under nitrous oxide or alcohol sedation being the only exception to this rule. A copy of the postoperative instructions should be given to the person escorting the patient home, and the important points stressed. Driving, operating machinery, drinking alcohol, and undertaking important business matters must be prohibited for the remainder of the day, protests from patients notwithstanding. No matter what the patient's assessment of his or her own condition may be, it is impossible to predict the degree and duration of sedative and amnesic after effects in individual patients. Medicolegally, strict observance of these instructions is very important, and should also be applied to nitrous oxide sedation if prolonged. It is this author's experience that it is far better to be overcautious than to take chances, and that patients respect this concern for their welfare.

Other postoperative precautions should include the avoidance of hot stoves, hot baths, and responsibility for the care of small children for several hours after treatment.

EQUIPMENT AND FACILITIES

In addition to having intelligent, highly trained, and responsible nursing assistance, the doctor must take care of certain other essentials before he undertakes intravenous procedures in the dental office.

1. Efficient, quiet suction is mandatory. This can only be provided by high-velocity motor-driven apparatus. Most water-operated suction devices are totally inadequate for the rapid removal of water, saliva, blood, and debris of cavity preparation.

2. Mouth packing must be completely effective, so that the airway is protected at all times against inhalation of the slightest trace of foreign material.[25] The best type for restorative procedures is a moistened cellulose sponge flange pack with a centrally tied tape which remains outside the mouth; e.g., "Metropack" (Metrodent Products, U. K.). The pack should be so positioned as to provide a complete barrier to the entry of water, saliva, and debris into the pharynx, and is generally used in conjunction with a suitable mouth prop; e.g., McKesson (Fig. 10–4).

Figure 10–4 Mouth packing. A moistened sponge pack is placed well back in the lingual sulcus to protect the pharynx from foreign material. The pack must be changed frequently and its position regularly checked. During treatment, an assistant supports the chin and operates a wide bore suction to remove water and debris (see Fig. 10–2). A divided suction attachment will also help evacuate water and saliva.

3. Resuscitation apparatus must always be immediately available, and the doctor and staff must be fully conversant with emergency procedures. Facilities for the administration of oxygen under pressure should be present in every dental office, and all cylinders must be checked regularly. I consider resuscitators based on the Elder Demand Valve greatly superior to those such as the AMBU: e.g., Robertshaw, Hudson.

4. Emergency drugs may include pressor agents, epinephrine, hydrocortisone, antihistamines, and narcotic antagonists. Drugs, however, should generally be regarded as aids to emergency procedures except in events such as acute allergic reaction or adrenal insufficiency. See the chapter on *emergency drugs*.

5. The dental chair should be of a type that allows the patient to be treated in a supine position and allows for the legs to be raised above the level of the head if necessary.

6. Proper sterilization facilities such as autoclaving or dry heat are essential. Boiling water is inadequate for the destruction of pathogens such as those of viral hepatitis. Disposables should be used where possible.

7. Pulse monitoring and blood pressure recording during treatment are advised; and careful attention to the airway, respiration, eye signs, and palpation of the carotid pulse is essential. Mechanical monitoring assumes greater importance with increasing depth of sedation or anesthesia. See the chapter on *monitoring*.

With most of the techniques outlined in this chapter, the patient is at a subanesthetic level and is able to hear and respond to the operator, but I still prefer to employ continuous pulse rate monitoring and intermittent blood pressure checking during treatment. A pulse monitor is an extremely useful and educational aid, warning the doctor of changes in pulse rates due to heavy-handed operating techniques, exogenous epinephrine effects, developing hypoxia, cardiac arrhythmias, etc. I have found the San-Ei pulsemeter one of the most useful and reliable types.

Blood pressure can be readily monitored by a trained dental assistant, and may be simplified by the use of an electronic sphygmomanometer such as the American Optical AO 1660.

8. Full and accurate treatment records should be kept for reference before subsequent appointments; these should include dosages administered, duration of operation, and the patient's behavior during and after treatment (Fig. 10–5).

9. Adequate recovery facilities must be provided. The patient must remain until a responsible person can take him home. Office and recovery area should be kept warm, particularly during winter months. As most anesthetic and sedative drugs produce peripheral vasodilatation, a blanket placed over the patient's legs will help prevent heat loss during long procedures.

SPECIAL MANAGEMENT OF THE HIGH RISK PATIENT

A major consideration in the management of high-risk patients is the avoidance of emotional and physiological stress. This is particularly important in patients with a history of cardiovascular disease, arterial hypertension, and

TREATMENT RECORD (OFFICE USE ONLY)

HISTORY RE-CHECK																
TREATMENT DATE																
DOSAGE																
DURATION																
PREMED																

COMMENTS:

Figure 10–5   Record of treatment, including dosage, duration of sedation or anesthesia, comments, etc.

cerebrovascular disease, in whom endogenous epinephrine production in response to stress may result in dangerously elevated blood pressure and cardiac arrhythmias. Stress must also be avoided in patients who have been receiving corticosteroid therapy, in whom an acute adrenal crisis may be precipitated.

Although high-risk patients may be hospitalized, for various reasons this is not always possible or desirable. When both physician and dental practitioner consider it in the best interests of the patient to perform treatment in the dental office, the following regimen is suggested, having first ensured that the patient is properly prepared and rested.*

(a) **When Effective Local Analgesia Can Be Obtained.**   Light diazepam sedation (without atropine) is, in my opinion, the safest method currently available for the management of high-risk dental patients, owing to the pronounced anxiolytic action of diazepam combined with its minimal cardiovascular and respiratory effects. Research suggests that diazepam dampens central pressor responses, which may be a further safety feature of the drug; for example, painful stimuli should be less likely to produce endogenous and possibly dangerous rises in blood pressure. Recent monitoring studies also confirm the safety of diazepam.[44, 45]

Once adequate sedation has been obtained by careful *slow* administration of diazepam to the supine patient, local injections are placed as required, using a gentle approach — topical agents, warmed solution, sharp needle, aspirating syringe, slow rate of injection. Local analgesics containing epinephrine may be avoided if preferred,[63, 64] or the amount utilized should be kept within the American Heart Association guidelines (see Chapters 2 and 15). Before and during treatment oxygen may be administered through a nosepiece or intranasal cannula. Pulse rate and blood pressure should be frequently monitored throughout, and the patient kept supine for an hour following the intravenous administration of diazepam. The duration of each appointment should be kept to a minimum.

(b) **When Effective Local Analgesia Cannot Be Obtained; e.g., Acute**

---

*In very apprehensive patients 5 to 10 mg of diazepam may be prescribed for oral sedation the night before treatment, and again as oral premedication on the day of treatment. See the chapter on *psychosedation, oral route*. Needless to say, it is perhaps even *more* important with anxious, poor risk patients to employ effective iatrosedation techniques.

Abscess. In this case, a short-acting light general anesthetic should be used if immediate surgery is indicated, provided the doctor administering the anesthetic is adequately trained and experienced in general anesthesia. At present, the most suitable drug for this purpose is methohexital sodium, which, with the exception of sinus tachycardia, is less likely to produce cardiac arrhythmias than other anesthetic agents.[61, 62]

When the patient is suffering from gross cardiac or respiratory disease and hospitalization is not possible, a decision must be made whether to administer a light general anesthetic or adopt the more conservative approach of instituting drainage and controlling acute infection with antibiotics, so that (a) can be employed at a later date. If immediate surgery is mandatory and in the best interests of the patient, a minimal sleep dose of methohexital sodium should be administered via a suitable intermittent set-up with additional increments as required.[14, 15] Slight response to painful stimuli may be accepted, providing that monitoring reveals no adverse cardiovascular effects. Oxygen should be administered as in (a) for a short period before induction and continued during anesthesia. The patient must again be rested following treatment, and the duration of anesthesia kept as short as possible.

Where the doctor has *not* been trained in general anesthesia and emergency treatment is necessary, (a) should be employed, even though it may not be possible to obtain completely effective local analgesia.

SUMMARY AND CONCLUSIONS

A number of intravenous techniques, most of which are used regularly in my own practice, have been briefly described. These techniques are now being more widely used in dentistry for the treatment of patients who are apprehensive of more traditional methods, and some have important implications in the management of high-risk patients. Other and better methods, incorporating newer drugs with additional safety features, will undoubtedly be developed in the future. However, those described already offer a useful range for the trained dental practitioner.

It must be stressed that a *brief* outline only of modern intravenous techniques is contained in this chapter, which will not substitute for proper training in these modalities. Doctors without extensive general anesthesia training should *not* utilize deep sedation or ultralight general anesthesia (intermittent methohexital and propanidid), but should limit themselves to techniques such as diazepam sedation and intravenous premedication (Jorgensen).

Adoption of intravenous methods entails considerable reorganization of surgery layout and routine, retraining of staff, and re-education of the doctor, particularly in the field of medical pharmacology. I personally feel that the doctor is more than compensated for these disadvantages by the increased satisfaction of providing a more complete dental service, a reduction in the nervous tension often associated with the practice of dentistry, and the development of new interests that show great promise for the improvement of the public image of the profession. Methods that allow for the safe, painless, effective, and efficient treatment of nervous patients and others will do much to improve this image.

Unfortunately, there are at present few training facilities for those interested in achieving proficiency in the use of intravenous procedures, although it is encouraging to see more comprehensive continuing education courses, which include supervised clinical experience, gradually replacing the shorter, mainly didactic courses of the past. Although still controversial in some quarters, it is evident that the growing acceptance and usefulness of intravenous techniques cannot be ignored, and it is the profession's responsibility to see that they are properly taught to those who wish to use them. It is my hope that future years will see widespread adoption of the teaching methods pioneered at Loma Linda, where the basic techniques are introduced at undergraduate level, and that continuing education courses leading to recognized qualifications will become available to the doctor who wishes to further his or her knowledge in this important and challenging area of dental practice.

REFERENCES

1. Aellig, W. H., Laurence, D. R., O'Neil, R., and Verrill, P. J.: Cardiac effects of adrenaline and felypressin as vasoconstrictors in local anaesthesia for oral surgery under diazepam sedation. Brit. J. Anaesth., 42:174, 1970.
2. Allen, G. B., Everett, G. B., Forsyth, W. D., and Kennedy, W. F. Jr.: The cardiorespiratory effects of epinephrine in local anesthetics for dentistry. Anesth. Prog., 20:152, 1973.
3. Ausinch, B., Malagodi, M. H., and Munson, E. S.: Diazepam in the prophylaxis of lignocaine seizures. Brit. J. Anaesth., 48:309, 1976.
4. Baird, E. S., and Hailey, D. M.: Delayed recovery from a sedative: correlation of the plasma levels of diazepam with clinical effects after oral and intravenous administration. Brit. J. Anaesth., 44:803, 1972.
5. Barron, D. W.: Clinical studies of induction agents. XXII: Effect of rate of injection on incidence of side effects with thiopental and methohexital. Anesth. & Analg., 47:171, 1968.
6. Beerman, H. M.: A controlled study of diazepam in psychiatric outpatients. Amer. J. Psychiat., 120:870 March 1964.
7. Berns, J. M.: "Twilight sedation": A substitute for lengthy office intravenous anesthesia. J. Conn. D. A., 37:4, 1963.
8. Bourne, J. G.: Deaths with dental anaesthetics. Anaesthesia, 25:473, 1970.
9. Bourne, J. G.: The common fainting attack. In Studies in Anaesthetics, Including Intravenous Dental Anaesthesia. London, Lloyd-Luke, Ltd., 1967, p. 131.
10. Bourne, J. G.: The teaching of dental anaesthetics — the problem of the operator-anaesthetist. In Studies in Anaesthetics, Including Intravenous Dental Anaesthesia. London, Lloyd-Luke Ltd., 1967, p. 154.
11. Bourne, J. G.: Whose thumb on the plunger? In Drummond-Jackson, S. L. (ed.): Intravenous Anaesthesia — S.A.A.D. 3rd ed. London, Society for the Advancement of Anaesthesia in Dentistry, 1967, p. 190.
12. Brandt, A. L., and Oakes, F. D.: Preanesthesia medication: Double blind study of a new drug, diazepam. Anesth. & Analg., 44:125, 1965.
13. Breimer, D. D.: Pharmacokinetics of methohexitone following intravenous infusion in humans. Brit. J. Anaesth., 48:643, 1976.
14. Brown, S. S., and Dundee, J. W.: Clinical studies of induction agents. XXV: Diazepam, Brit. J. Anaesth., 40:108, 1968.
15. Cadle, D. R., Boulton, T. B., and Swaine, M. S.: Intermittent intravenous anaesthesia for outpatient dentistry. A study using propanidid. Anaesthesia, 23:65, 1968.
16. Chambiras, P. G.: Evaluation of sedatives in dental practice: Preliminary report. Aust. D. J., 15:112, 1970.
17. Coleman, J., and Green, R. A.: Methohexital, a short-acting barbiturate. Anaesthesia, 15:411, 1960.
18. Corssen, G., Hayward, J. R., Gunter, J. W., and Groves, E. H.: A new parenteral anesthesia for oral surgery. J. Oral Surg., 27:627, 1969.
19. Cossham, P. S., and Dixon, R. A.: Subanaesthetic dosage of propanidid as a sedative for dentistry: a controlled clinical trial. Brit. J. Anaesth., 45:369, 1973.
20. Denhoff, E.: Drugs in cerebral palsy (Clinics in Developmental Medicine 16). Based on a

symposium from the American Academy for Cerebral Palsy. Dallas, William Heinemann, Ltd., 1964.

21. Dixon, R. A., Atkinson, R. E., Kenyon, C., Lamb, D., Thornton, J. A., and Woodhead, S.: Subanaesthetic dosage of Althesin as a sedative for conservative dentistry. A controlled trial. Brit. J. Anaesth., 48:431, 1976.
22. Dowell, T.: Diazepam premedication in pediatric patients. In Report of a Symposium: Diazepam in Anaesthesia. Bristol, John Wright and Sons, Ltd., 1968, p. 25.
23. Driscoll, E. J., Zale, J. S., Lightbody, P. M., and Fiorucci, R. D.: Sedation with intravenous diazepam. J. Oral Surg., 30:332, 1972.
24. Drummond-Jackson, S. L. (ed.): Minimal increment methohexitone. In Intravenous Anaesthesia — S.A.A.D. 3rd ed. London, Society for the Advancement of Anaesthesia in Dentistry, 1967, p. 153.
25. Drummond-Jackson, S. L.: The importance of safe mouth packing. Dent. Pract., 4:376, 1954.
26. Dundee, J. W., and Haslett, W. H. K.: The benzodiazepines. A review of their actions and uses relative to anaesthetic practice. Brit. J. Anaesth., 42:217, 1970.
27. Everett, G. B., and Allen, G. D.: Simultaneous evaluation of cardiorespiratory and analgesic effects of intravenous analgesia in combination with local anesthesia. J.A.D.A., 81:926, 1970.
28. Everett, G. B., and Allen, G. D.: Simultaneous evaluation of cardiorespiratory and analgesic effects of intravenous analgesia using pentobarbital, meperidine, and scopolamine with local analgesia. J.A.D.A., 83:155, 1971.
29. Foreman, P. A.: Control of the anxiety/pain complex in dentistry: intravenous psychosedation with techniques using diazepam. Oral Surg. Oral Med. Oral Path., 37:337, 1974.
30. Foreman, P. A.: Intravenous diazepam in general dental practice. New Zealand D. J., 65:243, 1969.
31. Foreman, P. A.: Intravenous sedation: A technique for the routine dental treatment of the apprehensive ambulant patient. Anesth. Prog., 13:218, 1966.
32. Foreman, P. A.: Intravenous sedation, a technique of pain control for conservative dentistry and minor oral surgery. Aust. D. J., 12:332, 1967.
33. Foreman, P. A.: Letter to the editor. Brit. Med., J., 2:178, 1969.
34. Foreman, P. A.: Pain control and patient management in dentistry — a review of current intravenous technics. J.A.D.A., 80:101, 1970.
35. Foreman, P. A.: Very light anaesthesia in dentistry. New Zealand D. J., 61:18, 1965.
36. Foreman, P. A., Neels, R., and Willetts, P. W.: Diazepam in dentistry. Anesth. Prog., 15:253, 1968.
37. Forsyth, W. D., Allen, G. D., and Everett, G. B.: An evaluation of cardiorespiratory effects of posture in the dental outpatient. Oral Surg. Oral Med. Oral Path., 34:562, 1972.
38. Francis, J. G.: Intra-arterial methohexitone; injection into the central artery of the rabbit's ear. Anaesthesia, 19:501, 1964.
39. Geifman, S. S., Gracely, R. H., Driscoll, E. J., et al.: Conscious sedation with intravenous drugs: a study of amnesia. J. Oral Surg. (in press) 1977.
40. Goldman, V., Astrom, A., and Evers, H.: A study of the interaction between a tricyclic antidepressant and some local anaesthetic solutions containing vasoconstrictors. Proceedings, 3rd Asian and Australasian Congress of Anesthesiology, Canberra, September 1970, pp. 517–523. Butterworths (Australia).
41. Guidelines for Postgraduate and Continuing Education in Pain and Anxiety Control. Anesth. Prog., 20:167, 1973.
42. Haslett, W. H. K., and Dundee, J. W.: Clinical studies of induction agents. XXIII: Reduction of respiratory complications by scopolamine and atropine. Anesth. & Analg., 47:174, 1968.
43. Healy, T. E. J., Edmondson, H. D., and Hall, N.: The use of intravenous diazepam during dental surgery in the mentally handicapped patient. Brit. D. J., 128:22, 1970.
44. Healy, T. E. J., Lautch, H., Hall, N., Tomlin, P. J., and Vickers, M. D.: Interdisciplinary study of diazepam sedation for outpatient dentistry. Brit. Med. J., 3:13, 1970.
45. Healy, T. E. J., Robinson, J. S., and Vickers, M. D.: Physiological responses to intravenous diazepam as a sedative for conservative dentistry. Brit. Med. J., 3:110, 1970.
46. Hellewell, J., and Hutton, A. M.: The use of methohexitone in the teaching of dental anaesthesia to undergraduates. Brit. D. J., 122:107, 1967.
47. Holden, G. G. P.: Letter to the editor, Brit. D. J., 127:5, 1968.
48. Jorgensen, N. B., and Hayden, J., Jr.: Premedication, local and general anesthesia in dentistry. Philadelphia, Lea & Febiger, 1967.
49. Keats, S.: The role of diazepam in the comprehensive treatment of cerebral palsied children. Western Med., 4:(suppl. 1) 22, 1963.
50. Kernohan, R. J.: Diazepam in cardioversion. Lancet, 1:718, 1966.
51. Langdon, D. E., Hartan, J. R., and Bailey, R. L.: Thrombophlebitis and diazepam used intravenously. J.A.M.A., 223:184, 1973.

52. Laskin, D. M. (ed.): Guidelines for the Teaching of Comprehensive Pain and Anxiety Control in Dentistry. Pain Control Conference, Columbus, Ohio, October 25–26, 1970. American Dental Association Council on Dental Education. Published May 1971.

53. Lawson, J. I. M., and Main, D. M. G.: Postgraduate and undergraduate teaching. Report of meeting held Feb. 3, 1966, Society for the Advancement of Anaesthesia in Dentistry. Digest Report 266, February 1966.

54. Lawson, J. I. M., and Main, D. M. G.: The use of intravenous anaesthesia by dentists. Brit. D. J., *122*:21, 1967.

55. Main, D. M. G.: "Pentazepam". S.A.A.D. Digest, *2*:232, 1975.

56. Malamed, S. F., and Pallasch, T. J.: U. S. C. School of Dentistry — Guidelines for the Control of Pain and Anxiety. Anesth. Prog., *21*:99, 1974.

57. Martin, R. T.: An exploratory investigation of the dentist/patient relation. Research investigation carried out by School of Applied Psychology, University of New South Wales, for the Dental Health Education and Research Foundation of the University of Sydney, 1965.

58. News Sheet NS 64/1168, Society for the Advancement of Anaesthesia in Dentistry, Nov. 1968, p. 69.

59. O'Neill, R., Verrill, P. J., Aellig, W. H., and Laurence, D. R.: Intravenous diazepam in minor oral surgery: Further studies. Brit. D. J., *128*:15, 1970.

60. Raffan, A.: Presidential address to Scottish Society of Anaesthetists, Annual Meeting, 1967.

61. Rollason, W. N., and Dundas, C. R.: Incidence of cardiac arrhythmia during dental anaesthesia. Proc. 4th World Congress of Anaesthesiologists, London, September 9–13, 1968, pp. 969–976. Excerpta Medica Foundation (Amsterdam).

62. Ryder, W.: The electrocardiogram in dental anaesthesia. Anaesthesia, *25*:46, 1970.

63. Sachs, S. A.: A survey of neuroleptanalgesia. Anesth. Prog., *16*:105, 1969.

64. Shane, S. M.: Intravenous amnesia for total dentistry in one sitting. J. Oral Surg., *24*:27, 1966.

65. Shane, S. M.: Intravenous amnesia to obliterate fear, anxiety and pain in ambulatory dental patients. J. Maryland D. A., *9*:94, 1966.

66. Waterson, J. G.: Anaesthesia as a dental problem. Aust. D. J., *12*:343, 1967.

67. Whitman, J. G.: Methohexitone (editorial). Brit. J. Anaesth., *48*:617, 1976.

68. Wilkinson, W. B., Foreman, P. A., and Neels, R.: The routine use of methohexital sodium in general dental practice. New Zealand D. J. *61*:12, 1965.

69. Wise, C. C., and others: Physiological responses to intermittent methohexitone for conservative dentistry. Brit. Med. J., *2*:540, 1969.

Part 2

TREATMENT OF SERIOUS MEDICAL EMERGENCIES

11

BASIC LIFE SUPPORT AND PARENTERAL DRUG ADMINISTRATION

JOHN HAGEN
and
STANLEY F. MALAMED

INTRODUCTION

This chapter is the first in the section on the treatment of serious medical emergencies. While subsequent chapters will discuss specific causes of medical emergencies and their treatment, we will review procedures which are essential to the management of most of these potentially life-threatening situations.

These procedures include the maintenance of a patent airway in the unconscious patient, techniques for delivering oxygen to conscious or unconscious patients, and monitoring of two very important vital signs, the blood pressure and the heart rate (pulse), which give us information concerning the functional status of the cardiovascular system. Taken together, these three procedures constitute the ABC's of basic life support; A for airway, B for breathing, and C for circulation. When all three procedures (ABC) are employed together the technique is termed cardiopulmonary resuscitation (CPR). It is only on rare occasions, fortunately, that the dental practitioner will be called upon to perform cardiopulmonary resuscitation within the dental office. (CPR is discussed in depth in Chapter 14.) However, the dental doctor will more than likely be presented with several occasions during his or her practice lifetime which will require implementation of the steps of basic life support.

With proper management most of these emergency situations will be readily correctable. Proper management is the vital key to success in most of these situations, and a thorough working knowledge of the procedures of basic life support is obligatory for proper management to occur.

This chapter will conclude with a description of techniques for parenteral drug administration. Two techniques for drug administration will be reviewed: the intramuscular and the intravenous routes. Specific drugs to be employed in the management of medical emergency situations will be discussed in later chapters. It must be stated clearly and be well understood that *the administration of drugs, in most medical emergency situations, should be secondary to the performance of the procedures of basic life support.* Once the ABC's have been satisfactorily accomplished the doctor can then give attention to the specific cause(s) of the emergency and give consideration to drug therapy to assist the patient's recovery.

MANAGEMENT OF THE UNCONSCIOUS PATIENT

Loss of consciousness is a common occurrence in the dental office. Whatever the precipitating factor, loss of consciousness always presents the practitioner with a potentially life-threatening emergency, demanding immediate and effective treatment if the victim is to be expected to recover. Loss of consciousness is assumed to represent cardiac arrest until proven otherwise.

Because of possible medicolegal implications, case reports of deaths during dental therapy are rarely observed in dental journals in the United States. However, much valuable information may be readily obtained from both dental and medical journals published in Great Britain. When these articles and reports are examined, an item which is seen to recur quite frequently is anoxia secondary to an obstructed airway, which goes unnoticed until permanent damage has occurred.[11, 12, 14, 19]

In response to these reports, the British Dental Journal published a letter which stated in part: ". . . at a lecture/demonstration a few years ago, not one dental surgeon participating knew how to give the 'kiss of life' correctly and, therefore, could not have resuscitated the patient. In reading accounts of death occurring under general anesthesia and that the 'kiss of life' was administered with no result in some of these cases, I hesitate, but wonder whether the method of resuscitation chosen was correctly applied."[17]

Loss of consciousness need not occur only in the patient receiving general anesthetic agents; indeed the most common cause of unconsciousness in dentistry is vasodepressor syncope (common faint) due to fear and apprehension, in unmedicated patients. The initial treatment in most circumstances of unconsciousness is essentially the same. One possible exception is the acute anaphylactic reaction, in which case the administration of epinephrine as soon as possible may well prove to be the single most important life-saving measure.

Unconsciousness is accompanied by muscular relaxation, and it is this muscular relaxation which is responsible for the associated problems of hypoxia and/or anoxia. In the unconscious patient, hypopharyngeal obstruction by the base of the relaxed tongue occurs always when the head is in the midposition (Fig. 11-1). As stated by Safar: complete airway obstruction leads to asphyxia and cardiac arrest within five to 10 minutes; while partial airway obstruction, through other more complex pathways, may lead to the same result.[18]

In all cases of unconsciousness, immediate treatment consists of the recognition of airway obstruction and the effective management of this problem. Once a patent airway has been secured, only then can the dental practitioner proceed to more definitive life-support measures (cardiac massage; drug administration). It is well to keep in mind the objectives of ventilation, as stated by Coryllos: life is continued as long as exchanges of oxygen and carbon dioxide in the tissues are carried on in a normal way.[9]

The establishment of a patent airway therefore becomes the primary objective of treatment in all cases of unconsciousness.

TECHNIQUES OF AIRWAY MAINTENANCE

Immediately upon the recognition of unconsciousness it is recommended that the following sequence be carried out until one is satisfied that a patent airway exists:

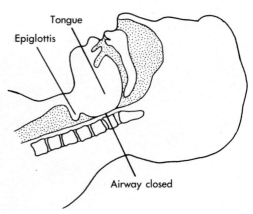

Figure 11-1 Airway obstruction. In flexed position, the tongue acts to produce obstruction, either partial or complete, in the unconscious patient. (From Malamed, S. F., Handbook of Medical Emergencies in the Dental Office. Saint Louis, C. V. Mosby, Co., 1978.)

Figure 11-2 Positioning of the unconscious patient. The unconscious patient is placed in a supine position with the chest and abdomen parallel to the floor, the head and legs elevated slightly. (From Malamed, S. F.: Handbook of Medical Emergencies in the Dental Office. Saint Louis, C. V. Mosby Co., 1978.)

1. Positioning of patient
2. Backward tilt of head
3. Check for airway, breathing
4. Forward displacement of mandible, if necessary
5. Check for airway, breathing, if necessary
6. Artificial ventilation, if necessary

1. Positioning of Patient (Fig. 11–2). An unconscious patient should be placed in the *supine* position. The chest and head should be horizontal to aid in delivery of blood to the brain, and the feet should be elevated slightly, aiding in return of blood to the heart.

Figure 11–3. Head tilt. The rescuer places one hand beneath the victim's neck, lifting the neck; the second hand, placed on the victim's forehead, pushes the forehead back.

Figure 11-4 Head tilt. Lifting the neck and pushing the forehead back serves to stretch the tissues in the pharynx, lifting the tongue off of the posterior pharyngeal wall. (From Malamed, S. F.: Handbook of Medical Emergencies in the Dental Office. Saint Louis, C. V. Mosby Co., 1978.)

    2. Backward Tilt of Head (Head-Tilt, Fig. 11–3). This is perhaps the single most effective step to take in the creation of a patent airway in an unconscious patient. One hand is placed under the patient's neck, lifting it, while the other at the patient's forehead pushes the head back. This simple maneuver stretches the tissues between the larynx and mandible (Fig. 11–4), lifting the base of the tongue from the posterior pharyngeal wall. Elevation of the patient's shoulders (achieved by placing a towel or pillow under the shoulders) may be a further aid in tilting of the patient's head.

    When properly carried out, this step alone provides an open airway in about 80 per cent of unconscious patients.

    3. Check for Airway Breathing. An evaluation of airway patency may rapidly be made by *looking* and *listening*.

    Look: look for movements of the chest and abdomen.

    Listen: listen and *feel* for air flow at the mouth and nose. This may be quickly accomplished by placing your ear one inch from the patient's nose and mouth and the palm of one hand on the upper part of the patient's abdomen. If no air exchange is immediately detectable, a gentle push will establish patency of the airway (Fig. 11–5).[8] This airway patency maneuver was first utilized by dental practitioners administering intravenous anesthesia in the early 1940's.

    Two types of airway obstruction may be evidenced: complete obstruction and partial obstruction. As mentioned above it takes only a period of between five and 10 minutes for complete airway obstruction to cause biological (non-reversible) death.

    Complete airway obstruction will be recognized by the inability to *hear* and *feel* air flow at the mouth or nose, and by *seeing* inspiratory retraction in the intercostal and supraclavicular areas. In the absence of spontaneous breathing movements (apnea), complete airway obstruction will be recognized by the inability to inflate the lungs during attempts at artificial respiration.

    Partial airway obstruction will usually be recognized by *noisy* air flow during spontaneous or artificial respiration. Depending upon the degree of obstruction present, retraction may or may not be present. Prolonged partial

Figure 11–5 Evaluation of airway maintenance. Maintaining head tilt, the rescuer evaluates the patency of the airway and spontaneous respiration by placing his or her ear approximately one inch from the victim's mouth and nose, hearing and feeling for respiration, and looking at the victim's chest, looking for spontaneous respiratory movement.

obstruction causes the respiratory center to become less sensitive to the usual stimulus from a buildup of carbon dioxide, leading ultimately to respiratory failure and cardiac arrest. In cases of partial obstruction, various degrees of noisy air flow may be elicited, depending upon the degree of obstruction and the cause of the obstruction. Table 11–1 lists several common causes of noisy respiration.

4. Forward Displacement of Mandible. In approximately one out of five patients, the previously described steps will not result in an open airway. In this instance, the mandible should be displaced forward. This may be accomplished by placing the thumbs on the posterior border of the ascending ramus and lifting the mandible anteriorly until a prognathic state is achieved (Fig. 11–6). This procedure may be made less fatiguing if the forearms are allowed to rest on the patient's shoulder.[2] Forward displacement may also be achieved by placing your thumb in the patient's mouth and pulling the mandible forward (Fig. 11–7).

TABLE 11–1 PARTIAL AIRWAY OBSTRUCTION – CAUSES

Sound Heard	Probable Cause
Snoring	Hypopharyngeal obstruction by tongue
Wheezing	Bronchial obstruction (as seen in asthma)
Crowing	Laryngospasm (partial)
Gurgling	Foreign matter (blood, water, vomitus) in the airway

Figure 11–6 Foreward displacement of mandible. The rescuer, positioned at the head of the victim, places his or her fingers on the posterior border of the ramus, pushing the ramus in a superior direction (arrow). Fingers placed in the corners of the mouth aid in maintaining a patent airway.

5. Check for Airway Patency and Breathing. Repeat procedure described in step 3. If the airway is now patent and the victim breathing spontaneously, the rescuer need only maintain the patency of the airway and proceed to the further diagnosis and treatment of the cause(s) of the unconscious state. In the absence of spontaneous respiratory movements the doctor must apply artificial ventilation.

Figure 11–7 Foreward displacement of mandible. The rescuer may grasp the anterior portion of the mandible. The mandible is pulled forward, lifting the tongue from the posterior wall of the pharynx. *Caution:* this procedure is employed primarily in edentulous patients; the rescuer risks self-injury when using it in patients with natural teeth.)

Figure 11–8 Monitoring of carotid pulse. The rescuer places his or her fingers in the groove on the lateral side of the neck. A minimum of 10 seconds is necessary to determine the presence, absence, and quality of the pulse.

ARTIFICIAL VENTILATION

In the absence of spontaneous respiratory movements (apnea) the rescuer immediately begins artificial ventilation of the victim. The goal of artificial ventilation is to supply oxygen to the blood in sufficient quantity to prevent cellular (biologic) death from occurring. Several techniques of artificial ventilation are available. These include exhaled air ventilation, atmospheric air ventilation, enriched oxygen ventilation, and positive pressure oxygen ventilation. Each of these will be discussed. The technique of exhaled air ventilation will serve as an example of airway maintenance and artificial ventilation.

Exhaled Air Ventilation

Following a determination of apnea, the rescuer maintains head tilt, pinches off the victim's nares, opens his mouth widely, sealing it securely over the victim's, and blows exhaled air into the victim's lungs. This first ventilatory attempt with exhaled air (which contains approximately 16 per cent oxygen) consists of four quick ventilations of the victim. Effective artificial ventilation is noted by observing the victim's chest rise with each ventilatory effort. Expiration is a passive procedure, the rescuer removing his mouth from the victim's, allowing the lungs to deflate.

Immediately following this initial ventilatory procedure the adequacy of the cardiovascular system must be assessed (C of the ABC's). The carotid artery, located in a groove on the side of the neck, is palpated for approximately 5 to 10 seconds (Fig. 11–8). If a palpable pulse is not found, external cardiac compression is commenced (see Chapter 14). In the more likely event that a palpable pulse is present, the rescuer continues to maintain a patent airway and administer artificial ventilation as indicated.

In the adult victim, artificial ventilation is applied at a rate of one ventilation every five seconds (12 per minute), while in younger victims the respiratory rate is more rapid (20 per minute, or one every three seconds). In all patients, regardless of age, adequacy of ventilation is indicated by elevation of the chest with each breath.

Following institution of the ABC's of basic life support the rescuer can seek to determine the cause of the emergency situation. If the victim does not recover spontaneously, then definitive therapy may be indicated. If the cause of the medical problem is known (e.g., hypoglycemia), then drugs may be administered (i.e., IV 50% dextrose or IM glucagon). The ABC's must still be carefully adhered to during this period of time. Should a diagnosis or drugs be unavailable, basic life support is maintained and medical assistance sought.

A variation of mouth to mouth ventilation is the mouth to nose technique. It is equally effective and is of use in instances in which mouth to mouth ventilation is difficult to perform, such as when the victim's mouth cannot be opened; when it is impossible to ventilate through the victim's mouth, and when it is difficult to achieve a tight seal around the victim's mouth. In this technique head tilt is maintained; however, the hand under the neck is moved so that it now lifts the victim's mandible upward, sealing the lips. The rescuer takes a deep breath, seals his lips around the victim's nose, and blows in until the victim's lungs expand. The rescuer removes his mouth and passive exhalation occurs.

Atmospheric Air Ventilation

Artificial ventilation with atmospheric air enables the rescuer to deliver approximately 21 per cent oxygen to the victim's lungs, an improvement over the 16 per cent delivered in exhaled air ventilation. To deliver atmospheric air to the victim, however, requires the utilization of adjunctive devices. These devices are not difficult to use, but they do require advanced training in order to be employed effectively. The device most often used to deliver atmospheric oxygen is the self-inflating bag-valve-mask unit (Fig. 11–9). Carden and Hughes[8] and Carden and Friedman[7] have tested those

Figure 11–9 Bag-valve-mask device. The self-inflating bag enables the rescuer to deliver atmospheric air to the victim. Enriched oxygen may be administered by attaching the oxygen tube to the opening at the back of the bag device (arrow).

Figure 11-10 Proper use of the bag-valve-mask device requires the rescuer to maintain head tilt and an air tight seal of the mask with but one hand.

devices which are currently being marketed and have concluded that the AMBU, PMR, Laerdal Resusci 2 Resuscitator and Hope 2 Resuscitator are acceptable devices.

In order for these devices to be effectively employed, the operator must be able to maintain a patent airway and maintain an airtight seal between the mask and the patient's face using but one hand. Two fingers, usually thumb and index finger, are used to hold the mask in position while the other fingers are hooked around the lower border of the mandible. The mask is held tightly against the victim's face, and the mandible is pulled backward, producing head tilt (Fig. 11-10). The opposite hand is used to squeeze the self-inflating bag at a rate of once every 5 seconds (adult) or once every 3 seconds (child). Adequate ventilation is ensured by observing the chest inflate with each ventilatory effort.

If the mask is not held securely, leakage will result which diminishes the volume of air reaching the victim's lungs.

Advanced training in the proper use of this and other adjunctive devices is strongly recommended. The face mask which is part of this device is available in a variety of sizes (Fig. 11-11). Several sizes should be avail-

Figure 11-11 Full face masks. Full face masks are available in a variety of sizes. They should be constructed of clear plastic so that the rescuer can observe the victim's mouth at all times.

able in the dental office for use in emergency situations. An additional factor concerning the face mask is the material from which it is manufactured. Until recently, face masks were solid, usually black rubber. While effective for ventilation, the use of solid masks made it impossible for the rescuer to see the victim's mouth for evidence of foreign materials, vomitus, blood, etc. Face masks are available today which are fabricated from clear plastics and rubber, which make it possible to view the victim's mouth during resuscitation efforts. These masks are highly recommended.

Enriched Oxygen Ventilation

Connecting a compressed gas cylinder of oxygen to a self-inflating bag-valve-mask device enables us to deliver oxygen concentrations in excess of atmospheric air to the victim. This is termed enriched oxygen ventilation, with concentrations ranging up to 100 per cent oxygen.

Oxygen is available as a compressed gas in cylinders. A wide range of cylinder sizes are available and are listed by letter according to their volume. An A cylinder contains 76 liters of oxygen, D cylinders 396 liters, E cylinders 659 liters, and an H cylinder 6931 liters. When used for resuscitation in enriched oxygen ventilation, a flow rate of approximately 10 to 20 liters per minute will be employed. However, when used as 100 per cent oxygen for positive pressure ventilation (see below) the flow rate will be increased to approximately 78 liters of oxygen per minute. For this reason the E size cylinder represents the minimal size of cylinder recommended for use in emergency situations. Empty oxygen cylinders are worthless. The larger cylinder (H) is too heavy to be portable. Canisters of oxygen produced by chemical reaction produce minimal flows and volumes of oxygen, are without merit, and ought not to be considered for use in emergency situations.

Specific devices such as pressure reducing valves, flow-rate controls, and connecting tubing must be added to the oxygen cylinder to adapt it for use with the self-inflating bag-valve-mask device. All of the recommended b-v-m devices have outlets for oxygen connectors (Fig. 11–9).

Positive Pressure Oxygen

For purposes of resuscitation, the delivery of 100 per cent oxygen is ideal. The Robertshaw Resuscitator (Fig. 11–12) and the Elder Demand Valve are devices operated by compressed oxygen which deliver oxygen on demand and also provide for intermittent positive pressure breathing. For positive pressure breathing, the face mask is held in the same manner as the self-inflating bag-valve-mask device. Positive pressure oxygen is then delivered by pressing a button on the mask. Oxygen is delivered at a flow rate of approximately 78 liters per minute. Overinflation of the lungs is prevented through an automatic cut-off when airway pressure of 54 cm of water is reached. Respiratory rates are 12 per minute for an adult, and 20 per minute for the child.

Figure 11-12 Positive pressure oxygen device. Full face mask attached to E-cylinder of oxygen. When properly employed, this device is capable of delivering 100 per cent oxygen to the patient.

If the patient is capable of maintaining his or her own respiratory cycle, positive pressure oxygen is not necessary, but supplemental oxygen can be used to assist the patient during any emergency situation in which he is physiologically depressed. With the mask placed over the patient's face, a minimal inspiratory effort of (−) 1 cm of water will trigger the device to deliver an oxygen flow adequate to ventilate the patient at rest. At (−) 3 cm H_2O the demand valve provides approximately 150 liters of oxygen per minute.

It must always be kept in mind that while higher percentages of oxygen are beneficial to our patients, the devices which operate from compressed gas cylinders will be effective only as long as oxygen remains in the cylinder. With the E cylinder this equates to approximately 30 minutes of positive pressure breathing. Once oxygen is depleted from the cylinder other methods of ventilation must be employed (atmospheric or exhaled air). Artificial ventilation must never be delayed while one seeks an oxygen cylinder. Commence mouth to mouth ventilation, switching to other techniques only when they become available and only if the rescuer is well versed in their use.

ADJUNCTIVE EQUIPMENT

Many devices are available to aid in the maintenance of a patent airway. All of these devices are used to supplement basic life support (ABC), therefore the ABC steps must not be delayed while seeking adjunctive equipment. The simplicity of basic life support, in that it requires no adjunctive equipment, is one of its most positive attributes. The more commonly used adjunctive devices will be reviewed. The use of these devices does entail a degree of risk and will require additional training of the doctor and staff members in order to become proficient in their use.

Artificial Airways

Artificial oral airways (Fig. 11–13) may become necessary to hold the base of the tongue forward and to maintain the teeth and lips in an open position. Oropharyngeal airways may be valuable adjuncts when prolonged airway maintenance is necessary. When it is difficult to open a patient's mouth, a nasopharyngeal airway may be inserted. The nasopharyngeal tube is less likely to stimulate vomiting in an unconscious patient than the oropharyngeal airway. In addition, an oral airway may, on rare occasion, extend beyond the pharynx and obstruct the air passage by forcing the epiglottis onto the trachea.

Artificial airways should be utilized *only* if maintenance of a patent airway without one is difficult, because unnecessary insertion may cause gagging, laryngospasm, and a delay in ventilation of the patient. Several sizes of oropharyngeal airway should be available to accommodate individual patient variation.

Esophageal Obturator Airway

The esophageal obturator is a plastic tube which is sealed at one end and which contains multiple small holes throughout its length (Fig. 11–14).

Figure 11–13 Oropharyngeal airways. Available in several sizes, oropharyngeal airways lie between the base of the tongue and the posterior pharyngeal wall, maintaining a patent airway. (*Caution:* proper use of this device requires specialized training.)

Figure 11-14 Esophageal obturator airway. The esophageal airway is a plastic tube sealed at one end (1), with multiple holes throughout its length (2). When the tube is properly placed in the esophagus, air delivered into the tube will enter the victim's trachea. A balloon (3) prevents the forcing of air into the esophagus. (Courtesy of Littel's Oxygen Inc. 13006 Saticoy, North Hollywood California.

In clinical practice the closed end of the obturator airway is inserted blindly into the patient's mouth and posteriorly into the esophagus. A cuff on the closed end of the tube is inflated, sealing off the esophagus and lower GI tract from the laryngeal area. Artificial ventilation is applied through the open end of the tube, air being forced through the openings along the tube into the oropharynx, trachea, and lungs.

Difficulties encountered in the use of this device include its inadvertent insertion into the trachea. This situation, which has been reported to occur in approximately 8 per cent of insertions, leads to total airway obstruction as air is forced into the esophagus and stomach. A second and more commonly observed adverse reaction is the disturbing propensity for regurgitation or vomiting to occur when the obturator airway is removed. Acidic stomach contents may produce airway obstruction, or might be aspirated into the trachea and bronchi, producing aspiration pneumonitis, which may be fatal. The esophageal obturator airway should not be used by untrained persons.

Endotracheal Intubation

Placement of a cuffed tube from the mouth into the trachea allows for an unobstructed airway. Endotracheal intubation isolates the airway, keeps it patent, prevents aspiration, and ensures delivery of a high concentration of oxygen to the lungs. However, because of the difficulties, delays, and complications in properly placing an endotracheal tube, the American Heart Association recommends that its use be restricted to medical personnel who are highly trained or who use endotracheal intubation frequently (anesthesiologists).[3]

MONITORING OF VITAL SIGNS

An integral part of the management of all medical emergency situations is monitoring the vital signs of the victim. One vital sign, respiration, has been evaluated previously during airway maintenance, with artificial ventilation being started, if needed. Following these ventilations the status of the cardiovascular system must be evaluated. Two vital signs aid in this evaluation: the pulse or heart rate and the blood pressure. The pulse allows for a rapid determination of cardiovascular function. Absence of pulse for a period of from 5 to 10 seconds is an indication for initiation of closed chest cardiac compression in the unconscious, apneic victim. Blood pressure may also be monitored in emergencies. Recordings on a patient should be compared to those observed prior to the emergency. These are termed baseline values and provide an indication of the severity of the problem faced.

PULSE (HEART RATE)

The arterial pulse may be recorded at any site in which an artery lies superficially under the skin. Several areas are readily available on the clothed

Figure 11-15 Brachial artery. The brachial artery is located on the medial aspect of the antecubital fossa.

Figure 11–16 Radial artery. The radial artery is located on the lateral aspect (thumb side) of the ventral surface of the wrist.

dental patient: the carotid artery, the brachial artery, and the radial artery. For routine (non-emergency) monitoring of the heart rate the brachial or radial arteries are suggested. In emergencies the carotid artery becomes of greater significance because a weak pulse is more likely to be detected at this site.

The brachial artery (Fig. 11–15) may be palpated in the antecubital fossa at the elbow. It is located on the mesial aspect of the fossa. This artery is not as superficial as the radial, so that more presssure must be applied to locate it.

The radial artery (Fig. 11–16) lies superficially on the lateral aspect (thumb side) of the ventral surface of the wrist. It may be located by placing the fingers on the radius (bone on the thumb side of wrist) and moving the fingers just slightly onto the wrist. The radial artery is located in a depression just medial to the radius.

The carotid artery is located in the neck in a groove located anterior to the sternocleidomastoid muscle. It is located by the doctor's placing two fingers on the thyroid cartilage (Adam's apple) and then sliding the fingers along the side of the neck until they reach the groove formed by the sternocleidomastoid muscle posteriorly. Gentle pressure is then applied (Fig. 11–17A and B).

Several important facts follow concerning pulse monitoring. The thumb should never be employed. The thumb contains a fair-sized artery which may easily be palpated and mistaken for the victim's pulse. It is suggested that the fleshy portions of the first two fingers be used for pulse monitoring. Pulse is recorded in beats per minute. Whenever possible (non-emergency situations), a full 60 seconds should be used to record the pulse. In emergency situations in which the primary objective is to determine if a functionally adequate pulse exists, not less than 10 seconds should be employed. In the absence of an adequate pulse, external cardiac compression must be started immediately. Evaluation of the pulse consists of determining not only the rate but also the quality of the pulse (thready, bounding, or weak) and the rhythm (skips, prematurities, flutters). Any deviation from a normal, full, regular pulse should be considered pathologic until a more explicit diagnosis is made.

Figure 11–17   Location of carotid artery. *A*, The rescuer places his or her fingers over the thyroid cartilage (Adam's apple) of the victim. *B*, The carotid artery is located in the groove on the side of the neck between the thyroid cartilage and the sternocleidomastoid muscle. (*Note:* head tilt must be maintained throughout this procedure.)

Evaluation of the Pulse

To better understand the more common cardiac irregularities, a description of the normal cardiac mechanism is presented for review.

The heart beat is initiated by stimulation of the sinoatrial node. The impulse spreads as a wave through the atrial musculature and is followed by contraction. When the impulse reaches the atrioventricular node it passes down the bundle of His, the bundle branches, and the Purkinje system into the ventricular musculature, resulting in a contraction. Disruption or impairment of this sequence will manifest as an irregularity in the heart beat which can at times be noted in the arterial pulse. See the conduction system diagram in the chapter on *monitoring*; also, further information on arrhythmias.

The following is a classification and description of the more common cardiac disturbances:

1. *Sinus arrhythmia.* This is noted in most healthy young patients and consists of an increase in the heart rate during inspiration and slowing during expiration.

2. *Premature beats.* These may arise in the atrium, the junctional tissues, or, more frequently, the ventricles. When occurring in the absence of organic heart disease, premature beats may be due to emotional stress, hypoglycemia, or excessive use of stimulants. The premature beat is usually recognized readily because it consists of a contraction before the next beat would normally occur, and is followed by a pause longer than the usual interval.

One special type of premature beat warrants mention. This is bigeminal rhythm, a state in which every alternate beat is premature. It should not be confused with pulsus alternans, a rhythmic disorder in which every alternate beat is feeble and which denotes a grave prognosis.

3. *Atrial fibrillation.* The paroxysmal form of this arrhythmia is most frequently seen in thyrotoxicosis, in rheumatic heart disease with mitral stenosis, or in senile heart disease. The attacks have the characteristics of all types of paroxysmal heart action, with the onset and end being sudden.

When the rate is rapid (120 or more) the diagnosis is made readily, because atrial fibrillation is the only common condition in which one has the combination of a well marked tachycardia with a gross irregularity.

Because of the complexity of the cardiac mechanism, many variables can arise, and the diagnosis and subsequent treatment must become the responsibility of the cardiologist. The pulse coupled with the blood pressure is essential for screening patients for possible cardiovascular disease.

BLOOD PRESSURE

The value of the measurement and recording of blood pressure as a means of preventing medical emergencies and as a valuable guide to the management of those that do occur within the practice of dentistry has been demonstrated by many authors[1, 5] and recognized by the American Dental Association.[15]

Physiology

The arterial blood pressure is the result of the discharge of a volume of blood by the heart into the arterial system which cannot all escape through the arterioles and capillaries into the venous system before the next heart beat occurs. Thus the arterial system is always overfilled and this causes the elastic peripheral vessels to be in a constant state of distention, creating a measurable pressure. This pressure will vary with beating of the heart, rising to a maximum during ventricular contraction (systole) and falling when the ventricles relax (diastole).

Maintenance of normal blood pressure is dependent on two main factors: cardiac output and the caliber of the peripheral vessels. An increased volume of blood discharged into the arterial system can only be accommodated by further stretching of the arterial walls, causing an increase in both the systolic and diastolic pressures. Likewise, constriction of the peripheral vessels will cause an increased arterial pressure by reducing the outflow of blood into the venous system. The pressure will rise until the quantity of blood entering the venous system equals the amount pumped into the arterial system by the heart. The opposite effect occurs when these vessels dilate. The pressure will fall until the arterial outflow is equalized by a proportionate inflow from the heart.

Aside from these factors, variances in the total blood volume, blood viscosity, and the elasticity of the arterial walls as a result of hemorrhage or disease will have varying degrees of influence on the blood pressure.

Under normal conditions these factors all interact in a reflexive compensatory manner to offset extreme changes in the blood pressure. For example, when there is a moderate reduction of cardiac output or blood volume, a reflex constriction of the small vessel walls occurs, and the peripheral resistance is increased. Conversely, when there is an increase in the blood volume or viscosity, the increased blood pressure is counteracted by vasodilatation.

Since arterial pressures cannot be measured precisely with a sphygmomanometer, it is important that this basic inefficiency not be increased by added error due to equipment or technique. Because normal blood pressure readings vary so widely between individuals, a base line or pretreatment determination should be established. This can be used as a comparison should an emergency arise with its attendant blood pressure changes.

Equipment

The sphygmomanometer consists of a compression bag surrounded by a cuff for application to the arm, a manometer by which the applied pressure is read, and an inflating bulb with a controllable exhaust.

In the selection of an instrument, certain points should be considered that will enhance the accuracy desired. The inflatable bag should be about 20 per cent wider than the diameter of the arm, and for an adult 12 cm is adequate. The aneroid type of manometer is preferred for dental office use because of the ease in storage and in reading the blood pressure.

To complete the apparatus requirements, a stethoscope with a diaphragm device is needed to determine blood pressure by auscultation.

For a more comprehensive discussion of the equipment used in recording blood pressure the reader is referred to Burch and DePasquale,[6] and to The American Heart Association's Recommendations for Human Blood Pressure Determinations by Sphygmomanometry.[4]

Figure 11–18   The stethoscope ear pieces are placed securely in the ears, facing anteriorly; the diaphragm is placed firmly against the skin over the medial portion of the antecubital fossa.

Technique

The patient may be either in a recumbent position or comfortably seated. The arm should be bared, slightly flexed, and abducted. In the sitting position the forearm should be supported at heart level.

The compression bag must be placed directly over the brachial artery, one inch above the antecubital fossa. After placing the cuff snugly, the radial pulse is palpated while the cuff is rapidly inflated until the pulse is no longer felt. Pressure in the cuff is now released. The point at which the radial pulse disappears is termed the palpatory systolic blood pressure.

After waiting 15 seconds to permit vascular congestion in the arm to diminish, the recorder places the ear pieces of the stethoscope in his ears. They should be placed facing anteriorly, creating a firm seal to block out extraneous sounds. The diaphragm of the stethoscope is now placed firmly against the skin on the medial portion of the antecubital fossa over the brachial artery (Fig. 11–18). If the diaphragm is not held securely against the skin sounds will not be magnified, and extraneous sounds will cause interference.

The pressure in the cuff is inflated to a level 30 mm Hg above that of the palpatory systolic blood pressure. The blood pressure recorder listens carefully for sounds. With the cuff inflated above the systolic blood pressure no blood will pass the cuff, therefore sounds will not be heard.

Release the pressure in the cuff so that the manometer is reduced approximately 2 mm per second. If the pressure is reduced too rapidly errors will appear in the measured blood pressure. When the pressure within the blood pressure cuff equals that of the systolic blood pressure, blood begins to squirt past the cuff into the artery, creating sounds which may be heard through the stethoscope. These sounds, which were first studied by Korotkoff, are called the Korotkoff sounds. Systolic blood pressure is recorded as the point at which these first sounds, a rhythmic tapping or thudding coincident with the heart beat, are heard. As pressure in the cuff is deflated further the sounds change in intensity until they disappear entirely. The point of disappearance is considered to be the diastolic blood pressure.

Following disappearance of the sounds, permit the cuff to deflate totally, and remove the cuff from the patient's arm.

Blood pressure is recorded as a fraction, systolic pressure over diastolic pressure, which is written as 130/80, for example. All blood pressures are measured in millimeters of mercury, mm Hg, but this need not be written. In addition there are no odd numbers on a manometer, so blood pressure readings are always recorded in even numbers.

Evaluation of Blood Pressure

For screening purposes, McCarthy and Malamed[13] have established four levels of blood pressure elevation. Category I is the patient with consistent measurements below 140 and 90 mm Hg. This represents the upper limit of normal blood pressure for adults. Pressures below these limits do not require additional monitoring, consultation, or precautions. Category II includes blood pressures between 140 and 160 mm Hg systolic and/or 90–95 mm Hg diastolic. It is recommended that blood pressures in this category be re-evaluated prior to each dental appointment. If three consecutive recordings occur above 140/90, medical consultation is indicated. Routine dental therapy may proceed with possible modification and special considerations.

Blood pressures between 160 and 200 mm Hg systolic and/or 95–115 mm Hg diastolic are Class III. The blood pressure should be retaken in approximately 5 minutes, and if still elevated medical consultation is indicated. In addition, modifications such as stress-reduction procedures (i.e., psychosedation, length of appointment) are warranted. See Chapter 2 regarding the USC physical evaluation system.

Class IV blood pressures include any systolic pressure in excess of 200 mm Hg and/or diastolic greater than 115 mm Hg. Recommended management includes medical consultation; no elective dental therapy until elevated blood pressure is corrected or found to be uncorrectable; emergency therapy (pain and/or infection) to be treated with medication and/or minimal operative intervention; and referral to hospital if immediate stressful dental therapy is indicated.

PARENTERAL DRUG ADMINISTRATION

Following the successful initiation of the ABC's of basic life support, the rescuer may now begin to consider the underlying cause(s) of the emergency situation being faced. If a cause is readily evident, if the problem is correctable through drug administration, and if the rescuer is knowledgeable in drug administration and pharmacology of the drug(s) to be administered, and is able to manage any adverse actions of the drugs, then parenteral drug administration is advisable. Should these criteria not be met, basic life support should be continued until medical assistance becomes available.

Two parenteral routes of drug administration are available: intravenous and intramuscular.

THE INTRAVENOUS ROUTE

The intravenous administration of drugs affords the dental practitioner an effective means of supportive treatment in many acute emergencies. Drugs administered intravenously act more rapidly than when given by other routes of administration, and their actions are far more predictable. However, venipuncture is an acquired skill which requires training to develop proficiency. Practice on normal, healthy patients is essential if success is to be expected in emergency situations. The dental doctor who is not experienced with the intravenous route should feel no moral or legal compulsion to attempt its use during an emergency.

Equipment

This suggested list of items is readily available and easily stored in the dental operatory:

1. emergency drugs for injection
2. sterile, disposable syringes (5 ml with 1 1/2", 20 gauge needle attached)
3. alcohol and gauze wipes
4. tourniquet
5. adhesive tape
6. optional — intravenous infusion (5% dextrose and water)
7. optional — intravenous tubing

Technique

The most convenient sites for venipuncture are usually located in the antecubital fossa and on the dorsum of the hand.

As a general rule it is best to select the largest vein available. The tourniquet is placed around the arm to obstruct venous flow and thereby distend the veins. Care should be taken not to stop arterial flow to the area. The patient should then open and close the hand several times and finally keep it closed until the venipuncture is complete (Fig. 11–19).

When veins are small, inadequate distention may occur. Gentle slapping of the vein or application of heat will induce a reflex dilatation of the vessel walls. Nitrous oxide/oxygen sedation will also assist dilatation.

After the injection site has been prepared with a skin disinfectant, the vein is ready for entry. This is achieved by placing the needle, with the bevel up, beside the vein with the needle parallel to the long axis of the vein. The thumb of the other hand is positioned so that with slight tension on the skin, the vein is stabilized (Fig. 11–20).

Figure 11-19 A tourniquet, impeding venous return to heart, is placed above the antecubital fossa. If arterial blood flow into the arm is unimpeded, the veins in the arm will distend.

The needle is placed at a 45 degree angle to the skin, and, with a gliding motion, is introduced into the vein. A backflow of blood into the syringe indicates venous entry. Now the needle is cautiously advanced well within the lumen of the vein (Fig. 11–21).

The tourniquet is released, the fist is unclenched, and the selected drug or drugs injected slowly. It is always well to titrate drugs into the blood stream while noting the patient's reactions. If an unfavorable reaction occurs before the entire dose is injected, stopping the procedure will minimize the untoward effects of the drug.

After the needle is withdrawn, firm pressure must be placed over the area to prevent the extravasation of the venous blood through the mechanically created rent in the vessel wall.

Figure 11-20 The needle is placed at a 45 degree angle directly over the vein. The bevel of the needle is facing up.

Figure 11–21 Blood flow into the tubing indicates successful venipuncture. The needle is carefully advanced into the vein while tourniquet remains in place.

If a continuous infusion is used the needle must be secured by tape (Fig. 11–22).

Complications

If the needle penetrates the vessel wall after entry into the vein and a portion of the drug is injected into the extravascular tissue, a wheal will form. The needle should be withdrawn and moist heat applied.

On rare occasions a superficial artery may be entered, and the operator

Figure 11–22 If the needle is to remain in the vein it must be secured. Tape is placed over each wing of the needle and across a loop of tubing.

will note a forceful backflow of bright-red blood into the syringe. Certain drugs, if injected, can cause a reflex arterial constriction with possible localized ischemia. If this occurs, the area distal to the injection site may become blanched and quite painful. An injection of 1 per cent procaine solution into the same needle will help to overcome the reflex mechanism.

Phlebitis may be a consequence of irritation by the needle (from prolonged position in the vein) or occur as a reaction to caustic drugs. The patient will complain of pain in the area for several days after injection, and, if the condition is allowed to continue, a thrombus may develop. The inflammation is best controlled by applications of moist heat three or four times daily. This is continued until the area is asymptomatic.

INTRAMUSCULAR ROUTE

When it is not feasible to utilize the intravenous route of administration because of vascular collapse, veins of poor quality, or lack of training, the intramuscular route offers an alternate choice for drug administration. Also, when prolonged action is preferred, a drug injected in a muscle will be more gradually absorbed into the blood stream.

Many sites are available, but the deltoid, gluteus maximus, and vastus lateralis muscles are the most commonly used.

Equipment

5 cc sterile disposable syringe; 20 to 23 gauge, 1 1/2 inch needle; cotton; alcohol; 2 × 2 gauze.

Technique

Deltoid Muscle. If the deltoid muscle is the site of choice, the skin is first cleansed with an antiseptic and allowed to dry. The muscle is then bunched with the thumb and fingers of the left hand, which will raise the muscle away from the underlying nerves, vessels, and bone. The syringe is held in the right hand by the thumb and first two fingers (Fig. 11–23). Entry into the muscle is made by a quick thrust with the needle perpendicular to the skin. The needle should be advanced only three fourths of its length, because, should the needle break, the cannula can be readily grasped with a hemostat. With the needle in the muscle, the syringe is held by the left hand, and negative pressure is applied to the plunger with the thumb and index finger of the right hand. If no blood appears in the syringe, the left hand is returned to its former position of raising the muscle, and the injection is made slowly. After the needle is withdrawn, the area is vigorously massaged to enhance absorption by greater distribution of the drug in the muscle.

Gluteal Area. The upper outer quadrant of the gluteal area is most commonly used for intramuscular administration, and the gluteus maximus is the muscle usually injected.

It is imperative that the upper outer quadrant be properly located, be-

Figure 11-23 Intramuscular injection into the mid-deltoid region.

GLUTEAL AREA

Iliac crest

Gluteus medius

Most frequently used site. Needle enters skin at 90° angle

Superior gluteal A. and V.

Piriformis

Sciatic N.

Gluteus maximus

Posterior view

Most frequently used site. Needle enters skin at 90° angle

Iliac crest

Site recommended by Hochstetter

Gluteus medius

Anterior superior iliac spine

Greater sciatic notch

Piriformis

Sciatic N.

Lateral view

Figure 11-24 The anatomical location of the "safe zone" for gluteal injections. (Redrawn from *Spectrum*, Winter 1964–65, Pfizer Laboratories.)

cause vessels and nerves (particularly the sciatic nerve) are abundant in the upper and lower inner quadrants, and nerve damage here could have grave effects on the extremity. It is recommended that the patient be lying face down with toes in. This position helps to obtain maximum relaxation, and the patient is less likely to see the approach of the needle.

D. J. Hanson[10] recommends that the point of insertion of the needle be lateral and superior to a line drawn from the posterior superior iliac spine to the greater trochanter (Fig. 11–24). Such a line would be lateral to and parallel with the course of the sciatic nerve and any injection lateral and superior to this line will be well away from the nerve.

Before injection, the skin is thoroughly cleansed with alcohol and a needle of adequate gauge and length must be chosen. It should be long enough to penetrate the belly of the muscle, thus avoiding injection into deep subcutaneous tissue which could result in persistent, painful nodules.

Hold the syringe by the index finger and thumb and with the other hand draw the skin of the buttock taut. With the needle perpendicular to the skin, drive the needle into the skin and muscle in a single movement, as though it were a dart. Aspiration should be continued for a few seconds, particularly if the needle has a narrow gauge.

Medications should be expelled slowly to allow time for distention of an accommodating space within the muscle and thereby to avoid pain from pressure-sensitive nerves within muscle tissue.

Vastus Lateralis. The area for injection is a narrow band extending from a handbreadth below the great trochanter to the same distance above the knee

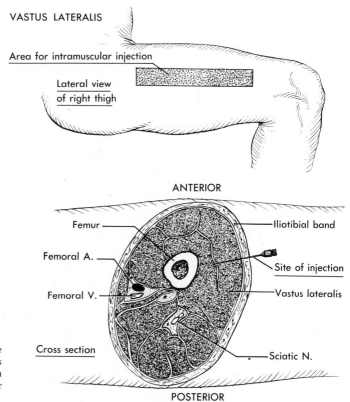

Figure 11–25 The injection site for drug administration in the vastus lateralis muscle. (Redrawn from *Spectrum*, Winter 1964–65, Pfizer Laboratories.)

(Fig. 11–25). It is readily available when the patient is either prone or supine. The needle is inserted to a depth of one inch parallel to the floor.

Serious complications are unlikely in this location, as there are no important nerves or vessels in the area. One other advantage in using this site is that it can readily accept larger quantities of fluid in a single dose than the gluteal muscles.

Wherever the injection is given and whoever gives it, careful training, a knowledge of anatomy, and awareness of the dangers are all prime essentials.

COMMENT

Loss of consciousness is assumed to represent cardiac arrest until proven otherwise. Every dental health professional is obliged to understand and be able to apply at a moment's notice the principles of basic life support. Included in basic life support are airway management, artificial ventilation, administration of positive pressure oxygen, cardiac compression, and monitoring of vital signs. Every dental practitioner must be capable of parenteral drug administration, at least by the intramuscular route. Drug administration is secondary to basic life support. Do not neglect to maintain life by the ABC's while shaking hands fumble with an ampule or a syringe.

REFERENCES

1. Abbey, L. M.: Screening for hypertension in the dental office. J.A.D.A., 88:563, 1974.
2. Allen, G.: Dental Anesthesia and Analgesia. Baltimore, Williams & Wilkins Co., 1972.
3. American Heart Association: Standards for Cardiopulmonary Resuscitation (CPR) and Emergency Cardiac Care (ECC). J.A.M.A., 227 (suppl):833, 1974.
4. American Heart Association: Recommendations for human blood pressure determinations by sphygmomanometry. 1967.
5. Berman, C. L., Guarino, M. A., and Giovannoli, S. M.: High blood pressure detection by dentists. J.A.D.A., 87:359, 1973.
6. Burch, D. E., and DePasquale, N. P.: Primer of Clinical Measurement of Blood Pressure. St. Louis, C. V. Mosby, 1962.
7. Carden, E., and Friedman, D.: Further studies of manually operated self-inflating resuscitation bags. Anesth. Analg., 56:202, 1977.
8. Carden, E., and Hughes, T.: An evaluation of manually operated self-inflating resuscitation bags. Anesth. Analg., 54:133, 1975.
9. Coryollos, P. N.: Mechanical resuscitation in advanced forms of asphyxia: A clinical and experimental study in different methods of resuscitation. Surg. Gynecol. Obstet., 66:698–722, 1938.
10. Hanson, D. J.: Intramuscular injection injuries and complications. Gen Pract., 27:109, 1963.
11. Legal Correspondent. Another death during dentistry. Br. Med. J., 2:352–354, November, 1974.
12. Legal Correspondent. Death during dentistry. Br. Med. J., 2:419–420, August, 1974.
13. McCarthy, F. M., and Malamed, S. F.: Physical Evaluation Manual. University of Southern California School of Dentistry, 1975.
14. Milner, L., Letter: Deaths During Dentistry. Br. Med. J., 2:225–26, October, 1974.
15. Minutes of the House of Delegates, ADA Trans. 1974:643.
16. Mulkey, T. F., and Hayden, C. L.: Monitoring. In McCarthy, F. M. (ed.): Emergencies in Dental Practice. 2nd ed., Philadelphia, W. B. Saunders Co., 1972, Chap. 3.
17. Nicholas, K. E., Letter: An unnecessary hazard in dentistry. Br. Dent. J., 1:83, February, 1975.
18. Safar, P.: Recognition and management of airway obstruction. J.A.M.A., 208:1008–1011, May, 1969.
19. Tomlin, P. J.: Death in outpatient dental anaesthetic practice. Anaesthesia, 29:551–570, 1974.

EMERGENCY DRUGS
AND ALLERGY

W. HOWARD DAVIS

This chapter is intended to present a practical and safe approach to the potentially serious reactions, primarily allergic, that may occur with drugs used in the dental office. It is felt that a dental practitioner should be prepared to cope with these reactions immediately, because occasions do arise when moments may mean the difference between life and death.

ALLERGIC REACTIONS

Introduction

Allergic reactions are usually caused by defects in the immune system. Knowledge in the field of immunology has greatly expanded, but significant gaps in the total picture are still present. The following seem to be important recent contributions: the identification and complex interaction of T and B lymphocytes in the production, utilization, and inhibition of antibodies; the molecular configuration of antibodies; biochemical pathways in the cell which influence mediating and inhibiting substances in allergic reactions;[37, 39] the identification of the elements and role of complement; the identification of more than one histamine type receptor;[3] etc.

Because allergic reactions are incompletely understood, it is not surprising that they are imprecisely defined. The term *allergy* (Greek *allos*, other, and *ergos*, action) seems appropriate to describe the response to a substance when that response is completely different from its usual effect (as penicillin allergy). The terms *sensitivity* and *hypersensitivity* are best used to describe a reaction wherein one responds or is "sensitive" to a substance to which the majority of the species is not responsive (as ragweed sensitivity). However, through custom, the terms *allergy* and *hypersensitivity* are often used interchangeably.

Semantics continues to be a plague when allergic reactions are subdivided, because the terms do not fit all situations. One classification is used that is based on the mechanisms of tissue damage, as suggested by Gell and Coombs[15] (see Table 12–1). Another commonly used classification has two categories based on the speed of onset of the reaction or the presence or absence of antibodies in the serum. One category is *delayed* or *cellular* or *bacterial* and the other is *immediate* or *humoral* or *atopic*.

The cellular (or delayed or bacterial) type reaction appears to be mediated by specifically sensitized lymphocytes reacting with the exciting substance and does not seem to require the presence of *circulating* antibody[4] (the antibodies appear to be attached to the surface of the lymphocyte).[30] The clinical lesions of cellular allergy may proceed from erythematous papules to serum-filled vesicles to oozing areas with crusting. Microscopically, these lesions show a highly cellular perivascular infiltrate of mononuclear cells. Histamine does not play a significant role in this process, and thus antihistamine drugs are not of specific value in cellular (or delayed or bacterial) type reactions. Many contact allergies fall into this category (as poison ivy) as well as bacterial skin tests (as tuberculin tests), graft versus host reactions, and viral exanthema. Because the cellular (or delayed or bacterial) type allergy is slowly progressive, it does not fall into the category of an emergency and will not be further discussed in this chapter.

The other gross category of allergic reactions is the humoral, immedi-

TABLE 12–1 CLASSIFICATION OF ALLERGIC REACTIONS BASED ON MECHANISMS OF TISSUE DAMAGE (AFTER GELL AND COOMBS)[29a]

Type	General Term	Immune Reactant	Suggested Mechanism of Tissue Damage
I	Anaphylactic	Reaginic antibody; primarily Ig E	Mediators from Ig E-sensitized mast cells cause increased vascular permeability, edema, and smooth muscle contraction
II	Cytotoxic	Ig G or Ig M antibody against cell-surface antigens	Antibody (generally with complement) reacting with cell-surface or cell-attached antigens results in cell destruction
III	Toxic antigen-antibody complex	Immune complexes	Immune complexes fix complement, which attracts leukocytes; mediators released from these cells produce inflammation
IV	Cell-mediated	Lymphocyte	Lymphocytes reacting with antigens release lymphokines, which produce cellular inflammation

ate or atopic. All the reactions in this category appear to be involved with appropriate antibodies, usually circulating in the serum.

Some diseases such as Arthus reactions, serum sickness, and possibly polyarteritis and glomerulonephritis, feature the deposition of antigen-antibody complexes in or near vessel walls and perivascular collections of polymorphs. These conditions are sometimes classified as humoral or immediate because of the relation of this category to antigen-antibody involvement, but they fall poorly within the classification of immediate reactions.

More appropriate to the classification of humoral or immediate are those reactions related to anaphylaxis. Anaphylaxis is not a well-defined term and is applied by some only to allergic (anaphylactic) shock, whereas by others it is broadly used to include local reactions. Among the conditions broadly included in anaphylaxis are anaphylactic shock, allergic rhinitis, gastrointestinal allergy, urticaria and angioedema (angioneurotic edema), and some aspects of serum sickness and bronchial asthma. Anaphylaxis in this chapter will be used broadly and anaphylactic shock as a specific. These lesions are characterized by perivascular serum accumulation with very few cells.

There are several mediating substances involved in anaphylactic reactions, such as skin-sensitizing antibody, histamine, slow-reacting substance of anaphylaxis (SRS-A), serotonin, bradykinin, and others.

Skin-sensitizing antibodies (reagin, atopic antibody) are immune globulins of the IgE class[20] which react with antigens and release histamine from mast cells[22] (and probably from basophils as well). Skin-sensitizing antibody (SSA) is so called because it can be detected in a patient's serum by passive skin tests (Prausnitz-Küstner test). It is probable that SSA interacts with other substances in an anaphylactic reaction.

The actions of histamine are probably responsible in part for many (but not all) of the manifestations of anaphylaxis, such as urticaria, angioedema, blood pressure fall, headache, and bronchial constriction.

Slow-reacting substance of anaphylaxis (SRS-A) is similar in action to histamine. Its action is slower and causes more bronchiolar constriction.[6] SRS-A is not antagonized by antihistamine drugs. Bradykinin and serotonin have questionable roles in human anaphylaxis. The precipitation of cardiac arrhythmias may be a part of anaphylactic shock.[5]

Some light has been shed on the mechanism of antigen formation. High molecular weight substances such as proteins and polysaccharides[1] can act as an antigen without modification. However, low molecular weight substances must fix themselves to a high molecular weight substance such as a protein to act as an antigen (haptenic reaction). Furthermore, more than one of these low molecular weight substances must combine with a protein (polyvalent) to act as an antigen.[7] As a matter of fact, if this low molecular weight substance is present without combining with a protein on a multiple basis, it will *block*[13] this specific antigen-antibody precipitation. Penicillin is a low molecular weight substance which seems unable to attach itself irreversibly to a protein, and thus it cannot act as a haptenic antigen.[12] But degradation products of penicillin can fix themselves to a protein and thus act as an antigen.[10] On this basis, reagents are being formulated to test for penicillin allergy using degradation products of penicillin. The most promising agents are penicilloyl-polylysine[27] and minor determinate mixture. Penicilloyl is a metabolite of penicillin, and when it is combined with polymerized lysine, penicilloyl-polylysine is formed. This substance seems to induce little or no allergenicity[27] and thus is acceptable as a testing agent.

TESTS FOR ALLERGY

Because testing for allergy is not completely reliable, a patient's history of allergic reactions becomes quite important. If a patient reports no allergic reaction to the medications that may be used, no further testing is required. If an allergic reaction is reported to a medication for which a substitute can be prescribed, no further testing is required. Fortunately, most medications used in dentistry have adequate substitutes. For example, erythromycin can usually be substituted for penicillin, and procaine can be substituted for lidocaine. Rarely a patient will report allergies to almost all medications or all local analgesic agents, etc. A careful history and investigation will often reveal that the patient is exaggerating or the patient has been told he or she is allergic to medications when the reactions were not true allergies. This is a common finding when a patient has had fainting episodes associated with local analgesia, or nausea with analgesic medications. However, when the history indicates that medications must be used to which the patient may be allergic, testing should be carried out.

A practical approach would be to begin the testing process using the radioallergosorbent test (RAST). This test is an in vitro assay of the patient's reagenic antibodies (IgE) to a specific antigen.[41] The RAST test is probably the most practical present day in vitro method to test for humoral (immediate, atopic) type allergies. A RAST panel would be appropriate, including several agents for the class of medications desired. For example, a local analgesic panel might include methylparaben (a common preservative), lidocaine, prilocaine, mepivacaine, procaine, etc., or an antibiotic panel might include penicillin G, ampicillin, phenoxymethyl penicillin (penicillin V), nafcillin, cephalexin, erythromycin, tetracycline, and clindamycin. Although the RAST test usually correlates well with the clinical response to a drug, it is not completely predictive. Thus, skin testing is a logical succeeding test after the RAST tests have suggested the least likely allergenic medications.

A scratch or prick test is done first. The scratch test involves making a shallow scratch through the epidermis (not drawing blood) of the volar surface of the forearm. A dilute solution of the agent to be tested is then applied to the scratch. The dilution of the solution should be related to the potential severity of a possible reaction. In the case of penicillin, for example, the dilution could be 5 to 1000 units/ml, related to the history and the RAST results. The prick test is favored by some over the scratch test.[19] The prick test is performed by placing a drop of the test solution on the forearm and puncturing the skin through the liquid. If the scratch or prick test is positive, a wheal and flare should occur within 20 minutes. If a systemic reaction occurs, a tourniquet may be applied proximal to the test site (although this has questionable value) and epinephrine and other drugs administered as described later in the chapter. If a very dilute solution was used initially, such as 5 units of penicillin per ml, and the test was negative, the test should be repeated with a more concentrated solution (10,000 units per ml of penicillin,[36] for example).

If the scratch or prick test proves negative, it would be appropriate to follow with an intracutaneous test. A minute amount of the test solution (about 0.02 ml) is injected in the epidermis of the forearm and the site observed for 20 minutes for the possible wheal and flare reaction.

A detailed description of a serial dilution method of subdermal testing is described by Incaudo, et al.[19a]

If the cutaneous tests are negative, it is reasonable to proceed with judicious administration of the drug, keeping in mind that skin tests are not completely reliable.

Skin testing may elicit misleading results in several ways. For example, if the *test* material is old and contains breakdown products of penicillin which readily fix with proteins (as discussed above), it may be easy to elicit a positive allergic response, whereas the actual *therapeutic* product may be fresh and not contain such breakdown products. Likewise the *test* material may contain an allergenic substance in the diluent[35] which is not present in the *therapeutic* material, or vice versa. A pure fresh product used as a test material may give a negative scratch test because no degradation products are present, but when placed in the body tissue it may break down and form antigenic material, giving a serious reaction. This is why it would be desirable to use substances such as penicilloyl-polylysine and minor determinate mixture intradermally[38] after a scratch test. From the above considerations, it is easy to see why a scratch test is not completely reliable.

Testing of drugs on mucous membranes is similar to scratch testing, but generally more dangerous, because most drugs are more readily absorbed from mucous membranes than from skin, and a tourniquet cannot be placed to limit circulation in mucous membrane areas.

The *indirect basophil degranulation* test is less commonly used since the advent of the RAST test, but its mechanism is as follows. In the presence of an antigen-antibody reaction, rabbit or human basophils will release granules which contain histamine.[32, 33] This change of the basophils can be roughly calibrated by someone with cytologic training. Unfortunately the reading of the basophilic degranulation is not simple, and the results are less than perfect. It does have a place in analyzing a patient who has had an allergic reaction while taking several drugs.[33]

A *passive transfer* (Prausnitz-Küstner) test is also useful for identifying an offending substance when there are several possibilities.[18] A nonallergic human or monkey is injected intradermally with the patient's serum. This area is later challenged with the substances to be tested, and usually will give a wheal and flare reaction to the offending agent. This test has obvious drawbacks for mass use.

Hemagglutination tests[40] require much time and are useful primarily for research.

MANIFESTATIONS OF IMMEDIATE (HUMORAL) ALLERGIES

Urticaria (hives) — a pruritic (itching) wheal.
Angioedema (angioneurotic edema) — an edematous swelling of localized area such as one eyelid. The eyelids, lips, tongue, and glottis are com-

mon sites, although most parts of the body can be affected.

Macular or *papular rash* or *flushing* accompanied by pruritis is suggestive of allergy.

Anaphylactic shock — a loss in vascular tone indicated by a fall in blood pressure usually caused by an injected allergen. Prodromal skin signs such as urticaria, flushing, or respiratory signs are often present.

Rhinitis — a pale, boggy swelling of the nasal mucosa with sneezing and watery discharge.

Nausea and/or *diarrhea* — when related to an immediate type allergy, the onset may be close enough to the ingestion of the allergen to help in the diagnosis. The diagnosis is otherwise often difficult to make.

Fever — fever related to an immediate type allergy is not common.

Blood dyscrasias — thrombocytopenic purpura or hemolytic anemia are uncommon with immediate allergies.

Cardiac dysrhythmias — may be a manifestation of allergy that is difficult to define owing to lack of initial diagnosis or spontaneous remission.

Certain allergenic drugs will be discussed in this chapter in varying degrees of detail according to the author's impressions in the light of today's usages and problems.

Aspirin and Angioedema

Aspirin, because of its ubiquitous use and its low incidence of allergic reaction, is commonly overlooked as a cause of allergy.[32] Allergy to aspirin may take several forms, but it is usually of the angioedema or asthmatic[29] type. Although edema of the glottis can be a primary lesion, it frequently follows edema of other areas, such as the lip or tongue. Because of the possible obstruction of the airway by a swelling of the glottis, angioedema must be recognized and promptly treated no matter where the primary lesion occurs.

Another interesting facet of angioedema is the ease with which the lip lesion can be confused with a periapical abscess of an adjacent tooth. When there is swelling of the lip because of a periapical abscess, one can palpate a continuous swelling from the lip to the apical area of the offending tooth; with angioedema, there will be no such swelling over the apex of the tooth.

A familial (autosomal dominant) variety of angioedema deserves attention because of the high incidence (about 30 per cent[24]) of death from laryngeal edema which may be precipitated by dental trauma. This form of angioedema appears to be related to an actual or functional deficiency of C1 esterase inhibitor which results in edema by complex mechanisms. Prophylactic treatment by epsilon-aminocaproic acid (EACA), tranexamic acid,[31] Danazol,[26] and fresh frozen plasma is usually effective, whereas treatment after the edema has occurred is often ineffective.[9a]

Penicillin and Anaphylactic Shock

Penicillin is a notoriously allergenic drug. At the present time, all the chemical variations of penicillin can still be lumped together as far as allergic potential is concerned, although ampicillin more commonly causes skin rashes than other penicillins.

The symptoms of penicillin allergy are extremely variable, but the most common sign is the skin lesion urticaria (hives). The skin lesions can rarely proceed to a dangerous exfoliative dermatitis. The respiratory tract may be affected with angioedema, as described above, or allergic bronchial asthma. The most serious problem is alteration of the circulatory system. Although any of the allergic manifestations can be serious, some warning is usually apparent before a patient is in extremis. This, however, may not be true with the circulatory system. A fatal drop in blood pressure may occur in seconds with no warning. This is anaphylactic shock, and must be dealt with immediately. It is a true medical emergency, in which proper treatment in the first few minutes may mean life or death.

With a condition as serious as anaphylaxis one must consider prevention. In the case of penicillin, an area of prevention worthy of consideration involves the mode of administration. Thousands of cases of anaphylactic shock have been reported after intramuscular injection of penicillin, whereas after oral administration only a relatively few cases have been reported.[23, 25] Using the oral route does not seem to decrease the total incidence of general allergy to penicillin — only the occurrence of anaphylactic shock. Because penicillin can be administered effectively by the oral route in most patients, intramuscular injection of penicillin should be discouraged unless an indication for this route is present.

Allergic nausea or diarrhea is very uncommon with penicillin, but may occur after oral administration and may herald anaphylactic shock, particularly if severe nausea or diarrhea occurs very shortly after orally administered penicillin.

Local Analgesic Agents

Procaine and related esters are capable of inducing the range of allergic reactions just discussed with penicillin. Local procaine reactions are discussed elsewhere in this book. Although systemic reactions to procaine are rare, they sometimes are manifest by such unusual signs and symptoms as prostration, nervousness, disorientation, etc. These unusual reactions to some local analgesics make the diagnosis of allergy to these drugs very difficult. Downs[11] reported a case of procaine reaction which seemed to be due to a lack of cholinesterase function. Kalow[21] and others reported the incidence of 1 in every 2820 persons in whom there is a poorly functional atypical cholinesterase. This results in an inability of these patients to normally hydrolyze the ester types of such local analgesics as procaine. Thus a relatively small dose may produce a toxic reaction.

The diagnosis of allergic versus toxic reactions to local analgesics is further complicated by the fact that the mouth is a very psychically charged area and therefore evokes many emotional episodes of syncope. Because syncope involves a derangement of the peripheral vascular system, it is not possible at first to differentiate syncope from other peripheral vascular disturbances arising from allergic or toxic causes. After having carefully questioned many patients who reported being allergic to various local analgesics, the author found that many times the symptoms and signs were indistinguishable from a marked episode of syncope. One should be very judicious before labeling a patient "allergic" on the basis of such inconclusive signs and symptoms. The probability of a patient's needing local analgesics is so high that a patient with a suspected allergy to a local analgesic agent should be carefully evaluated before a judgment is made.[19a]

Lidocaine and related amides cause rare allergic manifestations, such as angioedema or anaphylactic shock.

Vasoconstrictors

Allergy to the vasoconstrictors is unlikely. Since epinephrine is a normal hormone, allergic reactions should not occur but patients vary markedly in their susceptibility to this group of drugs.

Antibiotics Other Than Penicillin

Even though the reported incidence of allergic reactions to the sulfonamides is somewhat less than with penicillin, such reactions as blood dyscrasias, drug fever, and the common manifestations of allergy have occurred.

The tetracyclines have a low allergenicity, and reactions, when they do occur, usually are limited to mild skin eruptions. Erythromycin estolate (Ilosone) has rarely caused a disturbance of liver function, but only after prolonged use and returned to normal after discontinuance of the drug. This is similarly true of troleandomycin (TAO) except that after previous exposure, prolonged use is not necessary to cause liver dysfunction in those rare patients who are susceptible to this problem. Because it apparently occurs after previous exposure, it is postulated that the reaction may be on an allergic basis.

A cross allergy between penicillin and the cephalosporins (Keflex and Keflin) may occur.

Barbiturates

Relative to allergy, an interesting phenomenon occurs with the barbiturates: the shorter acting the drug, the less likely it is to cause allergy. Allergy to the ultra-short-acting barbiturates, such as thiopental sodium (Pentothal) and methohexital sodium (Brevital), is almost unheard of; allergy to such short-acting barbiturates as pentobarbital sodium (Nembutal) or secobarbital (Seconal) is rare; but allergy following prolonged use of phenobarbital is more common. The allergy to phenobarbital usually takes the form of a measles type rash.

Other Drugs

Some of the more common dental drugs that have demonstrated allergic problems are codeine and related compounds; meperidine (Demerol); morphine; antihistamines; corticosteroids; iodine; mercurials (Merthiolate, Metaphen, etc.); proteolytic drugs (Orenzyme, Chymoral, Ananase, Chymolase); ataraxics (Atarax, Compazine, Equanil, Librium, Miltown, Phenergan, Valium, Vistaril, etc.) Mentioning these drugs may seem superfluous, but it is easy to develop a contempt for their allergic potential when they are used day in and day out with no problems.

TREATMENT

Many signs arising from other causes resemble allergic signs, and rapid differential diagnosis between allergy and other causes may be impossible.[28] Therefore immediate treatment may be essentially symptomatic. Fortunately this is usually safe and effective.

When we discuss allergic phenomena we are frequently speaking of life-threatening reactions. Because some reactions are, may become, or may end as very serious problems, it is important to adopt procedures which will bear scrutiny. With this in mind, our approach will be to suggest therapy that will maximize safety. It goes without saying that many of the succeeding situations will require medical management after initial emergency treatment.

Anaphylactic Shock

Since circulatory failure takes precedence over other situations, it will be dealt with first. It may not be possible at first to distinguish syncope from the first stages of anaphylactic shock, and we will start our outline for treatment as if we were dealing with mild circulatory embarrassment, and then proceed as if the patient were not responding to therapy. The outlined steps should be followed expeditiously, utilizing a team, if possible, until the patient responds.

PALLOR

A common sign that suggests a failing of the circulatory system is pallor although a flush may be prodromal. This will be used as a starting point for treatment.

Place the patient in a supine position. Do not use the head between the knees technique as this could cause serious damage if, for example, cerebrovascular bleeding has occurred.

Next, test the patient's pulse. The carotid artery (just medial to the sternocleidomastoid muscle) is a better location than the radial pulse. If no pulse is present, cardiopulmonary resuscitation should be started immediately (as covered elsewhere in this book). If a pulse is present, proceed to the next step.

Elevate the legs above the torso. Considerable blood can be pooled in the great muscle tissue of the legs, and elevating the legs will return much of this blood to active circulation.

Administer oxygen. These first few steps can be accomplished within seconds by use of assistants.

If the patient is not responding well, the blood pressure should be taken. When the systolic pressure is above 80 mm of mercury and there is no suspicion of allergy, continuation of the above procedures is in order (except for the patient with pre-existing marked hypertension, as discussed below). However, if allergy is suspected as the cause of the fall in blood pressure because other signs of allergy are present, such as urticaria or wheezing respiration, *or* a notoriously allergenic drug was administered, then the immediate therapy for allergy must be instituted (as described below).

INADEQUATE CIRCULATION

If the systolic pressure is below 80 mm/Hg *or* allergic signs are present, consideration should be given to additional therapy. The figure 80 is rather arbitrary and debatable. An article by Cohn and Luria[9] suggests that cuff blood pressure readings which show little or no systolic pressure can be erroneous. They demonstrated this by comparing cuff readings with direct intra-arterial pressure using the femoral artery. One patient, for example, showed no peripheral pressure with a cuff reading, whereas a pressure of 110/70 was demonstrated in the femoral artery. Because it is not practical to measure intra-arterial pressure immediately, we must still rely on cuff readings, but we should probably be more cautious and less energetic in the use of vasopressors.

Notable exceptions to this caution are patients with marked arteriosclerosis or marked hypertension. These patients may require a blood pressure near their average to maintain vital functions.

For the patient with a systolic pressure of less than 80 or when allergic signs are present, the following therapy is suggested. Oxygen should be continued. Now is one of the few times we should depart from symptomatic treatment and make a differential diagnosis; that is, before the selection of a vasopressor.

If you feel that this drop in blood pressure is due to allergy (anaphylactic shock), because of the administration of an allergenic drug or the presence of allergic signs, epinephrine should be administered immediately. Epinephrine has three actions that are desirable in these circumstances: it is a vasopressor; it has an antihistaminic action; it is a bronchodilator. In addition, its action is quite rapid in onset. The dosage range for epinephrine in an adult will vary depending on the severity of the anaphylactic reaction. The drug may be administered intramuscularly or intravenously. When the intravenous route is used, it is probably best to inject fractionally. That is, inject slowly 0.05 mg for minimal blood pressure fall to 0.2 mg for severe blood pressure fall of a 1:10,000 dilution and wait two minutes to evaluate the effect. Repeat this procedure *if necessary* until the patient is improving or the cardiac status suggests the cessation of therapy by exceeding a rate of 150 beats per minute or becomes irregular. The effect of the

IV administration may last only a few minutes, so the IV epinephrine may be followed with 0.3 mg (1/3 ml of 1:1000) IM. The dosage range may be exemplified as follows. If a patient has a pressure of 70/40, an intramuscular dose of 0.3 mg or a slow titration of 0.05 mg per increment would be prudent. The other extreme of the dosage range would be exemplified by a patient who has little or no pulse or demonstrable blood pressure (CPR will be used concurrently if the patient is unconscious and there is *no* pulse). This patient should receive epinephrine intravenously, if possible, in increments of 0.2 mg or more; for various reasons, it might not be possible to use the intravenous route, so the next best thing is to give a 0.5 to 1.0 mg dose intramuscularly. Any accessible muscle mass is acceptable as a depot, including the tongue. If it is possible to enter a vein, it would be well to maintain this route by attaching a drip of 500 ml of 5 per cent dextrose in water, dripping at least 30 drops per minute or more in frank shock. Establishing such a drip while the patient still has adequate intravascular pressure will facilitate subsequent treatment, particularly if the patient's condition deteriorates to the point that intravascular pressure is very low and finding a vein will be difficult. The physician who follows your treatment will be especially appreciative of a patent intravenous infusion.

In treating circulatory dysfunction, it is important to be aware of the difference in treatment that is desirable if the cause of the fall in blood pressure is something other than allergy. As described, epinephrine has beneficial actions related to allergic problems, but its capacity to produce tachycardia and arrhythmia and to raise the blood pressure above normal is especially undesirable for many hypotensive conditions. For example, it is considered undesirable to elevate blood pressure above normal in myocardial infarction or cerebrovascular bleeding. Therefore, unless one is competent to manage the potent vasopressive drugs, it is probably wisest to use a mild vasopressor, such as mephentermine (Wyamine). It is less potent, but relatively safer because it will usually not raise blood pressure above normal. It may be given in doses of 15 to 30 mg intramuscularly or intravenously, depending on the degree of the circulatory problem. When blood pressure is severely depressed, it is usually desirable to use a rapid intravenous infusion of dextrose 5 per cent (and/or lactated Ringer's) in water until improvement is noted, then slow to approximately 60 drops per minute.

After the administration of epinephrine or mephentermine (Wyamine), a corticosteroid may be considered, for it is often beneficial in peripheral vascular problems. It is used secondarily because it may take as long as one hour to act[8, 17] and may not be efficacious. Cortisone is relatively safe for one-dose administration. A product should be used that can be given slowly intravenously or intramuscularly, such as methylprednisolone (Solu-Medrol), 125 mg, or dexamethasone (Decadron),[16] 4 to 20 mg.

An antihistamine may be beneficial in anaphylactic shock in combating histamine release. Chlorpheniramine maleate (Chlor-Trimeton), 10 to 20 mg., brompheniramine maleate (Dimetane) in 10 to 20 mg, or diphenhydramine (Benadryl), 25 to 50 mg may be given intramuscularly or slowly intravenously.

If at any time there is a complete loss of pulse or blood pressure, cardiopulmonary resuscitation should be instituted.

Respiratory Insufficiency Without Circulatory Failure

This usually involves bronchial or bronchiolar constriction owing to edema and/or spasm, and breathing is usually accompanied by an asthmatic, wheezing sound. Another cause of respiratory impairment is edema of the laryngeal area with resultant obstruction.

The strenuousness of treatment should be predicated on the degree of obstruction. If a mild respiratory wheeze is present, inhalation therapy is appropriate. Epinephrine, isoproterenol, and metaproterenol (Alupent) are commonly used. Metaproterenol[14] may be administered as follows: one inhalation is used; if a second inhalation is necessary, two minutes should be allowed before the second inhalation. No more than three inhalations should be used. This therapy is particularly effective for respiratory symptoms secondary to aspirin intolerance. If obstruction is marked, epinephrine is the drug of choice, with the dose of 0.3 ml (0.3 mg of 1:1000 solution) intramuscularly or subcutaneously and repeated every 10 to 15 minutes. If there appears to be complete obstruction of the glottic area by edema, an immediate coniotomy should be done. Because a coniotomy is done through the cricothyroid membrane, it is much more easily accomplished than an emergency tracheotomy. See the chapter on *emergency airway.*

Antihistamines are sometimes effective for glottic edema but may not be effective for bronchial constriction. If appropriate, diphenhydramine (Benadryl) may be used in a dose of 25 to 50 mg intravenously or intramuscularly, depending on severity.

A corticosteroid may be useful. Methylprednisolone (Solu-Medrol) 125 mg or a comparable product used slowly intravenously or intramuscularly is suggested.

Allergic rhinitis can be categorized with skin reactions relative to treatment.

Allergic Skin Reaction

The skin reactions that fall into the potential *emergency* category are those of the anaphylactic type, such as urticaria or flushing with pruritus or angioedema. These skin reactions should be treated promptly because if untreated they may progress to a serious problem such as exfoliative dermatitis, or more important, these lesions may be prodromal to anaphylactic shock, bronchial constriction, or obstructive glottic edema. Recognition and adequate treatment of skin reactions will usually abort these serious problems.

The most important element in evaluating the potential seriousness of an allergic reaction is the interval of time between the administration of the exciting substance and the appearance of the lesion. The shorter this time period, the greater the probability that the reaction will be heralding anaphylactic shock.

Treatment will be related to this criterion. A reaction which occurs over one hour after the administration of the allergen will usually, but not invariably,[2] be of a *nonemergency* nature. Always have the patient available for treatment for at least 24 hours and, if serious signs begin, treat as described under *rapid onset.* The usual treatment for slow onset allergy can be begun with an intramuscularly or orally administered antihistamine such as diphenhydramine (Benadryl) 25 mg intramuscularly or 50 mg orally every six hours. If additional therapy is needed, the patient's physician or allergist should probably be called upon for care.

A potentially serious reaction may be anticipated if the anaphylactic type lesions are produced within one hour (rarely longer[2]) of the administration of an allergenic substance. This situation demands immediate attention as it is a true medical emergency. Three tenths mg epinephrine (0.3 ml of a 1:1000 dilution) should be given intramuscularly or subcutaneously and repeated if necessary. No additional epinephrine should be used if the heart rate exceeds 150 beats per minute or is irregular. Intravenous titration of epinephrine may be used prior to IM administration by giving 0.05 mg (0.5 ml of 1:10,000) slowly with repetition every two minutes until signs are controlled. The intravenous infusion is maintained with dextrose 5 per cent in water.

Then an antihistamine, such as chlorpheniramine (Chlor-Trimeton) or brompheniramine (Dimetane), 10 to 20 mg or diphenhydramine (Benadryl), 25 to 50 mg is given intramuscularly or intravenously.

After the epinephrine and the antihistamine have been administered, a corticosteroid may be used. Eight mg of dexamethasone (Decadron), or 125 mg of methylprednisolone (Solu-Medrol), or a comparable dose of any similar adrenocorticosteroid prepared for intravenous use is acceptable.

Stimulation or Recurrent Convulsions

If during the course of an allergic reaction marked stimulation or convulsions occur, primary attention should be directed to the cardiorespiratory system wherein the cause of the convulsions probably lies. If convulsions persist, a short-acting or ultra-short-acting barbiturate or diazepam (Valium) may be used to control the convulsions.

It is important to use the sedative in a fashion that allows controlled dosage. Because a depressed, exhausted state may follow a series of convulsions, it is important to administer only enough sedative to control the convulsion and not incur the summation effect of drug sedation and the patient's depression. The most controllable form of administration of the sedative is by small incremental intravenous doses. If the intravenous approach is not possible, as will usually be the case during a convulsion, the intramuscular route should be used. To elucidate the intravenous route: diazepam (Valium) 5 mg is administered and a waiting period of 2 minutes is allowed. During this time the full degree of sedation is manifest. This procedure is repeated (5 mg being injected and a 2 minute waiting period) until the desired degree of sedation is achieved. If the intramuscular route is used 10 mg or more may be used.

Reassuring the patient who is excited is also highly important.

Emesis

If a patient vomits while unconscious, as in a convulsion, or in syncope just as he is lapsing into unconsciousness, the elimination of vomitus from the mouth and pharynx is an absolute must. Earlier it was stated that circulatory failure takes precedence over other situations; however, expelling the vomitus of an unconscious patient momentarily preempts even circulatory failure. See the chapter on *general anesthetic emergencies* for detailed treatment.

OUTLINE OF IMMEDIATE ALLERGIC TREATMENT

Keep a copy of this outline (or its equivalent) with your emergency drugs. Have a consultant follow your initial treatment when appropriate.

I. Circulatory problems: Because the etiology of circulatory depression may not at first be apparent, this outline allows a symptomatic approach to therapy
  A. Pallor — quickly do the following (utilize a team if possible)
    1. Supine position
    2. Elevate legs
    3. Pulse (at common carotid — medial to sternocleidomastoid muscle): if none, begin cardiopulmonary resuscitation
    4. Oxygen
    5. Blood pressure — if systolic pressure is above 80, continue this treatment except as follows: if blood pressure stays low for more than a few minutes *or* if allergy is suspected, *or* if there is a history of marked hypertension or arteriosclerosis, then use "inadequate circulation" treatment and seek consultation
  B. Inadequate circulation (have team member contact consultant)
    1. Continue oxygen
    2. Vasopressor
      a. Allergic cause probable (signaled by allergic signs or allergenic drug given moments before reaction)
      Use epinephrine first:
        If systolic pressure is above 60 mm Hg.
        If IV is possible, titrate dosage by giving slowly 0.05 mg (0.5 ml of 1:10,000) epinephrine. Follow with 0.3 mg (0.3 ml of 1:1000 epinephrine subcutaneously or IM for sustained effect. Stop administration if heart rate exceeds 150 or becomes irregular
        If IV is not possible, give 0.3 mg (0.3 ml) of 1:1000 solution IM.
      Systolic pressure below 60:
        If IV is possible, administer 0.2 ml (2 ml of 1:10,000) epinephrine and repeat every two minutes until patient is improving or heart rate exceeds 150 or becomes irregular. Concurrently use rapid IV infusion of dextrose 5 per cent in water until patient is improving, then slow to 60 drops per minute. Follow with 0.3 mg (1/3 ml of 1:1000) epinephrine IM or subcutaneously.
      Use antihistamine after epinephrine
        Depending upon severity, use 25 to 50 mg IV or IM of diphenhydramine (Benadryl) or equivalent
      b. Nonallergic cause probable
      If etiology of circulatory problem is known, be as specific as possible with treatment
      If etiology is unknown, use mephentermine (Wyamine). If the systolic pressure is 60 to 80, or *relatively* low in the hypertensive or arteriosclerotic patient, use 15 mg IM
      If the systolic pressure is below 60, use 30 mg IV or IM; also use rapid IV infusion of dextrose 5 per cent in water

3.   Establish and maintain infusion of dextrose 5 per cent in water at 30 drops per minute (except as noted above)

4.   Use corticosteroid —methylprednisolone (Solu-Medrol) 125 mg or dexamethasone, 8 to 12 mg slowly IV, if possible, or IM (or any equivalent product for intravenous use)

C.   Cardiac arrest — no pulse (use carotid artery to test). Immediately begin cardiopulmonary resuscitation. Use epinephrine early if allergic cause

II.   Respiratory insufficiency: Use oxygen and be sure of patient airway

A.   Mild

Use metaproterenol (Alupent) or equivalent, one inhalation, and wait two minutes. May repeat two more inhalations if necessary

B.   Severe

1.   Use epinephrine, 0.3 mg (0.3 ml of 1:1000) IM, and repeat as necessary

2.   Follow with antihistamine if impairment of airway is due to glottic edema — diphenhydramine (Benadryl) 25 to 50 mg IV or IM, depending on severity

3.   Follow with corticosteroid — methylprednisolone (Solu-Medrol) 125 mg, or dexamethasone (Decadron), 8 mg slowly IV or IM

III.   Skin reactions (urticaria or angioedema): Observe for many hours

A.   Slow onset — beginning one hour or longer after offending drug is administered

Use antihistamine — may begin with oral preparation, such as diphenhydramine (Benadryl) 50 mg every six hours, or begin with an intramuscular dose of diphenhydramine (Benadryl) 25 mg or equivalent, and follow with oral preparation

B.   Rapid onset — beginning within one hour (usually within 15 minutes) after administration of offending drug or whenever serious signs develop

1.   Use epinephrine, 0.3 mg (0.3 ml of 1:1000) IM or subcutaneously and repeat as necessary

2.   Follow with antihistamine — diphenhydramine (Benadryl) 25 to 50 mg IV or IM, depending on severity

3.   Follow with corticosteroid — methylprednisolone (Solu-Medrol) 125 mg or dexamethasone (Decadron), 8 mg slowly IV or IM

IV.   Marked excitement or recurrent convulsions

Allergic convulsions are usually due to circulatory and/or respiratory inadequacy. Treat these problems appropriately

When using a full face mask, continually check for emesis and patency of airway.

If these measures fail to control convulsions or marked stimulation must be controlled, use:

Diazepam (Valium)

If IV is possible, give 5 to 10 mg over one minute and wait two minutes before administering an additional 5 to 10 mg

If IV not possible, give 10 mg IM

Reassure patient who is excited

V.   Emesis while unconscious

Immediately lower patient's head and shoulders below waist, in a prone (not supine) position

Keep mouth open by elevating patient's forehead

A few pertinent notes:

Call a consultant whenever appropriate.

Doses listed are for adults. Proportionately smaller doses should be used for children.

It is helpful to read literature accompanying the drug and underline the part appropriate to your use. This then becomes a quick reminder of pertinent facts that can be reviewed at a glance.

EMERGENCY DRUG TRAYS

As one would suspect, there is no standardized drug regimen to manage emergencies. It, therefore, behooves each practitioner to select the drugs felt to be appropriate for emergency management. Thus, it follows that a commercial drug "kit" will not be applicable for everyone, or perhaps anyone.

It is anticipated that a patient may require emergency care in the office for up to one half hour until the patient can be transported to the hospital if necessary. With this in mind, two sample drug lists have been prepared: one for those practitioners who do not feel comfortable with intravenous medication and another for those who do.

A common indication is listed with each drug along with an average initial dose, but it is imperative that one should review in much greater detail the indications, dosage, and hazards of each drug.

It is helpful to read the literature accompanying a drug and underline the part that would be applicable in an emergency.

Drug doses are listed for adults, and proportionately smaller doses should be used for children.

Substitutions can be made for most of the medications with equivalent products.

Ideally, each practitioner should make an outline of the medications he or she would consider using for possible emergencies and keep this outline with the medications.

Figure 12–1   Illustrated is a set of emergency drugs which may be appropriate for a practitioner who does not feel comfortable with the use of the intravenous route. The drugs shown illustrate both the prefilled syringe type and the multiple dose vials. When the preloaded syringes are used, it is probably wise to keep a duplicate of the dose needed in case of accidental damage to one dose. This could easily happen considering the nervousness that might accompany a severe emergency. (Illustrated are: A, epinephrine; B, diphenhydramine; C, methylprednisolone; D, mephentermine; E, nitroglycerin; F, morphine; G, atropine; H, metaproterenol; I, tourniquet; J, alcohol sponges; K, needles, L, 3 cc syringe; M, 5 cc syringe.)

Figure 12–2   The above trays illustrate emergency drugs which may be appropriate for a practitioner who is proficient with the intravenous route. The drugs related to cardiac arrest are those recommended for Advanced Life Support by the American Heart Association in 1977.

A, A, epinephrine; B, diphenhydramine; C, methylprednisolone, D, sodium bicarbonate; E, atropine; F, lidocaine.

B, A, lidocaine; B, morphine; C, calcium chloride; D, isoproterenol; E, metaproterenol; F, theophylline; G, dopamine; H, nitroglycerin; I, diazepam; J, succinylcholine.

Illustration continued on the following page.

Figure 12–2 *Continued.*
    C, A, naloxone; B, dextrose 5% in water; C, dextrose 50%.
    D, A, tourniquets; B, alcohol sponges; C, 3 cc syringe; D, 5 cc syringe; E, 10 cc syringe; F, IV infusion sets; G, needles; H, IV catheter needles.

It is suggested that a standard be established within the office to routinely check the medications to be sure they are always present and not outdated. Many manufacturers of drugs will ~~~~~~~~~~~ ed medications at no charge.

Figure 12–1 ill~~~~~~~~~~~~~~~~~~~~~~~~~~~~ quipment for the *non-intra-venous* routes, wh~~~~~~~~~~~~~~~~~~~~~~~ enous capability.

Sample Drug List ~~~~~~~~~
the Intravenous R~~~~~~

1. Oxygen, 100 per ~~~~~
   With and with~~~~~
2. Epinephrine
   For anaphylaxi~~~~~
   Dosage, 0.3 to ~~~~~
   Have two doses ~~~~~~~~~~~~~~~~~~~~ on)
3. Diphenhydramine (~~~~~
   For anaphylaxis ~~~~~
   Dosage, 25 to 50 ~~~~~
   Have two doses a~~~~
4. Methylprednisolone ~~~~~
   For anaphylaxis, a~~~~~
   Dosage, 125 mg or ~~~~~
   Have two doses av~~~~~
5. Mephentermine (Wyan~~~~~
   For hypotension tha~~~~~
   Dosage, 15 to 30 mg~~~~~
   Have two doses avai~~~~~ ~~ mg/ml
6. Nitroglycerin (Nitrostat)
   For angina pectoris
   Dosage, 0.3 mg (1/200 grain) to 0.6 mg (1/100 grain) sublingually
   Have at least six fresh tablets available of 0.3 mg
7. Morphine
   For myocardial infarction
   Dosage, 10 mg intramuscularly
   Have at least three doses available of 10 mg/ml
8. Atropine
   For marked bradycardia, accompanied by hypotension, which is symptomatic
   Dosage, 0.5 mg intramuscularly
   Have at least three doses available of 0.5 mg/ml
9. Metaproterenol (Metaprel)
   For mild bronchial asthma
   Dosage, one inhalation 0.65 mg repeated every 3 minutes up to three inhalations
   Have available two inhalers
10. Syringes, needles, tourniquets, and alcohol sponges
11. Sugar packets
    For insulin reaction

Sample Drug List for Office Emergencies when the Intravenous Route Will Be Available

1. Oxygen, 100 per cent
   With and without positive pressure
2. Epinephrine
   For severe bronchospasm
   Dosage, 0.2 to 0.5 mg subcutaneously

For anaphylaxis
Dosage, 0.3 to 1.0 mg intramuscularly or titrate intravenously 0.05 mg every 2 minutes until signs controlled
For cardiac arrest
Dosage, 0.5 mg intravenously and repeated every 5 minutes as needed
Have two doses available of 1.0 mg/ml and two doses of 1.0 mg/10 ml

3. Diphenhydramine (Benadryl)
For anaphylaxis (not for asthma)
Dosage, 20 to 50 mg intramuscularly or slowly intravenously
Have two doses available for 50 mg/ml

4. Methylprednisolone (Solu/Medrol)
For anaphylaxis including asthma, aspiration, or shock generally
Dosage, 125 mg or more intramuscularly or intravenously
Have three doses available of 125 mg/vial

5. Sodium bicarbonate
For acidosis secondary to cardiac arrest
Dosage 1 mEq/kg as an intravenous bolus and repeated as appropriate
Have four doses available of 50 mEq/50 ml

6. Atropine
For marked bradycardia accompanied by hypotension which is symptomatic
Dosage, 0.5 mg as an intravenous bolus repeated as necessary
Have four doses available of 0.4 or 0.5 mg/ml

7. Lidocaine
For ominous ventricular dysrhythmias or ventricular fibrillation
Dosage, 100 mg as an intravenous bolus followed by IV drip of 1 to 4 mg/min
IV drip prepared by adding 2 gm of lidocaine to 500 ml of 5% dextrose in water giving 4 mg/ml
Have available:
2 doses of 100 mg/5ml
2 units of 2 gm/50ml

8. Morphine
For myocardial infarction or acute pulmonary edema
Dosage, 10 to 15 mg intramuscularly or 5 to 10 mg intravenously
Have available three doses of 10 mg/ml

9. Calcium chloride
For cardiac arrest when myocardial action is weak and patient is not digitalized
Dosage, 5 ml of 10 per cent solution
Have available two units of 10 ml of a 10 per cent solution

10. Isoproterenol (Isuprel)
For symptomatic third degree block or sinus bradycardia not responsive to atropine
Dosage, titrate at 2 to 20 µg/min until patient is asymptomatic
IV drip prepared by adding 1 mg of isoproterenol to 500 ml of 5% dextrose in water, giving 2 µg/ml
Have available two units of 1.0 mg vials

11. Metaproterenol (Metaprel)
For mild bronchial asthma
Dosage, one inhalation 0.65 mg repeated every 3 minutes up to three inhalations
Have available two inhalers

12. Theophylline (Aminophylline)
For severe bronchial asthma
Dosage, titrate at 12.5 mg/min intravenously until symptoms abate
Have available two units of 250 mg/20 ml (12.5 mg/ml)

13. Dopamine (Intropin)
For cardiogenic shock
Dosage, start infusion at about 400 µg/min, prepared by adding 200 mg dopamine to 500 ml of 5% dextrose in water. Titrate very carefully to restore peripheral blood pressure to about 90 mm Hg
Have available two ampules of 200 mg

14. Nitroglycerin (Nitrostat)
       For angina pectoris
       Dosage, 0.3 mg sublingually
       Have available at least six tablets
15. Diazepam (Valium)
       For status epilepticus or severe recurrent convulsions
       Dosage, 5 mg/min intravenously (if possible) until seizures controlled
       Have available 10 doses of 5 mg/ml
16. Succinylcholine (Anectine)
       For laryngeal spasm
       Dosage, 10 to 20 mg intravenously and repeated as needed
       Have available five doses of 20 mg/ml
17. Naloxone (Narcan)
       For reversing narcotic excess
       Dosage, titrate 0.1 mg intravenously every 2 minutes until desired effect
       Have available at least two doses of 0.4 mg/ml
18. Dextrose 50%
       For hypoglycemic coma
       For initial use in any seizure disorder
       Dosage, 50 mg intravenously
       Have available three doses of 25 mg/50 ml
19. Dextrose 5% in water
       For diluting drugs for slow intravenous dosage, for correction of hypovolemia,
       for maintaining a patent intravenous route
       Have available two units of 500 ml
20. Alcohol sponges, IV infusion sets, syringes, IV needles including IV catheter-
       needles
21. Tourniquets
       Have available four tourniquets long enough to use around limbs in acute
       pulmonary edema
22. Sugar packets
       For insulin reaction

ACKNOWLEDGMENT

I should like to acknowledge the assistance of Dr. Joseph Tulumello, Dr. Elaine Cooper, Frances Ishii, Janice Frembling, and Kathleen Incardona.

COMMENT

It is emphasized that each preceding sample list of emergency drugs and equipment is exactly that, a *sample* of what the clinician might choose. Neither list should be considered as a suggested standard of care, nor is it intended to be so considered. The intricacies and unknowns of emergency medicine, and the varying training and experience of practitioners, make standardization of drug kits both impossible and undesirable. The real consistencies of emergency medicine are constant change and the inability of experts to agree on standards.

The general practitioner is not expected to perform as a medical specialist in the event of a life-threatening emergency but *is* expected to act promptly in supplying non-drug life support (ABC's of resuscitation), followed by drug support as circumstances and individual training and experience allow.

The general practitioner, rather than choosing the drugs on the "non-intravenous sample" list, might feel more comfortable with a modification, such as: aromatic spirits of ammonia, sugar packets, nitroglycerin, oxygen (with and without positive pressure), epinephrine, and diphenhydramine.

REFERENCES

1. Austen, K. F.: Systemic anaphylaxis in man. J.A.M.A., *192*:116, 1965.
2. Barnard, J. H.: Nonfatal results in third-degree anaphylaxis from Hymenoptera stings. J. Allerg., *45*:94, 1970.
3. Black, J. W., et al.: Definition and antagonism of histamine H_2-receptors. Nature, *236*:385, 1972.
4. Bloom, B. R., and Chase, M. W.: Transfer of delayed-type hypersensitivity. A critical review and experimental study in the guinea pig. Progr. Allerg., *10*:151, 1967.
5. Booth, B. H., Patterson, R.: Electrocardiographic changes during human anaphylaxis. J.A.M.A., *211*:627, 1970.
6. Brocklehurst, W. E.: Slow reacting substance in anaphylaxis (SRS-A). *In* Wolstenholme, G. E. W., and O'Connor, C. M. (eds.): Ciba Foundation Symposium on Histamine. Boston, Little, Brown & Co., 1956, p. 175.
7. Campbell, D. J., and McCasland, G. E.: In vitro anaphylactic response to polyhaptenic and monohaptenic simple antigens. J. Immunol. *49*:315, 1944.
8. Cochrane, G. C., et al.: Evaluation of adrenal steroids administered intravenously, intramuscularly, and orally. J. Clin. Endocrinol., *13*:933, 1953.
9. Cohn, J. N., and Luria, M. H.: Studies in clinical shock and hypotension. J.A.M.A., *190*:113, 1964.
9a. Delfino, J., et al.: Management of a patient with hereditary angioneurotic edema. J. Oral Surg., *36*:890, 1978.
10. de Weck, A. L., and Eisen, H. N.: Some immunochemical properties of penicillenic acid. An antigenic determinate derived from penicillin. J. Exper. Med., *112*:1227, 1960.
11. Downs, J. R.: Atypical cholinesterase activity. J. Oral Surg., *24*:256, 1966.
12. Eisen, H. N., et al.: Elicitation of delayed allergic reactions with haptens: the dependence of elicitation on hapten combination with protein. J. Exper. Med., *95*:473, 1952.
13. Farah, F. S., et al.: Specific inhibition of wheal-and-erythema responses with univalent haptens and univalent antibody fragments. J. Exper. Med., *112*:1211, 1960.
14. Garra, B., et al.: A double-blind evaluation of the use of nebulized metaproterenol and isoproterenol in hospitalized asthmatic children and adolescents. J. Allergy Clin. Immunol., *60*:1, July 1977.
15. Gell, P. G. H., and Coombs, R. R. A.: Clinical Aspects of Immunology. 2nd ed., Philadelphia, F. A. Davis, 1968, p. 580.
16. Grater, W. C.: Cortical steroid choice analogy. Ann. Allergy, *21*:454, 1963.
17. Grater, W. C.: Intravenous hydrocortisone in allergy. Ann. Allergy, *13*:191, 1955.
18. Harris, M. C., and Shure, N.: Sudden death due to allergy tests. J. Allergy, *21*:208, 1950.
19. Imber, W. E.: Allergic skin testing: A clinical investigation. J. Allergy Clin. Immunol., *60*:47, July 1977.
19a. Incaudo, G., et al.: Administration of local anesthetics to patients with a history of prior adverse reaction. J. Allergy Clin. Immunol., *61*:339, May 1978.
20. Ishizaka, K., Ishizaka, T., and Hornbrook, M.: Allergen-binding activity of IgE, IgG and IgA antibodies in sera from atopic patients. In vitro measurements of reaginic antibody. J. Immunol., *98*:490, 1967.
21. Kalow, W.: Hydrolysis of local anesthetics by human serum cholinesterase. J. Pharmacol. Exper. Therap., *104*:122, 1952.
22. Keller, R.: Mast cells and anaphylaxis. Experientia, *18*:286, 1962.
23. Kern, R. A., and Wimberly, N. A., Jr.: Penicillin reactions: Their nature, growing importance, recognition, management and prevention. Am. J. Med. Sci., *226*:357, 1953.
24. Landerman, N. S.: Heredity angioneurotic edema. I. Case reports and review of literature. J. Allergy, *33*:316, 1962.
25. Maganzini, H. C.: Anaphylactoid reactions to penicillin administered orally. N. Engl. J. Med., *256*:52, 1957.
26. NIH: Male hormone prevents hereditary angioedema, corrects inherited abnormality which may be cause. J.A.M.A., *238 (19)*:2010, 1977.
27. Parker, C. W., et al.: Hypersensitivity to penicillinic acid derivatives in human beings with penicillin allergy. J. Exper. Med., *115*:821, 1962.
28. Prickman, L. E.: Anaphylactic reactions. Minnesota Med., *45*:905, 1962.
29. Salvaggio, J. E., et al.: Aspirin induced bronchial asthma. J.A.M.A., *188*:323, 1964.
29a. Schatz, M., et al.: Immunopathogenesis of hypersensitivity pneumonitis. J. Allergy Clin. Immunol., *60*:27, 1977.
30. Sell, S., and Asofsky, R.: Lymphocytes and immunoglobulins. *In* Kallos, P., and Waksman, B. A. (eds.): Progress in Allergy, White Plains, N.Y., Phiebig, 1968, Vol. 12, P. 135.
31. Sheffer, A. L., et al.: Tranexamic acid: preoperative prophylactic therapy for patients with hereditary angioneurotic edema. J. Allergy Clin. Immunol., *60*:38, July 1977.
32. Shelley, W. B.: Birch pollen and aspirin psoriasis. J.A.M.A., *189*:986, 1964.
33. Shelley, W. B.: Indirect basophil degranulation test for allergy to penicillin and other drugs. J.A.M.A., *184*:171, 1963.

34. Shelley, W. B.: New serologic test for allergy in man. Nature, *195*:1181, 1962.
35. Siegel, B. B.: Studies in penicillin hypersensitivity. V. J. Allergy, *33*:349, 1962.
36. Testing for penicillin allergy with aqueous penicillin, G. Medical Newsletter, *17*:84, Sept. 26, 1975.
37. Vane, J. R.: Inhibition of prostaglandin synthesis as a mechanism of action for aspirin-like drugs. Nature New Biology, *231*:232, 1971.
38. Voss, H. E., et al.: Clinical detection of the potential allergic reactor to penicillin by immunologic tests. J.A.M.A., *196*:679, 1966.
39. Walker, J. L.: The regulatory role of prostaglandins in the release of histamine and SRS-A from passively sensitized human lung tissue. Advances Biosci., *9*:235, 1973.
40. Watson, K. C.: Effect of various penicillin compounds on haemagglutination of penicillin-coated erythrocytes. Immunology, *5*:610, 1962.
41. Wide, L.: Clinical significance of measurement of reaginic (IgE) antibody by RAST. *In* Clinical Immunology — Allergy — in Paediatric Medicine. London, Blackwell Scientific Publications, 1973.

13

CARDIOVASCULAR AND OTHER MEDICAL EMERGENCIES

JOHN J. LYTLE

INTRODUCTION

A proper pretreatment physical evaluation will avoid most encounters with a medical emergency in the dental office. Nonetheless you must be prepared to cope with any emergency that may arise. The two most important requirements in the treatment of an office emergency are good judgment and an adequate supply of oxygen.

Certain broad groups of diseases will be discussed from the standpoint of pathologic physiology, symptomatology, and office treatment during acute episodes. A knowledge of various risk diseases seen in dental practice will allow you to provide a better service to your patient, and could prove to be lifesaving.

"Doctor, I'm feeling pain in my chest." Every dental practitioner should be prepared to respond intellectually, emotionally, and actively in an appropriate manner to that complaint.

Chest pain is not a clinical finding but a subjective symptom which may indicate that a life-threatening emergency is about to take place in your office. A rush of thoughts should flash through your mind, computing again the patient's age, previous history of cardiovascular disease, the apparent severity, onset, duration, and possible radiation of this pain. You will simultaneously be aware of the patient's skin and mucosal color, noting any developing pallor or diaphoresis (profuse sweating). Quite possibly you will be recalling the patient's preoperative blood pressure, or, more likely, be wishing that one had been obtained.

At this point you may remember that experienced older hands always said, "keep calm." Your composure and attitude toward the patient can markedly affect the progression of events. Keeping calm is usually a function of understanding the cause of the problem and the course of treatment to be undertaken. This requires preparation before the emergency arises, which is why you are reading this chapter.

BRONCHOPULMONARY DISEASES

PULMONARY EMPHYSEMA

The pulmonary emphysema patient who is ASA Class II or III (review the ASA classification in Chapter 2) will be treated in the office without special concern, except possibly for pharmacosedation. When using inhalation sedation, do not deliver less than 30 per cent oxygen; when supplying oxygen enrichment only, deliver 3 liters per minute via nasal cannula. *No* oxygen supplementation should be supplied to the ASA Class IV emphysema patient (rest dyspnea) if emergency dental care is given in the office.

An emphysema crisis is uncommon, but may occur. Should severe rest dyspnea with cyanosis and tachycardia occur, withhold oxygen if possible and call for assistance. The emphysema patient tolerates a very high arterial carbon dioxide tension. Lowering the carbon dioxide tension by administration of 100 per cent oxygen may cause cessation of breathing. If circumstances force the use of 100 per cent oxygen, be prepared to artificially ventilate the patient until transfer to competent paramedical or medical personnel.

BRONCHIAL ASTHMA

Bronchial asthma is a chronic reversible lung disease characterized by episodes of dyspnea produced by bronchospasm, mucosal edema, and the accumulation of secretions in the tracheobronchial tree. The patient's medical history will almost certainly reveal previous episodes of asthmatic attacks.

If a patient develops an acute asthmatic attack *without* a previous history of asthma the clinician should be thinking of a possible acute allergic reaction to medication and the possibility that the reaction will progress to anaphylaxis with circulatory collapse.

Clinical Findings

The patient will become aware of difficulty in breathing. Inspiration occurs without difficulty, but expiration will become prolonged and associated with characteristic "wheezing." The patient may become cyanotic and will want to sit up and perhaps lean forward to assist ventilation. The patient may become very restless and agitated if no remedial action is taken.

Treatment of a Severe Asthmatic Attack

1. Position the patient in a sitting position — leaning forward if that increases comfort.
2. Administer oxygen 100 per cent by an appropriate full face mask at a comfortable rate.
3. Begin monitoring blood pressure and pulse rate at frequent intervals.
4. Administer epinephrine, 0.3 ml of a 1/1000 aqueous solution subcutaneously.
5. If the patient fails to improve dramatically within 10 minutes of the epinephrine injection, transfer to an acute care hospital facility by ambulance.
6. Be prepared to support collapse of the cardiovascular system in the event the asthmatic attack represents the prodrome of an anaphylactic reaction.

CARDIOVASCULAR DISEASES

CONGESTIVE HEART FAILURE

Congestive heart failure (CHF) is that clinical syndrome occurring when the heart is unable to pump enough blood to meet the metabolic demands of the body. Usually the condition develops slowly and can result from a great variety of disease entities affecting the cardiovascular system. It may develop rapidly in the patient who suffers a myocardial infarction in your office. The prudent dental practitioner should not find himself treating the final decompensating stages of slowly developing CHF. Patients presenting with dyspnea, extreme fatigue, neck vein distention, pitting edema of the lower extremities, and rales in the lung bases on auscultation should be referred for medical management. Dental care should be deferred until the patient has been returned to a state of reasonable cardiac compensation.

During 20 years of dental practice, I have had two patients in serious stages of cardiac decompensation present for dental treatment. Both of these patients felt bad teeth was the cause of their extreme fatigue, dyspnea, and ankle swelling. One 38 year old woman with longstanding mitral valve incompetence tried, unconvincingly, to have me remove several grossly carious teeth. Her uncompensated congestive failure was so severe I urged immediate hospitalization for management of the cardiac problem. She expired the following day at home.

The other patient I vividly recall was a 67 year old man who had recently moved across the country to live with his family on the West Coast. He had a long history of coronary artery disease and had congestive heart failure requiring digitalis and diuretics. His selection of a physician in this new environment unfortunately resulted in one who attempted to manage the cardiovascular problem with diet and herbal preparations. During a six month period without his former medications he slowly decompensated and presented in my office short of breath, extremely fatigued, and concerned that an abscessed tooth was at the bottom of all his trouble. Pitting edema of the lower extremities, prominent neck veins, a positive hepato-jugular reflex, and basilar rales were present, and this patient was advised that the tooth was not the "root" of his problem. I referred him to an internist who reversed his decompensating cardiovascular status and one month later the oral problem was treated without incident.

Patients with a history of congestive failure who appear well compensated and adequately medicated, usually with a diuretic, a low sodium diet, and a digitalis preparation, can be managed very safely in the office environment. The well compensated patient does not suddenly and precipitously decompensate due to the stress associated with a dental procedure unless another problem such as an acute myocardial infarction supervenes. However, the borderline patient (ASA Class III) may decompensate in the office as a result of the emotional and physical stresses of dental treatment. See Chapter 2 for review of ASA classification.

Symptoms and Findings in Congestive Heart Failure

The well compensated patient with a history of previous congestive failure episodes usually can be managed uneventfully and will not present with the findings that follow. These findings may develop slowly as a result of chronic progressive cardiovascular disease or rapidly if this is an acute problem, such as a myocardial infarction affecting the heart's ability to pump blood.

The extreme fatigue that may be noted cannot be attributed to just one side of the heart but must be attributed to both. Decreased peripheral blood flow to the brain can produce mental confusion and stupor. Decreased circulation to the lower limbs can result in deep vein thrombosis. Decreased renal blood flow will result in blood chemistry alterations such as creatinine and blood urea nitrogen elevations. The chronically congested liver produces cardiac cirrhosis characterized by impaired liver function. Fibrosis of the liver occurs with the passage of time.

It is suggested that you review the pathologic physiology of congestive heart failure in Chapter 2 before proceeding.

Treatment of Congestive Heart Failure

Slowly developing congestive heart failure will respond favorably to the following:

1. *Bed rest:* This alone may correct any acute bout of CHF by reducing the demands on the heart.
2. *Low salt diet:* Since CHF initiates powerful sodium retaining mechanisms and these to some extent are responsible for the edema in the lungs and lower extremities, limitation of sodium intake greatly aids in the resolution of CHF.

3. *Diuretics:* Thiazide diuretics, mercurial diuretics, and Lasix (furosemide) mobilize edema fluid and aid in the excretion of sodium. Electrolyte imbalance is a potential complication of diuretic use which may be avoided by regular blood chemistry determinations.
4. *Digitalis:* This agent causes increased strength of myocardial contraction and improves cardiac output in low output failure. There are many different digitalis preparations available. They may be given intravenously, intramuscularly, or orally.

Treatment of Rapidly Developing Congestive Heart Failure

Rapidly developing heart failure occurring in the dental office should be managed as follows:

1. Administer oxygen 100 per cent by full face or nasal mask.
2. Apply rotating tourniquets to the four extremities. This bloodless phlebotomy can effectively reduce circulating blood volume by trapping as much as 700 ml in the extremities. Release one tourniquet for 5 minutes at a time, and continue this rotation.
3. Morphine sulfate 10 mg to 15 mg will specifically improve circulatory dynamics and reduce apprehension.

The decision on how far to carry treatment of rapidly developing CHF will be up to the individual clinician. It is appropriate to transport the patient with rapidly developing congestive heart failure to an acute hospital as quickly as possible. There, the underlying cause of pump failure can be determined and specific therapy directed toward the etiology as well as symptomatic treatment of the failing pump.

CORONARY HEART DISEASE

Angina Pectoris

In Chapter 2 angina pectoris and myocardial infarction were described and recommendations were made for managing the patient with a history of either disorder. Elderly individuals, known diabetics, and patients who describe previous anginal episodes, previous myocardial infarctions, and relief of chest pain with nitroglycerin are more likely to develop a cardiovascular emergency than are young people or those with no history of cardiovascular problems or diabetes. This does not mean that the latter do not develop cardiovascular emergencies, it is just less likely that they will. You will be much more concerned about the sudden onset of severe substernal pain in an elderly diabetic with a history of angina pectoris and a previous myocardial infarction than you might be if a 21 year old, healthy football player describes substernal (precordial) chest pain. We have all read accounts of sudden cardiovascular collapse in a previously healthy young individual, but it is far less likely than in the elderly, medically compromised patient.

The proper management of patients with a known history of cardiovascular disease must be individualized. These patients will benefit from careful preoperative assessment of cardiac reserve and control of preoperative anxiety with appropriate oral or parenteral sedation. Profound local analgesia, short, relatively atraumatic procedures, the availability of oxygen, and careful postoperative management of anxiety and pain are all important considerations. Even after carefully following these principles, a patient may develop chest pain and require immediate management.

MANAGEMENT OF CHEST PAIN OF SUSPECTED CARDIOVASCULAR ORIGIN

Any time chest pain develops before, during, or after dental treatment, one's attention should be focused upon obtaining pain relief for the patient. One of the most significant anxiety-producing factors for the distressed patient is an anxious attitude on the part of the clinician and his or her auxiliaries. It is imperative that you remain calm and stay with the patient until the immediate problem is resolved. An apparently calm doctor transmits confidence to staff and patient. This does not mean that the doctor should act unconcerned. One can demonstrate concern and still minimize anxiety-producing factors in the patient. The dental therapy should be interrupted until the anginal episode is past, and it might be unwise to proceed with elective treatment after the pain has subsided.

Loosen tight collars, coat buttons, scarves, corsets, or brassieres if present, and remove plastic aprons which may cause discomfort by retaining

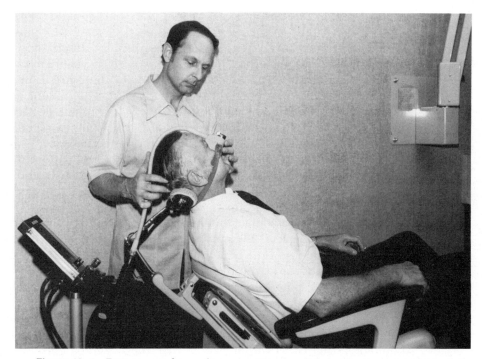

Figure 13-1 Patient seated in reclining position, head above chest, receiving oxygen by mask and being carefully observed.

body heat. Administer oxygen at a comfortable rate through an appropriate, comfortably fitting nasal hood, nasal cannula, or carefully held full face mask. This is comforting and reduces anxiety, and may in itself stop the pain. Be certain the patient is in a comfortable position. Generally, this is not lying flat, but is usually obtained by raising the head somewhat above the chest to a semi-reclining position (Fig. 13–1).

TREATMENT OF ANGINA PECTORIS

Give nitroglycerin from the patient's own fresh supply or from your emergency supply if the patient has none. In Chapter 2, it was suggested that the 0.30 mg strength be given from your fresh supply (not over six months old) if you are premedicating a patient to prevent angina. Once a full-blown anginal attack has occurred, 0.45 mg or 0.6 mg can be given. Two tablets from your office supply (0.30 mg), normally used for prophylaxis, can be safely given. If the patient is experiencing increasingly severe pain and your initial nitroglycerin dose is not effective within two to three minutes, amyl nitrite may be administered by inhalation. This is a potent vasodilator which can produce the side effects of headache, flushing, and occasionally syncope. I recommend reserving amyl nitrite for the most severe pain of unquestioned origin. If no relief is obtained within 10 to 15 minutes of your active intervention, including the administration of oxygen, you may assume that a myocardial infarction has occurred. Immediate transportation to the hospital is imperative. Further material on angina pectoris is included under Myocardial Infarction.

Myocardial Infarction

The patient with myocardial infarction usually describes severe, unremitting, crushing, substernal (precordial) pain. It is vise-like and may radiate down the left arm, up toward the jaw or to the neck. Less frequently, the pain radiates to the back or to the right side. The patient may become nauseated and weak and may express fear of imminent death. He or she should be placed in a position of comfort. All tight garments should be loosened and oxygen should be administered immediately.

The clinical signs become apparent quickly. The patient may develop an ashen pallor. The blood pressure may drop precipitously and an arrhythmia may develop. One should immediately call for outside assistance. If a well trained paramedic group is available in your community, this service is the best source to contact. An emergency telephone number should be available for instant use. Minutes are important in the early management of myocardial infarction. If an arrhythmia is present, the paramedics can begin immediate electrocardiographic monitoring, start an intravenous infusion, and continue the blood pressure monitoring and the oxygen administration which you initiated.

If paramedics are not available, it may be possible to develop a working agreement with a nearby physician who will respond to an emergency should it arise. However, it seems that these agreements are subject to many shortcomings. The most obvious is that the physician may not be available when you need him. According to a corollary of Murphy's Law, a severe cardiovascular emergency would be most likely to occur when the physician is unavailable.

An ambulance service without paramedic capabilities would be the second most effective agency to call for assistance in managing the problem of acute myocardial infarction occurring in the office. It is imperative that you stay with the patient to supervise supportive care and to continue monitoring until that responsibility can be transferred to an emergency room physician.

Each practitioner must decide how far he or she will go in the management of an acutely ill patient with suspected myocardial infarction. To monitor the pulse, blood pressure, and state of consciousness, to administer oxygen, and to be prepared to provide basic life support, ventilation, and closed chest cardiac massage are the *inescapable* basic responsibilities of all dental practitioners.

More advanced care, including the administration of pain relieving narcotic drugs, the support of blood pressure, and the management of arrhythmias may be beyond the scope of the general practitioner's expertise. However, the clinician who utilizes intravenous sedation and ultralight general anesthesia should be prepared to provide advanced life support. This will include the support of blood pressure, electrocardiographic monitoring, the treatment of arrhythmias with appropriate pharmacologic agents, and the management of cardiac arrest, including defibrillation of an electrically and functionally incompetent myocardium.

SUMMARY OF STEPS IN MANAGING ANGINA PECTORIS

1. Stop the dental treatment and direct your attention toward abolishing the pain.
2. Immediately administer nitroglycerin from the patient's own supply or from your fresh emergency supply. Give 0.6 mg (two 0.3 mg tablets).
3. Simultaneously administer 100 per cent oxygen by nasal cannula, through an appropriate nasal hood, or via a comfortable full face mask (Fig. 13–2).
4. Make certain the patient is comfortable, loosen restricting garments, remove plastic patient throws, rubber dam, etc.

This should resolve the anginal episode and you and the patient should decide whether or not to continue dental therapy. This is a judgment decision, and will depend upon the severity of the attack. If any doubt exists, do not perform further elective treatment at that appointment.

5. If the pain does not subside following the nitroglycerin administration within 3 to 4 minutes or, if the pain is very intense initially, an amyl nitrite ampule should be broken and the contents inhaled. This should produce pain relief within 30 seconds.
6. If relief is not obtained following these steps, you must assume that you are facing a more serious problem; perhaps a myocardial infarction has occurred and the patient should be removed as quickly as possible to a hospital emergency room facility.

Nitrous oxide in a concentration of 35 per cent has been shown to ame-

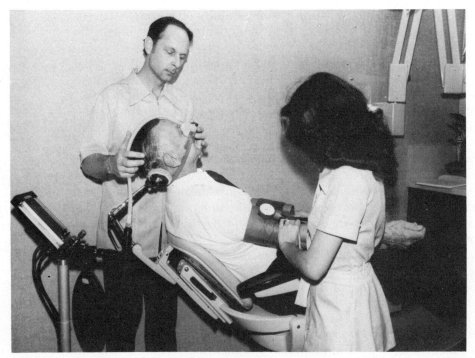

Figure 13–2   Patient seated in reclining position with oxygen being administered by nasal mask. Nurse checking blood pressure. Nitroglycerin may be easily administered with this arrangement.

Figure 13–3   Pitting edema of the lower extremities. Note that thumb pressure on the dorsum of the foot leaves a noticeable depression on the edematous foot which remains for several minutes.

liorate the pain of acute myocardial infarction. This use of nitrous oxide has not been accompanied by hemodynamic changes or significant adverse reactions. While this treatment is not a standard of care, it would be perfectly proper to utilize the agent in the dental office for relief of angina pectoris or acute myocardial infarction pain, the balance of the gas mixture being 65 per cent oxygen. It is my opinion that the favorable action of nitrous oxide in this instance results primarily from sedative rather than analgesic action.

SUMMARY OF FINDINGS AND MANAGEMENT OF MYOCARDIAL INFARCTION

Usually several, but not necessarily all, of the following are present:

1. crushing substernal (precordial) pain with or without radiation to arms, jaw or back
2. pain is not relieved by coronary artery vasodilators, oxygen, and rest
3. fear of impending death
4. nausea
5. ashen pallor
6. thready pulse
7. arrhythmia
8. drop in blood pressure
9. unconsciousness

EMERGENCY TREATMENT

1. Position patient comfortably, usually not supine, but with the head slightly elevated.
2. Monitor the pulse and blood pressure.
3. Give 100 per cent oxygen by mask.
4. Give nitroglycerin or amyl nitrite (nitroglycerin: two tablets, 0.3 mg size) (amyl nitrite, via ampule).
5. Transfer the patient to an acute emergency facility as soon as possible.
Optional treatment which may be indicated:
6. Begin an intravenous infusion of 5 per cent dextrose in water. Run very slowly just to maintain the intravenous route.
7. A narcotic can be given if pain is overwhelming and more than 10 to 15 minutes will elapse between onset and transfer to an emergency room. Demerol, 25 to 75 mg, or morphine sulfate, 6 to 10 mg, may be given IM.
8. Cardiopulmonary resuscitation may be necessary if arrest occurs, and one must be prepared to provide that treatment if required.
9. Stay with the patient until transfer to a physician's care in an appropriate emergency facility has been accomplished.

CEREBROVASCULAR DISEASES

CEREBROVASCULAR ACCIDENT

Patients may sustain a cerebrovascular accident or "stroke" in the dental office. Intracranial hemorrhage produces 25 per cent of cerebrovascular accidents. This emergency is most likely to occur while an individual is active during the day — perhaps visiting your office. The remaining 75 per cent of cerebrovascular accidents result for the most part from cerebral ischemia, have significantly different symptoms and findings, usually develop more slowly, and are not likely to present as a medical emergency in the dental office.

Intracranial Hemorrhage

The primary cause of this problem is hypertensive cerebrovascular disease. Other causes are atherosclerotic vascular disease, cerebral aneurysm, arteriovenous malformations, head trauma, and miscellaneous unusual causes such as ingestion of methamphetamine, or "speed," and blood dyscrasias. The untreated hypertensive patient beyond age 55 should be considered a potential candidate. Intracerebral hemorrhage classically presents with the onset of a sudden extremely severe headache. Nausea, vertigo, and severe neurologic deficit such as hemiplegia and/or coma may develop. The rapidity and severity of the developing neurologic symptoms is related to the amount and rate of intracranial bleeding.

The patient should be positioned as comfortably as possible, with slight elevation of the head and upper body. Tight garments should be loosened and oxygen via a full face mask should be given at a comfortable rate to an awake patient. If the patient loses consciousness, an oral airway should be placed and careful observation of respiration should be maintained and assisted ventilation instituted if respiration slows or stops.

These patients should be transferred to an acute care hospital facility as rapidly as possible by ambulance. As soon as you suspect the possible development of the sequence of events described above, a call should be made to obtain an ambulance. The practitioner should avoid giving medications to sedate the patient or to ease the pain if an intracranial hemorrhage is suspected because this may mask rapidly changing neurologic symptoms resulting from the hemorrhage.

This series of events is most likely to occur in older hypertensive patients; however, it may occur in young adults, suggesting rupture of a berry aneurysm, or in a child, suggesting bleeding from an arteriovenous malformation. Your primary responsibility as a dental practitioner is to recognize the potential seriousness of sudden onset of severe headache, nausea, and rapidly developing neurologic deficit, to protect the patient's airway if unconsciousness occurs, to support respiration, and to transport the patient by ambulance to a hospital as rapidly as possible.

Cerebral Ischemia

Ischemia of cerebral vessels makes up the vast majority (75 per cent) of cerebrovascular accidents. Neurologic deficit is usually slower in developing. Headache, nausea, and vomiting are not prominent. Frequently the patient awakens in the morning to discover the neurologic deficit which has resulted from ischemia occurring during the night.

Patients presenting for dental treatment with a history of weakness, change in gait, loss of speech, or any other serious neurologic deficit of very recent origin should be carefully evaluated prior to any dental treatment. Elective treatment should be deferred until there has been stabilization of deteriorating neurologic status.

Cerebral Embolism

This type of cerebrovascular accident makes up a very small per cent of problems. Sudden onset of deteriorating neurologic function usually occurs, without severe headache and with a systemic medical problem such as endocarditis; recent myocardial infarction, or congenital heart disease capable of producing a thrombus would lead one to suspect this possible cause of cerebrovascular accident.

Emergency treatment of both ischemic cerebrovascular disease and embolic cerebrovascular disease is the same. Should sudden deterioration of neurologic status occur in the dental office, support the vital functions of respiration and transfer the patient by ambulance as rapidly as possible to a hospital facility.

VASODEPRESSOR SYNCOPE

Vasodepressor syncope is defined as a transient loss of consciousness resulting from decreased cerebral blood flow following a drop in blood pressure evoked by anxiety or pain. This entity is the common faint and has also been called vasodepressor shock, hysterical reaction, and psychic reaction.

Syncope is a minor cardiovascular emergency that every dental practitioner will see on numerous occasions during his or her professional career. Diagnosis and treatment are straightforward and relatively simple. If fainting occurs during or after the administration of medications, the doctor should be concerned that what appears to be a syncopal episode may be a reaction to the medication. It is important to differentiate between syncope and toxic or allergic reactions. If an elderly patient with known cardiovascular or cerebrovascular problems experiences a syncopal episode, differentiation from cerebrovascular insufficiency of more serious etiology, such as cerebrovascular accident, must be considered.

In the minds of many persons anxiety and fear of pain are associated with dental treatment despite our efforts to minimize the discomforts associated with dental procedures. In offices where every effort is made to conceal all dental instruments, where patients never see blood and never are subjected to sounds or odors which may evoke syncope, a few patients still faint.

I have made every effort to minimize anxiety-producing factors in my practice, and I have the impression that a pleasant environment without the sights, sounds, and smells associated with pain does reduce the number of patients fainting, but it does not eliminate the problem entirely. Patients may be extremely fatigued or debilitated, or they may have fasted for an excessive period prior to their visit and sensitized their vasopressor mechanism to react to the slightest anxiety-producing factor such as entering a dental office.

Preoperative sedation, short or no preoperative waiting in the reception area, pleasant, concerned personnel, and complete pain control in a pleasant nonthreatening environment enable concerned clinicians to manage the syncope-prone individual once he or she has been identified.

Clinical Findings in Syncope

Pallor of the skin or oral mucosa is often the first indication of impending syncope. The patient may then volunteer that he feels weak, and perspiration may appear and is sometimes profuse. The patient may experience nausea, and some may regurgitate gastric contents.

If no corrective measures are taken the patient will become unconscious. Convulsions may accompany the lapse of consciousness. A marked drop in blood pressure will be noted. The pulse which initially may have been rapid and thready slows markedly (bradycardia). The pupils may be dilated. Cardiac arrest must be assumed until proven otherwise.

Treatment of Syncope

The patient should immediately be placed in a reclining position with his head at or slightly below the level of the heart. One hundred per cent oxygen should be administered via an appropriate full face mask. The blood pressure and pulse rate should be monitored, and aromatic spirits of ammonia may be inhaled intermittently. The patient should immediately begin to regain consciousness and may be momentarily confused (Fig. 13–4).

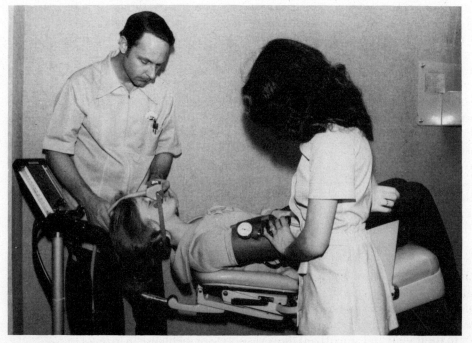

Figure 13–4   Patient in dental chair fully reclined with head at or below the level of the heart. Oxygen is being administered by mask, and blood pressure is being monitored.

The practitioner and auxiliaries should remain calm and reassure the patient that the situation is under control. The patient should be made comfortable by loosening tight or warm garments. A cool, moist towel applied to the forehead or to the back of the neck may be helpful.

The patient should not be allowed to stand quickly or walk unattended. If the faint has occurred in a location such as the reception room or in the doorway, he or she should be assisted to a more appropriate recovery area. The decision to proceed or to initiate planned dental treatment that day depends on the individual. In some instances, it will be possible to continue dental therapy but in others it may well be indicated to appoint the patient for another time and perhaps to utilize a different anesthetic approach or to suggest preoperative sedation. If syncope occurs before or during a sedative procedure, elective treatment should be discontinued. The cardiovascular system requires some hours to fully recover from complete syncope.

SUMMARY OF FINDINGS

1. The patient feels weak.
2. The patient may feel nauseated.
3. Perspiration appears on the brow.
4. Skin and mucosa are noticeably blanched.
   This is followed by:

5. Dilatation of the pupils.
6. Initial tachycardia which proceeds to bradycardia.
7. Marked hypotension.
8. Unconsciousness.
9. Occasionally convulsions precede or accompany the lapse of consciousness.

Differential Diagnosis

1. Orthostatic hypotension is an autonomic disorder in which syncope occurs when the patient assumes the upright position, as after a lengthy dental appointment in the semirecumbent position. There is a sharp fall in arterial blood pressure, followed by syncope, but there is no drop in pulse rate and no symptoms of pallor, sweating, and nausea. Consciousness quickly returns in the recumbent position.
2. Cardiac conduction defects such as the Adams-Stokes syndrome (pulse rate of 40 with short periods of asystole), reflex cardiac standstill, carotid sinus syncope, ventricular tachycardia, paroxysmal tachycardia, and ventricular fibrillation show no prodromal symptoms of vasodepressor syncope. Diagnosis is based upon sudden syncope, history, pulse evaluation, and other physical signs. Air hunger should be treated with oxygen. See the chapter on *cardiopulmonary arrest*.
3. Hyperventilation syndrome usually produces faintness, but not actual syncope, and is associated with acute anxiety. It is readily controlled by breath-holding or rebreathing into a paper bag or a reservoir (pressure) bag of the inhalation sedation machine.
4. Cough syncope follows a paroxysm of explosive coughing usually associated with bronchitis. Syncope is brief and there are no residua. It is caused by

Figure 13–5 Do not press the patient's head forward between the knees. This illustrates the incorrect way to treat syncope in the dental chair. The patient cannot be monitored, observed, or have respiration assistance with oxygen in this position.

a marked increase in intrathoracic and intra-abdominal pressures, causing a sharp elevation of cerebrospinal fluid pressure with resultant fleeting cerebral hypoxia.

5. Hysterical fainting is usually seen in young women with emotional illness. The attack commonly occurs in the presence of others, the patient gracefully crumpling to the floor without injury. There are no irregularities of pulse, blood pressure, or skin color.

6. Hypoglycemia. See insulin shock under diabetes mellitus.

MANAGEMENT OF PATIENT IN SYNCOPE

1. Position the patient in the supine position with the head at or slightly below the level of the heart. *Do not* press the patient's head forward between the knees in the sitting position (Fig. 13–5).

2. Administer 100 per cent oxygen by full face mask.

3. Monitor the blood pressure, pulse, and respirations. This is especially important if medications have been given immediately prior to syncope.

4. Intermittent administration of spirits of ammonia by inhalation during recovery may be useful.

5. Loosen tight clothing.

6. A cool, moist towel may be applied for patient comfort.

ENDOCRINE DISEASES

DIABETES MELLITUS

It is estimated that 5 per cent of the population are predisposed to diabetes mellitus. Two per cent are overt diabetics, 2 per cent are undiagnosed, and 1 per cent are undiagnosed and probably unrecognizable by available testing methods.

Diabetes is a heritable metabolic disease which most dramatically affects carbohydrate metabolism. Most commonly, insulin production by the beta cells in the islets of Langerhans of the pancreas decreases or stops entirely, and the classic clinical signs and symptoms of the disease are seen. In younger persons with rapid clinical expression of the disease process, weight loss, fatigability, excessive thirst (polydipsia), and excessive urination (polyuria), associated with a ravenous appetite (polyphagia) occur when alternate metabolic pathways, primarily for utilization of fats, are called upon to produce energy normally supplied by carbohydrate metabolism.

In older persons, diabetes is frequently associated with obesity, and the decreased insulin production is not as dramatic as in young individuals. In older diabetics the changes that take place in the cardiovascular system, the kidneys, the nervous system, and the eyes may be more distressing to the patient and of more concern to the dental practitioner. See Chapter 2 for diabetes classification.

The medical history obtained by the clinician and his or her auxiliary staff should uncover the known diabetic who presents for care. With current emphasis on education of the diabetic patient to enable him to understand and live with his disease, management of dental procedures in these patients should pose minimal problems for the knowledgeable practitioner.

Emergencies Associated with Diabetes Mellitus

The most frequent emergency the clinician is likely to encounter in treating diabetics is related to insulin overdose (hypoglycemic coma). A knowledgeable diabetic may take a normal dose of insulin and, owing to the fear or anxiety associated with impending dental treatment, fail to eat a sufficient amount of food. This individual may feel nervous, begin to perspire, become agitated, and become unconscious and convulse if not given carbohydrate in the form of sugar, orange juice, or candy, which can be quickly utilized.

Physicians treating patients who present unconscious in a hospital emergency room are impressed and gratified to see a patient respond dramatically to an intravenous dextrose bolus. You should have available a source of readily absorbable carbohydrate to prevent insulin reactions in anxious diabetic patients.

The second way a diabetic patient may become unconscious in your office is by developing diabetic (hyperglycemic) coma. This is extremely unlikely, but possible. A known diabetic, perhaps a teenager rebelling against an unwanted disease, may not take sufficient insulin to prevent ketoacidosis. This patient would probably be stuporous upon presentation in the dental office but may be seeking help for an acute infectious process which increases metabolic demands and leads the patient to think that dental treatment alone would improve his fatigue, lassitude, thirst, excessive urination, and acetone breath. It will not.

Treatment should consist first of recognizing that a potential medical emergency is developing in your office. The patient should be placed in a supine position, vital signs should be carefully monitored, oxygen should be administered, and a determination made as to the quickest way to transfer this patient by ambulance to an acute care hospital facility. If circulatory collapse seems imminent, based on low blood pressure, an intravenous route should be established if possible.

A frequent area of concern in managing the unconscious diabetic relates to the administration of glucose to a patient in diabetic coma, *not* one experiencing an insulin reaction. If you suspect that the problem may be related to hypoglycemia, give intravenous dextrose. This will not significantly adversely affect a patient in diabetic coma, but it will be immensely helpful in reversing an insulin overdose.

A final area of concern to the practitioner managing diabetics relates to the effects of the disease process on the cardiovascular system. Diabetic patients may develop occlusive vascular problems which predispose to premature myocardial infarction and to cerebrovascular accidents as well as to peripheral vascular problems. These patients should be managed more conservatively than the average patient. Follow the stress reduction protocol outlined in Chapter 2.

ADRENOCORTICAL INSUFFICIENCY

Hydrocortisone and aldosterone are two of the hormones produced by the adrenal cortex which are required for cardiovascular homeostasis (normal state). Patients presenting for dental care may have, either slowly or rapidly, lost the ability to produce these hormones for many reasons such as adrenal tuberculosis or idiopathic adrenal failure, or following adrenalectomy. These patients tolerate stress poorly and may decompensate under stress of dental treatment.

Recognizing the Patient with Adrenocortical Insufficiency

The medical history obtained by the clinician is the primary tool for establishing the presence of this problem. Patients with a well documented history of loss of adrenal function will under almost all circumstances be taking steroids on a regular basis. Generally these patients are managed without altering their regular steroid dose.

The most potentially serious problems are related to patients who have been given steroids for suppression of inflammatory responses associated with a multitude of metabolic, autoimmune, arthritic, or asthmatic conditions. The steroids are tapered off and discontinued as soon as practical, often leaving the patient with a suppressed endogenous steroid production mechanism. This patient may feel weak, tired, chronically nauseated and may relate all symptoms to bad teeth. Here again, the carefully taken medical history will alert the practitioner to the potential problem. After consultation with a physician, steroid supplements should be administered prior to dental procedures.

Treatment of an Acute Hypotensive Episode Related to Adrenocortical Insufficiency

1. Place the patient in a supine position with the head comfortably elevated.
2. The legs should be elevated at least to the level of the heart.
3. Monitor the vital signs and record the blood pressure and pulse rate at frequent intervals.
4. Administer 100 per cent oxygen via a suitable full face mask.
5. If possible, start an intravenous drip of isotonic saline and run in as rapidly as possible. Monitor the blood pressure response to intravenous fluids. Four to five liters of isotonic saline may be required to obtain a therapeutic response.
6. Administer hydrocortisone (Solu-Cortef) as an IV push or alternately dexamethasone (Decadron) immediately.
7. Transfer the patient by ambulance to an acute care hospital facility.

CONVULSIVE DISORDERS

GRAND MAL EPILEPSY

Epilepsy is characterized by spontaneously occurring clinical seizures resulting from abnormal neuronal discharge which spreads throughout the brain. It may develop without apparent cause, sometimes has a genetic link, and may follow brain injury, infections, or tumor.

Patients occasionally experience isolated convulsions as a result of a toxic amount of a drug such as lidocaine, occasionally during a syncopal episode, and occasionally with an intracerebral hemorrhage (rare). Children may experience a convulsion with a sudden temperature elevation associated with a systemic infection. These types of convulsions are not related to epilepsy.

The patient's medical history is the most important tool the dental practitioner has at his or her disposal to identify the patient with epilepsy. When a patient indicates that epilepsy is present, the clinician should be certain that the individual is taking an anticonvulsant agent on a regular basis. The most common agent in use is Dilantin, frequently used in combination with phenobarbital, but many other agents are also commonly in use.

Dental treatment should be planned so the patient is fully rested and perhaps sedated at the office visit.

Recognition of a Grand Mal Seizure

A grand mal seizure is characterized by a series of events which are certain to impress any first time observer. The patient may experience an aura, described as a visual, auditory, gustatory, or olfactory sensation which precedes the loss of consciousness. The patient falls to the ground if standing and becomes rigid in extension, the "tonic" phase. Classically, the patient under-goes a "clonic" phase in which rhythmic contraction and extension of the extremities occurs and the patient thrashes about uncontrollably and can sustain injury. The patient then enters a postictal, somnolent phase and may sleep for variable periods of time, sometimes hours. During the tonic and clonic phase the patient may bite his tongue, and a protective bite block, a gauze roll, or even a towel or washcloth placed between the teeth may be useful. The patient may appear cyanotic, and occasionally excess saliva appears as a frothing of the mouth.

Treatment of Grand Mal Seizure

1. Protect the patient from injury. This may include gently restraining the patient in the dental chair or on the floor. It will include protecting the tongue from injury during the active tonic and clonic phases with an appropriate bite block or other device (Fig. 13–6).
2. Oxygen administration may decrease central nervous system ischemia and reduce the partial neuronal death which accompanies every grand mal seizure to some extent (Fig. 13–7).
3. Intravenous diazepam (Valium) 5 to 10 mg may be given if the clinician is equipped to administer medications by this route and is able to treat any respiratory depression that could result.

Figure 13–6   Patient on the floor during seizure. The tongue should be protected from in-jury by teeth with the use of a mouth prop. In this illustration, a tightly rolled cloth towel is employed.

Figure 13–7 Patient on the floor with the airway supported and oxygen being administered through a full face mask.

4. Hospitalization may be indicated. It is suggested that you seek medical advice following the seizure.

OTHER TYPES OF EPILEPSY

There are numerous other types of seizure disorders which may occur. Petit mal disorders, or small seizures involving transient loss of consciousness or awareness of surroundings, are common and may actually go unrecognized. Focal, or jacksonian, seizures involving a single limb may occur during dental treatment. Patients with these disorders do not require emergency medical management, although it is important that the practitioner recognize these problems and refer the patient for proper management when required.

MANAGEMENT IN PREGNANCY

Treating the pregnant woman with dental disease can be extremely difficult. The dental problem itself is usually straightforward, complicated by temporarily altered physiology. Superimposed on this modestly more complicated circumstance is a group of factors, popular superstitions, governmental regulations, and legal precedents which collectively can make dental care of the pregnant female a harrowing experience.

Pregnancy is not a disease state. The condition normally persists for 10 lunar or nine calendar months. Nine of 10 pregnancies conclude successfully with the birth of a healthy offspring. For many reasons, approximately one of 10 pregnancies does not conclude successfully. Medications, maternal pathology, and other environmental factors can affect the developing fetus unfavorably.

The treating clinician must first assess the dental complaint. Is the problem one which requires definitive treatment immediately to protect or restore the patient's well being? What will the result of not treating the patient be? Can temporary treatment be undertaken and definitive therapy completed after delivery of the child?

Secondly, the practitioner must assess maternal health. Is the mother basically healthy? Is this a normal pregnancy uncomplicated by threatened abortion or other pathological processes which could result in fetal damage whether or not dental treatment is undertaken? Is this an unusually valuable pregnancy? I define an unusually valuable pregnancy as one occurring for the first time in a woman who has been attempting to achieve pregnancy for more than three years and who has finally developed this desired condition.

Having obtained favorable answers to the basic questions relating to the magnitude of the dental disease and the actual state of the pregnancy, I then want to assess the intangible factors which may cause the biggest problem in patient management.

Does the patient understand the facts of her pregnancy? Is she unusually fearful of the effects of anesthetic agents on the fetus? Has she been misinformed as to the effects of her dental disease on fetal development? Is she unusually apprehensive about the effects of dental treatment on the fetus?

If the patient has a significant dental complaint, such as a painful, abscessed tooth which requires extraction, and has an uncomplicated pregnancy and no unusual superstitions or anxieties which militate against treatment, I manage the patient exactly as I manage any other, non-pregnant woman.

Generally, a pregnant woman beyond the first trimester of pregnancy who has no history of previous abortions and who currently has no complications of pregnancy (spotting or cramping), can undergo needed dental treatment without the dental practitioner being open to criticism. Problems in management arise when the clinician finds himself or herself in a position to be criticized by the patient, her family, her physician, or her attorney if the pregnancy is unsuccessful and the dental treatment can be implicated, which it invariably can, since such a complaint is rarely based upon either facts or reason.

The medications commonly used in dentistry such as local analgesics, narcotics, barbiturates, and antibiotics do not produce problems in the developing fetus if used in reasonable therapeutic amounts for the short periods usually necessary to accomplish the goals of dental therapy.

Package inserts must indicate that safe use of a particular medication has not been established unless carefully controlled studies have proved that a particular drug has no effect on the developing fetus. Since these experiments have frequently not been done, an appropriate warning to that effect is included in the package insert. Food and Drug Administration regulations, coupled with a tremendous glut of eager professional liability attorneys, place the practitioner in a precarious position. Much anguish and harm has been visited upon patients and health practitioners by extrapolating animal experimentation to the human experience. One example of such fuzzy thinking is yogurt-induced cataracts in rats. Rats on a 100 per cent yogurt diet develop cataracts because they cannot tolerate galactose, which makes up 1.5 to 2 per cent of commercial yogurt. An occasional human cannot metabolize galactose. It has been suggested that a warning label be placed on yogurt containers.

The patient must be apprised of all potential problems and risks before treatment is instituted. It seems prudent to obtain a signed consent for treatment from pregnant patients which spells out the fact that potential risks have been explained prior to any planned dental procedure.

The practitioner should inquire into the patient's attitude about radiographs, medications, antibiotics, and regional or general anesthetics before embarking on a course of treatment. The patient who requests extraction of a difficult tooth, but who refuses radiographic study or antibiotic administration, places the clinician in a compromised position should these agents be required.

Generally, from a professional liability defense posture, elective dental procedures should be deferred until the patient delivers. If the practitioner and patient mutually decide to undertake an elective procedure, the treatment should be performed during the second trimester of pregnancy.

In summary, I would say that this area of dental practice can be successfully managed if the dental practitioner carefully evaluates the patient and her family's attitudes toward dental care. The patient should make the decision as to whether a procedure should be undertaken. If the doctor perceives that the patient may not be willing to accept all of the necessary aspects of the procedure, such as radiographic studies and/or antibiotic therapy, these facts should be carefully discussed and documented on the record, and it might be wise to refuse treatment. The patient cannot give up her rights to legal redress by agreeing to care which the practitioner feels is substandard.

Further views on the perplexing problem of management in pregnancy are given in Chapter 5.

COMMENT

Laryngeal, bronchial, and esophageal foreign bodies are reviewed in Chapter 2; the Heimlich maneuver is presented in both Chapters 17 and 19, while tracheotomy is covered in Chapter 19 and cricothyrotomy in Chapter 17. Allergic manifestations are reviewed in Chapter 12, with emphasis upon anaphylactic shock and surgical shock. Chapter 11 is devoted primarily to basic life support, while Chapter 14 covers cardiopulmonary resuscitation in depth. Other chapters are devoted exclusively to complications of regional and general anesthesia.

Certain other diseases are not covered in this chapter because the possibility of an attendant life-threatening emergency in the dental office is so remote. For example, a sickle cell crisis or polycythemia vera CVA will be treated symptomatically until the patient is transported to the hospital. Good judgment, a calm attitude, and judicious utilization of oxygen will help the practitioner to hold the fort until the patient can be moved. The reader is reminded to refrain from administering 100 per cent oxygen to the emphysema patient with rest dyspnea.

420 CARDIOVASCULAR AND OTHER MEDICAL EMERGENCIES

SUGGESTED READING

1. Cahill, G. F.: Diabetes mellitus. *In* Beeson, P. B., and McDermott, W. (eds.): Textbook of Medicine. 14th ed., Philadelphia, W. B. Saunders Co., 1975, Chap. 806, pp. 1599–1618.
2. Crevasse, L.: Congestive heart failure. *In* Conn, H. F. (ed.): Current Therapy 1977. Philadelphia, W. B. Saunders Co., pp. 197–201.
3. Dack, S., Acute myocardial infarction. *In* Conn, H. F. (ed.): Current Therapy 1977. Philadelphia, W. B. Saunders Co., 1977, pp. 221–226.
4. Earp, H. S., and Ney, R. L.: Adrenal insufficiency. *In* Conn, H. F. (ed.): Current Therapy. Philadelphia, W. B. Saunders Co., 1977, pp. 487–488.
5. Forcheimer, L. L.: Yogurt induced cataracts in rats, J.A.M.A., *217*:1113, 1971.
6. Glasser, G. H.: The epilepsies. *In* Beeson, P. B., and McDermott, W. (eds.): Textbook of Medicine. 14th ed., Philadelphia, W. B. Saunders, 1975, Section 16, pp. 723–743.
7. Heyman, A.: Syncope. *In* Beeson, P. B., and McDermott, W. (eds.): Textbook of Medicine. 14th ed., Philadelphia, W. B. Saunders, 1975, Chap. 353, pp. 626–629.
8. Innes, I. R., and Nickerson, M.: Norepinephrine, epinephrine and the sympathomimetic amines. *In* Goodman, L. S., and Gilman, A. (eds.): The Pharmacological Basis of Therapeutics. 5th ed., New York, Macmillan, 1975, Chapter 24, pp. 477–511.
9. Lyon, L. Z., and Wishan, M. S.: Management in pregnancy. *In* McCarthy, F. M. (ed.): Emergencies in Dental Practice. 2nd ed., Philadelphia, W. B. Saunders Co., 1972, pp. 487–488.
11. Skelton, C. L.: Angina pectoris. *In* Conn, H. F. (ed.): Current Therapy 1977. Philadelphia, W. B. Saunders Co., 1977, pp. 168–172.
10. Ojemann, R. G.: Intracerebral and intracerebellar hemorrhage. *In* Youmanns, J. R. (ed.): Neurological Surgery. Philadelphia, W. B. Saunders Co., 1973, Vol. 2, Chap. 38, pp. 844–851.
11. Skelton, C. L.: Angina pectoris. *In* Conn, H. F. (ed.): Current Therapy 1977. Philadelphia, W. B. Saunders Co., 1977, pp. 168–172.
12. Thompson, P. L., and Lown, B.: Nitrous oxide as an analgesic in acute myocardial infarction. J.A.M.A., *235*:924–927, 1976.

14

CARDIOPULMONARY ARREST

THOMAS W. QUINN

INTRODUCTION

Cardiac arrest can occur in the dental office. It is imperative that *all* dental practitioners and their assistants be familiar with the emergency measures associated with cardiopulmonary resuscitation. This chapter will review the proper management of cardiac arrest in the office.

For the clinician who does not utilize the intravenous route, basic life support is in order. For those practitioners who administer intravenous agents for sedation or general anesthesia, a program of advanced life support will be outlined.

DIAGNOSIS OF CARDIAC ARREST

When a patient collapses in the dental office, emergency resuscitative efforts must be instituted immediately. It is mandatory to differentiate between cardiac arrest and other forms of the unconscious state, such as vasodepressor syncope (common faint) or profound hypotension.

The patient who is in a state of cardiac arrest has an ashen-gray appearance. The skin is cold and clammy, and there is an absence of pulsation in the large arteries. There is also an absence of heart sounds and respiration. Observation of the eyes later in the arrest indicates that the eyes are fixed with pupils dilated. The signs of cardiac arrest can appear when the heart is in complete standstill (asystole), when the heart is in ventricular fibrillation, or when the heart rate is so slow and ineffective that there is inadequate perfusion of vital organs.

BASIC LIFE SUPPORT

Basic life support is an emergency first aid procedure that consists of recognizing respiratory and cardiac arrest and starting the proper application of cardiopulmonary resuscitation. The basic life support procedure maintains life until the victim recovers sufficiently to be transported or until advanced life support is available. The ABC steps of cardiopulmonary resuscitation refer to the following: A= airway, B = breathing, C = circulation.

Because of the extreme importance of the ABC's of basic life support, there will be some duplication of material on airway management, artificial ventilation, and oxygen therapy which has been presented in Chapter 11. The reader is invited to review that section at this time.

AIRWAY AND BREATHING

When respiratory arrest occurs, gas exchange between the blood stream and lungs ceases. This produces an immediate accumulation of carbon dioxide, resulting in respiratory acidosis. The lack of oxygen and tissue hypoxia leads to anaerobic metabolism and lactic acidosis (i.e., metabolic acidosis). At the same time the body responds with increased sympathetic nervous system activity which results in an increase in the pulse rate, peripheral vasoconstriction, and restlessness. Hypoxia and acidosis depress the heart, reducing cardiac output, and eventually produce cardiac dysrhythmias which can lead to cardiac arrest.

The dental chair should be positioned so that the patient is supine with the feet slightly elevated. It is recommended that an emergency oxygen source that has been regularly checked be available in all offices. Also there should be an oral airway and a full face mask available to administer oxygen under positive pressure. A mask attached to a self-inflating reservoir bag, intermittently compressed by hand, is also acceptable. No time should be lost in assisting respiration. The clinician or assistant should immediately initiate ventilation of the lungs by the mouth-to-mouth technique. It is imperative to elevate the mandible, thereby drawing the tongue away from the posterior pharyngeal wall to provide a patent airway. A solid obstruction of the airway may be dislodged by a forceful thrust upward into the epigastrium, as in the Heimlich maneuver, which is described in Chapters 17 and 19.

If vomiting has occurred, it is necessary to remove the vomitus by placing the patient's head to one side and by using fingers, gauze and suction, drawing out all foreign material in the oropharynx. Following removal of the vomitus, adequate ventilation can be carried out.

Figure 14-1 The head in a position of maximum backward tilt.

Mouth-to-Mouth Ventilation

The practitioner or assistant responsible for respiratory assistance places one hand behind the patient's neck to maintain the head in a position of maximum backward tilt (Fig. 14–1). The patient's nostrils are pinched together with the thumb and index finger while pressure is exerted on the forehead to maintain the backward tilt (Fig. 14–2). The patient's mouth is opened as widely as possible, the resuscitator takes a deep breath, makes a tight seal with the lips around the patient's mouth, and then blows

Figure 14-2 The nostrils are pinched together while pressure is exerted on the forehead to maintain maximum backward tilt.

into the patient's mouth. The patient is allowed to exhale passively. Observation of the chest to determine adequate respiratory movement is essential.

In some cases mouth-to-nose ventilation is more effective than mouth-to-mouth ventilation. Mouth-to-nose ventilation is recommended for the small child or in those cases where it is impossible to ventilate the patient through the mouth.

Resuscitation with Positive Pressure Oxygen

Oropharyngeal Airway. When an oxygen source is available, an oral airway should be inserted and a tight-fitting, full face mask applied. The oropharyngeal airway is a semicircular-shaped apparatus made of plastic or rubber. It is curved to fit over the back of the tongue, and in this position it will hold the tongue away from the pharynx. It is more easily inserted into the mouth upside down. As the airway approaches the posterior wall of the pharynx near the back of the tongue, it should be rotated into its proper position. If the oropharyngeal airway is not inserted properly, it is possible to push the tongue posteriorly, thus obstructing the airway. Proper head position must be maintained even with the use of a properly positioned airway.

One hundred per cent oxygen is administered to the patient, whose head is in the same backward tilt position with the mandible forward. Observation of the thoracic cage to determine effective ventilation is mandatory. A clear, full face mask to observe the presence of vomitus is recommended. As mentioned previously, a resuscitator bag with atmospheric air as the inflating gas, or attached to an oxygen source, can also be utilized.

Esophageal Airway. Another method of ventilating the patient is with an esophageal airway. The esophageal airway is a tube approximately 15 inches long which is open at the top and has a blind end at the bottom. The lower end is inserted into the esophagus. An inflatable cuff is located just above the blind end. There are several side holes located near the upper end which allow air from the interior of the tube to enter the pharynx. Pressurized air enters the upper end of the esophageal airway and exits through the side holes in the pharynx. The inflated cuff prevents air from entering the esophagus and allows the air to pass into the trachea, inflating the lungs. See Chapter 11 for further information on the esophageal obturator.

CIRCULATION

As mentioned previously, the mechanisms leading to cardiac arrest are ventricular standstill, ventricular fibrillation, and cardiovascular collapse.

Examples of ventricular standstill in patients undergoing dental treatment are: vagal stimulation with increased parasympathetic activity, drug overdose, or absence of electrical activity in patients with diseases of the conduction system of the heart.

Ventricular fibrillation may be seen in patients with acute myocardial infarction, hypoxia, or digitalis toxicity.

Cardiovascular collapse could occur when there is inadequate mechanical strength of the heart (cardiogenic shock) or inadequate filling of the heart (vasomotor collapse).

In all cases, external cardiac compression is initiated in an attempt to restore cardiac output. Although the cardiac output may be only one fourth or one third that of normal, it can be lifesaving.

Precordial Thump

A sharp blow to the mid-sternum has traditionally been recommended to establish a normal heart beat in cases of ventricular tachycardia, ventricular fibrillation, or heart block of recent onset. It is now questionable as to the value of the precordial thump as one of the initial steps in basic life support.

The precordial thump has been successfully employed to terminate ventricular tachycardia in the monitored patient. However, in studies on experimental animals, no beneficial effects resulted from the precordial thump to correct ventricular fibrillation or asystole. Precordial thumping of an hypoxic myocardium, whether active or in asystole, may produce ventricular fibrillation, a situation that is apparently irreversible in the absence of a defibrillator and is not recommended as a routine procedure on the unmonitored patient.

External Cardiac Compression

The patient is in a supine position in the dental chair. If the chair does not have a firm backrest, it is recommended that a 12″ × 24″ board be placed under the patient's back (Fig. 14–3). *Do not move the patient to the floor!* It is extremely awkward to attempt resuscitation when the patient is on the floor. Most dental operating rooms are small, and the dental chair occupies most of the room. It is much easier to carry out adequate CPR with the patient in the dental chair, provided there is adequate back support.

To effectively carry out external cardiac compression, it is essential that the lower sternum be depressed from 1½ to 2 inches. The individual responsible for cardiac compression is positioned on the side of the patient and places the heel of one hand over the lower half of the sternum. To determine the exact position, it is essential to palpate the xiphoid process and then advance the heel of the hand superiorly about 1½ inches. The other hand is now placed on top of the first one; the shoulders are directed over the patient's sternum. The arms remain straight, and a downward vertical pressure is exerted to compress the sternum 1½ to 2 inches. The compressions are continuous, regular, and at a rate of approximately 60 to 80 per minute. The heel of the first hand should remain in contact with the chest wall during relaxation when the sternum returns to a normal resting position between compressions.

After each 5 compressions of the sternum, one breath of air by mouth-to-mouth or oxygen under positive pressure is administered. If the practitioner or assistant is alone when cardiac arrest occurs, the following outline is suggested:

One-Person Resuscitation

Artificial ventilation and compression must be accomplished utilizing a 15 to 2 ratio. This consists of two quick lung inflations followed by 15 chest compressions. The two full lung inflations must be delivered in rapid succession within a period of five or six seconds, without allowing full exhalation between the breaths. If the time for full exhalation were allowed, the additional time required would reduce the number of compressions and ventilations that could be achieved in a one-minute period.

Infants and Children

The cardiac compression technique is similar for children (ages two to 10 years) except that only the pressure of the heel of one hand is required. The ventricles of small children lie higher in the chest, and external pressure should be exerted over the mid-sternum. Young children require 3/4 to 1½ inch compression of the sternum. The compression rate should be 80 to 100 per minute with breaths delivered as quickly as possible after each five compressions.

EMERGENCY SERVICES

It is important that at the time of any cardiovascular collapse, the following be adhered to:

1. The time of collapse must be recorded and an emergency flow chart activated. This flow chart is a modified form of a CPR chart that can be used in the dental office (Fig. 14–10).

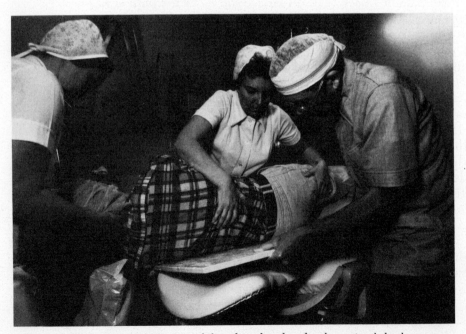

Figure 14–3 A 12 × 24 inch board is placed under the patient's back.

Figure 14-4 A clear, full face mask with oral airway is applied to administer positive pressure oxygen.

2. An emergency ambulance service with appropriate CPR equipment and qualified personnel should be called immediately. The emergency room of a local hospital should be instructed that a patient who has collapsed is being transported to the emergency room for immediate care.

ADVANCED LIFE SUPPORT IN THE OFFICE SETTING

The following is an outline for advanced life support prior to transportation to a hospital.

In the offices of those practitioners who utilize IV sedation or general anesthesia, an intravenous line is standard procedure. If a catastrophe should occur under local analgesia, or in cases where an IV is not in place, it is important that an intravenous line be established if possible; this should not interfere with cardiac compression and ventilation. A continuous drip of 5 per cent dextrose in water or lactated Ringer's should be administered. If the patient can be adequately ventilated by means of a full face mask with oral airway, there is no need for endotracheal intubation (Fig. 14-4). If this method does not provide adequate respiratory exchange, then endotracheal intubation is recommended. The endotracheal tube should be attached to a non-rebreathing valve with a source of oxygen supplied for resuscitation.

EMERGENCY DRUGS

Oxygen. Oxygen is considered an essential in resuscitation. An increase in arterial oxygen tension is required; and, therefore, oxygen must

Figure 14–5 External cardiac compression with ventilation. The anesthesia assistant is checking the carotid pulse while the surgical assistant attempts to obtain the blood pressure.

Figure 14–6 Electrocardiogram leads are applied without interrupting cardiac compression and ventilation.

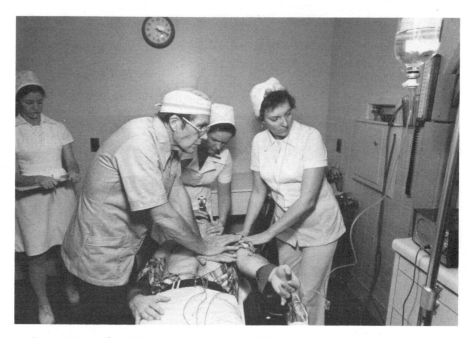

Figure 14–7 The CPR team observing the ECG monitor while the circulating nurse records all necessary information on the emergency flow chart.

Figure 14–8 Administration of emergency drugs by an assistant under the direction of the leader of the CPR team.

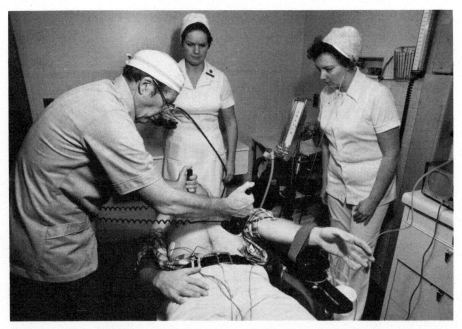

Figure 14-9 Application of defibrillator paddles; 4 × 4 inch gauze pads are dampened with saline and placed under the paddles.

be administered in the presence of suspected hypoxemia of any cause and especially in cardiopulmonary arrest.

Na Bicarbonate.   Profound metabolic acidosis occurs within a few minutes in circulatory collapse. To overcome this acidosis, 44.5 mEq of sodium bicarbonate or 1 ampule (50 ml) of the disposable syringe type should be administered intravenously if the heart has not resumed rhythm approximately 30 seconds after arrest. This dose should be repeated every 5 minutes prior to transportation to the hospital. The maintenance of a normal pH renders the myocardium more responsive to circulating and administered catecholamines.

Epinephrine.   Epinephrine is the most effective drug used in cardiopulmonary resuscitation. The immediate intracardiac injection of epinephrine in the dental office is not recommended. This drug should be administered intravenously in dilutions of 1:10,000, approximately 5 ml every 5 minutes.

MONITORING

In offices where general anesthesia is used, an ECG or cardioscope should now be applied in such a way as to not interfere with cardiac compressions or ventilation (Fig. 14-6). The only evidence for effective circulation is a readily palpable carotid or femoral pulse, a satisfactory blood pressure, and reactive pupils. Rhythmic electrical activity alone does not indicate effective circulation. The ECG, however, will allow differentiation between asystole, ventricular fibrillation, or dysrhythmia resulting from ineffectual

Name:_____

Date: _____

Time CPR started:_____
Time ambulance called: _____
Time ambulance arrived: _____
Time hospital called:_____
Time patient left office:_____

TIME

	0	5	10	15	20	25	30	35	40	45	50	55	60		
BP															
Pulse															
Respiration															
EKG															
Pupils															
Epinephrine															
NA Bicarb.															
Lidocaine															
CA Chloride															
Solu-cortef															
Defibrillation															

Comments: _____   Personnel: _____

Figure 14–10   Emergency flow chart.

heart action. If fibrillation is diagnosed, defibrillation should be carried out as soon as possible. In all offices utilizing general anesthesia, a defibrillator should be avaialble.

DEFIBRILLATION

The defibrillator paddles are applied using electrode jelly or preferably 4″ × 4″ gauze pads dampened with saline. One electrode is placed just below the right clavicle at the right sternal border and a second is placed just beyond the cardiac apex below the left breast (Fig. 14–9). The optimum amount of electrical energy for defibrillation of the adult patient is usually in the area of 400 joules, or watt seconds, for cases of ventricular fibrillation. Lower settings are frequently effective in converting ventricular fibrillation and ventricular tachycardia and produce less myocardial damage. The damage resulting from the defibrillator shocks is usually proportional to the energy used; and maximal settings, where not required, may further impair an already damaged myocardium. All monitoring devices attached to an electrical wall outlet should be disconnected prior to defibrillation. All personnel should avoid contact with the patient or chair during defibrillation.

A single defibrillatory shock does not produce serious functional damage to the myocardium, so there is no reason to withhold it in the unconscious, apneic, pulseless adult when a direct-current defibrillator is available, *even though the patient is unmonitored.* In these circumstances, unmonitored defibrillation with a single shock may be performed by the practitioner or assistant; but it is emphasized that this single shock must not delay the prompt application of basic life support measures in any way. Unmonitored defibrillation is not recommended for children.

In cases where there is an apparent cardiac arrest secondary to prolonged anoxia or drug overdose, CPR for a period of two minutes or more is recommended with re-evaluation prior to the delivery of an unmonitored defibrillator shock.

ADJUNCTIVE DRUGS

Atropine.   Atropine sulfate is a parasympatholytic drug which reduces vagal tone and thereby accelerates the rate of discharge of the SA node. It may also improve atrioventricular conduction by this vagolytic action. It is useful in treating severe bradycardia with hypotension. Dosage is 0.5 mg intravenously every 5 minutes until the desired rate of around 60 beats per min is achieved. The total dose should not exceed 2.0 mg.

Lidocaine.   Lidocaine is used to reduce the irritability of the myocardium. Fifty to 100 mg of lidocaine is administered intravenously and may be repeated every 5 minutes. This is useful to control multifocal, premature beats and episodes of ventricular tachycardia.

Calcium Chloride (Adults Only).   Calcium chloride is a cardiotonic stimulant that is given slowly by the intravenous route, and this drug is used to increase the amplitude of organized electrical complexes on the ECG. The usual recommended dose of calcium chloride is 2.5 ml to 5 ml of a 10 per cent solution. This is injected intravenously as a bolus at intervals of 10 minutes. Calcium gluconate provides less ionizable calcium per unit value. Large doses of calcium may elevate calcium blood levels with detrimental effects. Calcium must not be administered together with sodium bicarbonate, since this mixture results in the formation of a precipitate.

TRANSPORTATION TO HOSPITAL

Other vasoactive compounds plus diuretics and steroids can be administered when the patient has been transferred to a local hospital. Monitoring of urine output, central venous pressure, blood gases, and electrolytes is more effectively carried on in this type of advanced care facility.

The practitioner should always accompany the patient to the hospital, and the new life support team should be informed as to the type and amount of emergency drugs that have been administered.

TERMINATION OF BASIC OR ADVANCED LIFE SUPPORT

The decision to terminate resuscitative efforts depends upon the assessment of the cerebral and cardiovascular status of the patient. It is important to continue CPR procedures until the patient is transported to a hospital setting where a final decision is made to continue with the CPR treatment or to terminate resuscitative efforts.

SUMMARY

It is important to recognize that a cardiac emergency in the dental office presents a serious problem that requires immediate resuscitative efforts in an attempt to restore adequate, spontaneous circulation. This includes basic life support with utilization of the fundamental ABC's of resuscitation, alerting a nearby hosptial or advanced life support unit, and arranging transportation of the patient to this facility as rapidly as possible. When advanced life support is carried out in the dental office, there should be a greater chance for success because of the introduction of essential drugs as well as adequate cardiopulmonary resuscitative efforts. Monitoring of cardiac rhythms is also an advantage to enable the practitioner to determine which emergency drugs are essential. The utilization of defibrillators to reverse ventricular fibrillation should increase the chance of survival. Even though advanced life support procedures are carried out in the dental office, it is also imperative that a local hospital be advised that a patient has collapsed in the office and cardiopulmonary resuscitative efforts are being carried out; and the patient should be transferred to the intensive care unit immediately.

SUGGESTED READING

1. Dripps, R. D., Eckenhoff, J. E., and Vandam, L. D.: Introduction to Anesthesia. Philadelphia, W. B. Saunders Co., 1977.
2. Heimlich, H. J.: A life-saving maneuver to prevent food choking. J.A.M.A., 234:398, 1975.
3. Pennington, J. E., Taylor, J. and Lown, B.: Chest thump for reverting ventricular tachycardia. N. Engl. J. Med., 283:1192–1195, 1970.
4. Sprone, C. W., and Mullanney, P. J. (eds.): Emergency Care: Assessment and Intervention. St. Louis, C. V. Mosby Co., 1974.
5. Standards for cardiopulmonary resuscitation (CPR) and emergency cardiac care (ECC). J.A.M.A., 227:833–868, 1974.
6. Yakaitis, R. W., and Redding, J. S.: Precordial thumping during cardiac resuscitation. Crit. Care Med., 1:22–26, 1973.

15

COMPLICATIONS FROM LOCAL ANALGESIA

JESS HAYDEN, JR.
and the late
NIELS BJORN JORGENSEN

INTRODUCTION
LOCAL COMPLICATIONS
SYSTEMIC COMPLICATIONS

DISCUSSION
PROPHYLAXIS AND TREATMENT
SUMMARY AND CONCLUSIONS

INTRODUCTION

The purpose of this chapter is to set forth in a classified form and to discuss the complications which may accompany or follow the injection of local analgesic solutions.* The classification is that of the writers, and the discussion relates to our observations made in the course of the clinical practice of dentistry.

The basic format and information in this chapter were prepared in co-operation with the late Niels Bjorn Jorgensen. Over the years of his associa-tion with Loma Linda University's Schools of Medicine and Dentistry, Dr. Jorgensen established a model program for the teaching of local analgesia, and inhalation and intravenous sedation to the candidates for a degree in dentistry. A man of great humility, his teaching nevertheless brought inter-national recognition both to him and to the University he devotedly served. It is a great tribute to his foresight that a majority of the concepts which he pioneered were incorporated in the American Dental Association's "Guide-lines for Teaching the Comprehensive Control of Pain and Anxiety in Den-tistry."[19] The title of one of his films, "The Comfort of the Patient," sig-nified the thrust of his academic and professional achievement. The story of his struggle to realize the goals he envisioned are revealed elsewhere.[21, 24]

In the United States, local analgesia undoubtedly is the most used mo-dality for the control of pain during dental treatment. In fact the use of local analgesia in dentistry has become such a routine procedure that one is

---

*In the United States, the term local anesthesia is generally employed rather than the precise term, local analgesia.

apt to ignore possible hazards in its employment. Although it does appear to be without dangers, local or systemic complications occasionally do happen. These complications have been classified below as: I. Local, and II. Systemic.

A more extensive bibliography is readily available in *Accepted Dental Therapeutics*,[1] which is conveniently divided into sections concerning: (1) the general principles of medication, including emergency treatment and sterilization; (2) therapeutic agents, which includes suggestions for certain clinical problems; (3) preventive agents; and (4) indexes.

LOCAL COMPLICATIONS

A. *Bacterial contamination* occurs when a needle tip inadvertently touches any tissue or object without the oral cavity, usually the clinician's or assistant's finger or the patient's lip. If the needle is used for deep injections, a serious infection may result. Bacterial contamination always occurs when the needle touches the mucous membrane in a relatively dirty mouth.

Since all mouths contain myriad bacteria, and it is not feasible to assess the patient's (host's) resistance to these, a routine preparation of the tissues should precede each injection. Such a preparation is described in connection with the inferior alveolar injection. Aerosols from the area of treatment are spread some distance from the oral cavity, depending on the techniques of dentistry employed and the immediate physical environment. Therefore, a routine must be established to insure the continued sterility of needles, syringes and cartridges, and ampules or vials of local analgesics. For instance, in the Pediatric Dental Clinic, Dental Science Building of the University of Iowa, random samples, which were then cultured, revealed that on the average, one out of 10 diaphragms of local analgesic cartridges were contaminated. For test purposes, the cartridges were left in their original container, with the lid removed, sitting on the operatory bench. Thereafter, immediately before insertion into a cartridge syringe, the diaphragm of each cartridge was swabbed with merthiolate and rubbed dry with a sterile gauge 2 × 2 sponge. The usual sequela of contamination is a low-grade infection, whether confined to the area of the attached periodontal tissues, or deeply situated in the pterygomandibular space. Improper techniques of sterilizing and storing needles or methods of handling by the assistant or doctor lead to varying degrees of contamination.[2] *Chemical deposits* on the needle are due to sterilizing solutions, or perhaps to chemical vapor sterilization. Inflammation and pain are frequent after-effects.

B. *Local reactions to topical or injected solutions* are usually seen as *epithelial desquamation* following the application of topical analgesics. Such desquamation usually results from too long an application of the topical analgesic, but may be due to a heightened sensitivity of the tissue. All local analgesics are toxic. The after-effects usually are transitory. *Sterile abscesses* or gangrene may result owing to ischemia resulting from injecting an excess of analgesic solution, with its contained vasoconstrictor, into the firm, hard tissue of the palate. *Local allergic reactions,* such as blisters on the oral mucosa or lips, are to be considered as a sign of warning, and further use of the causative agents should be accompanied with suitable precautions and a change to a local analgesic of different chemical structure.[2] Emphatically, clinicians are not immune to contact dermatitis. *Trismus and pain* follow the injection of solutions into muscles and tendons, and they are among the variety of local tissue changes produced by local analgesics. Much of the soreness frequently attributed to post-surgical operative causes is simply the result of improper administration of solutions.

The anatomical structures basic to local analgesia were incorporated into clinical textbooks shortly after the discovery of the benefits of local analgesia. As Allen[25] in his foreword wrote, "There is no substitute for the correctly placed needle tip for achieving local anesthesia". Improper placement in one instance led to a patient's inability to open the mouth following a mandibular (inferior alveolar?) block and resulted in a $75,000 award to the patient.[29] A further complication, similarly related in some instances to failure to adhere to principles of injection based on morphology, is post-injection anesthesia, *paresthesia* and/or *neuritis* caused by the needle's penetrating the nerve.[18, 39] Steiner and Thompson[37] (p. 511–512), as additional sequelae of "repeated and inaccurate plunging of the needle into a helpless patient," list: exhausted buffering capacity, myositis, hemorrhage with hematoma or ecchymosis, fibrosis, and edema.

C. *Breakage of needles* is seldom a problem. Needles available today possess physical qualities which should prevent such a mishap. When breakage does occur, it usually is the result of the needle's impaling muscular tissue or passing beneath the periosteum and being snapped off during sudden closure of the mouth. Kennett, Curran, and Jenkins[27] describe such needle breakage in a five year old. The needle was a "short 27 gauge." Although many advocate short 27 gauge needles as being less painful, and have not experienced needle breakage, reason would appear to dictate the use of long hubs and long needles for deep injections. See the chapter on *surgical emergencies* for treatment of broken needles.

D. *Lip-chewing* is a complication caused by the use of long-acting local analgesics for children. The after-effects can be most unpleasant for the child, his parents, and the practitioner. Many clinicians routinely employ long-acting analgesics in order to obtain profundity of effect. The child should always be premedicated prior to the injection if dismissal from the dental office long precedes the dissipation of the analgesic action. For brief appointments, the use of short-acting solutions for block analgesia should be routine. Even so, a cotton roll should be placed between the lips, or tied in the vestibule by means of dental floss or sutures passed through the dental embrasures if analgesia exists at the time of dismissal. Verbal warnings should be given to the child or accompanying adult, but may be futile if not reinforced by the cotton roll. A small, oval, self-adhesive, red luminescent sticker warning "WATCH ME PLEASE, MY LIPS AND CHEEK ARE NUMB" may be affixed to the child's forehead. *

E. *Emphysema uncommonly occurs after an injection.*[44] An example is that of a 10-year-old boy who received an inferior alveolar injection. Within two hours of his dismissal, he returned to the office exhibiting homolateral swelling and crepitation in the anterior triangle of the neck and the face.

---

* Professional Education Products, 4116 Farnam Street, Omaha, Nebraska 68131.

His consulting pediatrician shared the amazement at this dental treatment sequela, and prescribed antihistaminics on the basis of a possible allergic response. Questioning revealed that the boy had been blowing up balloons immediately after his dental treatment. The manner in which the symptoms subsided suggested that air in the fascial planes, rather than allergy, was the cause.

F. *The trauma of injection* comprises the vast majority of local complications. Reactions from the supraperiosteal technique generally are minor, consisting of edema, after-pain, and sometimes slight ulceration of the puncture point. The former are due to infection, too rapid injection, or injecting too large a volume; the latter is due to an infection. The unpleasantness generally passes in a few days. Hematomas may result from nicking an artery. Usually the effects are seen in connection with the posterior superior alveolar artery, and less commonly the facial. Obviously, any of these local complications can result in swelling and pain. Two common techniques of administration often cause pain, the first because of lack of skill of administration; the second is irrevocably tied to morphology and physiology: the complications from palatine injections are mostly immediate pain from the needle insertion; subperiosteal injections may result in lifting the periosteum from the bone, causing after-pain and even infection. From a physiologic standpoint, this injection probably is contraindicated.

The use of long beveled, thin, pointed disposable needles predisposes to hematomas and trismus, for arteries, nerve trunks, and muscles or tendons are easily penetrated with these much too flexible instruments.

G. *Bleeding due to hemophilia* or anticoagulant therapy is always a hazard. The first is readily recognized by both the patient and clinician. The latter is much more prevalent, but is not as well recognized. It is a particular danger when deep block injections are required for the relief of pain in an active ambulatory patient. See the chapter on *physical evaluation* for further information on handling of the anticoagulant-treated patient.

SYSTEMIC COMPLICATIONS

A. *Allergic reactions* are extremely uncommon. *Anaphylaxis* presents the gravest challenge, for the opportunity to render support to the patient is so fleeting that death usually results. Fortunately, anaphylactic shock is known by the rarity of its response to analgesic solutions. *Skin eruptions* occasionally may be a manifestation of allergy. Methylparaben, a preservative in many local analgesics, may cause an allergic or hypersensitivity reaction.[14, 28] See the chapter on *emergency drugs and allergy* for more information on anaphylactoid and toxic reactions.

B. *Toxic reactions* are expressed systemically if too large an amount of an analgesic drug is absorbed too rapidly into the system. Shane, et al.[34] reported that 12 cartidges of 2 per cent lidocaine with epinephrine 1:100,000 were injected into a four year old child. The child became lethargic and required artificial ventilation with oxygen for 55 minutes before recovering. We know of other instances in which the death of a child ensued and local analgesia toxicity was evident. (The recommended dose of an amide local analgesic with vasoconstrictor is approximately 7 mg per kg, or 3 mg per lb. It is incumbent in the administration of a local analgesic to be familiar with the doses recommended by the manufacturer.) Absorption is increased when too much solution is injected too rapidly into the highly vascular circumoral tissues. Further, "If a doctor accidentally injects a cartridge of procaine intravenously over a period of five seconds, the rate is fifteen times that which is considered safe, or over two hundred times more toxic."[2] It is noteworthy that all the amide local analgesics, used in the same concentration as procaine, are more toxic than procaine. Further, two reactions may simultaneously occur, those caused by (1) the local analgesic and (2) the vasoconstrictor. Adriani and Campbell[3] reported that spray or paste topical analgesics may simulate the effect of intravenous injection. Spray products apparently are no more effective in producing analgesia than those applied with a swab; but sprays do have several disadvantages which may introduce unnecessary hazard in their use.[2] In any case, the toxic reaction sequence may take the form of stimulation, convulsions, and depression.

In addition, the report of Allen and co-workers[4] indicates that the amount of epinephrine 1:100,000 in a 1.8 ml cartridge is sufficient to affect the heart's stroke volume. Epinephrine effects are directly dose related and care should be taken to inject minimal quantities.

C. *Psychic reactions* are exhibited by most patients, but clinicians usually notice only those signs which immediately precede *syncope.* Certainly catecholamine levels are elevated in the very anxious or phobic patient.[15] Fortunately, first-aid procedures for syncope are so ingrained into most people, and the recuperative powers of the body are such that shock seldom ensues.

Acute asthmatic attacks may follow the administration of a local analgesic. Such attacks are considered to be due to allergy or emotional stress.

D. *Viral Hepatitis.* From our reading of the literature and consultation with dental and medical doctors, it presently appears that viral hepatitis is caused by at least two immunologically distinct infectious agents: virus A, the etiologic agent of infectious, epidemic, or short incubation hepatitis (HA), and virus B, which is responsible for serum hepatitis, or long-term incubation hepatitis (HB). In the case of acute viral hepatitis it may be impossible to make a specific diagnosis, and it is therefore designated type unspecified. Several other viral agents are now being classified as "non-A, non-B" if the distinction can be made.

The prevalence of hepatitis A (HAV) is decreasing, while that of hepatitis B (HBV) is increasing. Virus B (HBV) is of the greatest concern to the staff of a dental office. The "carrier" rate in the United States among the general population is about 0.5 per cent. Among health care workers it is 1 to 2 per cent. It is estimated that general dental practitioners have two to four times the risk of acquiring type B hepatitis than do persons not in the health care professions. The risk is higher among oral surgeons. In the United Kingdom, the "carrier" rate of the hepatitis B surface antigen (HB_SAg) ranges from 1 in 500 to 1000 among Europeans to as high as 1 in 5 for Afro-Asians. The "carrier" state occurs after some 5 to 10 per cent of acute infections. The groups that pose the highest risk of transmitting HBV when they present to the dental practitioner for treatment are: those undergoing chronic renal hemodialysis; the mentally retarded and institutionalized, particularly those with Down's syndrome; leukemics (and some other dys-crasias); individuals treated with radiation and immunosuppressives; hemo-philiacs or others who receive large volumes of blood or its derivatives, or those transfused with blood from paid donors; drug addicts, particularly those who share syringes for parenteral inoculation of illicit drugs; male homosexuals and prostitutes; the tattooed; and individuals who have been transfused in or recently returned from countries with a high background prevalence of hepatitis B. The list is not exhaustive. Perhaps the greatest cause of exposure to HBV for the clinician and staff is puncture of the skin with contaminated instruments. The risk of developing hepatitis B after an accidental puncture by a hepatitis B contaminated needle is 6 to 7 per cent.

It now appears that "carriers" of type B hepatitis do not present as great a risk to casual contacts as was believed in the late 1960's. Nevertheless, for the practitioner or staff member who acquires hepatitis B, the result is 100 per cent. Therefore, care should be taken to minimize exposure. There is a voluminous literature concerning hepatitis A and B. For an informative survey related to dental practice see the recommendations in the reports and publications of the American Dental Association's Council on Dental Thera-peutics, the Dental Health Committee of the British Dental Association, and the report of surveys by Mosley and White.[5, 10, 31]

DISCUSSION

To better illustrate what may happen during the deep injection of local analgesic solution, the path of the needle during deep injections is de-scribed:

A. When administering the *inferior alveolar* injection the mucous membrane at the area of the needle insertion should be wiped clean with sterile gauze, and an antiseptic, such as tincture of merthiolate, applied. If saliva flows copiously at the time of needle insertion, bacteria may be in-troduced into the deeper structures, and though these may be relatively harmless to the host, low-grade infection and after-pain may result. To pre-vent this invasion, a roll of sterile gauze should be placed in the upper vestibule blocking the parotid duct, and a second pad of gauze placed un-derneath the tongue over the salivary caruncula. Bacteria of a more harmful nature also may be introduced by the inadvertent touch of the needle point to any foreign object, such as a finger, the lips, etc. As mentioned before, a serious infection within the pterygomandibular space may result.

1. The path of the needle is through loose areolar tissue. If the needle is inserted or directed too far medially, it will enter the medial pterygoid muscle, resulting in trismus, after-pain, and probably incomplete or no an-algesia.

2. If the needle is directed too far laterally, it will penetrate the deep tendon of the temporalis muscle. Trismus and after-pain may be expected. Furthermore, if the needle is continued in this too-lateral path, it will be rammed against the periosteum, and the result will be pain and a reflex action by the patient which may result in needle breakage.

3. If the needle is directed in a path diverging inferiorly from a plane through the coronoid notch, the deepest point of the concavity of the an-

terior border of the ramus, it will have to penetrate the sphenomandibular ligament, which covers the mandibular sulcus. If the entire bevel of the needle is not lateral to the sphenomandibular ligament, solution is deposited along its medial aspect, and incomplete anesthesia is the result.

The inferior alveolar nerve or the lingual nerve may be traumatized by the needle. These nerves, if accidentally rammed by the needle, do not slide away, as is generally supposed, since they are both attached firmly to the interpterygoid fascia, a structure which continues forward from the anterior border of the sphenomandibular ligament to the lateral pterygoid lamina. As the inferior alveolar nerve runs downward toward the foramen it is attached to the lateral surface of this fascia. The lingual nerve is attached to the medial surface, but farther anteriorly. When the mouth is kept wide open, the interpterygoid fascia is stretched and holds the two nerves quite firmly, as if on a trellis.[25]

To avoid injury to the lingual nerve the needle must be inserted at the proper level, relative to the coronoid notch, kept close to the medial aspect of the deep tendon of the temporalis muscle and lateral to the pterygomandibular raphe. It must be clearly understood that injury of a nerve does not necessarily indicate a fauly approach but may be related to the long, beveled, pointed thin needles which are now in vogue and demand, and which make it impossible to detect and follow necessary anatomical landmarks.

As the needle advances toward the mandibular sulcus, it may easily injure or penetrate the inferior alveolar nerve. To avoid this, the needle should enter the sulcus over the lingular notch; it should touch the periosteum just before reaching the notch, and then slide gently over this saddle-like bony surface into the anterior part of the sulcus. A heavy, rigid needle with a short bevel is required if this is to be easily accomplished. If the lingual and inferior alveolar nerves are injured, paresthesia or post-analgesic neuritis may result. If the needle is advanced posteriorly into the mandibular sulcus, the inferior alveolar artery or vein may be punctured and injected into. The result may be a local hematoma or a systemic toxic reaction from the injected drug. This can be avoided by confining the needle tip to the anterior part of the sulcus. Injection into the vessel must be avoided by aspirating before injecting.[23, 25, 35]

B. *The posterior superior alveolar nerve block* is a simple and effective injection that recently has been abondoned by many practitioners because of the frequent occurrence of hematomas. These are due to the characteristics of thin, usually disposable needles (see above). From just distal of the zygomatic process the needle point must be advanced medially, superiorly, and posteriorly along the periosteum toward the foramina located halfway between the upper and lower borders of the maxilla. Here the tuberosity makes a sharp turn medially, and if the needle advances farther the pterygoid venous plexus or the maxillary artery may be punctured. If the syringe and needle are kept in a plane parallel with the sagittal plane, the maxillary artery and/or the lateral pterygoid muscle may be invaded. Obviously, trismus and hematoma are possible complications of this injection if the needle deviates from the proper path, and it will with a thin flexible needle. Only with a heavy rigid needle with a short bevel can the correct anatomical pathway routinely be followed, as with a probe.

C. When the *maxillary nerve* block is administered through the pterygopalatine canal, care must be exercised that the needle does not penetrate the thin medial wall of the canal and enter the nasal cavity. Not only will there be no anesthesia, but infection also may result. When directed laterally, the needle and solution may through the pterygomaxillary fissure enter the infratemporal space and the pterygoid muscle. Trismus will result. If the needle is in the correct path but advanced too far, the orbital cavity may be entered. Solution injected here may temporarily paralyze the muscles of the eyeball; even the optic nerve may be anesthetized, resulting in temporary blindness. In checking the path through the pterygopalatine canal in approximately 200 skulls, bony obstructions were found in 15 per cent of the cases. If obstructions are encountered when giving this injection, the needle should not be forced, or needle fracture may result. The alternative path is along the tuberosity. The commonest complication will be severe hematoma if the maxillary artery is punctured. Also, the orbit might be entered if the needle is advanced too far. These complications can be avoided by following Smith's[36] and Jorgensen's[22, 25] technique for a determination of the depth of needle insertion.

A most serious complication is post-injection infection; asepsis must be maintained when using this technique.

D. The treatment of patients with *hypertensive, cardiovascular,* or *cerebrovascular* disease is increasingly common. Specific considerations regarding evaluation, routine management, and precautions are covered in detail in Chapter 2.

Hypertensives are a special problem because they exhibit a great lability of blood pressure. The anticipation of dental treatment causes an initial elevation of their blood pressure, which may be heightened by the stimulus of an injection or dental treatment.

Patients with a history of cardiovascular or cerebrovascular disease suffer an elevation in blood pressure after any noxious stimulus. Obviously, any rise in blood pressure may be dangerous for these patients. The reports of Cheraskin and Prasertsuntarasai,[12] McCarthy,[30] and observations of dental clinic patients at Loma Linda University since 1955 confirm that the blood pressure is not elevated by the small amount of epinephrine (1:100,000 to 1:50,000) contained in the most commonly employed dental analgesic solutions unless they are injected intravenously. In addition, a special report of the New York Heart Association in 1954 concluded that there is no hazard for the cardiac patient if no more than 0.2 mg of epinephrine is utilized at a single dental appointment.[41] The total maximum dose of 0.2 mg of epinephrine is equal to 20 ml of local analgesic solution containing epinephrine in the amount of 1:100,000 (0.01 mg per ml). It is stated that 0.5 mg of epinephrine is the effective dose for positive or pressor effects in man when injected subcutaneously.[43] This is two and one-half times the maximum amount of epinephrine advised by the New York Heart Association, and it represents 50 ml of epinephrine 1:100,000.

Warnings against the use of vasoconstrictors such as epinephrine are still heard. Many of these are repetitions based on early teaching, such as those expressed by Berlove.[7] However, it is recognized that some hypertensive patients are extremely sensitive to epinephrine, and recommendations are seen in the literature against the use of epinephrine in such cases.[11] One reported death that occurred in the dental office was due to a burst cerebral aneurysm following sedation and the injection of four 2.2 ml ampules of lidocaine with 1:80,000 noradrenaline.[42] Still it is our belief that the hypertensive patient who is so sensitive that as little as 0.02 mg of epinephrine (2 ml of 1:100,000 solution) could not be administered is rare indeed, if he exists at all. We continue to recommend the routine use of epinephrine for sedated hypertensive patients in order to achieve the deepest level of analgesia. Inadequate analgesia resulting from a local analgesic solution without epinephrine results in the pain-produced release of significant amounts of endogenous epinephrine, thus subjecting the patient to the risk of a hypertensive episode. Again it must be remembered that very anxious patients will exhibit similar outpourings of catecholamines.[15] It is our belief that considerable research is needed on the effect of epinephrine in the dental patient.

Adequate *sedation* is the single most important prophylactic measure in preventing adverse systemic responses in the hypertensive patient during dental treatment. Proper administration of the local analgesic solution is mandatory: 25 gauge or larger needle, aspirating syringe or cartridge, and *slow* administration.

With regard to aspiration, Harris'[20] classic paper is still significant. Harris remarked that aspiration was not universally practiced because (1) "It is evidently thought by some that, when a needle point is in a blood vessel, blood will enter, or can be 'teased,' into a nonaspirating cartridge," (2) "So little has been said about it in the literature that many dentists believe the incidence of puncturing blood vessels is insignificant in dental injections." (3) "The hazards of intravascular injection are not sufficiently appreciated by the profession." A final quotation is warranted: "One of the most insidious dangers in therapeutics is the complacency which develops when undesirable reactions are infrequent. . . . If any of these deaths might have been prevented by ordinary or even extraordinary precautions, that they occurred at all seems inexcusable." It is not easy to ascertain the prevalence of deaths due to local analgesia, but they have not ceased,[9, 38, 42] and Harris' statement is still valid.

Slow administration of minimal amounts of local analgesic 0.5 to 1 ml over 1 to 2 minutes permits the tissues to adequately buffer the local analgesic solution; greater profundity and duration of effect is obtained and the risk of toxic or allergic reaction to the local analgesic, vasoconstrictor, or preservative is minimized. A review of fundamental biochemical phenomena such as the Henderson-Hasselbalch equation will substantiate the efficacy of the injection of minimal amounts of local analgesia over a maximal time.[14]

Another facet of the epinephrine controversy has arisen with the introduction of the monoamine oxidase inhibitors. It has been suggested that patients taking these agents should not be given epinephrine-containing compounds because of the possibility of increased sensitivity to epinephrine.[11] Monoamine oxidase inhibitors are true antidepressants and are utilized in the treatment of melancholia and depressive states. The monoamine oxidase inhibitors include Nardil, Niamid, Parnate, and Marplan. They inhibit monoamine oxidase, the enzyme which destroys neurohormonal substances such as serotonin and norepinephrine. The mode of antidepressant action is not understood.

Diverse side effects from monoamine oxidase inhibitors have been reported, among which are postural hypotension, potentiation of CNS depressants, and hypertensive episodes.[6, 32] While hypertensive episodes are uncommon, it is recognized by us that great care should be taken when administering epinephrine in local analgesic solutions to the hypertensive or cardiac patient who is taking a monoamine oxidase inhibitor. Since reports of these side effects are sparse and conflicting at this time[14] we do not feel that the use of epinephrine should be flatly discontinued in such patients for the same reasons already enumerated regarding alleged epinephrine hypersensitivity. We suggest the continued use of epinephrine, the usual precautions of administration, and that extreme caution be used in the administration of sedative drugs due to potentiation by the MAO inhibitors.

PROPHYLAXIS AND TREATMENT

The treatment and prophylaxis of many of the local complications have been altered by the introduction of disposable needles. For instance, if the precautions outlined under *Bacterial contamination* (p. 435) and *Inferior alveolar* injection (p. 439) are followed, then bacterial infections will be noted for their uncommon rarity. The best practical prophylaxis is the establishment of a precise routine for the handling of cartridges, needles and syringes, and the preparation of the tissues of the patient for a meticulously administered injection. Trauma from tearing of the tissue would seem a thing of the past. At the same time, however, the extraordinary sharpness of the needles does increase the hazard of inadvertently entering tissues that should be avoided. The passage for the needle in deep injections such as the inferior alveolar, the tuberosity, or the infraorbital, is through loose, fatty, areolar tissue. In our opinion, thin needles with long, pointed bevels cannot be used as probes, and may easily invade a muscle, artery, or nerve. Trismus and after-pain, hematoma, paresthesia, or post-anesthetic neuritis may follow.

A brief discussion of needle bevels, gauges and lengths is appropriate to the foregoing and following remarks regarding prophylaxis. Smith[36] (p. 306, Fig. 178) depicted for block injections the "correct" needle, with a short bevel, and the "incorrect" needle, with a long, pointed bevel. Today, manufacturers distribute similar long, pointed bevels. A "Status report on dental anesthetic needles and syringes"[13] provides photographs of long, pointed bevels deformed by barbs or burrs following inferior alveolar and long buccal nerve blocks. A deformed or burred needle may cause damage as it is withdrawn from the area of deepest penetration. The type and angle of the needle bevel must be considered in relation to the needle tip strength, and what the needle tip is expected to perform. Reportedly,[33] a short, 45 degree bevel offers strength, is sharp, and will offer a full diameter cutting surface with drag-free insertion and withdrawal of the cannula. The long, tapered, multibeveled point, such as is designed for venipuncture, not only has reduced wall thickness and is prone to hook and burr when striking bone but also fails to incise the full diameter of the cannula; therefore, dragging and tearing of the tissues may result when it is used for dental block injections.

Lumen size, of course, is related to the caliber of the needle and therefore affects both the strength of the needle and the probability of aspiration. The Hagen-Poisuelle law of laminar flow in tubes states that the flow rate is proportional to the fourth power of the diameter. A small increase in the diameter of the lumen of the cannula will markedly increase the flow and the possibility of aspiration.

The reported prevalence of aspiration of blood following intravascular injection varies from 2.4 to 5 per cent, and may be greater.[8] However, it is not infrequently observed that a 21 gauge or larger needle in a hand or arm vein may not permit aspiration, although fluid administered via the needle indicates that the needle is in the vein. For this reason, it seems logical to propose that the smaller the gauge of the dental needle tip, the greater the possibility of similar occlusion.

The length of the needle is related to its strength; longer needles are stronger. At present, needle lengths are not standardized; for example, the length of a needle designated as ¾, 1, or 1¼ inch may vary widely (Council report, p. 1173).[13] A longer needle provides a desirable margin of safety; that is, it prevents penetration up to the hub. If there is breakage, the portion remaining outside of the oral tissue may be grasped and the broken remains extracted.

The rigidity of a needle is a combination of caliber size and length. A heavier gauge or conical needle will not deflect, whereas a thin needle may deviate up to 3 millimeters.[13] Thus, if the needle tip is not placed precisely at the lingula for an inferior alveolar injection, a deviation of from 6 to 10 mm from the lingula to the needle tip may result, enough to place the needle in the medial or lateral pterygoid muscle. Although the intimate relation of the pterygoid muscles to the mandibular foramen is not generally recognized by the clinician, it has long been depicted in adults in anatomical atlases, such as those by Kampmeier, Cooper and Jones[26] and Truex and Kellner.[40] The relationship in a child is depicted by Jorgensen and Hayden (Fig. 8-5, p. 117).[25]

There is at present no complete set of standards for the needles, cartridges, and syringes used in dentistry. However, the American Dental Association, in cooperation with the American National Standards Institute, has established a subcommittee to propose such standards.

The *prophylaxis for trismus* is to adhere strictly to the correct anatomic route for the needle, which we find is impossible without the use of a heavy rigid needle with a short bevel.

In regard to needle size, it will be noted from Table 15-1 that a disposable 25 gauge needle has an outside diameter only 0.10 mm greater than the 27 gauge, which is too flexible for deep injections. Thus, by using the 25 gauge needle, the dental practitioner gains the advantages of far greater rigidity and an increase of approximately 0.05 mm (one fifth larger) in inside diameter, which may enhance the opportunity for positive aspiration.

However, in our opinion, for deep injections of the mouth, the needle of choice is either the Mizzy, Inc., conical needle or the 23 gauge needle, even though these needles require sterilization by autoclaving. If a well trained staff is available, a large gauge needle may be cleaned, sterilized, and reused;[16] if not, the needles may be sterilized preoperatively, used once and discarded; this is probably the most practical approach when cir-

TABLE 15-1 APPROXIMATE DIMENSIONS OF SEVERAL CARTRIDGE TYPE NEEDLES*

Size Gauge	Length mm	Dimensions of Cannula Outside Diameter Limits mm	Inside Diameter Minimum at point	Length ≅ Inches
30	25	0.30–0.31	0.13	1
27	25	0.39–0.41	0.19	1
27	35	0.39–0.41	0.19	1¼
25	25	0.49–0.52	0.24	1
25	35	0.49–0.52	0.24	1¼
23	41	0.62–0.64	0.32	1⅝
Conical	41	0.62–0.64 0.41–0.44**	0.24	1⅝

*Dimensions from drafts proposed by the Subcommittee on Needles, Cartridges, and Syringes Used in Dentistry of the American National Standards Committee MD-156, and by courtesy of Ernst Fanta, Mizzy, Inc. Clifton Forge, VA. (For this table the lengths are given to the nearest millimeter.)
** at point

cumstances permit. The outside diameter at the tip of the very rigid 23 gauge needle is only 0.23 mm greater than the outside diameter of the tip of the disposable 27 gauge needle, but the inside diameter is 0.13 greater. At the tip the outside of the conical needle is about the same size as that of a 27 gauge needle, while the inside diameter is about the same as that of a 25 gauge needle.

The *proper treatment for trismus and neuritis,* in our experience, is infrared irradiation. The paresthesia which may follow the injury to the nerve will pass in 2 to 8 weeks, though we are now observing paresthesia lasting for several years associated with the use of long, pointed bevels. We are convinced that hematomas can largely be avoided by the use of a heavy, rigid needle with a short bevel which will transmit a sensation if it touches the resistant wall of an artery. The needle can then be slightly withdrawn and a new path taken. A vein may also be entered, but this does not result in hematoma. However, aspiration must be done to avoid systemic reactions.[1, 2, 23, 25, 35] If the technique is careless, infection may result. This can be serious and at times very difficult to control. Mizzy conical needles were used by dental students in the Oral Surgery Department of Loma Linda University for approximately ten years, during which time only one hematoma was observed. When disposable needles became mandatory for student use, seven hematomas occurred during the first trial period of 500 injections. The disposable needles were 23 gauge, with a *long, pointed bevel.* The treatment of a *hematoma* in the region of the maxillary tuberosity starts with control of the bleeding by placing gauze, packed under pressure, in the buccal vestibule, and extraoral pressure over the swollen area. Later treatment includes the use of infrared rays.

As mentioned, *allergic* reactions to local analgesics may happen, though rarely.

Careful questioning of the patient who is to receive the injection of a drug may either reveal a history of allergy or raise the suspicion that one may exist. In the first instance, the patient may be aware of the drug causing the reaction; in the second instance skin testing may be indicated. There is often expressed uncertainty as to the value of such procedures. In such an instance it is of value to consider the opinion of DeJong:[14] "While skin testing may give a high yield of false positives (due to the irritancy of anesthetics such as tetracaine) it has been convincingly demonstrated that subjects not reacting to intracutaneous testing may be given the local anesthetic with reasonable impunity."

The first treatment for a fall in blood pressure is the administration of oxygen, followed, if necessary, by pressor drugs and a suitable corticosteroid intravenously. Antihistamines are also to be administered. Subsequent analgesics should be of a different chemical structure[14] (see the chapter on *emergency drugs and allergy*).

The treatment for *syncope, convulsions* or *shock* is to place the patient in a horizontal position and to administer oxygen, with positive pressure if necessary. If the convulsions do not cease when this method is employed, intravenous injection of diazepam should be made slowly, using just barely enough to stop the convulsion. Because of the usual depression which follows the convulsion, it is advisable to continue the administration of oxygen for some time. If the blood pressure has dropped and does not come back by this method, then a pressor drug such as mephentermine or phenylephrine should be administered intravenously. It has also been suggested that the administration of a corticosteroid is useful.

Worth noting is the possibility that syncope, or all of these untoward events, may often be prevented by positioning the patient in a semi-supine position in the dental contour chair during the time of injection and treatment. The report of Forsyth, Allen, and Everett,[17] in regard to the effects of posture on the cardiorespiratory system warrants careful study and further evaluation. Some patients may become syncopic as a result of hypoglycemia induced by fasting, drugs, ethanol, or other cause. The prophylaxis is simply a preoperative high carbohydrate meal. Two to four ounces of honey may also be administered preoperatively. The point is that prevention is simple, and treatment of hypoglycemic syncope is time consuming. Shane and co-workers[34] reported a classic example of this presumed complication, based on elicited history.

Acute asthmatic attacks should be treated with epinephrine. The drug should be slowly and cautiously administered, either intramuscularly or intravenously.

The prophylaxis for dental patients with *hypertension, cardiovascular,* or *cerebrovascular disease* is to control, by careful sedation, the rise in blood pressure caused by endogenous epinephine.[12, 15, 30, 42] Only light sedation is induced, but the elevated blood pressure reverts to the patient's usual level and does not subsequently rise after the use of local analgesic solutions with vasoconstrictors and the surgical or restorative treatment. At Loma Linda University, dental patients with these diseases are *always* sedated.

The transmission of hepatitis B (HBV) is most likely to occur during those procedures in which blood may be transferred from patient to clinician or assistant, patient to patient, and clinician to patient. With regard to parenteral injections of local anesthetics for sedation the most likely carrier of HBV will be the needle, and/or needle-tracked drug abuser.

Hepatitis B can be prevented by thoroughly cleansing and then sterilizing instruments which penetrate the soft tissues. Needles should be autoclaved at 121° C, for 15 to 30 minutes, or by exposure to dry heat at 160°–

170° C (320° F.) for one to two hours. The Council on Dental Therapeutics of the American Dental Association has further recommended that if blood may inadvertently, or as a result of positive aspiration, be drawn into a non-disposable syringe, the syringe should be exposed to boiling water (100° C.) for 30 minutes. Individual dose cartridges or ampules of local analgesic solutions are recommended, which in the words of the *Accepted Dental Remedies* of 1966, ". . . of course, should never be used for more than one patient" (p. 38)! Neither needles, syringes nor carpules or ampules should be stored in disinfectant solution which might become contaminated with pathogenic microorganisms through careless handling. Rather the articles should be kept in the containers in which they were sterilized.[1]

Care should be taken to avoid accidental puncture of the skin with used needles when cleaning the instrument tray. The discarded needles should be in a container which does not permit their inadvertent sticking of individuals disposing of the container.

SUMMARY AND CONCLUSIONS

Much patient distress could be avoided by the use of 25 gauge or heavier short-bevel needles, aspirating syringes, or cartridges, and the slow administration of minimum volumes of local analgesic solution. In the treatment of toxic or psychic reactions, the administration of oxygen usually is best. No dental office is adequately equipped unless the dentist can immediately administer oxygen under pressure. If the patient does not recover rapidly, medical assistance should be summoned. The spread of serum hepatitis can be prevented in the dental office by the use of sterilized needles and syringes and by never using a portion of any one analgesic cartridge on more than one patient.

Finally, the best way to prevent local complications, such as trismus, neuritis, or cellulitis, is to adhere strictly to the principles of asepsis and anatomy. An understanding of human physiology, coupled with a careful history and observation of the patient's vital signs, can minimize or prevent complications ranging from mild allergy to total collapse.

REFERENCES

1. Accepted Dental Therapeutics. 37th ed. Chicago, American Dental Association, 1977.
2. Accepted Dental Therapeutics, 36th ed. Chicago, American Dental Association, 1975.
3. Adriani, J., and Campbell, D.: Fatalities following topical application of local anesthetics to mucous membrane. J.A.M.A., *162*:1527, 1956.
4. Allen, G. D., et al.: The cardiorespiratory effects of epinephrine and local anesthetics for dentistry. Anesth. Prog. *20*:152, 1973.
5. American Dental Association Council on Dental Therapeutics: Type B serum hepatitis and dental practice. J.A.D.A., *92*:153, 1976.
6. Ayd, F. J., Jr.: The treatment of everyday depressive patients with nialamide. Clin. Med., *6*:1569, 1959.
7. Berlove, I. J.: Dental-Medical Emergencies and Complications. Chicago, Year Book Publishers, Inc., 1959, p. 128.
8. Bos, A. L., Coppes, E. J., et al.: Aspiration control in the administration of local anesthesia in dentistry. Netherlands D. J. (Supp. 6), *78*:24, 1971.
9. Bourne, J. G.: Deaths with dental anesthetics. Anesthesia, *25*:473, 1970.

10. British Dental Association, Dental Health Committee: The prevention of transmission of serum hepatitis in dentistry. Br. Dent J., *137*:28, 1974.
11. Burch, G. E., and DePasquale, N. P.: Arterial hypertension and the dental patient. J.A.D.A., 73:102, 1966.
12. Cheraskin, E., and Prasertsuntarasai, T.: Use of epinephrine with local anesthesia in hypertensive patients. IV. Effect of tooth extraction on blood pressure and pulse rate. J.A.D.A., 58:61, 1959.
13. Council of Dental Materials and Devices and Council on Dental Therapeutics of the American Dental Association, Joint Report. J.A.D.A. 89:1171, 1974.
14. DeJong, R. H.: Local Anesthetics, 2nd ed., Springfield, Ill., Charles C Thomas, 1977.
15. Edmondson, H. D., et al.: Biochemical evidence of anxiety in dental patients. Br. Med. J. 4:7, 1972.
16. Feinberg, Larry. Personal communication, 15 July 1978.
17. Forsyth, W. D., Allen, G. D., and Everett, G. B.: An evaluation of cardiorespiratory effects of posture in the dental outpatient. Oral Surg. Oral Med. Oral Path, 34:562, 1972.
18. Gibilisco, J. A., et al.: The differential diagnosis of atypical facial pain. Lancet, 85:450, 1965.
19. Guidelines for teaching the comprehensive control of pain and anxiety in dentistry. Chicago, Council on Dental Education. American Dental Association, 1971.
20. Harris, S. C.: Aspiration before injection of dental local anesthetics. J. Oral Surg., *15*:299, 1957.
21. Hayden, J., Jr.: The limits of excellence: What one man can do. 1st Annual N. B. Jorgensen Memorial Lecture, 29 February, 1976, Loma Linda University, Loma Linda, Calif. Anesth. Prog. *25*:75, 1978.
22. Jorgensen, N. B.: Measurements for intra-oral block of the maxillary nerve. J. Oral Surg., 6:1, 1948.
23. Jorgensen, N. B.: Accidental intravenous injection of procaine in dentistry. J. South. California Dent. Assoc., *20*:17, 1952.
24. Jorgensen, N. B.: Pain Control. *In* Royer, R. Q. (ed.): Current Therapy in Dentistry. St. Louis, C. V. Mosby Co., 1970, Vol. IV, p. 371.
25. Jorgensen, N. B., and Hayden, J., Jr.: Sedation, Local and General Anesthesia in Dentistry. 2nd ed. Philadelphia, Lea and Febiger, 1972.
26. Kampmeier, O. F., Cooper, A. R., and Jones, T. S.: A frontal section anatomy of the head and neck. Urbana, University of Illinois Press, 1957, Frontal Section 9.
27. Kennett, S., Curran, J. B., and Jenkins, G. R.: Management of a broken hypodermic needle: Report of a case. Anesth. Prog., *20*:48, 1973, and J. Can. Dent. Assoc., *38*:414, 1972.
28. Larson, C. E.: Methylparaben — an overlooked cause of local anesthetic hypersensitivity. Anesth. Prog., *24*:72, 1977.
29. Litigation California jury awards $75,000 to patient with locked jaw. J.A.D.A., *89*:983, 1974.
30. McCarthy, F. M.: Clinical study of blood pressure responses to epinephrine-containing local anesthetic solutions. J. Dent. Res., *36*:132, 1957.
31. Mosley, J. W., and White, E.: Viral hepatitis as an occupational hazard of dentists. J.A.D.A., *90*:992, 1975.
32. Parker, S.: Effect of nialamide when used alone and with other therapies in the treatment of depression. Dis. Nerv. System, (Sec. 2), *20*:591, 1959.
33. Personal Communication. Mizzy Corporation, Clifton Forge, VA.
34. Shane, S. M., et al.: Intravenous Amnesia — an appraisal after seven years and 10,500 administrations. Anesth. Prog., *21*:36, 1974.
35. Sicher, H., and DuBrul, E. L.: Oral Anatomy. 5th ed. St. Louis, C. V. Mosby Co., 1970, p. 420.
36. Smith, A. E.: Block Anesthesia and Allied Subjects. St. Louis, C. V. Mosby Co., 1920.
37. Steiner, R. B., and Thompson, R. D. (eds.): Oral Surgery and Anesthesia. Philadelphia, W. B. Saunders Co., 1977.
38. Tomlin, P. J.: Death in outpatient dental anesthetic practice. Anesthesia, *29*:551, 1974.
39. Trieger, N.: Pain Control. Chicago, "Die Quintessenz," 1974.
40. Truex, R. C., and Kellner, C. E.: Detailed Atlas of Head and Neck. New York, Oxford University Press, 1948, Fig. 111a, p. 103.
41. Use of epinephrine in connection with procaine in dental procedures. J.A.D.A., *50*:108, 1955.
42. What may happen. . . ? SAAD Digest, 2:75, 1973 (London).
43. White, J. C., Smithwick, R. H., and Simeone, F. A.: The Autonomic Nervous System. New York, The Macmillan Co., 1952, p. 98.
44. Worth, H. M.: Principles and Practice of Oral Radiologic Interpretation. Chicago, Year Book Publishers, Inc., 1963, p. 212.

16

GENERAL ANESTHETIC EMERGENCIES AND COMPLICATIONS

JOHN B. McVEIGH

INTRODUCTION

This chapter is concerned with the safe administration of general anesthetics to ambulatory patients. It is widely recognized that the administration of general anesthesia entails certain risks, some of which are life threatening. The reader should notice that emphasis is placed first on the prevention of emergencies and complications associated with general anesthesia, and second on the prompt recognition and proper treatment of such undesirable occurrences.

Outpatient anesthesia for dental patients enjoys an enviable safety record (See mortality records in Chapter 2).[18, 41] The low incidence of mortality and morbidity demonstrates the safety and acceptance of this procedure. Unexpected, serious events sometimes occur, however, and will continue to do so. Those who are concerned with general anesthesia are aware of this fact and dedicate themselves to the prevention of such occurrences.

Emergencies in anesthetized patients are directly related to the survival of vital body organs. Irreversible brain damage occurs after four to five minutes of cerebral anoxia. Prompt recognition of adverse changes and immediate corrective therapy are essential to prevent brain damage or death. While anesthetized the patient's normal physiology is altered, and protective reflexes are reduced or abolished, leaving him or her relatively defenseless. It is incumbent, therefore, upon those involved with the safety of the patient to exercise the greatest care until he or she has completely recovered from the anesthetic.

Successful anesthesia and surgery or operative dentistry demand coordinated teamwork. Each member of the anesthesia team has definite responsibilities and must be alert to recognize any abnormal signs. It must be stressed that prevention of emergencies and complications is much to be preferred to their treatment. Impending emergencies or complications may be avoided or at least diminished in severity by early recognition and immediate application of corrective measures.

RESPIRATORY EMERGENCIES AND COMPLICATIONS

RESPIRATORY OBSTRUCTION

Most general anesthetic emergencies are related to respiratory tract obstruction. The respiratory tract, including the anatomic dead space, extends from the lips and nares to the pulmonary alveolar membrane. Obstruction of the flow of air or gases can occur at any level within these limits. The usual sites of obstruction are the lips, oropharynx, nasopharynx, glottis, vocal cords, trachea and large bronchi, bronchioles, and alveoli. *The prevention of respiratory obstruction by the maintenance of a patent airway is the greatest single factor in the administration of a safe and satisfactory general anesthetic.*

Respiratory obstruction is characterized by any or a combination of the following signs:

1. Reduced or inadequate gaseous exchange, as evidenced by weak expansion of the anesthetic reservoir bag or weakness in respiratory sounds.
2. Noisy respiration, unless obstruction is complete.
3. Cyanosis. (See under Respiratory Emergencies, *Apnea.*)
4. Strong diaphragmatic activity and excessive abdominal movement.
5. Exaggerated activity of the secondary muscles of respiration.

Respiratory obstruction prevents adequate gaseous exchange, resulting in hypoxia and, if not corrected, will ultimately lead to cardiac arrest. *It has been estimated that 90 per cent of deaths associated with general anesthesia are related to improper management of the airway.*[14]

Anatomic and Mechanical Considerations

The Lips. During general surgery hindrance of air flow past the lips may occur in patients whose dentures have been removed or in patients with thick, full lips. The use of an oral or nasal airway or endotracheal tube in more difficult instances will correct this obstruction. In operations within the oral cavity the lips are not a significant factor in airway obstruction, as the mouth is held open by a mouth prop and the lips are retracted.

The Oropharynx. The oropharynx is the most frequent site of upper airway obstruction. When the tongue and jaw relax under anesthesia they tend to fall backward and may occlude the space between the base of the tongue and the posterior pharyngeal wall. This is corrected by supporting the angle of the mandible and properly positioning the oropharyngeal pack to elevate the tongue. These procedures will bring the tongue forward and away from the posterior pharyngeal wall. This type of obstruction is extremely dangerous if unrecognized, as the airway is almost completely occluded. If obstruction persists, a pharyngeal airway or endotracheal tube should be placed.

The Nasopharynx. Obstruction at this level is usually due to one of the following: edema of the nasal mucous membrane, deviated nasal septum, enlarged turbinates, or hypertrophied adenoid tissue. With nasopharyngeal obstruction an oropharyngeal or oroendotracheal tube should be placed; as in dental procedures the mouth is open and the oropharynx is packed.

The Glottis. Restriction of air flow at the glottis is most often due to obstruction by foreign bodies too large to enter the larynx. These may be gauze sponges, fragments of broken dentures, dental bridgework, and so forth. All removable appliances should be removed prior to induction of anesthesia. A properly positioned oropharyngeal pack will help prevent this form of obstruction.

The Larynx. Interruption of air flow in the larynx may be due to the presence of teeth, parts of teeth, dental materials, or other small foreign bodies in the area, or to partial or complete adduction of the vocal cords (laryngospasm). Reflex adduction of the vocal cords in response to an irritant is a protective mechanism to prevent contamination of the lower respiratory tract. (See under Respiratory Emergencies, *Laryngospasm.*)

The Trachea and Large Bronchi. Obstruction at this level is usually the result of aspiration of foreign matter such as vomitus, whole teeth or tooth fragments, dental materials or devices, etc.

The Bronchioles. The smooth muscle of the bronchioles may contract, resulting in bronchospasm. This may occur in some patients while under light anesthesia, particularly those with a history of asthma, or contraction may be precipitated by the use of certain sensitizing drugs. (See under Respiratory Emergencies, *Bronchospasm.*)

The Alveoli. Emphysematous changes or atelectasis (lung collapse) will result in obstruction of the alveoli. With alveolar obstruction there will be an increase in the pulse rate, lag of the chest wall on the affected side, and progressive cyanosis. Assisting respiration with 100 per cent oxygen under positive pressure will aid in oxygenating the blood.

Laryngospasm

Laryngospasm is a reflex protective mechanism to prevent contamination of the lower respiratory tract. In laryngospasm there is partial or complete adduction of the vocal cords. With partial adduction, a crowing sound will be heard and a moderate hypoxia will result from the impaired airway. If this partial adduction is not promptly and properly treated, it will often develop into complete adduction of the vocal cords and result in complete obstruction of the airway, severe anoxia, and cyanosis. Complete obstruction must be relieved promptly to prevent cardiac arrest. Laryngospasm is an infrequent complication in the properly prepared patient receiving a well-administered ultralight general anesthetic.

CAUSES

1. Irritation of the vocal cords by blood, mucus, or debris.
2. Improper administration of parasympathomimetic drugs, such as a barbiturate, particularly in the unpremedicated patient.
3. Sudden high concentrations of inhalation anesthetic agents.

PREVENTION

1. Many premedicate with atropine or scopolamine, unless contraindicated; others do not feel it is necessary.
2. Properly position the oropharyngeal pack to prevent irritation of the vocal cords by blood, mucus, or debris passing beyond the pack.
3. Maintain adequate depth of anesthesia to obtund reflex mechanisms that may be stimulated during surgery.
4. Maintain a patent airway and provide adequate oxygenation.

TREATMENT

Frequently this respiratory emergency is improperly managed. It is not uncommon to see the inexperienced anesthetist who is confronted with a patient experiencing laryngospasm to reach hurriedly for succinylcholine, administer 20 to 40 mg intravenously, and follow this with 100 per cent oxygen via a full face mask without attempting to determine the cause of the spasm. While doing this, any blood, mucus, or debris in the pharynx will either be aspirated when the vocal cords relax or will remain to act again as an irritant and set up a second spasm.

Laryngospasm can be properly managed in the following manner:

1. Grasp the tongue with gauze and draw forward.
2. Using a tonsil tip, suction the pharynx and oral cavity free of all debris.
3. Replace the soiled pack with a fresh oropharyngeal pack.
4. Administer 100 per cent oxygen via nasal mask.
5. If surgery is completed, lighten the level of anesthesia; if more surgery

is contemplated, some anesthetists prefer to slightly deepen the anesthetic level; others do not.

These measures will suffice to alleviate the laryngospasm in nearly all instances. If the spasm persists, however, administer 10 to 20 mg of succinylcholine slowly intravenously (succinylcholine chloride should be injected slowly to minimize muscular fasciculations and resultant postoperative muscle pain). After the laryngospasm is broken, respiration should be assisted if necessary by manual compression of the thorax or by intermittent positive pressure applied by hand to a bag of oxygen connected to a tight-fitting nasal mask. Intubation should not be attempted while the patient is in laryngospasm as the cords will be tightly adducted and the intubation procedure would be extremely difficult and unduly traumatic. The time wasted in attempting intubation with the cords adducted would increase the hypoxia and no doubt result in unfortunate sequelae. Artificial respiration is ineffective in severe laryngospasm and should be avoided until the airway is established, as it would tend to evacuate the remaining oxygen from the lungs. Air will not enter the lungs on the release of pressure on the chest wall until the airway is clear. Succinylcholine should not be used indiscriminately and without adequate resuscitative drugs and equipment on hand. Its administration is certainly justified in relieving severe laryngospasm that does not respond to the treatment measures outlined above. Even here, however, the minimal effective dose should be employed. If a general anesthetic is properly administered to a properly prepared patient, and the causes of laryngospasm are clearly understood and appreciated, respiratory obstruction in this area will rarely occur.

Bronchospasm

Bronchospasm is a condition of partial or complete contraction of the bronchiolar musculature. Partial bronchospasm is not uncommon in patients under general anesthesia, and it is not difficult to control. Total bronchospasm, which fortunately is rare, is a very serious emergency. Its treatment will be described below. It is most frequently encountered in patients with a history of bronchial asthma or chronic bronchitis. When there is contraction of the bronchiolar musculature, and a resulting hypoxia, the patient is said to have a bronchospasm. The chest is fixed in a position of inspiration.[26] In partial bronchospasm an expiratory wheeze, such as is heard in bronchial asthma, will be heard. In total bronchospasm, usually no sounds are heard from the lungs.

CAUSES

Bronchospasm may be due to several factors:

1. Vagal stimulation by mucus, blood, aspirated gastric contents, or surgery.
2. Histamine release.
3. Mechanical stimulation by an endotracheal tube.
4. Irritating vapors.

PREVENTION

1. A careful medical history is important. Those individuals with chronic bronchitis or bronchial asthma are more susceptible to bronchospasm.
2. The parasympathetic nerves cause constriction of the bronchiolar musculature. Premedication with atropine, a parasympatholytic agent, may help to prevent bronchospasm in susceptible patients.
3. Provide a smooth induction of anesthesia.
4. Avoid irritating inhalation agents.

TREATMENT

Epinephrine is an excellent bronchodilator in normal individuals. The moribund asthmatic, however, is invariably resistant to epinephrine and isoprenaline. In the event of severe bronchospasm Gold[26] and others[15, 53] recommend the slow IV injection of 250 to 500 mg of aminophylline (i.e., given over a 5 minute period). Aminophylline must be injected slowly, as a marked hypotension will result with rapid administration. Hydrocortisone, 100 mg, IV, remains the most effective treatment of a severe and protracted bronchospasm. In total bronchospasm, cyanosis appears very rapidly, and one's natural inclination is to force oxygen into the lungs at any cost. Dickson[15] feels that this is wasted effort, and, more important, wasted time. Every second is important, and even if some oxygen is forced into the lungs it will at best relieve the hypoxia and cyanosis only momentarily. It will still be impossible to remove carbon dioxide from the lungs, and cardiac arrest may follow rapidly. If hydrocortisone and aminophylline are administered in the dosage given above immediately after the diagnosis is made, the chances for recovery are good.[53]

Aspiration of Vomitus

Vomiting under anesthesia, particularly with the use of inhalation agents, is not an uncommon occurrence. Fortunately the material is rarely aspirated and the only problem is one of debridement. However, if vomitus is aspirated, one is confronted with a most serious emergency. In addition to the obvious hazard of airway obstruction, which results in anoxia and possible death if treatment is mismanaged, there is the often unrecognized sequence of events leading to aspiration pneumonitis. Aspiration of gastric contents constitutes a grave emergency, the frequency of which can be minimized by appropriate preventive measures. The most obvious preventive measure is to avoid general anesthesia in a patient who is suspected to have food in the stomach. Nearly all dental or oral surgical procedures can be delayed for some time if necessary. If emergency surgery is needed, a local analgesic technique should be employed if the patient has recently eaten. It usually requires about 4 hours for most food to pass through the stomach, but if the patient is quite apprehensive or in considerable pain, 10 to 12 hours or longer may be required. Other preventive measures include insuring adequate oxygen levels being supplied to the patient to prevent nausea and maintaining meticulous observation from the point of induction to the time of complete recovery from the anesthetic. The patient should not be moved from the surgery room to the recovery room until protective reflexes are present.

INCIDENCE

Deaths from aspiration were reported soon after the introduction of ether and chloroform for surgical anesthesia. The first death reported to be related to aspiration was in 1848. Historically, aspiration into the tracheobronchial tree was recognized early as a cause of morbidity and mortality. Aspiration of vomitus has been reported[34] as the primary cause of death in 0.03 to 26.3 per cent of anesthetized patients. The incidence is higher in obstetric patients, apparently because of relatively poorer preparation and greater likelihood of a full stomach as compared with general surgical patients. Edwards et al.,[20] in a report on 1000 anesthetic deaths, considered 110 to be due to aspiration of vomitus. In a recent paper by Cameron et al.,[10] the clinical records of 47 patients with documented aspiration were reviewed. The overall mortality was 62 per cent. If only one lobe was involved on x-ray, mortality was 41 per cent. If two or more lobes on one or both sides were involved, mortality increased to 90 per cent.

DIAGNOSIS

The diagnosis of aspiration of vomitus requires a high index of suspicion, as the original episode may have gone unnoticed, or its immediate effects may have been masked by the anesthetic state. If vomitus appears in the mouth or pharynx, the possibility of aspiration should be considered and investigated. Aspiration may cause immediate circulatory collapse and respiratory apnea or spasm of reflex origin, but the onset of severe illness may be more subtle and occur after a latent period; sometimes even 6 to 8 hours after the initial features have subsided or passed unobserved. Aspiration of solids is diagnosed by the presence of obstruction of the airway or by signs of lung collapse. Liquid aspirate is not always easily diagnosed. Cyanosis, tachycardia, and tachypnea, possibly associated with bronchospasm or respiratory distress, may occur immediately or at a variable interval. If, during anesthesia, there is difficulty in maintaining the patient's color and there is an increase in the inflationary pressure, aspiration must be suspected. Endotracheal aspiration may be diagnostic. Acute pulmonary edema in a severe case of aspiration is revealed by a profuse serosanguinous froth pouring from the airway. X-ray examination may show widespread infiltration of the lung, more often affecting the right side and the lower lobes, but changes are usually more marked 24 hours later. Progressive hypotension with low venous pressure, a rising hematocrit, hypoxemia, and acidosis may lead to a state of shock and death.[44] Stetson[60] emphasizes the importance of pre-anesthetic evaluation and preparation along with scrupulous observation of the patient to prevent this disaster.

Aspiration Pneumonitis. Except for the situations of obvious asphyxiation which lead to sudden death, there was little significance attached to the aspiration of small quantities of vomitus that did not cause sudden death, but that later resulted in aspiration pneumonitis. In these cases death was usually attributed to secondary pulmonary infection. In the

1860's it was finally realized that something besides infection was going on in the lungs. Winternitz[67] injected HCl into the bronchi of anesthetized rabbits and unknowingly described what is now accepted as the typical picture of acute aspiration pneumonitis. Other studies, for example, those of Mendelson[45] in 1946 and Teabeaut[62] in 1952, clarified the pathologic sequence of events occurring in the lungs after aspiration. The pulmonary reaction to the aspiration of gastric contents is directly related to the nature and volume of the aspirated material. Experimental studies evaluating the significance of what is aspirated, such as enzymes, pH, bacteria, blood, fecally contaminated gastric juice, alcohol, and various combinations thereof, including the addition of solid food, have been conducted using experimental animals. From these studies the pH of the material aspirated was considered the most important factor in determining the degree of pneumonitis. Normal gastric juice is acidic and ranges from pH 1.5 to 2.4. When the pH was less than 1.2, patchy atelectasis and hemorrhagic areas with occasional frank necrosis occurred in the lungs as well as air leaks from the lung surface and pulmonary edema. In experimental studies using isolated perfused ventilated lungs, gastric juice containing methylene blue, after being introduced into the trachea, appeared on the lung surface within 12 to 18 seconds. When we realize the rapidity of distribution of material within the lungs, it follows that the treatment of aspiration must be rapid and correct. Aspiration can occur from two distinct sources caused by two different mechanisms. These are vomiting and regurgitation. A distinction between these two actions should be made before describing prevention and treatment. One is an active phenomenon; the other is passive. Regurgitation is a passive act with a high and often unrecognized incidence during anesthesia. It occurs when the intra-abdominal pressure exceeds the intrathoracic pressure and there is an associated incompetence of the gastroesophageal closing mechanism. If the patient is in the supine position and someone inadvertently exerts pressure on the abdomen, there is the possibility that regurgitation, which is silent, may occur. There is no retching or other muscular movement which would warn the surgeon or anesthesiologist of the regurgitation episode. Vomiting, however, is an active phenomenon caused by a different mechanism and is equally as hazardous as regurgitation. Nausea, which precedes the act of vomiting, may be masked by the anesthetic state. The alert anesthetist, however, can recognize such objective signs of an impending vomiting episode as increased salivation, sweating, repetitive swallowing, increased pulse rate, and variations in the character of respiration. Recognizing these signs may allow as much as a minute's advance warning of vomiting. Bannister and Sattilaro[4] described the microscopic findings following the aspiration of matter with a low pH. After 24 hours there is usually a peribronchial infiltration of polymorphonuclear leukocytes, followed later by mononucleated cells predominating. If the aspirated material is contaminated, lung abscesses will also be evident.

TREATMENT

Successful treatment of this emergency depends on prompt recognition. Once the diagnosis is made, treatment is begun immediately. The patient should be placed in the Trendelenburg position with the head down at least 15 degrees. The patient is then rolled onto his right side to aid in the drainage of vomitus from the mouth and to help confine any aspirated material to the dependent right lung. The right lung is more often affected because of the configuration of the main bronchi. This position will, therefore, tend to localize the aspiration to the right side while the airway is being cleared and the patient is being oxygenated. The oropharynx should be cleared digitally with gauze placed over the fingers and by the use of suction. When the pharynx is clear, roll the patient onto his back and intubate. A rapidly acting muscle relaxant, such as succinylcholine, 20 mg IV, may be helpful if needed. Intubation will facilitate the administration of high oxygen concentrations and tracheobronchial irrigation and suction, and will prevent additional aspiration of any material inadvertently left in the mouth. Following intubation, the patient is placed in a slight Fowler position, that is, with the head above the horizontal plane. Normal saline in 5 to 10 cc increments is introduced through the endotracheal tube to facilitate the removal of particulate matter. This is followed by suction and ventilation with oxygen. *This procedure should be reserved for selected cases as the instillation of saline could conceivably force aspirated material deeper into the pulmonary tree.* The main advantage of introducing saline is that it tends to dilute and thereby elevate the pH of highly acidic vomitus. Lavage using large volumes of fluid has been shown to increase the spread of acid and, therefore, is contraindicated. Maintenance of a patent airway for adequate ventilation with oxygen is of primary importance. Within the last decade numerous authors have advocated the use of corticosteroids to combat pneumonitis.[4, 31, 42] A satisfactory dosage schedule would be 100 mg of hydrocortisone (Solu-Cortef) given intravenously as soon as practicable, then 100 mg every eight hours for three days, followed by 25 mg every six hours for an additional two days.[16] It should be pointed out that since hydrocortisone may reduce the patient's defense mechanisms against bacterial infection, adequate doses of antibiotics should be considered. In addition, there should be symptomatic treatment for other complications such as vasopressors to support circulation, bronchodilators such as aminophylline (250 mg given IV in 500 ml of dextrose and water every eight hours), and digitalis for heart failure and pulmonary edema.[4] Tracheostomy should be considered in severe cases in which continued support of respiration is deemed advisable. Nicholl et al.[50] encourage treacheostomy also in that it reduces the anatomic dead space. See the chapter on *maxillofacial injuries.*

The paper of Mucklow and Larard[48] lends additional support to the treatment described above. They based their technique on experience gained from working in a busy casualty department where many patients were admitted in coma caused by drug overdosage, trauma, or diabetes, together with seven cases in which aspiration of vomitus was associated with anesthesia. They used lavage in 40 cases, six of which were patients under anesthesia, with apparent clinical success. They further advocated the intravenous administration of aminophylline, 250 mg slowly, to reduce or prevent the element of bronchospasm which is frequently present. Hydrocortisone was also employed in the same dosage schedule mentioned above. After the patient has sufficiently recovered from this initial treatment, he or she should be hospitalized for further indicated treatment and observation.

RESPIRATORY ABNORMALITIES

Alterations of the normal respiratory pattern are most often encountered during the induction phase of anesthesia. Respiratory abnormalities include the following:

Tachypnea. Usually associated with light anesthesia, particularly with the inhalation agents, and with surgical stimulation before adequate anesthesia is achieved. The tidal volume is reduced and ventilation becomes inadequate. This results in respiratory acidosis, hypoxemia, and hypercapnia.

Shallow Breathing. Sometimes seen with deep anesthesia, halothane use, muscle relaxants, etc. Respirations should be assisted until the normal respiratory pattern returns.

Slow Breathing. Slow, deep breathing is characteristic of overdosage of opiates.

Apnea. Apnea is a state of "no breathing" characterized by an increase in the pulse rate, progressive hypoxia, and cyanosis. If breathing is not promptly restored, hypoxia will become severe and result in irreversible brain damage or death.

Apnea may be caused by any of the following:

1. High concentration of inhalation agents.
2. Irritating vapors.
3. Overdosage of anesthetic agents.
4. Depletion of carbon dioxide.
5. Muscle relaxants.

Simple breath-holding is frequently seen during induction by "pushing" a high concentration of inhalation agents, or by stimulation from irritating vapors. Smooth induction will most often prevent breath-holding. When apnea occurs, the mask should be removed from the patient's face and the gas machine flushed promptly with oxygen to remove the irritating agent. The mask should then be reapplied snugly and respirations assisted by rhythmic contraction of the bag. If you are unable to ventilate the patient by this procedure, remove the mask and examine the patient for a possible obstruction in the airway. Laryngospasm or bronchospasm should also be considered as possible causes of inability to inflate the lungs. These conditions have been discussed earlier in this chapter.

If the lungs can be inflated but the patient's condition does not improve, there may be a mechanical failure in the anesthetic machine or an incorrect hookup of the oxygen and gas tanks. Fatalities have occurred in some instances when nitrous oxide was administered instead of the intended oxygen. In this situation the anesthetic machine should be discarded and mouth-to-mouth resuscitation performed until the error can be detected. The pulse should be monitored to determine if the circulation is still intact, as artificial respiration is useless unless the circulation is maintained.

Apnea resulting from an overdosage of anesthetic agent can occur for several reasons. Premedication with meperidine, morphine, or barbiturates will result in a certain degree of expected respiratory depression. Intravenous anesthetic agents also have a depressant effect on respiration. The combination of premedication and intravenous anesthesia has an additive effect, and may lead to respiratory depression and apnea. This problem is infrequently encountered in anesthesia for the ambulatory patient, as minimal premedication and light planes of anesthesia are usually employed. The goal in outpatient anesthesia is a safe anesthetic with a level no deeper than the surgical stimulus requires. Overdosage sometimes occurs in elderly patients as their metabolic rate is lower and their circulation time is somewhat longer than in younger individuals, and additional increments of intravenous agents may be mistakenly administered when the effect of the initial injection is not readily realized. Overdosage may occur also in patients with impaired liver function.

Apnea resulting from a depletion of carbon dioxide is seen rarely, but may be encountered in the induction phase of inhalation anesthesia in a child. No treatment is indicated, as carbon dioxide accumulates during the apneic state, and respirations will resume quickly.

Apnea may occur as the result of painful stimulus in light planes of anesthesia. The anesthetic level should be deepened and respiration assisted, using 100 per cent oxygen.

Apnea is commonly seen when muscle relaxants are employed. This can be minimized by using the minimal effective dose for the purpose desired. Treatment here is to manually assist respirations with 100 per cent oxygen until normal breathing returns.

As apnea, if allowed to persist, will lead to hypoxia and cyanosis, it is felt that the problem of cyanosis should be discussed. The appearance of cyanosis of the skin or mucous membranes will, in the absence of certain heart diseases or blood dyscrasias, indicate either peripheral vascular stasis or inadequate oxygenation of arterial blood in the lungs. Cyanosis may result from airway obstruction, incorrect gas-oxygen mixture, deficient pulmonary ventilation, or interruption of oxygen transfer from the alveoli to the pulmonary capillaries. Since the appearance of cyanosis depends on the presence of a minimum of reduced hemoglobin (approximately 5 gm), it may be late in onset or absent in states associated with anemia. Furthermore, there is an appreciable element of observer's error involved in its recognition. Its *absence* is therefore of little value for judging the state of the circulation. When it suddenly develops, however, it is a sign of the greatest importance. Whether its primary cause is circulatory or respiratory, its continuance is an indication that insufficient oxygen is reaching the vital body organs. The sudden appearance of cyanosis warns of the existence of an emergency situation requiring immediate action to restore a normal circulation and assure a patent airway and normal pulmonary gaseous exchange. It should be noted that the disappearance of cyanosis following ventilation with 100 per cent oxygen does not necessarily imply an adequate oxygen supply to the body, as the blood may be fully oxygenated but not have sufficient flow to provide an adequate amount of oxygen to the vital organs.

Coughing. Coughing may be initiated by irritating vapors during induction with inhalation agents. Coughing may also be encountered during intravenous anesthesia in heavy smokers or those with inflammation of the air passages. Adequate premedication and a smooth induction will reduce excessive mucus flow, a factor in reflex coughing. If marked coughing develops during anesthesia and persists afterward, the patient may have aspirated and should be referred for thoracic consultation without delay.

Hiccup. Hiccup is a state of intermittent spasm of the diaphragm accompanied by sudden closure of the glottis. Respiratory exchange is diminished to some extent and may lead to hypoxia. Jerking movements accompanying hiccup often make surgery difficult or impossible. Hiccup usually will respond to the administration of 10 to 20 mg of succinylcholine followed by ventilation with oxygen under positive pressure.

DECREASED OXYGEN CONCENTRATION

Oxygen is essential to life, but, unfortunately, there is no store of oxygen in the body to be drawn upon in an emergency. The brain is particularly sensitive to oxygen lack, and irreversible brain damage occurs after 4 to 5 minutes of oxygen deprivation. An excellent practice is to administer 30 to 100 per cent oxygen to the patient immediately after starting intravenous anesthesia and to continue to do so during the procedure to increase the oxygen saturation of the blood. If a respiratory emergency should later arise, precious time is added for treating the problem.

Decreased oxygen concentration usually results from one or more of the following:

1. Any cause of respiratory obstruction, as noted above.
2. Incorrect oxygen-to-gas ratio resulting from an improper mixture setting of the gas machine, accidental crossing of anesthetic lines or tanks, or depletion of oxygen at the tank.
3. Inadequate flow of oxygen from the gas machine to the patient.

CARDIOVASCULAR EMERGENCIES AND COMPLICATIONS

ALTERATIONS OF PULSE RATE

Tachycardia. Tachycardia signifies a pulse rate greater than 100 beats per minute. Sinus tachycardia is more common than ventricular tachycardia. The rate is usually 100 to 180 beats per minute, with normal P-R intervals and QRS complexes. It is important to distinguish between supraventricular (atrial) tachycardia and ventricular paroxysmal tachycardia, as the treatment and prognosis of each are different. Electronic monitoring of cardiac rate and rhythm is a matter of routine in many offices. An atrial tachycardia will often respond to vagal stimulation (carotid sinus or eyeball pressure) and to methoxamine, phenylephrine, or neostigmine. Tachycardia is generally well tolerated in the absence of myocardial disease. Treatment is indicated when hypotension develops or there is cardiac failure. Ventricular tachycardia, particularly when accompanied by multiple premature ventricular contractions (PVCs), may lead to ventricular fibrillation.

Bradycardia. Bradycardia is characterized by a pulse rate less than 60 beats per minute with normal P-R intervals and QRS complexes. It is most often due to an increase in vagal tone. Vagal tone may be increased reflexly by pain, or by pressure on the carotid sinus, the eyeballs, or the posterior pharyngeal wall. Uncomplicated bradycardia produces no symptoms unless it is extreme, when it may lead to syncope or convulsions. Bradycardia may be treated by atropine, 0.4 to 0.8 mg intravenously.

CARDIAC ARRHYTHMIAS

An arrhythmia is any deviation from the normal cardiac rhythm. Minor arrhythmias, usually arising in the S-A node, such as sinus tachycardia, sinus bradycardia, or sinus arrhythmia, in the absence of other symptoms, do not preclude general anesthesia. Other arrhythmias, arising in the atria, the conduction system, or the ventricles should be pursued and corrected prior to the administration of a general anesthetic. Cardiac arrhythmias seen in patients under general anesthetic are the result of multiple factors acting on the pacemaker, the conduction system, and the myocardium. Arrhythmias may produce an emergency situation if cardiac filling is so impaired that there is a sharp decrease in cardiac output. In such a case hypotension would follow and the resultant myocardial hypoxia would further reduce the force of cardiac contraction.

Predisposing Factors

Factors contributing to arrhythmias during general anesthesia and surgery include the preoperative condition of the heart, length of surgery, type of surgery, type and duration of anesthesia, age of patient, metabolic considerations, and, most important, duration and degree of hypoxia.

Ventricular arrhythmias may be insignificant, such as an isolated PVC, or they may be of sufficient magnitude to cause death. Patients with serious ventricular arrhythmias obviously are not candidates for general anesthesia. Fatal arrhythmias may be prevented by recognition and prompt treatment of prefatal disturbances.

Four ventricular arrhythmias are considered prefatal: Ventricular bigeminy or trigeminy, multiple (more than six per minute) PVCs, R on T phenomena, and multifocal PVCs.

Bigeminy. This is a rhythm in which every other beat is premature, so that each two beats appear coupled. In *trigeminy,* two premature beats follow each normal beat, or two normal beats are followed by a premature beat. These beats can lead to other ventricular dysrhythmic problems. When bigeminy is suspected, surgery should be discontinued and a diagnosis established. If the coupled beats do not disappear and the patient's condition continues to worsen, lidocaine, 1 mg per kg, should be administered intravenously along with oxygen under positive pressure.

Multiple PVCs. This arrhythmia can lead to ventricular tachycardia, a potentially fatal arrhythmia. More than five PVCs per minute is a matter of concern. Ventricular tachycardia is frequently followed by ventricular fibrillation. Ventricular tachycardia may also result in a sudden loss of blood pressure and shock. Restoration of blood pressure with vasopressors and fluids along with 400 watt-seconds of countershock to the precordium may be suitable treatment for this problem.

R on T Phenomena. The R on T phenomenon relates to ventricular contraction while the heart is repolarizing and is in its most vulnerable period. A cardiac contraction during the vulnerable period can initiate ventricular fibrillation.

Multifocal PVCs.   These are initiated from different areas of the ventricles. These may also lead to ventricular fibrillation.

Prevention and Treatment

When alterations of cardiac rhythm are accompanied by cardiovascular changes such as hypotension, they require prompt diagnosis and corrective therapy. The usual treatment consists of discontinuing anesthetic administration, hyperventilating the lungs with oxygen under positive pressure, followed by measures to correct hypotension, and, in the small number of patients who fail to respond to these primary measures, administration of an antiarrhythmic drug. There are several useful drugs available for the prevention and treatment of arrhythmias. Tolas and Allen[63] in a controlled study involving 124 patients demonstrated rather conclusively that the beta-adrenergic drug propranolol (Inderal) was effective in the prevention of cardiac arrhythmias associated with anesthetic induction. They warned, however, because of the potency of the beta blockade, that it be used with caution. Fukushima et al.[25] studied the effects of propranolol on blood pressure, heart rate, and cardiac rhythm during ventricular arrhythmias initiated by hypercarbia on 13 patients. Propranolol was considered effective in all subjects. The successful use of propranolol suggests the mechanism of ventricular arrhythmias produced by hypercarbia to be related to beta-adrenergic receptors. Blockade of these receptors by propranolol decreased the sensitization of the myocardium to sympathetic stimulation. Morrow[47] suggests the intravenous administration of lidocaine, 1 to 2 mg per kg. Harrison et al.,[30] in discussing the antiarrhythmic properties of lidocaine, stated that lidocaine is effective and also has little effect on systemic arterial pressure and little or no effect on the contractile force of the heart. Underhill and Tredway[64] feel it futile to attempt to control arrhythmias in the presence of hypotension. They stated further that ventricular and atrial arrhythmias which failed to respond to cardiac depressants often reverted when the blood pressure was raised to normal levels with norepinephrine. Presumably the increased coronary flow results in improved myocardial stability. The value of pressor amines in the control of ventricular tachycardia appears to lie in their ability to accelerate the basic idioventricular pacemaker, thereby suppressing ectopic activity. Payne[51] stated that Pronethalol blocks the cardiac effects of both catecholamines and sympathetic activity. When given in moderate doses of 2.5 to 10 mg intravenously, it is capable of completely abolishing extrasystoles associated with respiratory acidosis and catecholamine release. One per cent procaine administered intravenously frequently has been used to control arrhythmias. Quinidine lactate injected intravenously in doses of 100 to 300 mg often will correct some ventricular arrhythmias refractory to procaine. The external electrical defibrillator is sometimes effective in reversing ventricular fibrillation if the myocardium is well oxygenated. Premedication with appropriate dosages of atropine is useful in inhibiting reflex vagal activity. Drugs which act as general depressants of cardiac irritability may aid materially in protecting the heart from arrhythmias. They are useful also in restoring an irregular rhythm to normal.

See the chapter on *monitoring* for discussion of the cardiac conduction system and of the cardioscope.

HYPOTENSION

Hypotension occurring during anesthesia, regardless of cause, may develop into an acute emergency. When hypotension exists to a mild degree preoperatively there is little concern if the patient is asymptomatic. If the patient presents with a more marked preoperative hypotension, a medical consultation is deemed advisable. With the patient under anesthesia, the anesthetic team must be constantly aware of his condition, as it has been demonstrated often the morbidity and mortality resulting from severe hypotension are directly related to the length of time the patient is in shock. Therefore, prompt recognition of a hypotensive state and immediate corrective therapy are required to prevent cardiovascular collapse. Hypotension has been reported in anesthetized patients who previously had been receiving antihypertensive therapy,[11, 49] and adrenal insufficiency with marked hypotension is sometimes seen in anesthetized patients who have previously been receiving corticosteroids.[58] Miscellaneous causes of hypotension would include excessive blood loss, air embolism, severe hypoxia, and overdosage of an anesthetic agent.

Shock may be regarded as a state of cardiovascular collapse often associated with insufficient venous return to the heart and complicated by a persisting deficiency of blood flow to the peripheral tissues. Various forms of shock are well known. In this chapter, however, we are concerned only with shock as a complication associated with the use of a general anesthetic. Certain anesthetic agents such as halothane may cause peripheral vasodilation and a resultant fall in systemic blood pressure. In general, the miscellaneous causes of hypotension listed above may result in shock in the anesthetized patient.

Rauwolfia Alkaloid Therapy

Reserpine and similar drugs are commonly used in the treatment of hypertension and psychiatric disorders. Reduction of blood pressure produced by intramuscular reserpine is gradual in onset and usually moderate, but significant. In addition, the drug possesses a behavioral effect, causing sedation which allows the patient to rest and yet be easily aroused for nursing care.[2] The action of reserpine depends on its ability to lower the level of catecholamine and serotonin content in all organs where these mediators are normally stored. The major storage areas, central and peripheral, include the lower centers of the brain, the adrenal medulla, sympathetic ganglia and nerves, cardiac muscle, and vascular and intestinal walls.[68]

The onset of hypotensive effect is one to two hours after intramuscular administration, after which the blood pressure falls gradually over a period of an hour and then slowly returns to pretreatment levels over a widely variable period of several hours to as much as several days.[24] At times the reduction of blood pressure achieved with reserpine alone is not sufficient to control the blood pressure at the desired level. In such instances hydralazine may be added. Parenteral hydralazine should be given only when the drug cannot be given orally.[52] The initial dose recommended is 10 mg, t.i.d., and is gradually increased to 100 mg t.i.d., over a period of four weeks. It is well known that the surgical and anesthetic risk is higher in the hypertensive patient.

There have been differences of opinion over the years regarding the delay of surgery in patients who are or have been recently receiving antihypertensive drugs. Freis[24] feels that surgery should be delayed until the blood pressure has been controlled for at least several days and symptoms of heart failure have cleared entirely. Others[68] are of the opinion that reserpine is potentiated by anesthetic agents and that extreme hypotension may result if the catecholamine level has previously been lowered. They feel that elective surgery should be delayed for two weeks after the drug is discontinued, this being the time required to return the catecholamine level to near normal in most patients. Present thought is that patients on reserpine therapy present few problems that are fundamentally new and would not be encountered in nontreated hypertensives. As an example of this concept, Morrow and Morrow[47] carried out corrective cardiac operations in five normotensive males, aged 16 to 35, each of whom had received oral reserpine for 38 to 68 days preoperatively up to the day preceding operation. None of the patients had significant changes in blood pressure or heart rate when anesthesia was induced, at the time of endotracheal intubation, or during maintenance of anesthesia. No patient required a vagolytic or vasopressor compound during operation. All had uncomplicated postoperative courses. The results of this study provide at least indirect evidence that the difficulties encountered in the anesthetic management of hypertensive patients receiving reserpine are attributable to their underlying hypertensive cardiovascular disease rather than to the pharmacologic effects of reserpine. In addition, Munson and Jamicek[49] stated that hypertensive individuals not receiving reserpine may have unstable blood pressures. They felt that this was commonly due to the loss of cardiovascular homeostatic mechanisms secondary to arteriosclerotic changes. Hamelberg[29] points out that no essential difference exists in the incidence of hypotension during anesthesia between the treated and nontreated patients. Opinion now tends to favor maintaining patients on their antihypertensive medication. No matter by which view one chooses to abide, he should be aware of the fact that catecholamine-depleted tissues are sensitive to exogenous catecholamine.[9] Bosomworth[6] states that his personal experience indicates that phenlyephrine and norepinephrine are the most reliable vasopressors when hypotension occurs in the reserpine-treated patient. The general feeling currently held regarding patients receiving antihypertensive drugs is that careful attention to anesthetic technique and an understanding of the pharmacologic action of these drugs make the postponement of surgery unnecessary.

Steroid Therapy

Patients receiving steroids or who have previously been on steroid therapy are being seen more frequently in practice today. In the patient with organic adrenal insufficiency any stressful procedure, such as surgery or anesthesia, was frequently fatal prior to the introduction of desoxycortisone acetate and adrenal cortical extract.[29] Steroids combined with careful attention to electrolyte balance increased the patient's chance to survive surgical procedures and anesthesia. Although a blessing for patients with adrenal cortical insufficiency, corticosteroids became a hazard when used for other diseases. Several men[33, 58] reported unresponsive hypotension and fatalities in this group of patients. There is evidence that this state of shock is the outcome of adrenal cortex depression induced by corticosteroid therapy.[40, 55] In one study[58] shock was successfully treated in 80 per cent of patients by further administration of cortisone.

It has been suggested that cortisone be administered to any patient about to undergo surgery who has had parenteral corticosteroid therapy within six months to a year.[8] Brown states that the usual course of therapy employed for the patient who is on maintenance or who has a history of having been on cortisone is to change the patient's daily dose to 200 mg of cortisone orally, beginning on the day prior to operation.[8] Cortisone or hydrocortisone, 150 mg diluted in 1000 ml. of 5 per cent glucose, is slowly infused. This infusion is discontinued in the recovery period if no signs of adrenal crisis appear. Maintenance on 200 mg of steroid per day is continued for two to three days postoperatively, and the dose is gradually reduced to the previous maintenance level. Close cooperation between the dental practitioner and physician must be maintained when confronted with these patients.

Although the prophylactic preparation of patients on steroids at the time of surgery is still recommended, one author questions this concept in those patients who have discontinued their steroids.[54] He based his remarks on recent studies measuring the plasma levels of 17-hydroxycorticosterone. In his study steroid therapy was discontinued, and within 48 hours normal values of 17-hydroxycorticosterone were present. Further, these patients responded to stressful situations without difficulty. It should be mentioned that caution must be exercised in this concept, because in the early reports of mortalities from iatrogenic adrenal insufficiency the cardiovascular instability did not occur until some six to twelve hours after the operative procedure.[40] It has been suggested that in patients whose steroid therapy has been discontinued steroids should be administered because of an unexplained cardiovascular instability. In these patients, 200 mg of hydrocortisone is given in one injection, followed by 100 mg by intravenous drip every eight hours. This dose is large enough to fully saturate the binding properties of transcortin and should correct the cardiovascular instability of adrenal insufficiency.[56] No one appears to have exact data which would indicate how long a patient must be receiving steroids before significant adrenal depression results. Also, Bosomworth[6] feels that it cannot be stated with certainty how long after discontinuance of cortisone therapy adrenal function can be considered normal. The consensus today appears to be that steroid therapy be adjusted and continued in those patients receiving steroids at the time of surgery, but reinstitution of therapy in patients who have discontinued therapy for some time is not routinely required.

Miscellaneous Causes of Hypotension

As with most emergency situations, prevention is the best cure. This is particularly true in the prevention of hypotension from miscellaneous causes. If heavy bleeding is expected, the patient should be hospitalized and replacement blood ordered. A dramatic hypotension may follow air embolism; therefore extreme care should be exercised during intravenous administration of drugs. If sufficient air is inadvertently injected, the patient becomes cyanotic, gasps for breath, and usually develops hypotension. Once this condition is recognized, the patient should be immediately placed on his left side to confine the air to the right side of the heart where it may gradually be absorbed. Anesthetic errors that may precipitate marked hypotension are severe hypoxia and overdosage of anesthetic agents.

HYPERTENSION

Hypertension carries with it the danger of increased bleeding, rupture of cerebral vessels, and pulmonary edema. It therefore follows that the surgical and anesthetic risk is high in patients with severe hypertension. Hypertension is usually a chronic disease for which patients can be treated with oral medication. Occasionally, however, crises arise during anesthesia whereby the patient's blood pressure rises acutely to dangerously high levels, and prompt treatment with parenteral medication is necessary to prevent serious complications. Physiologically, acute regulation of arterial pressure is effected primarily in the nervous system, the shift of fluid between interstitial space and blood, and the stress-relaxation mechanism of the vascular system. However, these factors, even including the nervous system, seem to be unimportant for the long-term regulation of arterial pressure. Long-term regulation has been found to depend almost entirely on the kidneys.[28] In the case of a hypertensive crisis Baldini[3] suggests intermittent intravenous injections of 2.5 mg of chlorpromazine at intervals of two to four minutes with frequent repeated determinations of blood pressure until the desired reduction of blood pressure is achieved. Other men[2, 24, 68] feel that reserpine is the drug of choice for most hypertensive emergencies. Scherbakova[57] states that patients with marked hypertension must receive a preliminary course of antihypertensive drugs (reserpine, dibazole, or euphylline). Whenever potent antihypertensive drugs are being administered, a solution of levarterenol or a similar drug should be available for immediate use should excessive blood pressure drop occur. Elective surgery should be delayed until the blood pressure level has been controlled for at least several days.

CARDIAC ARREST

Cardiac arrest is the most urgent general anesthetic emergency. Circulatory arrest occurs with both ventricular fibrillation and asystole, and the clinical picture is essentially the same.

Clinical Picture [17]

1. Absence of carotid or peripheral pulse.
2. Sudden pallor and cyanosis.

3. Absence of heart sounds.
4. Wide dilatation of the pupils *later* in the arrest.
5. Absence of bleeding.
6. Dark blood in operative site.
7. Loss of consciousness.
8. Convulsion.
9. Electrocardiographic evidence of asystole or ventricular fibrillation.

Cause

Circulatory arrest is usually due to one or a combination of the following:[13]

1. Progressive hypoxia leading to anoxia of the myocardium.
2. An accumulation of certain chemicals in the heart, such as carbon dioxide, potassium, epinephrine, or agents which depress the myocardium.
3. Cardiac reflexes.

Prevention

A thorough preoperative evaluation of the patient is essential as the first step in the prevention of cardiac arrest. Serious arrhythmias that may lead to ventricular fibrillation or asystole might be expected to develop in the following individuals: (a) those in the older age group; (b) those with a past history of ectopic rhythms; (c) patients with advanced heart disease; (d) those with coronary artery disease; and (e) patients with W-P-W syndrome, A-V heart block, or bundle branch block.

Anesthetics that predispose to the development of ventricular fibrillation should be avoided. Lidocaine increases the ventricular fibrillation threshold and is considered the drug of choice in treating premonitory arrhythmias. There are many offices where electronic monitoring is performed. By early detection and correction of less serious arrhythmias, fatal ventricular arrhythmias may be prevented. Adequate oxygenation of the patient from induction to complete recovery from the anesthetic must be insured.

Treatment[5]

1. Start cardiopulmonary resuscitation immediately.
2. Oxygen under positive pressure.
3. If ventricular fibrillation is identified by ECG, immediate defibrillation should be tried using 400 joules (watt-seconds).
4. Sodium bicarbonate, one ampule (44 mEq), intravenously every 5 minutes or so during CPR.
5. Calcium gluconate or calcium chloride, one ampule intravenously, if indicated.
6. Epinephrine 5 to 10 ml of 1:10,000, intravenously, prior to repeated cardioversion.

The patient should be transferred to the hospital as soon as possible for observation and additional care.

For more information see chapter on *Cardiopulmonary Arrest*.

ACCIDENTAL INTRA-ARTERIAL INJECTION

The accidental injection of intravenous anesthetic agents into an artery may lead to gangrene and ultimate amputation of tissue supplied by the injured artery. Many theories[1, 12, 35, 36, 61] have been proposed in regard to the pathologic response to intra-arterial barbiturate injections. These theories include arterial spasm, intimal damage and thrombosis, blockage of the lumen of arterioles by acid crystals, and release of norepinephrine. The necrosis was first thought to be a result of severe arterial spasm, possibly from the high alkalinity of the barbiturate, but there is little laboratory evidence to support this theory. Kinmonth and Shepherd[35] found that the period of vasoconstriction following injection is too short to produce the resulting necrosis. Waters[66] discounted thrombosis as a cause because thrombosis is a slow process and could not effect the changes that occurred shortly after injection. He reported that crystals of thiopental separated out in arterial blood and could block arterioles mechanically on reaching them, and could be responsible for the initial symptoms seen. The stagnation could lead to subsequent thrombosis. The mechanism of thrombosis is controversial, but biopsy has shown that, regardless of cause, thrombosis develops in all cases where tissue necrosis occurs.

Incidence

The true incidence is unknown, having been reported from a high of 1:3500[19] to a low of 1:200,000.[18] Many cases cause only minor injury and go unreported.

Clinical Picture

After intra-arterial injection of barbiturate there is a sudden onset of severe burning pain extending peripherally from the injection site. This severe pain may continue or gradually subside after a few minutes and usually will persist as a burning sensation for several hours. The involved extremity may become edematous and cyanotic. The prognosis is poor if these changes develop rapidly.[27]

Prevention

Most often accidental intra-arterial injection occurs in the antecubital fossa. Engler[23] suggested that the lateral aspect of the antecubital fossa be selected over the medial aspect, where the branches of the ulnar and brachial arteries are more superficial and close to the vein and are easily entered. One must be particularly careful when reinserting a needle in an anesthetized patient, as intra-arterial injection would not elicit pain and the emergency might go unrecognized. An excessively tight tourniquet and hypotension might mask arterial pulsations. Dependence cannot be placed on the color of the blood; arterial blood may sometimes be darker than expected. Release of the tourniquet may allow arterial pressure to push back the plunger. If there is still doubt, a very small amount of medication may be injected at first, waiting for any untoward reaction or pain before completing the injection.

Treatment

Intra-arterial injection constitutes a serious emergency. Any but emergency surgery should be cancelled. Treatment aimed at preventing thrombosis should begin immediately. Efforts to re-establish circulation are rarely successful after thrombosis has occurred.[12] No single treatment has been consistently successful. It is almost universally agreed, however, that injection of 1 to 2 per cent procaine, several milliliters through the same needle in place, may be of value. Immediate heparinization is advocated by many writers.[27, 35, 39] In experiments using rabbits Kinmonth and Shepherd[35] showed that heparinization reduced the area of gangrene. They reported the most critical factor regarding tissue loss was the concentration of the barbiturate injected. A concentration of 10 per cent caused an area of gangrene averaging 14.8 cm^2, one of 5 per cent resulted in an area of 10.4 cm^2, and a concentration of 2.5 per cent produced an area of only 0.15 cm^2. Stellate ganglion block or general anesthesia with halothane may be tried to promote vasodilation. Other measures include arteriography, to determine the extent of injury, and thrombectomy, to re-establish pulses. Amputation of areas of tissues necrosis may be necessary. The patient should be hospitalized as soon as possible for the above treatment by a vascular surgeon. In spite of therapy, some patients have developed gangrene and suffered amputation, particularly with higher concentrations of agent. Awareness of the possibility of this complication and a careful intravenous technique should do much to prevent this tragic accident.

NEUROLOGICAL EMERGENCIES AND COMPLICATIONS

CONVULSIONS

Convulsions contributed significantly to the anesthesia associated death rate in the past, but with better understanding of their causes and with the introduction of intravenous anesthetic agents this emergency is infrequently encountered today.

Clinical Picture

Convulsions are characterized by sudden involuntary tonic and clonic contractions of the arms and legs. In addition, the patient exhibits forced expiration and a rigid rib cage, and sometimes experiences laryngospasm.

Causes

Cerebral hypoxia is the most frequent cause of convulsions in the anesthetized patient. Other common causes are carbon dioxide retention, overdosage of local analgesic agents, epilepsy, or air embolism.

Prevention

Proper premedication to allay fear and apprehension in the overly anxious patient, along with a smooth induction and a well-administered anesthetic, will keep the incidence of this emergency at a minimum.

Treatment

Artificial respiration while the patient is convulsing is ineffective in inflating the lungs. Treatment consists of stopping the convulsion, relieving laryngospasm if present, maintaining respiration, and supporting the circulation, which soon fails in the untreated patient. Any drug used to control convulsions may lead to respiratory depression; therefore, it is advisable to use only the smallest effective dose. Intravenous barbiturates have been used to control convulsion, but they augment the depression seen following convulsions and may produce a difficult problem in managing the depressed state. Small doses of succinylcholine (10 to 20 mg), intravenously, are usually sufficient to control the convulsing patient. Respiration must be supported with 100 per cent oxygen.

TREMORS

Occasionally a pronator spasm may occur in the arm receiving an injection of barbiturate. This is usually eliminated by deepening the anesthetic and adding nitrous oxide and oxygen. Minor jactitations are often associated with hypoxia and are easily controlled by supporting respirations with 100 per cent oxygen.

MISCELLANEOUS EMERGENCIES AND COMPLICATIONS

Malignant Hyperthermia

Malignant hyperthermia is a rare emergency associated with general anesthesia, having an incidence of about 1:75,000. It was seen by Lee in the mid 1930s in some patients under ether anesthesia.[38] Most of today's cases involve children who have received halothane and succinylcholine. It is a condition in which the body temperature rises progressively and will terminate in death in the absence of adequate treatment. In susceptible individuals, any potent inhalation anesthetic agent such as methoxyflurane, halothane, diethyl-ether and cyclopropane, or any skeletal muscle relaxant such as succinylcholine, decamethonium, gallamine, and d-tubocurarine can precipitate an acute crisis characterized by fever, often malignant. Temperatures of 111.2° F (44° C) have been reported.[32]

Cause

The exact cause of malignant hyperthermia is unknown, but recent studies strongly suggest it is most likely to occur in a patient with an inherited sarcoplasmic defect.[59, 65] The inheritance is as an autosomal dominant. Members of susceptible families have minor muscle abnormalities such as ptosis, squint, or kyphoscoliosis and may have moderate elevation of creatine phosphokinase and serum aldolase levels, possible evidence of a subclinical myopathy.[22] This relationship between malignant hyperthermia and inherited muscular defects was demonstrated in a report by Ellis.[21] It was shown that musculoskeletal abnormalities and surgery to correct them are common in patients with myopathy. Many patients who developed malignant hyperthermia have had surgery for squints, ptosis, hernias, or orthopedic abnormalities. Triggering agents appear to release stored calcium to the cytoplasm. This, in turn, causes sustained myofibrillar contraction, mobilization of glycogen from the liver, and acceleration of lactic acid and carbon dioxide production. Once this rapid process resulting in malignant hyperthermia has started it is almost impossible to halt. The overall mortality rate is about 64 per cent and is unchanged in recent years in spite of aggressive therapy.[56]

Clinical Signs

Often the first indications of developing trouble are violent fasciculations followed by skeletal muscle rigidity after the administration of succinylcholine. The most consistent early sign is a ventricular arrhythmia-tachycardia. Other early findings are rapid, deep respirations, hot skin, profuse sweating, rigidity, and a mottling cyanosis.[7]

Late events of ominous prognostic significance are hemolysis, consumption coagulopathy, acute left heart failure, and decerebration. The latter is characterized by fixed and dilated pupils, loss of deep tendon reflexes, convulsions, coma, and loss of central temperature regulation. Returning consciousness and hyperactivity of deep tendon reflexes are favorable signs.

Prevention

Unexplained deaths associated with anesthesia should be investigated with the malignant hyperthermia syndrome in mind. Relatives should have their creatine phosphokinase levels determined. Normal levels are less than 100 units per liter in males and less than 60 in females.[38] If the history and investigations indicate a patient is likely to develop malignant hyperthermia, careful thought must be given to the planning of anesthesia or sedation. Local analgesia should be used wherever possible, but lignocaine should not be used; the local analgesia of choice is procaine HCl. If general anesthesia is unavoidable, inhalation agents, particularly halothane, are contraindicated in conjunction with succinylcholine and atropine. Sodium pentothal, Brevital, promethazine and diazepam are probably safe, as are nitrous oxide and a nondepolarizing relaxant technique.[22] The patient should be hospitalized for general anesthesia when the probability of this condition exists.

Treatment

Treatment must be aggressive if the patient is to survive. Should this emergency occur in the office, anesthesia and surgery must be terminated immediately. Give 100 per cent oxygen by positive pressure while arrangements are being made to transfer the patient to a hospital. The patient should be transferred to the hospital as soon as possible. The present position with regard to treatment is as follows:

1. Hyperventilate with 100 per cent oxygen (8 to 10 L O_2 flow), if necessary by IPPV.
2. Actively cool the patient by aggressive methods.
   a. IV iced saline (not Ringer's lactate) 1000 ml/10 minutes for 30 minutes.
   b. Lavage of stomach, bladder, rectum, peritoneal and thoracic cavities with iced saline.
   c. Extracorporeal circulation and heat exchange (femoral to femoral).
   d. Surface cooling with ice and hypothermia blanket.
3. Administer sodium bicarbonate, 100 mEq stat, and up to 600 mEq over time, guided by arterial pH and pCO_2. Since increasing the blood pH drives potassium into cells, sodium bicarbonate is highly effective in reversing the severe hyperkalemia.
4. Maintain urine output. Mannitol should be given IV to dislodge myoglobin from the renal tubules.
5. Procine amide 15 mg/kg over 5 to 10 minutes with ECG control.
6. Administer insulin to shift potassium back into cells and to improve glucose uptake.
7. Support circulation with isoprenaline, using blood pressure and ECG monitoring.
8. Discontinue cooling when the temperature reaches 101° F.

AIR EMBOLISM

Accidental entrance of air as a complication of general anesthesia could occur during intravenous infusion or during intravenous injection.

Clinical Picture

When air enters a vein in sufficient quantity, it travels to the right heart and lung and may set up an obstruction within the pulmonary artery. This may be followed by a loud precordial murmur. A precordial stethoscope will elicit the characteristic bubbling or so-called "mill wheel murmur" sounds. A sudden cyanosis will develop, followed rapidly by hypotension, tachycardia, engorged neck veins, and irregular, gasping respiration, progressing through tachypnea and hypopnea, and if not treated promptly will lead to cardiac arrest.

Treatment

1. Prevent further entrace of air into the vein.
2. Tilt the chair back steeply and lower the head to keep air out of the cerebral vessels.
3. Turn the patient onto the left side so that bubbles of air are carried away from the pulmonary artery.
4. Give 100 per cent oxygen and stop nitrous oxide. N_2O is more soluble than nitrogen in blood and would thus increase the size of the emboli.
5. Infuse large volumes of intravenous fluid to wash out froth.
6. Papaverine, 30 to 60 mg to dilate pulmonary vessels.
7. Vasopressors.[38]

Prevention here, as elsewhere, is stressed. Strict observance of proper technique will prevent this complication.

INJURIES TO SOFT TISSUES AND TEETH

Ocular Injury

Corneal abrasion is a painful injury usually resulting from careless application of the face or nasal mask. In the hospital, with the patient supine and covered with drapes, the eyelids are usually taped shut. This precaution is not necessary in outpatient procedures where the head is not covered with drapes. Care should be taken, however, to insure that there is no drying of the cornea, which may contribute to ulceration, and that masks are properly applied.

The eyes should be checked after surgery for any inadvertent injury. If any injury is found, the patient should be referred for ophthalmic consultation. If corneal abrasions are treated promptly, they usually re-epithelialize within 24 hours.

Extravascular Injection

Extravasation of injected medication is a common complication of intravenous anesthesia. It is due either to a faulty intravenous technique or to displacement of the needle during anesthesia. Extravasation is followed by pain and swelling at the site of injection. The pain is intense if the solution is alkaline, acid, or hypertonic. In the anesthetized patient extravasation can only be detected by careful observation, and could go unnoticed.

TREATMENT

1. Remove the needle immediately.
2. Inject 5 to 10 ml of 1 per cent procaine into the involved area to dilute the barbiturate. Sloughing has occurred with such medications as Levophed or Pentothal. Brevital rarely produces a slough.
3. Massage the area to disperse the irritant.
4. Heat application may be dangerous if skin circulation is poor.

Chipped or Loosened Teeth

The upper anterior teeth are particularly prone to injury by the laryngoscope blade during intubation. The teeth should never be used as a fulcrum for the laryngoscope blade. It is wise to protect the anterior teeth with a thin lead strip such as can be fashioned easily from the lead backing in an occlusal film packet. Another source of injury to anterior teeth is the damaged mouth prop. Whenever the internal metal portion of the mouth prop shows through the rubber it should be discarded immediately. Here, as with most other injuries, prevention is the key.

Injuries to the Tongue and Lips

Injuries to the tongue are most often due to impingement of the tongue between the mouth prop and teeth. Injuries to the lips are frequently the result of impingement of the lips between the teeth and a dental forceps or the laryngoscope blade. Both the operator and the surgical assistant must be aware of the problem and prevent pressure on the soft tissues by instruments and teeth.

POSTOPERATIVE EMERGENCIES AND COMPLICATIONS

RESPIRATORY

Airway Obstruction

Airway obstruction in the postoperative period is most often the result of the tongue falling back against the posterior pharyngeal wall when the patient is in the supine position and the jaw is relaxed (Fig. 16–1). Examination of the patient reveals hyperactivity of the secondary muscles of respiration, flaring of the nares, and little or no elevation of the thoracic wall. Auscultation will demonstrate inspiratory stridor or, in some cases, no sounds at all. While the patient is in the supine position, simple elevation of the mandible is usually sufficient to draw the tongue away from the posterior pharyngeal wall and thus clear the airway (Fig. 16–2). A gauze pack in the mouth to aid in clot formation is also a potential source of airway obstruction. It is suggested that the gauze pack be large enough to protrude from the mouth for easier observation. Although the procedure described will relieve obstruction in the supine

Figure 16–1 Head not extended, mandible retruded. This position causes the tongue to fall backward against the posterior pharyngeal wall, occluding the airway.

patient, obstruction will recur unless the patient is constantly being helped. It is far better to turn the patient onto his side, flex the knees, and place a pillow behind the back to maintain the side position. In this position the jaw does not tend to fall back and, in fact, tends to fall forward, opening the airway. In any case, close observation of the patient is essential in the postoperative period.

Laryngospasm.   Laryngospasm may develop in the postoperative period and is usually caused by irritation of the vocal cords by mucus or blood. Oxygen under positive pressure should be administered after suctioning the mouth and pharynx and changing the oropharyngeal pack. This will usually relieve the spasm. If the spasm persists, small doses of succinylcholine, 10 to 20 mg, should be given intravenously. The mouth should then be resuctioned and the patient ventilated with 100 per cent oxygen under positive pressure.

Bronchospasm.   Bronchospasm in the postoperative period is most likely to be the result of irritation of the airway or misplacement of the endotracheal

Figure 16–2 Head extended, mandible drawn upward. This maneuver elevates the tongue away from the posterior pharyngeal wall and opens the airway.

tube. Heavy smokers and those with chronic bronchitis are more prone to postoperative bronchospasm. Aminophylline will relieve the problem but entails a certain risk in the hypoxic or hypercarbic patient. Isoethrane may be effective as an aerosol. In severe instances of bronchospasm, intravenous isoproterenol or epinephrine should be effective, whereas an aerosol would not.

Aspiration of Vomitus. This subject is discussed elsewhere in this chapter; however, a few remarks are in order here. The patient should not be removed from the surgery room to the recovery room until protective reflexes are present. If the patient in recovery is placed onto his side, as described above under postoperative airway obstruction, the danger of aspirating after vomiting is greatly reduced. A reliable source of suction and oxygen should be immediately available in the recovery room for both emergency use and for the prevention of emergencies. Many offices have seat belts attached to the recovery bunks to prevent undue movement and falling.

Hypercarbia

Postoperative hypercarbia can result from an inadequate respiratory drive or increases of CO_2. Inadequate respiratory drive may result from the residual effects of the anesthetic agent or depression of respiration from premedication with narcotics. Increased CO_2 production is seen with shivering or emergence delirium. Respiratory depression due to the residual effects of anesthetic agents is best combatted by controlled ventilation with oxygen until the anesthetic agents are detoxified and the patient is able to control his own respirations. If the depression is due to narcotic medication, intravenous injection of a narcotic antagonist such as naloxone 0.2 to 0.4 mg will result in immediate elimination of respiratory depression followed by arousal and awakening. The patient must be carefully observed, as the narcotic's duration of action may be considerably longer than that of naloxone. Naloxone may have to be repeated once or twice to maintain wakefulness.

CARDIOVASCULAR

Hypotension

Postoperative hypotension constitutes one of the most common complications encountered in the recovery room and may result from various causes.[43] A mild hypotension in the early postoperative period is frequently due to a change in position or to physical movement during transport to the recovery area. This postural hypotension is a result of a lack of efficiency of the patient's compensatory mechanisms caused by the effects of anesthetic, analgesic, tranquilizing, or antihypertensive drugs. The underlying mechanism appears to be pooling of blood in the lower extremities or other peripheral regions with subsequent reduction in arterial pressure.

CLINICAL SIGNS

Clinical signs of hypotension are as follows:

1. The skin is pale or gray.

2. The skin is cold, clammy and diaphoretic (profuse sweating).
3. The pulse is rapid and thready.
4. Respirations are rapid and shallow.
5. There are signs of cerebral ischemia which include disorientation, restlessness and anxiety.

These clinical signs are often difficult to recognize as they may be masked by residual anesthetic drugs.

TREATMENT

When hypotension is recognized, corrective therapy is started immediately. Therapy includes parenteral administration of fluids, oxygen under positive pressure, and a vasopressor agent. If the patient is sitting, he should be layed down and placed onto his side. The blood pressure should be checked at frequent intervals until stable.

Arrhythmias

Serious arrhythmias may occur after surgery and anesthesia. Often these disappear without treatment. If a serious arrhythmia persists, it may lead to a reduction of cardiac output and severe hypotension. For treatment of the various more common arrhythmias see *Cardiac Arrhythmias,* in this chapter.

MISCELLANEOUS COMPLICATIONS

Emergence Delirium

Emergence delirium is a condition of muscular activity and excitement during the immediate postoperative period. It is most often seen in healthy teenagers recovering from an intravenous barbiturate anesthetic. There may be uncontrolled thrashing about accompanied by loud vocalization. Although the problem is not dangerous, it is most troublesome. It is well known that barbiturates possess no analgesic properties and are therefore unable to dull the pain of recent surgery. This and the lingering effects of the anesthetic on cortical function result in a patient who is restless, confused, and unable to cope with any pain following surgery. Local analgesia given to prevent postoperative pain will often avert this problem. Narcotics in conservative doses may be helpful in stubborn cases. It is important to prevent injury to the patient, but mechanical restraints often do more harm than good. A reassuring voice along with minimal control of movement is frequently helpful.

Shivering

Shivering after operation may occur with most anesthetic agents but is most common with halothane and is frequently seen after anesthesia with barbiturates. Pyramidal tract signs mimicking convulsions may sometimes be seen. This condition usually responds to the administration of methylphenidate (Ritalin), 20 mg.

Pain

Some pain is inevitable after operation. Its effects are exaggerated in the unstable patient. Opiates must be given with caution in the immediate post-operative period, as there is danger of hypotension and hypoventilation. Morphine, 5 mg, or meperidine, 50 mg, given intramuscularly, is generally satisfactory for the average adult.

Prolonged Recovery

Prolonged recovery from dental or oral surgical procedures is an infrequent complication. When it does occur it is usually related to overdosage of anesthetic agents or premedication agents, or it occurs after relatively lengthy procedures. Clinical observation leads me to believe that Orientals are more prone to prolonged recovery than others. Some experts feel that prolonged recovery may be minimized by supplementing general anesthesia with local analgesia; others do not.

DISCHARGING THE PATIENT

Before discharging the patient, oral and written post-operative instructions should be given to the patient and the individual accompanying the patient home. Under no circumstances should the patient be allowed to drive himself. He should be driven home by a competent adult. The patient is never discharged until vital signs are stable, until all bleeding is controlled, and until he can walk without difficulty.

EMERGENCY EQUIPMENT

The life-endangering nature of general anesthetic emergencies requires that the necessary drugs and equipment be readily available. The emergency tray should be checked at least monthly to be certain that batteries and lights for the laryngoscope are functioning properly and that all drugs are within their date limit.

Electronic monitoring equipment is now found in many offices, and no doubt electronic monitoring will become standard practice. It should be recognized that the cardioscope only registers electrical activity of the heart and does not indicate adequacy of circulation. The pulsemeter, however, requires the presence of a pulse to function and thus gives evidence of circulatory perfusion.

Emergency situations may arise suddenly and require immediate action. For this reason it is strongly urged that periodic "emergency drills" be practiced to familiarize each member of the anesthesia team with emergency treatment and equipment.

* * * * * *

Perhaps the most valuable result of all education is the ability to make yourself do the thing you have to do, when it ought to be done, as it ought to be done, whether you like to do it or not.

THOMAS HUXLEY

REFERENCES

1. Albo, D., Jr., et al.: Effect of intra-arterial injection of barbiturates. Am. J. Surg., *120*:676, 1970.
2. Alper, M. H., Flacke, W., and Krayer, O.: Pharmacology of reserpine and its implications for anesthesia. Anesthesiology, *24*:524, 1963.
3. Baldini, E., and Lincoln, J. R.: Treatment of acute hypertensive crises in surgical patients. J.A.M.A., *190*:157, 1964.
4. Bannister, W. K., and Sattilaro, A. J.: Vomiting and aspiration during anesthesia. Anesthesiology, *23*:251, 1962.
5. Benson, D. W., Jude, J. R., and Kouwenhoven, W. B.: External cardiac massage. Anesth. Analg., *42*:132, 1963.
6. Bosomworth, P. P.: Discussion of reference 29. Anesth. Analg., *43*:107, 1964.
7. Britt, B. A.: Recent advances in malignant hyperthermia. Anesth. Analg., *51*:841, 1972.
8. Brown, E. S.: Steroids and the anesthesiologists. Connecticut Med., *26*:227, 1962.
9. Burn, J. H., and Rand, M. J.: The action of sympathomimetic amines on animals treated with reserpine. J. Physiol. (Lond.), *144*:314, 1958.
10. Cameron, J. L., Mitchell, W. H., and Zuidema, G. D.: Aspiration pneumonia. Clinical outcome following documented aspiration. Arch. Surg., *106*:49, 1973.
11. Coakley, C. S., Alpert, S., and Boling, J. S.: Circulatory responses during anesthesia of patients on rauwolfia therapy. J.A.M.A., *161*:1143, 1956.
12. Cohen, S. M.: Accidental intra-arterial injection of drugs. Lancet, *2*:409, 1948.
13. Collawn, T. H.: Causes and prevention of cardiac arrest. North Carolina Med. J., *23*:336, 1962.
14. Cullen, S. C.: Anesthesia. 6th ed. Chicago, Year Book Medical Publishers, 1961, p. 48.
15. Dickson, D. N.: Total bronchospasm. So. Afr. Med. J., *38*:108, 1964.
16. Dines, D. E., Baker, W. G., and Scantland, W. A.: Aspiration pneumonitis — Mendelson's syndrome. J.A.M.A., *176*:229, 1961.
17. Dripps, R. D.: Introduction to Anesthesia. 5th ed., Philadelphia, W. B. Saunders Co., 1977, p. 452.
18. Driscoll, E. J., and American Society of Oral Surgeons Committee on Anesthesia. ASOS anesthesia morbidity and mortality survey. J. Oral Surg., *32*:733, 1974.
19. Dundee, J. W.: Thiopentone and Other Barbiturates. London, Livingston Ltd., 1956.
20. Edwards, G., Morton, H. J., Pask, E. A., and Wylie, W. D.: Deaths associated with anaesthesia. Anaesthesia, *11*:194, 1956.
21. Ellis, F. R.: Malignant hyperpyrexia. Anaesthesia, *28*:245, 1973.
22. Ellis, F. R., Keaney, N. P., and Harriman, D. G.: Histopathological and neuropharmacological aspects of malignant hyperpyrexia. Proc. Roy. Soc. Med., *66*:66, 1973.
23. Engler, H. S., et al.: Gangrenous extremities resulting from intra-arterial injections. Arch. Surg., *94*:644, 1967.
24. Freis, E. D.: Hypertensive emergencies. Med. Clin. North Amer., *46*:353, 1962.
25. Fukushima, K., et al.: Effect of propranolol on the ventricular arrhythmias induced by hypercarbia during halothane anesthesia in man. Brit. J. Anaesth., *40*:53, 1968.
26. Gold, M. I.: Treatment of bronchospasm during anesthesia. Anesth. Analg., *54*:783, 1975.
27. Goldsmith, D., and Trieger, N.: Accidental intra-arterial injection: A medical emergency. Anesth. Prog. *22*:180, 1975.
28. Guyton, A. C., et al.: Physiologic control of arterial pressure. Bull. New York Acad. Med., *45*:811, 1969.
29. Hamelberg, W.: Current concepts on antihypertensive drugs and steroids. Anesth. Analg., *43*:104, 1964.
30. Harrison, D. C., Sprouse, J. H., and Morrow, A. G.: The antiarrhythmic properties of lidocaine and procaine amide. Clinical and physiologic studies of their cardiovascular effects in man. Circulation, *28*:486, 1963.
31. Hausmann, W., and Lunt, R. L.: Problem of treatment of peptic aspiration pneumonia following obstetric anesthesia. Obstet. Gynaec., Brit. Emp. *62*:509, 1955.
32. Hawthorne, A. T., Richardson, M. E., and Whitfield, G. T.: Fulminating hyperthermia and general anesthesia. Brit. Med. J., *4*:750, 1968.
33. Hays, M. A.: Surgical treatment as complicated by prior adrenal cortical steroid therapy. Surgery, *36*:945, 1956.
34. Heironimus, T. W.: Regurgitation and aspiration during anesthesia. Virginia Med. Monthly, *90*:162, 1963.
35. Kinmonth, J. B., and Shepherd, R. C.: Accidental injection of thiopentone into arteries; studies of pathology and treatment. Brit. Med. J., *2*:914, 1959.
36. Klatt, E. C., Brooks, A. L., and Rhamy, R. K.: Toxicity of intra-arterial barbiturates and tranquilizing drugs. Radiology, *92*:700, 1969.

37. Lee, J. A.: A Synopsis of Anaesthesia. 7th ed., Chicago, Year Book, 1976, p. 801.
38. Lee, J. A.: A Synopsis of Anaesthesia. 7th ed., Chicago, Year Book, 1976, p. 825.
39. Lindell, T. D., Porter, J. M., and Langston, C.: Intra-arterial injection of drugs. N. Engl. J. Med., 287:1132, 1972.
40. Lundy, J. S.: Cortisone problems involving anesthesia. Anesthesiology, 14:376, 1953.
41. Lytle, J. J.: Anesthesia morbidity and mortality survey of the Southern California Society of Oral Surgeons. J. Oral Surg., 32:739, 1974.
42. Marshall, B. M., and Gordon, R. A.: Vomiting and aspiration in anesthesia. II. Canad. Anaes. Soc. J., 5:438, 1958.
43. Marx, G. F., et al.: Postoperative hypotension. New York J. Med., 67:1893, 1967.
44. McCormick, P. W.: Immediate care after aspiration of vomit. Anaesthesia, 30:658, 1975.
45. Mendelson, C. L.: The aspiration of stomach contents into the lungs during obstetric anesthesia. Am. J. Obstet. Gynecol., 52:191, 1946.
46. Morrow, D. H., and Logic, J. R.: Management of cardiac arrhythmias during anesthesia. Anesth. Analg., 48:748, 1969.
47. Morrow, D. H., and Morrow, A. G.: The responses to anesthesia of nonhypertensive patients pretreated with reserpine. Brit. J. Anaesth., 35:313, 1963.
48. Mucklow, R. G., and Larard, D. G.: The effects of the inhalation of vomitus on the lungs: Clinical considerations. Brit. J. Anaesth. 35:153, 1963.
49. Munson, W. M., and Janicek, J. A.: Effect of anesthetic agents on patients receiving reserpine therapy. Anesthesiology, 23:741, 1962.
50. Nicholl, R. M., Holland, E. L., and Brown, S. S.: Mendelson's syndrome: Its treatment by tracheostomy and hydrocortisone. Brit. Med. J., 2:745, 1967.
51. Payne, J. P.: Pronethalol in treatment of ventricular arrhythmias during anesthesia. Brit. Med. J., 1:603, 1964.
52. Physician's Desk Reference.
53. Rees, L. T.: Bronchospasm during anaesthesia. Anaesthesia, 18:103, 1963.
54. Robinson, B. H., Mattingly, D., and Cope, C. L.: Adrenal function after prolonged corticosteroid therapy. Brit. Med. J., 1:1579, 1962.
55. Salassa, R. M., Bennett, W. A., and Keating, F. R.: Postoperative adrenal cortical insufficiency: Occurrence in patients previously treated with cortisone. J.A.M.A., 512:1509, 1953.
56. Sandberg, A. A., and Slaunwhite, W. R.: Transcortin, a corticosteroid binding protein. J. Clin. Invest., 38:384, 1959.
57. Scherbakova, L. S.: Anesthesia for hypertensive patients. Eksp. Kchir. Anest. (Russian), 3:67, 1964.
58. Slavey, G., and Brooke, B. N.: Post-operative collapse due to adrenal insufficiency following cortisone therapy. Lancet 1:1167, 1957.
59. Steers, A. J. W., Tallach, J. A., and Thompson, D. E.: Fulminating hyperpyrexia during anaesthesia in a member of a myopathic family. Brit. Med. J. 2:341, 1970.
60. Stetson, J. B.: Patient safety: Prevention and prompt recognition of regurgitation and aspiration. Anesth. Analg., 53:142, 1974.
61. Stone, H. H., and Donnelly, C.: The accidental intraarterial injection of thiopental. Anesthesia. 22:995, 1961.
62. Teabeaut, J. R.: Aspiration of gastric contents. Experimental study. Am. J. Path., 28:51, 1952.
63. Tolas, A. G., and Allen, G. D.: Comparison of effects of methods of induction of anesthesia on cardiac rhythm. J. Oral Surg., 25:54, 1967.
64. Underhill, W. L., and Tredway, J. B.: Treatment of paroxysmal tachycardia with isoproterenol. Ann. Int. Med., 60:680, 1964.
65. Wang. J. K.: Acute hyperthermia with anesthesia. Minn. Med. 55:618, 1972.
66. Waters, D. J.: Intra-arterial thiopentone: A physiochemical phenomenon. Anaesthesia. 21:343, 1966.
67. Winternitz, M. C., Smith, G. H., and McNamara, F. P.: Effect of intrabronchial insufflation of acid. J. Exper. Med., 32:199, 1920.
68. Ziegler, C. H., and Lovette, J. B.: Operative complications after therapy with reserpine and reserpine compounds. J.A.M.A., 176:916, 1961.

17

ESTABLISHING AN EMERGENCY AIRWAY

LEO KORCHIN

RECOGNITION OF OBSTRUCTION
NONSURGICAL MANEUVERS TO RE-
LIEVE OBSTRUCTION
Abdominal and Chest Thrust
Mouth-to-Mouth Breathing

ESTABLISHMENT OF AN EMERGENCY
AIRWAY
Cricothyroid Membrane Puncture
Anatomic Considerations
Surgical Considerations
Technique

There is no provision for the storage of oxygen in the body, and oxygen deprivation is tantamount to strangulation. Permanent brain damage or death will be produced by total airway obstruction lasting three to five mintues. Partial airway obstruction is not so critical, yet it too will produce permanent brain damage and even death unless early and rational treatment is instituted. Preparation for this unhappy situation could place one in the position of saving a life which, in the absence of a preconceived plan, might be lost.

Many substances placed in a patient's mouth during a dental procedure can be aspirated. Since pharyngeal reflexes are abolished during general anesthesia, the ease of aspiration is greater than when local analgesia or no anesthesia is used. It might be well to state at this time that the type of emergency situation with which this chapter is concerned is that which might occur to a patient who receives treatment under local analgesia or no anesthesia. While the treatment of acute foreign body obstruction is the same for a patient under general anesthesia, there are other considerations involved that are beyond the scope of this presentation. The subject material is applicable, however, to patients who are recovering from general anesthesia. Following are some of the materials that might be aspirated and produce obstruction: vomitus, fragments of teeth or whole teeth, amalgam fillings or particles of amalgam, gold inlays, crowns, prosthetic appliances, impression material, sponges, packs, drains, cotton rolls, broken instruments, etc. A convulsive seizure may occur in the waiting room or operatory, and one of the hazards of this circumstance is the aspiration of vomitus.

Aspiration most frequently does not produce acute respiratory obstruction. After initial symptoms of choking, coughing, gagging, and wheezing, the material is expelled or passed through the larynx to lodge in the trachea or a bronchus. Unless present in massive amount, the complications produced by a foreign body in the deeper air passages do not become manifest at once. If the fragment is not soon removed, however, tracheobronchial or pulmonary disease subsequently becomes evident. When a foreign body disappears from the oral cavity and is accompanied by signs of laryngeal and bronchial irritation, it must be presumed to have passed into the respiratory passage until proved otherwise. These patients should be referred at once to a physician. However, if total airway obstruction occurs, immediate definitive treatment should be rendered with equipment at hand. An airway must be reestablished within three to five minutes from onset in order to avoid permanent brain damage. See chapter 2 for further information on laryngeal, bronchial, and esophageal foreign bodies.

There are three basic steps for the restoration of ventilation in critical airway emergencies: (1) prompt recognition of obstruction; (2) nonsurgical maneuvers to relieve obstruction; and (3) establishment of an emergency surgical airway. This plan of action is rational and provides an orderly series of steps for the emergency treatment of airway obstruction in the dental office.

RECOGNITION OF OBSTRUCTION

A patient gasping for breath with great effort, possibly clutching his throat or chest, demonstrating suprasternal retraction, and unable to obtain air exchange is presumed to have an upper respiratory tract obstruction, and nonsurgical maneuvers to relieve the obstruction should be initiated.

The clinician faced with an apneic patient must determine whether this is a late effect of obstruction or whether there is some other cause. Ordinarily this is not difficult, because if there is obstruction the foreign body might have been seen to disappear into the pharynx, the patient will be unable to speak and/or the patient will have demonstrated signs of respiratory distress. However, the apnea of anxiety-induced hyperventilation, particularly if accompanied by cyanosis,[3] might be puzzling until its true nature was determined. This and other respiratory disturbances, such as those which might follow the intravascular injection of a local anesthetic agent, or the depressant effect of barbiturates and other depressant drugs on the respiratory center, can be distinguished from obstructive phenomena because resistance to air or oxygen during resuscitative efforts is not encountered.

NONSURGICAL MANEUVERS TO RELIEVE OBSTRUCTION

When respiratory obstruction occurs in the conscious patient, protective mechanisms are activated which attempt to eject the obstructing object. The patient will cough, wheeze, gag, choke, and make great efforts to expel the respiratory block. Attempts at removal by the doctor might be actively resisted. Nevertheless such an attempt should be made, although force must not be used. If the obstruction is large, the attempt at removal may be successful. A general anesthetic should not be administered, because removal of the voluntary respiratory effort may result in immediate asphyxia.

ABDOMINAL AND CHEST THRUST

If the attempt to manually remove the obstruction is not successful, a rapid series of thrusts to the upper abdomen (Heimlich maneuver[6]) is done. This maneuver can be accomplished with the patient seated while turned in the chair, standing, or lying supine. In the seated and standing positions, the doctor places himself behind the patient. He grasps one fist with his other hand, the thumb side of the fist against the patient's abdomen, between the xiphoid and the umbilicus, and the other hand placed on top of the first (Fig. 17–1). If the patient is in the supine position with the doctor kneeling beside or astride him, the heel of the doctor's one hand is placed between the xiphoid and the umbilicus and the other hand is placed on top of the first (Fig. 17–2). Now pressure is exerted upward into the epigastrium by means of a quick upward thrust. The sudden elevation of the diaphragm compresses the lungs and increases the air pressure within the tracheobronchial tree. This pressure is forced out through the trachea and acts to eject a foreign body occluding the airway. If the patient is grossly obese or in a state of advanced pregnancy, the same maneuver can be perfomed by means of a backward thrust with the arms around the lower chest. In this position, the thumb side of the fist should be on the lower sternum, not on the xiphoid process.[2]

The possibility of a rib fracture and damage to the internal organs, such as rupture or laceration of the abdominal viscera, is a significant consideration in performing these maneuvers, but the possible iatrogenic effects

Figure 17–1 Abdominal thrust. Position of hands when the patient is seated or standing.

Figure 17-2 Abdominal thrust. Position of hands when patient is supine.

should not be a deterrent when a life can be saved. However, it is important to stress that pressure must never be placed on the xiphoid process of the sternum or on the lower margins of the rib cage.

If this maneuver is unsuccessful, the unconscious patient should be placed in a head-down position, fluid aspirated, and the mouth and pharynx explored with the fingers, removing any foreign bodies encountered. (If not attempted on the conscious patient, the Heimlich maneuver can now be performed.) The mandible should be held forward to prevent occlusion of the pharynx by the tongue. This also can be accomplished by grasping the tongue with a gauze sponge and pulling it forward. Many obstructions will be relieved at this time, and respiration may begin spontaneously. The airway should remain supported until the patient is conscious. If respiration cannot be started, mouth-to-mouth resuscitation should be initiated at once.

See also Chapter 19 on the Heimlich maneuver. This life-saving technique is so valuable that two independent presentations are made for emphasis and clarity.

MOUTH-TO-MOUTH BREATHING

If obstruction is not complete, it is possible for enough air to reach the lungs by means of mouth-to-mouth breathing so that life can be maintained. Mouth-to-mouth breathing should be continued until the patient is in the hands of a professional person capable of accepting responsibility for the further conduct of the case, or until the patient recovers. During this procedure it is important to support the mandible in a forward position so that the airway is not further obstructed by the base of the tongue. If resuscitative efforts are successful, the chest will be observed to rise and fall rhythmically as the rescuer breathes into the patient's mouth and allows for passive exhalation, about 12 to 18 times a minute. See observations on the same subject under *maxillofacial injuries.*

It is important to check the carotid arterial pulse and the pupils of the eyes. If a pulse is absent and the pupils are dilated, closed chest cardiac massage must be instituted concurrently with mouth-to-mouth breathing. See the chapter on *cardiopulmonary arrest.*

Inability to inflate the lungs because of complete obstruction or absence of expiration owing to a check-valve type of obstruction will become evident after a few breaths. Without delay an emergency surgical airway must be established.

ESTABLISHMENT OF AN EMERGENCY SURGICAL AIRWAY

CRICOTHYROID MEMBRANE PUNCTURE

Anatomic Considerations

The cricoid cartilage lies directly below the thyroid cartilage, forming a complete ring around the larynx below the vocal cords. It is the only complete cartilaginous ring in the respiratory passage and can be palpated in the midline of the neck as the smaller protuberance below the thyroid cartilage. Posteriorly the cricoid becomes wider and thicker, a safety factor impeding accidental posterior perforation into the esophagus during cricothyroid membrane puncture. The thyroid and cricoid cartilages are connected anteriorly by the cricothyroid membrane. This membrane is superficial, covered only by skin and thin layers of adipose tissue and fascia. It is elliptical in shape, and its average useful dimensions are 0.5 to 1.2 cm vertically at the midline, and 3 cm transversely.[4] An instrument passed through the skin and cricothyroid membrane immediately enters the space of the larynx below the vocal cords. Since no important blood vessels overlie the membrane, it can be pierced with little or no bleeding. Some practice is required to locate the cricothyroid membrane quickly. This can best be done with the neck in the normal or slightly flexed position. In men, where the thyroid cartilage is prominent, the palpating finger is placed on this structure and carried down the midline to the soft depression between the thyroid and cricoid cartilages. In women and children, where the thyroid cartilage is not so prominent, the palpating finger is carried superiorly along the midline from the suprasternal notch to the prominent cricoid cartilage.

Surgical Considerations

Technically, the approach to the tracheal space through the cricothyroid membrane is influenced by the character of the skin, the mobility of the larynx, and the direction of the fibers in the elastic membrane.

The skin is loose, tough, and resistant. Forceful attempts at penetration by a sharp, pointed object and sudden release might transfix the posterior shield of the cricoid cartilage, overcoming this protective barrier and producing a perforation into the esophagus. Extreme upward or downward position might also produce esophageal perforation. If a trocar and cannula are used, the cannula edge is apt to catch on the skin. Since the skin is loose, the manipulation used to free the cannula might change its direction and result in a sudden, forceful penetration of the tissues lateral to the trachea. These complications can be avoided by incising the skin over the cricothyroid membrane with a scalpel or by pinching the skin and snipping through with scissors.

The cricothyroid membrane is also resistant to penetration, although considerably less so than the skin. Since the larynx is not firmly fixed, it must be stabilized while the cricothyroid membrane is punctured.

The objective of cricothyroid membrane puncture is to provide an opening, a stoma large enough to restore normal ventilation. This is accomplished by spreading the fibers of the membrane at right angles to their course with the blades of the instrument used for the initial penetration. The dilation of the stoma in the transverse plane is the maneuver that opens the trachea to the outside. If the instrument is held in position to prevent collapse of the stoma, the objective of providing an opening to restore normal ventilation will have been attained. Refinement of the procedure provides for the passage of a firm rubber, plastic, or metal tube between the blades of the dilating instrument into the tracheal lumen. The dilator is then withdrawn.

Technique

Because they are time consuming, and since each second is of life-saving importance, normal surgical requirements of aseptic technique, local analgesia, and hemostasis are disregarded.

The patient is placed in a head-down position and the neck is moderately hyperextended. This can be accomplished easily in the dental chair by lowering the headrest. In those dental chairs without a movable headrest the neck is hyperextended by placing a roll behind the shoulders. To produce extension of the neck when the patient is on the floor, he is placed on his back and his shoulders are supported and elevated by means of a roll. The chin and sternal notch are held in the median plane. A 2-cm. incision through skin only is made over the cricothyroid membrane. A scissors can be used to make this incision by pinching the skin and snipping through (Fig. 17–3). The larynx is stabilized by grasping it between the left thumb and middle finger. The left index finger is pressed into the cricothyroid membrane through the incision. A fine-pointed hemostat or scissors is passed along the fingernail and forced through the membrane into the tracheal space. An episode of coughing usually accompanies entrance into the trachea. After the membrane is perforated, the beaks of the instrument are spread and the airway dilated transversely (Fig. 17–4). A tube is inserted between the beaks of the dilating instrument (Fig. 17–5), and the instrument is removed (Fig. 17–6).

Figure 17-3

A   B

Figure 17-4

Figure 17-3 Skin pinched and snipped through with scissors.
Figure 17-4 Blades of instrument spread to dilate membrane.

To prevent dislodgement of the tube by coughing or movement, and also to prevent its aspiration into the trachea, it must be held firmly in place. A firm rubber or plastic tube can be sutured to the skin or secured with adhesive tape. A metal tube can be made with a flange which serves the double purpose of preventing its aspiration and providing anchorage for tapes which are tied around the neck (Fig. 17–7). This approach is essentially the same as that recommended by Ruhe, Williams, and Proud,[7] who have designed special instruments to facilitate the procedure (Fig. 17–8).

Figure 17-5

Figure 17-6

Figure 17-5   Tube inserted between blades of scissors into trachea.
Figure 17-6   Tube extending into trachea through the cricothyroid membrane.

Figure 17–7   **Figure 17–8**

Figure 17–7   Tube with oxygen adaptor designed for use in cricothyroid membrane puncture.

Figure 17–8   Commercial instruments designed for cricothyroid membrane puncture. (Storz Instrument Co., St. Louis, Mo.)

The complications that may result from cricothyroid membrane puncture are infection and pressure necrosis of the cricoid cartilage. Some degree of laryngeal stenosis may occur if the tube is not removed within 48 to 72 hours.

COMMENT

For many years needle puncture through the cricothyroid membrane with a 13-gauge needle has been advocated as an emergency procedure, and would appear to be a simple and direct method of providing an airway.

Figure 17–9   **Figure 17–10**

Figure 17–9   Opening into trachea obtained rapidly by incising the cricothyroid membrane.

Figure 17–10   Stoma maintained by placing handle of scalpel between the cricoid and thyroid cartilages.

A large bore needle of this type, however, is not ordinarily available in a dental office. If required for more than a very short time, one 13 gauge needle will not permit adequate air exchange,[1] and the rapid accumulation of secretions probably would limit the effectiveness of two or even three such needles.

In an extreme emergency, an airway can be produced within a few seconds by making an incision through the cricothyroid membrane and then placing the handle of the scalpel or some other flat object between the thyroid and cricoid cartilages to keep the wound open (Figs. 17–9 and 17–10). This method, while rapid, is apt to produce damage to the cricoid cartilage, and may cause subsequent laryngeal stenosis. The possibility of this complication is minimized if a low tracheostomy is performed as soon as the patient's condition permits. See the chapter on *maxillofacial injuries* for technique.

SUMMARY

The approach to a patient with acute airway obstruction should consist of an orderly series of steps: (1) Prompt recognition of obstruction. (2) Nonsurgical maneuvers to relieve obstruction. 3) Establishment of an emergency surgical airway.

Under emergency conditions an airway can be established rapidly, safely, and easily through the cricothyroid membrane. If it is necessary for an artificial airway to remain in place, a low tracheotomy should follow within 48 to 72 hours so that laryngeal stenosis will be avoided.

REFERENCES

1. Allison, M. L.: Personal communication.
2. American Heart Association: Statement on first aid for foreign body obstruction of the airway (Interim Recommendations), April 9, 1976.
3. Best, C. H., and Taylor, N. B.: The Physiological Basis of Medical Practice. 6th ed. Baltimore, Williams & Wilkins Co., 1955, p. 413.
4. Caparosa, R. J., and Zavatsky, A. R.: Practical aspects of the cricothyroid space. Laryngoscope, 67:577, 1957.
5. Chipps, J. E.: The dentist's role in the management of foreign bodies. Dent. Clin. North Amer., July 1957, p. 393.
6. Heimlich, H. J.: A life-saving maneuver to prevent food-choking. J.A.M.A. 234:398, 1975.
7. Ruhe, D. S., Williams, G. V., and Proud, G. O.: Emergency airway by cricothyroid puncture or tracheotomy: Comparative study of methods and instruments. Trans. Am. Acad. Ophthalmol., 64:182, 1960.

Part 3

PREVENTION AND TREATMENT OF SURGICAL AND OPERATIVE EMERGENCIES

SURGICAL EMERGENCIES

Robert B. Shira

Surgical emergencies and complications are encountered in every dental practice that includes surgical procedures in its scope. While many of these emergencies and complications are of little consequence, others may assume major proportions. No dental practitioner should include surgery in his or her practice unless prepared to cope with emergencies and complications when they arise and unless possessed of the knowledge and skill to manage the problems successfully.

This discussion will cover the surgical emergencies and complications associated with intraoral procedures.

PREVENTION OF SURGICAL EMERGENCIES AND COMPLICATIONS

Val Peterson, former Director of Civil Defense, once said, "The best way to survive an atomic attack is not to be there when the bombs go off."

Figure 18–1   *Left,* Severe blood loss following removal of a maxillary molar from a hemophiliac.
Right, Soft friable clot with seepage of blood around margins at the extraction site.

By the same reasoning, the best way to treat an emergency or complication is to prevent its occurrence.[10]

Before undertaking any surgical procedure, a thorough preoperative evaluation of the patient should be made. While most patients receiving dental treatment are ambulatory and presumably in good health, constant vigilance is necessary to discover associated or concomitant conditions that may have a distinct bearing on the problem at hand. The evaluation should include a careful history, a thorough clinical examination, adequate roentgenograms, and any necessary laboratory procedures. The findings may point to some local or systemic condition which would result in an emergency or complication if the planned surgical procedure were carried out. See the chapter on *physical evaluation.*

An excellent example of the importance of the preoperative evaluation is the serious bleeding problem that arises when extractions are performed on an unprepared hemophiliac or a patient with leukemia. (Fig. 18–1). When the bleeding problem is recognized by a proper preoperative evaluation, the patient usually can be prepared for surgery in such a manner that

Figure 18–2 Pathology at the apex of a residual root that could only be discovered by adequate roentgenograms.

Figure 18-3 Roentgenogram reveals the distal root of the third molar to be curved buccally or lingually, adding to the difficulty of removing this tooth.

no serious bleeding problem will occur.[32, 48] See the chapter on *hemorrhage* for evaluation procedure.

To prevent emergencies and complications, no surgical procedure should be performed on the teeth or supporting structures until adequate roentgenograms are available. The roentgenogram is an indispensable aid to the practitioner, for it furnishes additional information on the over-all problem and frequently assists the operator in his surgical approach. Adequate roentgenograms will reveal pathologic conditions (Fig. 18–2), operative complications (Fig. 18–3), and involvement of adjacent structures (Fig. 18–51). They also provide an accurate record of the preoperative conditions, which is so essential if any medical-legal problems should arise. Procedures carried out without roentgenograms may result in fractured roots, fractured alveolar process, involvement of the maxillary sinus, nerve injury, etc., which possibly could have been avoided by utilization of the information furnished by the roentgenogram.

As a further step in prevention of emergencies and complications, the clinician should possess the knowledge to properly evaluate the surgical problem *before* treatment. If the preoperative evaluation reveals a concomitant systemic condition, he must know the effect of this condition on the local problem. Likewise, he must be able to evaluate the technical difficulty of any specific problem as revealed by the clinical and roentgenographic examination. Not all procedures are of the same magnitude, and complications may arise when an operator attempts procedures that are beyond his capabilities. Prevention of these complications calls for an honest appraisal of the problem and referral of those problems that are beyond the comfortable range of operating ability of the practitioner. Adherence to the old adage, "A good doctor knows what he can't do as well as what he can do," will pay large dividends in preventing emergencies and complications of operative origin.

The information derived from the above considerations should lead to a surgical plan. Emergencies will be minimized if a well thought out, well regulated surgical plan is formulated before the procedure is started. It should be flexible enough to cope with any operative complications that were anticipated as the result of the preoperative evaluation, or any emergencies that might arise during surgery. By adherence to a set plan, the procedures can be systematized and the operation carried through to a successful conclusion with a minimum of trouble.

Adherence to sound surgical principles at time of surgery is essential to reduce further any risk of emergencies and complications. These principles include asepsis, complete and profound anesthesia, anxiety control, adequate exposure of the operative field, hemostasis, adequate but conservative removal of bone when indicated, use of controlled force, careful debridement and closure of the wound, and the conservative manipulation of tissue at all times. These principles have stood the test of time and, if followed meticulously, may be relied upon to minimize complications.

While it is realized that adherence to the above considerations will reduce the number of emergencies and complications, the fact remains that unavoidable situations will still occur. These must be treated properly. It is obviously impossible to cover all the emergencies and complications of exodontia and oral surgery in this discussion; therefore, our attention here will be limited to the more common surgical emergencies seen in a busy dental practice.

INFECTIONS

ACUTE INFECTIONS

One of the most commonly encountered surgical emergencies is the acutely infected tooth. It is manifested by a swollen face, an elevated temperature, and varying degrees of pain (Fig. 18–4). The patient usually has spent one or more sleepless nights, is dehydrated, and may have eaten little since the onset of the condition. Local examination reveals an extremely tender, sore, loose tooth. There may or may not be fluctuation in the soft tissues, signifying localization of the infectious process.

Figure 18–4 Cellulitis resulting from acute periapical abscess. Antibiotic therapy was initiated and tooth extracted one hour later.

Figure 18–5 *A*, Facial infection involving an anatomic space. *B*, Intraoral incision and drainage of space abscess with insertion of a drain.

In the past, this condition was usually treated in a conservative manner by delaying extraction of the tooth until the inflammatory process had subsided. Older textbooks[32] recommended this therapy on the premise that extraction of the tooth during the acute stage might cause an increase in the inflammatory process with spread of the infection to surrounding bone, soft tissues, and blood vessels. An old adage frequently quoted is: "Never extract a tooth until the condition is improving." This conservative therapy was often supplemented by applications of heat in an attempt to localize the infection in the soft tissue, so that an incision could be accomplished to establish drainage (Figs. 18–5 and 18–6). After drainage was established and the swelling had subsided, the tooth was then extracted. During this course of treatment, the patient was in continual pain, was spending sleepless

Figure 18–6 Intraoral incision and drainage of infection.

Figure 18-7 Patient in Figure 18–4 forty-eight hours later. Note complete resolution of the infectious process.

nights, and was unable to eat a normal diet — all of which led to exhaustion and lowering of resistance.

It is now realized that many of these old beliefs are open to question,[20, 37] and some of the conditions which were once considered dangerous may now be treated with safety.[26] Most oral surgeons now believe that the conservative treatment of the acutely infected tooth is no longer indicated and that immediate extraction of the involved tooth is the procedure of choice. Experience has shown that this treatment may be carried out with minimal danger to the patient. By using adequate pre- and postoperative antibiotic therapy and extracting the offending tooth by an atraumatic surgical procedure under general or regional block anesthesia, early resolution of the infectious process may be expected. Removal of the tooth produces immediate relief from pain, and usually results in reduction of the swelling by the following day, with complete resolution of the suppurative process without untoward complications (Fig. 18–7). Immediate extraction satisfies the basic surgical principle of "removal of the cause" and permits drainage of the original focus through the socket.[19] Any collection of pus in the soft tissue may be evacuated at the same time by adequate incision and drainage. This permits rapid healing, and postoperative complications are practically unknown. If the procedure should lead to any adverse sequelae, it is safe to say that the sequelae would probably have occurred anyway, and extraction of the tooth should not be held responsible.

SPACE INFECTIONS

Unfortunately, all patients with acute odontogenic infections do not seek early treatment. In these instances the infection may spread along fascial planes and localize in anatomic spaces (Fig. 18–8).[23] When this occurs, removal of the offending tooth or teeth is still indicated; however, addition-

Figure 18–8 Peritonsillar abscess due to infection progressing along a fascial plane and localizing in an anatomic space. Incision and drainage with insertion of a drain are indicated.

al therapy is usually necessary to bring about a resolution of the infectious process.[49]

Several therapeutic measures are indicated. Heat should be applied to the involved area to hasten the localization of the infection. Antibiotics should be utilized to combat the infectious process. General supportive measures to enhance body defense mechanisms should be instigated. These include restoration of physiologic fluid balance and maintenance of an adequate nutritional intake. Analgesics should be prescribed to relieve pain to enable the patient to obtain adequate rest. Finally, surgical intervention consisting of incision into the involved space to establish drainage and insertion of a drain to maintain the drainage is essential (Fig. 18–9).[28]

PERICORONAL INFECTIONS

Pericoronal infection is another surgical emergency that is frequently encountered. It usually occurs in young people during the eruption process

A   B

Figure 18–9 *A*, Space abscess secondary to a dental infection. *B*, Extraoral incision and drainage with insertion of a rubber drain.

Figure 18–10   Acute pericoronitis. Symptoms of pain, trismus, elevated temperature, edema, sore throat, and difficulty in swallowing.

of the third molars, with the mandibular teeth being the most frequent offenders. The oral mucosa is broken by a cusp of the erupting tooth. This produces an ideal situation for the development of infection under and about the pericoronal flap. The region is hot, moist, and dark, and contains decomposed food products in which rapid growth of bacteria may occur.[16] This infectious process develops rapidly and often spreads to contiguous structures, resulting in trismus, pain, sore throat, swelling, and difficulty in swallowing (Fig. 18–10). At times the infectious process may be of sufficient severity to produce hyperpyrexia, chills, rapid pulse, and general malaise.

Management of this condition presents a formidable problem, and considerable controversy exists regarding the proper therapy. Some feel that treatment should include the immediate removal of the involved tooth,[26] whereas others[16] believe that surgery is almost never indicated in the initial treatment of this infectious condition. The correct answer probably lies midway between these two extremes and depends upon a thorough evaluation of each case. If the infectious process is more or less limited to the immediate surrounding soft tissue, and if the offending tooth is so situated that its removal could be accomplished by a simple surgical procedure with minimal trauma to the surrounding tissue, then the immediate removal of the tooth, with indicated supportive measures consisting of antibiotics and strong analgesics, would be the treatment of choice. If, however, the infectious process is diffuse and the causative tooth is in such a position that its removal would require a complicated, prolonged procedure, necessitating the formation of soft tissue flaps and removal of osseous structures and sectioning the tooth, it would be best to treat the pericoronal infection until it resolves before undertaking removal of the tooth.

In treatment of the pericoronal infection before extraction, drainage and irrigation of the pericoronal pocket are the important factors. This can be accomplished by passing a blunt instrument under the flap and displacing the flap upward. This usually permits the escape of a small amount of purulent discharge from the pocket. If this does not permit adequate drainage, the mucosa overlying the tooth should be incised. The area is then irrigated with normal saline or a comparable solution, using a 10 ml syringe

Figure 18–11 Irrigation of pericoronal area with syringe and 13-gauge needle.

with a blunt, curved, 13-gauge needle (Fig. 18–11). This mechanical lavage washes out accumulated debris and facilitates drainage of the area. A small segment of iodoform gauze or a rubber drain may then be placed under the flap and extended back into the pericoronal pocket. The drain prevents further accumulation of debris and infectious material in the pocket and allows for continuous drainage. Following treatment of the pericoronal infection, it should be determined if the maxillary third molar is impinging on the swollen tissue surrounding the mandibular tooth. If this occurs, it is good judgment to extract the maxillary tooth during the first visit. Since the tooth is usually free of infection, it may be safely extracted without fear of complications.

Following these procedures, the patient should be maintained on antibiotic therapy and strong analgesics and examined frequently for further irrigation and treatment. This therapy usually controls the pain, and rapid recovery from the infection may be anticipated. See the chapter on *drugs* for a review of antibiotics and analgesics.

Following resolution of the infection, serious consideration should be given to the advisability of retaining the involved tooth. The tooth is usually only partially erupted, and frequently there is insufficient room in the arch for its complete eruption (Fig. 18–12). Such teeth are potentially dan-

Figure 18–12 Resolution of infection. Tooth should now be extracted because there is insufficient space in the arch for its complete eruption.

gerous because they easily become re-infected with resulting complications. Therefore, if, in the evaluation, it is found that there is insufficient room in the arch for complete eruption with elimination of the pericoronal pocket, the tooth should be removed.

ALVEOLAR OSTEITIS

Alveolar osteitis, dry socket, necrotic socket, and alveolitis are synonyms used to describe a painful postoperative condition produced by disintegration of the clot in a tooth socket. Since this painful condition is the result of a surgical procedure and correct management is so important, it warrants discussion in this chapter.

Many conditions have been implicated as causative factors in producing this condition; however, it is in reality a loss of the blood clot which acts as a bandage to protect the underlying osseous tissue. With loss of the clot, nerve endings in the bone become exposed to the oral cavity, resulting in varying degrees of pain. Thus, any condition that would interfere with formation and maintenance of a healthy clot in the socket can be incriminated as causing the condition. It is a very common postoperative complication and is known to any practitioner who extracts teeth.[52]

Prevention is, of course, the ideal solution to the problem and many writers have advocated various means of preventing the condition. Insertion of some type of space obliterator such as Gelfoam or Surgicel, perforating the cortical bone surrounding the socket to insure a more adequate blood supply, general supportive care, vitamin therapy, systemic antibiotic therapy, etc., are among the measures utilized. In spite of these measures, however, alveolar osteitis is still encountered and must be treated to relieve the patient of the persistent pain associated with the condition.

Treatment should be directed toward relief of the pain and stimulation of normal repair of the extraction wound. For the most part, a dressing containing an obtundent to relieve the pain and an antiseptic to combat any infection that may be present is used. Before applying the dressing, the socket should be cleansed of all remaining disintegrated clot so the medication may come in direct contact with the bone. This can be accomplished by irrigation and/or by light curettage. The bone should then be dried and a dressing containing one of the many analgesics and antiseptic drugs in a liquid or paste form should be applied. This dressing should give relief from pain within a few minutes and keep the patient comfortable for longer than 24 hours. A dry socket should not be dressed every day.[53] If the dressing is changed daily, the manipulation of the socket will interfere with the proliferatiion of repair tissues and prolong the recovery period. Thus, a dressing should contain ingredients that have a prolonged effect and that require changing only every second, third or fourth day. One dressing that meets these criteria is:

Eugenol   46 per cent
Balsam Peru   46 per cent
Chlorobutanol   4 per cent
Benzocaine   4 per cent

The dressing should be placed on iodoform or plain gauze and applied loosely in the socket, covering all the exposed bone. The socket should be repacked as often as necessary to keep the patient comfortable and continued until the bone is covered by the proliferating repair tissues.

Other preparations that fill the above criteria are also available.[2]

Curettement of the exposed bone has been advocated as a means of stimulating bleeding and causing a new blood clot to form in the socket. Experience has shown that this procedure is of little value and its use should be condemned.[43]

INJURIES TO SOFT TISSUE

Lack of control of instruments used in surgical and operative procedures occasionally results in lacerations, tears, or other injuries to adjoining soft tissues. Elevators or forceps may slip from tooth structure and be forced into the soft tissues of the lip, cheek, tongue, floor of the mouth, or palate. During exodontia the alveolar bone adjacent to teeth may be fractured and dislodged, resulting in ragged tears of the overlying mucosa. Furthermore, disks, burs, and other rotating instruments utilized in restorative dentistry may inadvertently slip from tooth structures, injuring adjacent soft tissues.

These soft tissue injuries usually are preventable. Careful attention to detail and utilization of surgical techniques that insure proper application of instruments and adequate hand support to limit the movement of instruments if they slip from tooth structure will minimize the problem.

MUCOSAL TEARS

These wounds should receive immediate attention, and the majority can be treated by primary suture without debridement. Hemorrhage usually can be controlled by pressure, although it may occasionally be necessary to clamp and tie larger severed vessels or active bleeding points. Lacerations and tears limited to the mucosa are seldom of sufficient depth to warrant closure of the tissues in layers. Repositioning of the mucosa and suturing with interrupted or continuous sutures is all that is required (Fig. 18–13). Mucoperiosteum that has been stripped from bone should be repositioned and sutured without delay.

Figure 18–13 Soft tissue lacerations produced when an elevator inadvertently slipped from the tooth during extraction.

DEEP SOFT TISSUE WOUNDS

Deep wounds may be produced when disks, burs, or exodontia instruments slip from the teeth and lacerate or tear the soft tissues. Larger vessels occasionally are severed, and profuse hemorrhage results. Fortunately such emergencies are rare, but when they occur prompt action is necessary. The operator must remain calm and immediately begin measures to arrest the hemorrhage. This usually can be accomplished by maintaining hard digital pressure on a piece of gauze inserted over the bleeding area. Occasionally hard bimanual pressure is required, one hand being held intraorally over the bleeding point while counterpressure is applied extraorally with the other hand. If this method does not arrest the bleeding, strong suction should be employed to cleanse the mouth of blood. The margins of the wound should then be retracted and the severed vessels and large bleeding points visualized, clamped, and tied. In deeper wounds, where it has been possible to arrest the hemorrhage by pressure, the margins of the wound also should be retracted, and any severed vessels or large bleeding points that can be visualized should be clamped and tied to prevent secondary hemorrhage.

Following hemostasis, these deep wounds should be closed in layers. The deeper tissues should be closed to eliminate all dead space, and the submucosal layer closely approximated to minimize tension on the mucosal sutures.[29] While absorbable sutures are most frequently utilized in tying vessels and closing the deeper layers, cotton or silk nonabsorbable sutures also may be used since they are well tolerated by the tissues.

THERMAL BURNS

Heated instruments utilized in the mouth produce painful burns when allowed to come in contact with the mucosa. Overheated handpieces or rotating instruments coming in contact with the skin or mucosa are other causes of thermal burns (Fig. 18–14). Such wounds seldom require treatment. Suturing is not indicated, and the wound usually will heal rapidly by secondary intention.[46] If pain is a problem, it may be relieved by covering

Figure 18–14 Wound on face and oral mucosa produced by overheated handpiece utilized to remove bone and section tooth during removal of impacted third molar.

the wound with a protective medicament, such as Bucrylate, Orabase, or tincture of benzoin. When utilizing hot instruments or rotating instruments that may become overheated, the operator should exert every precaution to keep them from contacting the skin and mucosa to prevent this type of soft tissue wound.

ELECTRICAL BURNS

While in the past electrical burns involving the oral structures have been rare, their incidence is increasing.[14] Most electrical burns in the oral area result from accidents involving electric outlets or electric cords and usually produce injuries to the lips or tongue, or both (Fig. 18–15). These injuries are more common in young children and occur when the child bites through an electric cord or projects the tongue into an electric outlet. The extent of the injury varies with the intensity of the current, the efficiency of the grounding, the amount of tissue exposed, and the length of time the tissues are exposed to the current.[13] The injuries are produced when heat is generated as the current passes through areas of high resistance with resultant thrombosis of the vessels and ischemia of the tissues. While local tissue destruction is usually severe, the extent of the damage is initially difficult to determine. Soft tissue, bone, and teeth may be involved. Soft tissue injury results in ulceration, sloughing, and scarring with severe contraction that decreases the mobility of the involved tissues. Varying degrees of deformity may result. Injury to bone may result in devitalization with ultimate sequestration of the devitalized bone.[5] Injury to teeth, if severe, may result in devitalization and subsequent exfoliation unless proper treatment is instigated.

Early treatment is essential. Antibiotic therapy and prophylaxis against tetanus should be instituted. Analgesics to control pain should be administered. Initially, conservative debridement of the burned areas is indicated until the full extent of the injury is determined. If possible, the wound

Figure 18–15 Flash electrical burn of the lip caused by child chewing through the insulation of an electric extension cord.

should be covered with a Furacin type dressing; however, if this is not practical the wound may be left open. If feasible, positive splinting of the involved tissues should be provided to minimize scar contraction and prevent deformity.[12] Involved teeth should be carefully evaluated and, if devitalized, appropriate pulpal therapy should be provided if and when feasible.

PUNCTURE TYPE SOFT TISSUE WOUNDS

A type of soft tissue wound which has received little attention in the literature is the puncture type wound. Such wounds usually are the result of falls or accidents while some hard, pointed object is held in the mouth. However, similar wounds are produced when pointed dental instruments are accidentally forced into the soft tissues. When the lips, cheek or soft palate are involved, an actual perforation may be produced (Fig. 18–16).

The wounds resulting from these injuries are more alarming than dangerous. The puncture wound seldom bleeds profusely, and the tissues usually collapse or contract to obliterate the defect when the penetrating object is withdrawn. Suturing is seldom necessary; in fact, it is contraindicated, for this procedure favors the growth of anaerobic pathogenic bacteria which may have been implanted. Treatment consists of examining the wound to insure that no foreign body remains, flooding the defect with an antiseptic solution, and allowing the wound to heal by granulation.[45] Steps also should be taken to prevent the development of a secondary infection.

All intraoral wounds are produced in a contaminated area, and secondary infection is an ever-present possibility. Every effort should be expended to prevent infection or to eliminate it should it develop. These preventive measures should include strict adherence to sterile techniques, thorough cleansing of the wound, complete hemostasis, and accurate closure. While antibiotic coverage is not essential in the management of superficial wounds, it is definitely indicated when the deeper structures are involved. Antibiotics, when indicated, should be administered in sufficient

Figure 18–16 Puncture wound of the soft palate produced by an elevator.

quantity and for sufficient time to prevent or control infection and to prevent the emergence of resistant organisms.

Prophylaxis Against Tetanus

Prophylaxis against infection by *Clostridium tetani* must be considered in all contaminated wounds. It is particularly important when puncture type wounds are produced by contaminated objects which force dirt or debris deep into the wound.

Tetanus infections are so catastrophic and have such a high mortality rate that active prophylaxis must be provided if there is any question of a wound's being contaminated. A patient who has been immunized with tetanus toxoid and who has received booster injections at the indicated intervals should receive an additional booster injection of 0.5 ml of tetanus toxoid aluminum hydroxide, USP (Alhydrox).[1, 54] If a patient has not been inoculated against tetanus or if there is doubt about the adequacy of the patient's active immunity, passive immunity should be provided by the administration of 250 to 500 units of tetanus immune globulin (human) (Hyper-Tet) by deep intramuscular injection. At the same time, but in a different extremity and with a separate syringe, 0.5 ml of tetanus toxoid aluminum hydroxide, USP (Alhydrox), is administered followed by a second dose in four weeks and a booster dose of 0.5 ml in six to twelve months.[17] Administration of tetanus prophylaxis is in the realm of medical practice; so referral of the patient requiring this therapy is indicated.[35]

INJURIES TO BONE

Fractured Alveolar Process

During difficult extractions portions of the alveolar bone overlying the teeth may inadvertently be fractured. This fractured bone may remain attached to the extracted tooth or it may remain behind in the wound. If the fractured bone is removed with the extracted tooth, the remaining alveolar bone about the socket is left in a rough, jagged condition (Fig. 18–17). When this condition exists, a small mucoperiosteal flap should be reflected to gain access to the area, and the rough, irregular bone margins smoothed with rongeurs and bone files.

When the fractured segment of alveolar bone remains in the wound, two possible methods of treatment exist. If the fragment is small, and particularly if it has been separated from its periosteal attachment, it should be removed and the remaining rough bony socket treated as described above. However, if the segment is large, and if its periosteal attachment is undisturbed, the fractured segment should be repositioned by digital pressure and held in place by sutures placed through the overlying soft tissue.

This problem occasionally is encountered in removal of impacted mandibular third molars, when large segments of the lingual plate may be fractured. Removal of the fragment is a difficult procedure and results in a large residual defect accompanied by marked postoperative pain, edema,

Figure 18–17 Fractured alveolar process removed with extracted tooth. Resulting rough, jagged alveolar bone should be smoothed with rongeurs or bone files.

and trismus. The problem is best managed by leaving the fragment in position where it will reattach and heal in a short time.

FRACTURED MAXILLARY TUBEROSITY

Fracture of the maxillary tuberosity is occasionally encountered. The problem results most frequently from the application of uncontrolled force when extracting a maxillary second or third molar or from the injudicious

Figure 18–18 Sectioning maxillary molar to prevent fracture of the maxillary tuberosity. *A*, Soft tissue flap and removal of buccal bone to obtain access for sectioning of the two buccal roots. *B*, The crown and lingual root removed in one segment. *C*, Removal of the buccal roots with elevators.

Figure 18-19 Flap has been elevated, buccal bone removed, and buccal roots separated from the crown and lingual root to facilitate removal of the maxillary molar.

use of elevators in removing firmly attached teeth. Frequently the broken segment is quite large and may include one or more teeth and the floor of the maxillary sinus as well as the maxillary tuberosity.

Proper preoperative planning usually will prevent this emergency. Any time a tooth is to be removed from the tuberosity area, particularly if the roentgenogram reveals a large maxillary sinus extending close to the crest of the alveolar ridge, it should be realized that fracture of the tuberosity is an ever-present possibility. By reflecting a mucoperiosteal flap and removing a small portion of the buccal bone, the tooth can then be sectioned by burs and removed in segments (Fig. 18–18). This procedure, while it may consume slightly more time than a forceps extraction, will enable the operator to avoid the embarrassing emergency of a fractured tuberosity (Fig. 18–19).

If a tuberosity is fractured it should be preserved if at all possible. An attempt should be made to remove the tooth from the fractured tuberosity without avulsing the bone. If possible, it is best to delay extraction of the tooth for several weeks to allow the fracture of the tuberosity to heal. If mobility of the fractured tuberosity is minimal, no fixation is needed; but if gross movement is present, it should be stabilized by use of splints or fracture appliances. After the fracture has healed, a mucoperiosteal flap may be elevated, the buccal bone removed, and the tooth sectioned with burs and removed in sections. This procedure usually will allow removal of the tooth without recurrence of the fracture.[18]

An alternate procedure is indicated if it is necessary to remove the tooth immediately. In these instances the operator should stabilize the tuberosity as well as possible and proceed with the surgical removal of the tooth as described above. Following removal of the tooth the fractured tuberosity should be repositioned manually and held in place by accurate reapproximation and suturing of the overlying soft tissue.[8]

On occasion it is necessary to remove the entire segment of bone. It may be impractical or impossible to remove the tooth or teeth from the fractured segment (Fig. 18–20). On other occasions large mucoperiosteal flaps may have been formed before the fracture occurred. Such flaps jeopardize the blood supply of the bone, and in these instances it is best to re-

Figure 18–20 Fractured maxillary tuberosity involving two teeth and the maxillary sinus. It was impractical to attempt removal of the teeth from the thin bone, so the entire segment was removed.

move the tuberosity. Removal is accomplished by carefully elevating the mucoperiosteum from all aspects of the body segment until it is completely free. The fractured tuberosity and the involved teeth may then be removed with little or no difficulty.[50] The resulting defect usually is quite large and often involves the maxillary sinus. Utilization of an absorbable hemostatic agent to fill the defect and to reposition the soft tissues to their original position will mimimize the residual deformity. Accurate reapproximation and careful suturing of the soft tissue usually will prevent the development of an oroantral fistula.

FRACTURED MANDIBLE

The accidental fracturing of the mandible during the tooth removal is rare, but does occur. While most fractures of this type result from over-

Figure 18–21 *Top*, Fracture of mandible resulting from excessive force applied with elevators. *Bottom*, By sectioning the crown and removing the tooth in segments the need for excessive force is usually eliminated.

zealous use of elevators (Fig. 18–21) or from the use of uncontrolled force with forceps, the fact remains that well trained operators who follow careful and accepted surgical techniques occasionally will fracture a mandible. This problem, even though rare, should be considered a normal hazard of exodontia, and its occurrence does not necessarily imply negligence on the part of the operator. The problem is most frequently encountered in older people when deeply embedded teeth are being removed from thin, atrophic mandibles; however, it may occur at any time.

A fracture occurring during the extraction of a tooth usually is accompanied by an audible crack, with associated abnormal mobility at the site of fracture. If the tooth remains firmly attached to the bone, the extraction procedure should be abandoned and the patient treated by one of the recognized methods for treating a fractured mandible. However, if the tooth has been luxated and can be removed with minimal additional trauma, it should be removed before proceeding with treatment of the fracture.

This problem usually can be prevented by adhering to the accepted surgical principles of obtaining adequate access, creating an unimpeded path of removal for the tooth, and use of controlled force.

INJURIES TO TEETH

INJURIES TO ADJACENT TEETH

Injudicious use of forceps or elevators may accidentally luxate, avulse, or fracture teeth adjacent to the one being removed. Removal of a crowded, malposed tooth becomes a difficult problem because of the difficulty of seating a forceps or elevator without impinging on adjacent teeth (Fig. 18–22). Rotary luxating movements with a forceps may bring the beaks of the

Figure 18–22 Cuspid to be removed for orthodontic purposes. Note the lateral incisor is in contact with the first bicuspid. Extreme care must be exercised in removal of the cuspid to prevent injury to the adjacent teeth.

Figure 18–23 In removal of the right central incisor for orthodontic reasons, extreme care must be exercised to prevent injury to adjacent teeth.

forceps in contact with adjacent teeth, causing injury; the injudicious use of elevators may dislodge a tooth adjacent to the one being extracted (Fig. 18–23).

Emergencies of this type can be avoided by careful preoperative evaluation of the problem and by careful surgical techniques that avoid force being imparted to adjacent teeth at time of surgery.

When adjacent teeth are injured, treatment depends on the severity of the injury. If a tooth is loosened and mobility is minimal, no treatment is indicated, since the tooth usually will reattach. If movement is excessive, the tooth should be splinted with an arch bar or some type of splint. When a tooth is completely avulsed, careful evaluation of the problem is necessary. If the tooth is of little value or is extensively involved by disease processes, nothing should be done. However, if it is a healthy, important tooth, it should be immediately repositioned in the socket and splints applied for stabilization. When reattachment has occurred, endodontic therapy may preserve the tooth.

When small portions of the crown of an adjacent tooth are fractured, the crown may be recontoured and polished. If larger segments are involved, temporary coverage should be provided and a permanent restoration placed at a later date. If the fracture involves the pulp, pulp capping or immediate endodontic procedures are indicated.

DISLODGED AND BROKEN FILLINGS

Another regrettable emergency of exodontia is the dislodgment of a filling from an adjoining tooth. This is encountered most frequently in the removal of an impacted third molar when the adjoining second molar has a distal restoration. It is possible, however, to dislodge any filling from an adjacent tooth by the inaccurate placement of forceps or elevators.

Prevention is the best treatment for this problem. Careful use of instruments with attention to protection of the adjacent teeth should prevent this complication. However, the most careful operators will on occasion dislodge a filling. If this possibility has been explained to the patient prior to surgery, it usually is accepted without question. When it occurs, the operator should

Figure 18–24 Amalgam filling which fell undetected into an open socket at time of surgery. If healing has occurred, removal of these metallic fragments is seldom indicated.

proceed with removal of the tooth and then place a temporary filling in the adjacent tooth. A permanent restoration should be placed at a later date.

Broken fillings or other debris may fall into open sockets, where they may escape detection and become closed in the wound. This is not a serious problem, but should be avoided if possible. Routine use of postoperative roentgenograms before closure of wounds would prevent this problem, but this is not always practical or desirable due to radiation hazards. In instances where a tooth or filling has been shattered during extraction or when the procedure has been particularly difficult, roentgenograms may be utilized to see if any foreign body has been left in the wound. If discovered, debridement prior to closure is indicated.

Another simple measure to minimize this problem is the sequence of removal of teeth. When maxillary and mandibular teeth are to be removed at the same appointment, removal of the maxillary teeth before the mandibular teeth should be considered. When mandibular teeth are removed first, dislodged fillings, tooth fragments, and other debris resulting from the removal of the maxillary teeth may fall into the open mandibular sockets and remain undetected. It is much less likely that debris generated from the extraction of the mandibular teeth would fly up and lodge in the maxillary sockets.

Metallic fragments discovered by routine roentgenograms in normal alveolar bone need not be removed (Fig. 18–24). They seldom produce symptoms, and may be retained for years without trouble. The surgical procedure to recover these fragments can be traumatic and destructive, and seldom is indicated.

EXTRACTION OF THE WRONG TOOTH

Extraction of the wrong tooth is a regrettable emergency for which treatment obviously is most unsatisfactory. Fortunately this emergency is easily avoided if the operator is alert and adheres to certain important principles. First, he must have a clear understanding of the tooth or teeth to be removed. It is well to ask the patient if he is aware of the teeth that are to be removed. In a referral practice, if any doubt exists, the referring practitioner should be contacted before proceeding. Next, properly processed and oriented roentgenograms must be available and the clinical problem correlated with the roentgenographic findings. Finally, the operator must give his individual attention to the problem at hand and not allow distractions to interfere with the management of the case. When removing sound teeth for orthodontic reasons, it is well to mark the crowns of the teeth to be removed with an indelible pencil or some similar marking agent to insure removal of the proper teeth (Fig. 18–25).

On occasion the injudicious use of elevators may dislodge a tooth adjacent to the one being extracted. This most frequently occurs when the roots of the adjacent tooth are cone shaped and a dislodging force is applied to the crown by an elevator blade (Fig. 18–26). It is best avoided by a careful evaluation of the problem with extreme care being exercised to see that no force is imparted to the adjacent tooth during instrumentation (Fig. 18–27).[24]

Once a wrong tooth has been removed, the extracted tooth may be man-

Figure 18-25 Teeth to be removed for orthodontic reasons have been marked with indelible pencil to insure removal of the correct teeth.

Figure 18-26 Cone shaped roots of the second molar. This tooth could easily be forced from its socket if an injudicious dislodging force were applied by an elevator to the crown during removal of the third molar.

Figure 18-27 An elevator may inadvertently apply a dislodging force to a second molar. While the superior edge of the elevator is engaging the third molar, the inferior edge may dislodge the second molar unless care is exercised. (From Hayward, J. R., and Costich, E. R.: The Use of Elevators. *In* Practical Dental Monographs. Chicago, Year Book Medical Publishers, Inc., 1957. Used by permission.)

aged as described earlier under the treatment of accidentally avulsed teeth. However, when it is not feasible to replace the extracted tooth, the operator is faced with the problem of making the best of a bad situation and attempting to avoid any legal entanglement by treating the patient in an honest, concerned, and humane manner.

FRACTURED ROOTS

While fractured roots which are allowed to remain in the alveolar bone may occasionally produce a pathologic process, more frequently they may be retained for years without creating problems. This is not meant to imply that fractured roots should be allowed to remain, for, with very few exceptions, they should be removed immediately.

Although it is often possible to prevent the fracture of roots by the utilization of radiographs and proper preoperative planning, many teeth present conditions that make their removal without fracturing the roots extremely difficult. Root breakage may be anticipated if any of the following conditions are present:

1. Slender roots
2. Curved roots
3. Divergent roots
4. Ankylosed roots
5. Devitalized teeth
6. Dense overlying alveolar bone
7. Use of excessive force
8. Failure to grasp tooth properly

Of the above, only the use of excessive force and failure to grasp the tooth properly are under the control of the operator. Therefore, root fracture should be considered a normal hazard of exodontia and it should not be looked upon as an indication of improper technique or lack of skill. When a root is fractured, in most instances it should be removed at once, because the removal does not entail a difficult surgical procedure.

Closed Removal

The removal of roots must be divided into several categories. In single rooted teeth in which the crown has been fractured and the entire root remains, the root may sometimes be removed by forceps technique. However, it is usually difficult to seat the forceps properly on the fractured root without sacrificing considerable bone. Therefore, the use of a straight elevator inserted between the root and the alveolar bone is usually indicated (Fig. 18-28, center). Efficient utilization of an elevator depends on establishing a firm place of application on the root and having an adjacent bone wall of sufficient thickness to offer a strong point of resistance. When these factors are present, forcing the elevator apically between the root and alveolar bone and rotating it clockwise and counterclockwise will usually dislodge the single fractured root (Fig. 18-28, bottom).

Figure 18–28   *Top*, Fractured single root. *Center*, Elevator inserted between root and alveolar bone. *Bottom*, Elevator forced apically and rotated to dislodge the root.

Figure 18–29   *Top*, Fractured multirooted tooth. *Center*, Roots separated with bur. *Bottom*, Roots removed individually with straight elevator.

When the crown is fractured from a multirooted tooth, a different approach is indicated. Although occasionally the roots may be grasped with a forceps, it is usually impossible to obtain sufficient "purchase" on the roots to insure their removal. Consequently, it is usually indicated to separate the roots by means of burs or chisels and to remove them as single roots as described above (Fig. 18–29).

Open Removal

When attempts at removal of roots by the closed method are not successful in a reasonable length of time, this method should be abandoned and the open method utilized. This procedure consists of reflecting a mucoperiosteal flap from the labial or buccal surface of the alveolar process and removal of sufficient bone to permit access and direct visualization of the root. Removal of interseptal bone is sometimes indicated. Removal of the root with elevators or forceps usually becomes a simple matter after access has been obtained, hemostasis is secured, and the root visualized under a good light.

Root Tips

In removal of root tips, the root surface of the extracted tooth should be carefully examined before any attempt is made to remove the fragment. This

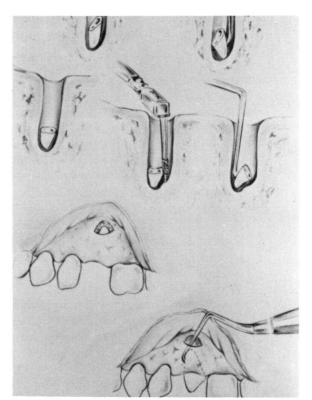

Figure 18–30 *Top,* Elevator inserted between bone and angled fractured root to displace root into the socket. *Center,* Bur used to enlarge socket to facilitate removal of root. *Bottom,* Window prepared in alveolar bone to permit insertion of elevator to dislodge fractured root.

may give a clue which will simplify the procedure. If the root has been fractured at an angle, many times a sharp pick elevator can be inserted between the bone and the sharp angle of the fractured surface to dislodge the root (Fig. 18–30, top). In some instances a bone drill may be utilized to enlarge the socket around the root tip until the root becomes loosened. Its removal with a small elevator or forceps is then possible (Fig. 18–30, center). If these procedures fail, or if access and visibility into the socket are difficult, attempts to remove the root through the socket should be abandoned. The root should then be exposed by reflection of a mucoperiosteal flap and removal of sufficient buccal and intraseptal bone to permit direct visualization. Occasionally, it is advantageous to make a bone window over the apex of the root to allow the insertion of an elevator to displace the root down into the empty socket (Fig. 18–30, bottom). This is particularly advantageous in removal of the buccal root of the upper first biscuspids. In any event, removal of the root with elevators or forceps is usually a simple matter after adequate access has been obtained.

Should All Root Tips Be Removed?

While the removal of fractured roots is indicated in most situations, there are rare occasions when sound surgical judgment dictates that they should be allowed to remain in the alveolar process. Some root tips are in such a position that removal would entail a difficult, time-consuming, traumatic operation which would require the removal of large amounts of overlying bone. Such loss of bone could conceivably jeopardize the support of adjacent teeth. Extensive surgery to remove root tips in close relationship with the mandibular canal may produce injury to the inferior alveolar nerve with resultant troublesome paresthesia.[21] To prevent such complications it is good judgment to allow the root fragments to remain.

In other instances fractured roots of mandibular teeth may be so situated that attempts at removal may force them through the lingual plate of the mandible into the sublingual or submandibular space. This possibility exists because the mandible is wider at the superior surface than at the inferior margin. This loss of width is always at the expense of the lingual side, and the roots of the molar teeth often are in close proximity to the lingual plate. Pressure exerted on a root tip may force the root through the lingual plate. If this occurs, the position the root occupies is determined by the location of the insertion of the mylohyoid muscle (Fig. 18–31). If the attachments of this muscle are below the apices of the tooth, the root will be in the sublingual space. If the mylohyoid muscle attaches superior to the apices of the tooth, the root will be in the submandibular space (Fig. 18–32).

In a similar manner, maxillary teeth may be so situated that attempts to remove fractured roots may force them through the thin maxillary bone into the maxillary sinus.

Removal of displaced roots from the area lingual to the mandible and from the maxillary sinus involves extensive surgery which should be avoided if possible. Once a root has been fractured, the operator should carefully consider the possibility of the root's being forced into an adjacent space at time of its removal. If this possibility exists it is good judgment to allow the root to remain undisturbed in the alveolar bone. In these cases the mere existence of a

Figure 18–31   **Figure 18–32**

Figure 18–31   Relationship of the attachment of the mylohyoid muscle to the apices of the mandibular molars.

Figure 18–32   *Above,* Third molar to be removed. Note the increased density just above the apices of the teeth. This represents the mylohyoid ridge. *Below,* Distal root broken and forced through the lingual plate of mandible below the attachment of the mylohyoid muscle. The root is in the submandibular space.

residual root does not imply negligence; it often is the indication of sound surgical judgment.

The prevalence of retained root fragments in the general population was demonstrated in the 1969 ADA Health Screening Program, where panoramic x-rays were taken of 2251 dental practitioners; retained root tips were found in 46 cases, an incidence higher than 2 per cent.[3] This is a relevant finding, particularly when one considers that small root fragments are often not observed with panoramic radiography.

When it is decided that a root should not be removed, the situation should be discussed with the patient with the explanation that the aftermath of the surgical procedure might be more severe than the effects of leaving the root in the alveolar bone, or, that the cure might be worse than the disease. If a root is allowed to remain, the patient should not be told that it will resorb or exfoliate. He should be told that the area will be reexamined periodically by roentgenograms and, if pathologic changes become evident, the condition will be reevaluated. A statement that the root has been allowed to remain and that the situation has been fully explained to the patient should be entered on the patient's record.

If a fractured mandibular root has been forced through the lingual surface of the mandible it should be removed. This is accomplished by reflecting a large mucoperiosteal flap from the alveolar ridge on the lingual side of the

mandible and recovering the root with small curved curets. Removal is frequently facilitated by maintaining extraoral counter pressure over the involved
area to prevent additional displacement of the root during manipulation of the
tissues.

Removal of roots which have been displaced into the maxillary sinus will
be discussed in another section of this chapter.

TEETH FORCIBLY DISPLACED

Injudicious application of force occasionally will displace an entire tooth
into an adjoining anatomic space. The problem is encountered most frequently
in removal of impacted third molars, when a maxillary third molar may be
forced into the infratemporal fossa (Fig. 18–33) or the maxillary sinus, or a
mandibular third molar forced through the lingual side of the mandible into the
submandibular space (Fig. 18–34). The latter problem is caused most fre-

Figure 18–33   Tooth displaced into the infratemporal fossa during attempted removal.

Figure 18–34   Tooth forced through lingual side of
mandible during attempted sectioning of the tooth.

quently when an attempt is made to split the tooth with a chisel after it has been loosened from its attachments. The blow of the mallet converts the chisel into a pile driver, forcing the loosened tooth through the lingual plate of the mandible. Improper application of force with elevators is responsible for displacement of the maxillary third molar.

The displaced mandibular third molar should be removed immediately. It invariably can be recovered through an intraoral approach. By turning a large lingual mucoperiosteal flap from the crest of the alveolar ridge, the tooth can be retrieved without much difficulty by curved curets or elevators. Removal of a tooth from the maxillary sinus also should be carried out immediately by wide exposure through a Caldwell-Luc approach. Removal of a maxillary third molar displaced into the infratemporal fossa presents a real problem and calls for a different approach. Access is very difficult and, because of the limited access, the tooth is hard to grasp once it is visualized. Attempts to grasp the tooth with an instrument often force the tooth deeper into the tissues, compounding the problem. To avoid this complication, it is good judgment to delay surgery and to allow the tooth to remain in the infratemporal fossa for several weeks. This delay allows the soft tissue to fibrose about the displaced tooth. Fibrosis tends to immobilize the tooth and prevents its movement deeper into the tissue when subsequent surgery is performed. After the proper interval, the area may be widely exposed and, with good hemostasis and brilliant illumination, removal may be accomplished by grasping the tooth with a serrated instrument.[55]

BROKEN NEEDLES AND INSTRUMENTS

With the introduction of disposable needles into dental practice, the hazard of broken hypodermic needles was largely eliminated. Although the problem of broken hypodermic needles is rarely encountered, the breakage of suture needles still occurs with some regularity. Breakage of elevators and other surgical instruments also occurs; so the management of broken needles and instruments must be considered in any discussion of surgical emergencies.

BROKEN NEEDLES

It is easy to understand why some general practitioners become alarmed and greatly concerned when a needle is broken during a dental procedure. Much of this reaction stems from the misconception that broken needles migrate, become infected, or produce cicatrization of the tissues which may cause masticatory dysfunction. In reality, these complications rarely occur.[33] There is little evidence to indicate that broken needles migrate; in fact, they are usually imprisoned in situ by the scar tissue that forms rapidly around the needle (Fig. 18–35). In those cases in which needles have migrated they are usually pushed into the new position by aborted attempts at removal. Infections caused by retained needles are extremely rare and the scar tissue that forms about the needle is so minimal and so localized that interference with function is an extremely remote possibility. In fact, the cicatrization that results from the extensive, prolonged, and traumatic surgical procedures that are usually necessary to remove a broken needle may produce more dysfunction than leaving the needle undisturbed in the tissues.

Figure 18-35 Broken needle that has remained in the soft tissue for 24 years. There have been no associated complications.

When a needle is broken, consideration should be given to its immediate removal. If it is located in superficial tissues and if it can be easily localized by clinical and radiographic examination, its removal by a competent surgeon is usually possible. However, in spite of the superficial location, some needles are difficult to remove, even by competent surgeons. If the attempt to remove the needle is not successful in a reasonable length of time, the wise surgeon will abandon the procedure and allow the needle to remain. If the needle is broken in the deeper tissues, or if it is difficult to localize, serious consideration should be given to allowing it to remain with no attempt being made at removal.

There is ample precedent to justify the retention of broken needles. In medicine and surgery, it is considered good practice to allow metallic foreign bodies that have been accidentally or intentionally placed in the tissues to remain. Soldiers with shrapnel or other missile wounds frequently have multiple metallic fragments scattered throughout the tissues. Removal of all the fragments, short of complete resection of the entire area, is impossible. Hence, they are allowed to remain and they have produced no problems. The old military adage of "A bullet ceases to cause damage when it ceases to move" is applicable here. Metallic plates, wires, and pins are frequently utilized in the treatment of fractures, and there is no hesitancy in allowing them to remain in the tissues. Thus it is accepted that metallic foreign bodies, with the possible exception of those in the eye and the heart, cause no harm and should be allowed to remain. In fact, most surgeons are reluctant to attempt their removal.

The same principles should apply to the broken needle. The surgical procedure to remove a needle is frequently time consuming and traumatic and often fails. The resulting morbidity, manifested by pain, trismus, scar formation, and dysfunction, may produce a condition that is worse than the one that existed prior to the procedure. In these instances in which the "cure is worse than the disease" the patient should not be subjected to the surgical procedure. Therefore, a conservative approach is indicated and the best interest of all will be served if the needle is allowed to remain.

If the decision is to leave the broken needle alone, the problem should be explained to the patient and the fact that the patient was told of the situation should be clearly indicated in the records. The patient should be reassured that the needle will undoubtedly cause no harm and that an extensive surgical procedure to recover the needle is not justified. It might be well to show the patient similar cases in which broken needles and other metallic foreign bodies have remained in the tissues for many years without causing adverse complications. This will reassure him of the wisdom of the decision.

As in all emergencies, prevention is the best treatment. Robinson[36] suggests the following steps to be taken to prevent needle breakage and the actions that should be taken if a needle breaks.

Prevention:
1. A disposable needle of at least 25 gauge and 1¼ inches in length should be used.
2. The needle should not be inserted to the hub.
3. Once the needle is inserted to the desired depth, no attempt should be made to redirect the point without first withdrawing the needle almost completely, then redirecting the point.

At the moment of breakage:
1. Remain as calm as possible; *don't panic*.
2. Instruct the patient not to move, and do not remove your hand from the mouth. Keep the mouth open; a bite block may be inserted if one is available.
3. See if the fragment is protruding. If so, remove with cotton pliers, or a small hemostat.

If the above instructions are followed, most broken needles can be removed if they are not inserted to the hub.

If the fragment is lost:
1. Do not proceed with incision or further probing if the fragment cannot be seen.
2. Inform the patient calmly; allay his fears and apprehension.
3. Note the incident on your records. Save the remaining needle fragment, and inform your insurance carrier.
4. Refer the patient to an oral surgeon for consultation — *NOT* for removal of the needle.

BROKEN INSTRUMENTS

The principle of the management of broken needles also applies to broken surgical instruments. If the broken fragment is large and easily localized, its removal is indicated (Fig. 18–36). If, however, the fragment is small or if it is

Figure 18–36 Fractured end of elevator in tooth socket. Its size and location facilitated its removal.

Figure 18-37 Small fragment of surgical instrument displaced on lingual side of mandible. Its removal is not indicated.

deeply displaced in the tissues where its removal would be a traumatic, time consuming procedure, it should be left alone (Fig. 18–37). The condition should be explained to the patient and a suitable entry noting the decision and the fact that the patient was apprised of the situation should be entered in the record.

EMERGENCIES INVOLVING THE MAXILLARY SINUS

Because of the proximity of the maxillary sinus to the roots of the maxillary bicuspids and molars, the extraction of these teeth frequently involves the sinus. While some of the openings into the sinus may result from carelessness, inadequately planned procedures, or ignorance on the part of the operator, the maxillary sinus is occasionally violated by the most experienced operators who follow correct surgical principles and carefully planned operative techniques.[9] Thus, involvement of the maxillary sinus must be accepted as another normal hazard of exodontia, and the operator should be prepared to cope with the emergencies and complications associated with this structure.

Perhaps the most frequently encountered maxillary sinus complication is the accidental opening of the sinus during extraction of the maxillary posterior teeth. This happens frequently, and may occur without the operator being aware it has occurred. The problem is of little consequence, and the socket usually heals without postoperative complication. Sacrifice of bone to permit apposition of the soft tissue is seldom indicated. A sterile gauze pad should be placed over the socket and held in place for sufficient time to enable a clot to form and to prevent saliva and infectious material from gaining access to the sinus. The socket should be allowed to fill with a normal blood clot, and the use of absorbable hemostatic agents or other space obliterators is not indicated. These procedures usually will result in primary healing.[30] If an oroantral fistula develops following the accidental opening of the sinus during the routine extraction of a tooth, it probably is the result of a concomitant sinus infection, and the opening of the sinus should not be held responsible.[9]

An emergency associated with the maxillary sinus which occurs less frequently is the accidental forcing of a tooth or root into the sinus. While this problem most often can be avoided by a careful preoperative study of the problem, together with employment of a careful operative technique and the judicious use of forceps and elevators, the fact remains that occasionally it cannot be avoided. It has been the accepted belief for many years that roots and other foreign bodies forced into the maxillary sinus should be removed immediately or as soon as practical.[11, 25, 34, 50] Yet root tips which obviously are causing no difficulty occasionally are discovered in the maxillary sinus during routine roentgenographic examinations. In these cases the alveolar ridge usually is intact with no opening into the maxillary sinus. The patient seldom has complaints, and often cannot recall when the root was displaced into the sinus. Experience has shown that root tips and other foreign bodies can be tolerated in the maxillary sinus for long periods without causing symptoms and that they usually do not lead to infection of the sinus unless associated with an oroantral fistula.[9]

Due to the work of Sprague,[47] it is obvious that the problem of removing root tips from the maxillary sinus must be reevaluated in light of present knowledge. He reviewed the dental and otolaryngeal literature from 1858 to 1952, a period of 94 years, and found references to 161 root tips and other foreign bodies in the accessory sinuses, of which 151 were in the maxillary sinus, eight in the nasal cavity, one in the frontal sinus, and one in an undetermined site. The foreign bodies reported included root tips, teeth, dental impression material, tube drains, a knife blade, shell fragments, a straight pin, an iron bolt, an automobile spark plug, and a full-grown centipede. If such foreign bodies can be tolerated in the accessory sinuses, then the presence of root tips in the maxillary sinus cannot be considered a serious problem.

In the reported cases, 145 patients presented symptoms while 16 had no complaints. Of the cases of roots in the maxillary sinus, 67 had symptoms and 10 were asymptomatic. From these data, it would appear that a cause and effect relationship exists between the foreign bodies and the symptoms. However, when the reported symptoms are critically evaluated, a different conclusion is justified. The symptoms that were reported are acute and chronic sinusitis, oroantral fistula, polyposis, pain, facial neuralgia, rhinorrhea, feeling of fullness, headache, toothache, and osteomyelitis. These are the symptoms of maxillary sinusitis, which is a well known clinical entity that may have multiple causative factors.[39] In the reported cases no attempt was made to determine if the patients had any evidence of preexisting disease before the foreign bodies gained entrance into the accessory sinuses. It is well recognized that root tips in the maxillary sinus seldom produce the symptoms of maxillary sinusitis and, on the evidence presented in Sprague's study, it is erroneous to implicate them as the causative agents in producing the reported symptoms. Until some well controlled and well documented study is presented which conclusively indicates that root tips are responsible for these symptoms, it is safe to conclude that most of them are well tolerated and produce a minimum of symptoms.

As a result of his survey, Sprague drew the following conclusions:

1. Foreign bodies displaced into the accessory sinuses are not reported in the literature in any significant degree.
2. They may be retained for years without producing serious problems.
3. They do not produce serious complications.
4. They do not evoke a "foreign body reaction."

5. They do not interfere with regeneration of the antral membrane.
6. They do not evoke neoplasia or a fulminating inflammation.
7. They apparently do not act as foci of infection.

Is it then necessary to remove all root tips and other foreign bodies from the maxillary sinus? In light of the above, the decision to remove or not to remove a root tip should be based on a critical evaluation of each individual case. With the paucity of evidence that severe or serious complications result from their retention, it would seem that a conservative approach is justified. If a root tip that is producing no symptoms and obviously has been in the maxillary sinus for some time is discovered during a routine roentgenographic survey, good judgment dictates that nothing should be done. If, on the other hand, the patient presents with the classic symptoms of maxillary sinus disease, and roentgenograms and other diagnostic procedures reveal that an infection exists along with a concomitant root in the sinus, it should be treated. If it is not necessary to resort to surgery to bring the infectious process under control, there is little need for the root tip to be removed. If surgery is required to eradicate the infection, it is logical that the root tip should be removed at the same time.

If an entire tooth or a fractured root tip is inadvertently forced into the maxillary sinus during a surgical procedure, a somewhat different approach is justified. Most authorities[11, 25, 50] agree that since the wound is open and the

Figure 18-38   Localization of tooth displaced into maxillary sinus. *Left,* Lateral view. *Right,* Posteroanterior view. These two views accurately localize the tooth in the anterior medial aspect of the sinus.

Figure 18-39   Stereo-Waters view confirms location of tooth. The cloudy appearance of the sinus indicates hemorrhage into the sinus. Note the tooth in the anterior, medial aspect of the sinus.

area is anesthetized, removal of the tooth or root is indicated. In competent hands this is not a difficult procedure. However, in inexperienced hands it can become a formidable procedure and should not be attempted by operators in this category.

When a root or tooth disappears into the sinus, the usual extraction procedure should be discontinued immediately and the new problem explained to the patient in clear, understandable terms. The inexperienced operator should then refer the patient to a competent oral surgeon for further evaluation and treatment. If, on the other hand, the operator has had sufficient experience in the management of this type of problem, he may immediately proceed to remove the tooth or root.

In removal of a tooth or root from the sinus its position should first be determined by clinical and roentgenographic examination. In this localization it is important to ascertain if the tooth or root is actually within the sinus. Little difficulty is encountered in visualizing a tooth that has been displaced into the sinus (Figs. 18–38 and 18–39) but small root fragments frequently present a problem. A root fragment may occasionally be merely displaced between the alveolar bone and the sinus membrane, while the sinus itself remains intact. Rupture of the sinus membrane can be determined by gentle probing or by holding the patient's nose and having him blow gently. Evidence of air escaping through the tooth socket is ample proof that the membrane has been pierced and that the root fragment lies within the sinus.

If the root cannot be located by clinical and roentgenographic examination, no attempt at removal is indicated. Roentgenograms should be taken from several angles and if, after careful viewing under a strong light, the root cannot be visualized, the wound should be closed and the patient dismissed. There is always the possibility that the root tip did not go into the sinus but fell into the mouth and was expelled by the patient. If strong suction is being used, the root may have been drawn into the suction apparatus. To continue the search for a root that cannot be visualized by either clinical or roentgenographic examination often results in mutilating surgery that may cause permanent deformities of the alveolar ridge. Such surgery is not justified and should be condemned.

When the root is visualized and definitely localized, the operator may proceed with the removal. If the root is found to be in close proximity to the open socket, an exploratory procedure to attempt removal through the point of entry is justified. By making a generous flap and utilizing the principles of adequate access, a good light, direct visibility, hemostasis, and patient cooperation, removal of the root is occasionally possible by slightly enlarging the bone opening and engaging the root with a small hook or mosquito forceps. Frequently the root tip will catch on the tip of the suction and be delivered from the sinus in this manner. When the root has been delivered through this approach, sufficient buccal and lingual bone should be removed to allow approximation of the soft tissue which is then carefully sutured over the defect. The patient should be placed on antibiotic therapy and warned against blowing the nose for several days. When these procedures are followed, the wound usually heals by primary intention without fistulization.

If the foregoing efforts to remove the root through the tooth socket are not immediately successful, this approach should be abandoned and an approach through the canine fossa utilized. Prolonged attempts to remove the root through the socket frequently require gross enlargement of the bony opening,

Figure 18–40 Exposure of canine fossa to remove root tip or tooth from maxillary sinus. *Upper left,* Large mucoperiosteal flap is formed from area of cuspid to third molar. *Upper right,* Mucoperiosteal flap reflected from necks of teeth exposing anterolateral surface of maxilla. *Lower left,* Opening made through anterolateral wall of maxillary sinus through canine fossa high over the roots of the bicuspid teeth. *Lower right,* Following removal of foreign body, mucosal flap is returned to its original position and sutured.

and predispose to fistulization. The canine fossa is exposed by extending the existing mucoperiosteal flap high into the buccal sulcus, and an opening is made into the sinus through its anterolateral wall, above the apices of the bicuspid teeth (Fig. 18–40). This opening should be high enough to avoid damage to the teeth and of sufficient size to permit visualization of the sinus (Fig. 18–41). Hemostasis is obtained, and by use of a small, bright spotlight, the

Figure 18–41 Opening in canine fossa for removal of root tip from maxillary sinus.

Figure 18-42   **Figure 18-43**

Figure 18-42 Following removal of root tip, mucoperiosteal flap sutured in its original position.

Figure 18-43 Exposure of the anterolateral wall of the sinus to remove the displaced tooth shown in Figures 18-38 and 18-39. Note the excellent access that has been obtained and the clear visualization of the tooth.

root can usually be visualized and removed by curets or a mosquito hemostat. In securing hemostasis, it is important to utilize a clean suction apparatus, since the root frequently is withdrawn by the suction. If gauze sponges are used, they should be carefully examined on removal from the wound, because the root may become engaged in the gauze. Following removal, if the sinus membrane is normal, the wound is closed primarily as previously outlined (Figs. 18-42 and 18-43). However, if the sinus membrane is thickened by chronic infection, or polypoid tissue is noted, an antrostomy with construction of an antral-nasal window is indicated before closure. This procedure is in the field of the rhinologist and, when indicated and possible, should be carried out in conjunction with a specialist in this field.

Occasionally other foreign bodies are found within the sinus. These usually result from the foreign body gaining access through a preexisting oroantral opening. Impression material, various filling materials, surgical packs, food, and chewing gum are among the objects that have been found in the sinus. A chronic sinusitis may accompany the condition, and removal of the object, prior to closure of the oroantral fistula, is indicated.

OROANTRAL FISTULA

As mentioned previously, most openings between the oral cavity and the maxillary sinus will heal spontaneously. However, when the opening is large or when an acute or chronic sinusitis is present, an oroantral fistula may develop. These fistulas should be closed.[34]

Of prime importance in the successful closure of an oroantral fistula is the elimination of all infection from the maxillary sinus. This can usually be accomplished by repeated irrigations of the sinus and administration of the appropriate antibiotic. On rare occasions, these measures are not sufficient to eliminate the infection, in which case the sinus must be surgically exposed to permit the removal of all the infectious material. This procedure, known as an antrostomy, is usually combined with the procedure to close the fistula.

Figure 18-44 Gold, 36 gauge, 24 carat, utilized in closure of oroantral fistula.

Several surgical procedures have been developed to close the oroantral-nasal fistula. A pedicle palatal flap, a broad-based buccal flap, and a combination of buccal and lingual sliding flaps have been described. All are successful, provided the infection is eliminated from the sinus, the flaps are large enough to cover the bony defect, and the flaps are sutured without tension. These procedures are so well known that they need not be reemphasized in this discussion.

In recent years, a very simple and highly successful method of closing the oral-antral fistula has been developed. It consists of placing a gold plate under the gingival tissues and over the bony defect. The gold plate acts as a barrier between the oral cavity and the sinus. It also acts as a stent and allows the soft

Figure 18-45 *Upper left*, Oroantral fistula. *Upper right*, Flap reflected. *Lower left*, Gold plate inserted and flaps sutured. Note the flaps do not completely cover the gold plate. *Lower right*, Gold plate removed. Note proliferation of tissue which closed the fistula.

tissues on the antral side of the plate to proliferate and "bridge the gap," thus closing the opening.

The use of metal foil or plates to close antral defects was first suggested in 1951. Several articles[6, 7, 31] described the technique of placing tantalum foil or tantalum plate over the bone and under the mucosa to accomplish permanent closure of the opening. Owing to the difficulty in adapting the tantalum to the bony defect, this procedure was soon abandoned. The procedure did not become popular until gold plate was substituted for the tantalum.[15, 22]

The surgical procedure is simple, practical, and effective. It can often be accomplished under local analgesia on an outpatient basis. After the infection has been eliminated from the sinus, the soft tissues around the fistulous tract are excised. An incision is then made along the crest of the alveolar ridge and generous buccal and lingual flaps are reflected, exposing all aspects of the bony defect. A disc of 36 gauge, 24 carat gold plate (Fig. 18–44) that is large enough to cover the entire bony defect is prepared. It is important that all margins of the disc rest on bone. The gold is then inserted over the defect and carefully burnished to insure accurate adaptation of the margins to the underlying bone. The soft tissue flaps are then returned to their original positions and sutured without tension. Since the defect is closed by the proliferation of the soft tissues under the plate, there is no reason for concern if the soft tissue flaps do not completely cover the gold (Fig. 18–45). In fact, the gold plate is often visible in the center of the operated area.

Use of prophylactic antibiotic therapy to prevent infection and a nasal spray to maintain good nasal drainage is indicated.

There is little postoperative edema or pain associated with the procedure. The tissues tolerate the metal well and healing is usually uneventful (Fig. 18–46).

Figure 18–46   Closure of oroantral fistula. *Upper left,* One week following insertion of gold plate. *Upper right,* Four weeks after insertion of gold plate. Note how well the tissue tolerates the metal. *Lower left,* Immediately following removal of plate. Note that the tissues on the antral side have proliferated to close the fistula. *Lower right,* Four weeks following removal of plate. The fistula is closed and there has been no loss in height of buccal sulcus.

Figure 18-47   Roots of bicuspids and molars in close proximity to the maxillary sinus. Infections arising in these teeth may simulate primary maxillary sinus disease.

DENTAL INFECTIONS INVOLVING THE MAXILLARY SINUS

Because of the proximity of the teeth to the maxillary sinus, infections of the teeth may simulate infections of the maxillary sinus (Fig. 18–47). It is important to differentiate this condition from primary maxillary sinus disease, for the treatment of the two conditions is different.

The symptoms are those of an acute or chronic maxillary sinusitis. Pain and tenderness in the cheek area, pain in the upper teeth on the involved side, a feeling of fullness in the maxillary area, fever, malaise, a purulent nasal discharge and edematous tissues in the region of the turbinates are the common findings. Roentgenograms of the accessory sinuses reveal clouding of the involved sinus.

Dental treatment consists of management of the infected tooth. It should be extracted or treated by endodontic therapy. The patient should be referred to an otolaryngologist for treatment of the maxillary sinus problem.

PRIMARY MAXILLARY SINUS DISEASE MANIFESTED IN THE ORAL CAVITY

Several disease processes that originate in the maxillary sinus occasionally manifest themselves in the oral cavity and may be misinterpreted as dental emergencies. Of these, maxillary sinusitis is the most common. It is an inflammation of the mucosal lining of the sinus which may be caused by infection, allergy, trauma, or by cyst or tumor formation which interferes with the normal

Figure 18–48 Facial asymmetry resulting from malignant tumor involving maxillary sinus.

Figure 18–49 Enlargement of alveolar process produced by tumor shown in Figure 18–48.

Figure 18–50 Flange of denture had been removed to accommodate for the enlarging tumor.

drainage of the sinus. The sinusitis may be acute or chronic. The symptoms are the same as listed in the preceding paragraph.

Treatment is in the realm of the otolaryngologist. Essentially, it consists of shrinkage of the mucosa and suction to facilitate drainage; analgesics to control pain; and antral puncture and lavage to remove the purulent exudate. If these measures do not correct the problem, surgical intervention to remove the diseased tissues is indicated.

Cysts and tumors originating in the maxillary sinus may cause swelling and pain in the oral cavity. Differentiation from a problem of dental origin that might be interpreted as a surgical emergency is important. The tumors may be benign or malignant. They usually present as a slowly expanding mass that eventually erodes through the maxillary bone and produces an enlargement in the oral cavity (Fig. 18–48). This enlargement may produce pain and interfere with function. If located in a denture-bearing area, the mass may interfere with the proper seating of the denture (Figs. 18–49 and 18–50).

Cysts and tumors originating in the maxillary sinus are treated by the otolaryngologist; however, it is essential that they be differentiated from dental problems to insure that proper therapy is administered.

INJURIES TO NERVES AND BLOOD VESSELS

INJURIES TO NERVES

Intraoral surgical procedures may produce injuries to nerves supplying areas of the face and oral cavity. The inferior alveolar and mental nerves are most frequently involved, but, on rare occasions, the lingual nerve may be injured. Some of these injuries are unavoidable; others may be prevented by utilization of careful operative techniques.[21]

Third molar roots may form around the mandibular nerve in such a manner that extraction of the tooth will cause injury to the nerve (Fig. 18–51). Injudicious curetting, blind use of elevators, or removal of deeply placed roots that impinge on the nerve are other causes of injury to this nerve.[51]

The relationship of the mandibular nerve to its associated structures usually can be demonstrated on preoperative roentgenograms. When the possibility of injuring the nerve exists, this should be explained to the patient

Figure 18–51 *Left,* Mandibular canal constricted by root of third molar. Removal of tooth will possibly result in injury to the nerve. *Right,* Third molar has not produced a constriction of the mandibular canal. Removal of tooth probably will not result in injury to the nerve.

prior to surgery. There is thus less chance of undue alarm should residual numbness or paresthesia persist.

In most instances injury to the mandibular nerve is not serious, since the nerve usually regenerates and sensation returns in six weeks to one year.[44] When altered sensation persists beyond this time, careful examination may reveal that the bony walls of the mandibular canal have been displaced and are impinging on the nerve. In such instances, removal of the bone and decompression of the nerve often will be followed by nerve regeneration and return of normal sensation.

The mental nerve may be injured by injudicious use of instruments in the region of the mental foramen or by improper flap design when surgery is carried out in this area. When surgery is required in the mandibular bicuspid area, the possibility of injury to the mental nerve should be kept constantly in mind, and extreme care should be exercised to prevent injury to the nerve. When soft tissue flaps are required, they should be formed in such a manner that the mental nerve is reflected in the flap. While this procedure may produce trauma to the nerve and result in a residual loss of sensation, the condition will be transient, and normal sensation will return in a short time. However, if the mental nerve is cut or accidentally severed, the probability of a return of normal sensation is remote.

The lingual nerve may be traumatized or severed in mandibular third molar surgery. Fracture of the lingual plate, penetration of the lingual bone with a bur during removal of bone or sectioning a tooth, and utilization of a lingual soft tissue flap are procedures that could possibly traumatize the lingual nerve.[40] It is also conceivable that the lingual nerve may be traumatized by the needle utilized in obtaining lingual nerve anesthesia. Furthermore, any intraoral surgery involving the floor of the mouth, such as removal of calculi from the submaxillary gland or duct, may induce trauma to the nerve.

The lingual nerve usually lies in the floor of the mouth in the area medial to the mandibular third molar. However, it occasionally follows an aberrant course and assumes an abnormally high position in the soft tissues medial to the mandible. Hence, as mentioned above, any surgery in the area, including the removal of third molars, may result in trauma to the nerve with resultant paresthesia. This may occur regardless of how carefully and meticulously the surgical procedure is carried out and must be considered a normal hazard of the surgery.

Knowledge of the location of the lingual nerve together with careful surgical technique will help prevent this emergency.

If the lingual nerve is merely traumatized, it will regenerate; but if it has been completely severed the chance of return of normal function is remote unless the severed ends are sutured.[44]

Injury to the nasopalatine nerve is of no consequence and results in no residual deficit of sensation. Removal of palatally placed impacted teeth and enucleation of cysts of the incisive canal often require the avulsion of the nasopalatine nerve, but patients seldom if ever complain of any loss of sensation in the involved area.

INJURIES TO BLOOD VESSELS

Injury to blood vessels is a common emergency in intraoral surgery. Fortunately the majority of vessels in this area are small in caliber, and, when they are severed, the resultant hemorrhage usually may be controlled by pressure. However, a few large vessels are present and, when hemorrhage originates from this source, it is necessary to clamp and tie the severed vessel.[29]

Injuries to blood vessels result from trauma which may involve the soft tissue or bone. Injury to vessels in soft tissues has been discussed earlier. Hemorrhage arising from vessels located in bone presents a different problem, since these vessels are inaccessible and cannot be grasped and tied.

Extraction of teeth or other surgery involving the maxilla or mandible may produce vigorous hemorrhage. This is most frequently encountered when the vessels in the mandibular canal are traumatized or when nutrient vessels located in the bone are involved in the surgical field.

Bleeding originating from bone is easily controlled by pressure. Packing of the cavity with gauze or an absorbable hemostatic agent invariably will arrest the bleeding. If gauze is utilized, the packing should be left in place for five or ten minutes and then carefully removed. This pack will arrest the vigorous hemorrhage, but oozing of blood may persist. If this occurs, the cavity may be repacked with gauze, which should be left in place for several days. However, it is more convenient to control the oozing by packing the cavity with an absorbable hemostatic agent which can be sutured in the wound and does not require removal.[42]

When bleeding arises from nutrient canals, the vessels may be compressed and the hemorrhage arrested by crushing the overlying bone with a blunt instrument or by placing bone wax in the orifice of the bleeding nutrient canal.[38]

ASPIRATION OR SWALLOWING OF A FOREIGN BODY

One of the dreaded operative emergencies in dental practice is the aspiration or swallowing of a foreign body. The object most frequently involved is a tooth; however, any object — a root tip, gauze pack, inlay, crown, bridge, or partial denture — may be aspirated or swallowed (Figs. 18–52 and 18–53). The problem is encountered during surgical procedures when teeth that are being removed suddenly and unexpectedly become dislodged, or when portions of crowns or fillings broken from adjacent teeth fall uncontrolled or undetected into the pharynx.

Every precaution should be taken to prevent this emergency. The throat should always be packed when any dental procedure is carried out under general anesthesia. When working under local analgesia, the possibility of teeth or other foreign bodies being accidentally dislodged should be kept in mind and extreme caution exercised to prevent these objects from getting out of control.

Once a foreign body has escaped into the throat, the patient usually will cough or gag and expel the object. When an object disappears into the posterior area of the mouth, the patient should immediately be placed in the supine position, with head dependent, to assist in expelling the foreign body. Should this not be effective, and if coughing persists, direct visualization of the pharynx and removal of the foreign body with instruments or the fingers is indicated. The Heimlich maneuver may be successful at this time. Review the

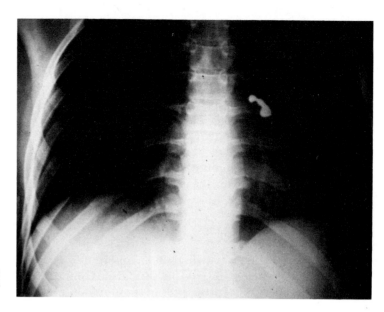

Figure 18-52 Dental bridge aspirated into the lung during a dental procedure.

technique in Chapters 17 and 19. Any foreign body in the pharynx either will be expelled or will pass into the respiratory or alimentary tract.[27]

A foreign body may also lodge in the larnyx, where it can produce an acute respiratory obstruction. This problem is recognized by a change in the respiratory pattern — gasping for breath, laryngeal stridor (harsh, high-pitched respiratory signs) with the patient becoming restless and cyanotic and eventually passing into unconsciousness. When these signs are present, the tongue should be grasped and pulled forward and the pharynx cleared of all foreign matter by means of the fingers, instruments, or suction. If this procedure does not relieve the obstruction, and if the Heimlich maneuver fails, an emergency airway must be created without delay. See the chapter on *establishing an emergecy airway*.

Figure 18-53 Partial denture swallowed into the gastrointestinal tract.

Once the emergency airway has been established, the patient should be referred to a physician for removal of the foreign body.

When a foreign body disappears into the throat and cannot be expelled by the patient or removed by mechanical means, a different problem is created. If the patient is not in respiratory distress it may be assumed that the foreign body has passed into the respiratory or alimentary tract. If it has lodged in the alimentary tract, no treatment is necessary as it usually will pass harmlessly through the body. However, if it has lodged in the respiratory tract, it must be removed.

When a foreign body has been aspirated, the patient should be referred immediately for localization and any indicated treatment.

CONCLUSION

"The best way to treat an emergency is not to have it happen." Most of the emergencies covered in this discussion are preventable. Adherence to the sound surgical principles of thorough preoperative planning, adequate access, careful manipulation of tissues, use of controlled force, and, above all, concentration and undivided attention to the problem at hand will keep surgical emergencies to the minimum.

In spite of this care, emergencies do occur in the best regulated practices. Therefore, it behooves every dental practitioner who includes surgery in his practice to have the knowledge and skill to permit him to cope successfully with emergencies when they arise.

REFERENCES

1. American College of Surgeons, Committe on Trauma: Prophylaxis against Tetanus; Management of Fractures and Soft Tissue Injuries. 2nd ed., Philadelphia, W. B. Saunders, 1965.
2. American Dental Association: Accepted Dental Therapeutics. 37th ed: Chicago, 1977, p. 265.
3. American Dental Association Council on Dental Therapeutics: Health Screening Program 1969. A. D. A. Transactions, 1970. p. 95.
4. Archer, W. H.: Oral Surgery. 5th ed., Philadelphia, W. B. Saunders Co., 1976, p. 1620.
5. Ballinger, W. F., et al: The Management of Facial Trauma. Philadelphia, W. B. Saunders Co., 1973, p. 704.
6. Budge, C. T.: Closure of antraoral opening by use of tantalum plate. J. Oral Surg., *10*:32, 1952.
7. Budge, C. T.: Edentulous antraoral opening closed by tantalum plate. Dent. Surv., 27:953, 1951.
8. Burch, R. J., and Morris, C. R.: Complications in oral surgery. Dent. Clin. North Am., Nov., 1959, p. 655.
9. Chipps, J. E., and Budetti, J. A.: Fractured tooth roots in the maxillary sinuses. U. S. Armed Forces, Med. J., 3:899, 1952.
10. Clark, H. B., Jr.: Practical Oral Surgery. 3rd ed., Philadelphia, Lea & Febiger, 1965, p. 152.
11. Clark, H. B., Jr.: Practical Oral Surgery. 3rd ed., Philadelphia, Lea & Febiger, 1965, p. 237.
12. Colcleugh, R. G., and Ryan, J. E.: Splinting electrical burns of the mouth in children. Plast. Reconst. Surg., 58(2):239, 1976.
13. Converse, J. M.: Reconstructive Plastic Surgery. Philadelphia, W. B. Saunders Co., 1964, p. 255.
14. Crikelair, G. F., and Dhaliwal, A. S.: The cause and prevention of electrical burns of the mouth in children. Plast. Reconst. Surg., 58(2):206, 1976.

15. Crolius, W. D.: Use of gold plate for closure of oro-antral fistulas. J. Oral Surg., 9:836, 1956.
16. Dingman, R. O., and Hayward, J. R.: Oral Surgery in general practice, J.A.D.A., 35:607, 1947.
17. Douglas, B. L.: Hospital Dentistry. 2nd ed., St. Louis, The C. V. Mosby Co., 1970, p. 139.
18. Douglas, B. L., and Casey, G. J.: A Guide to Hospital Dental Procedure. Chicago, American Dental Association, 1964, p. 49.
19. Feldman, L., and Trace, I. M.: Subacute bacterial endocarditis following removal of teeth or tonsils. Ann. Intern. Med., 11:2124, 1938.
20. Forbes, I.: Defense mechanisms of the body. J. Oral Surg. Oral Med. Oral Path., 42:231, 1976.
21. Frank, V. H.: Paresthesia: Evaluation of 16 cases. J. Oral Surg. Anesthesiol. & Hosp. D. Serv., 17:27, 1959.
22. Frederics, H. S., Scopp, I. W., Gerstman, E., and Morgan, F. H.: Closure of oro-antral fistula with gold plate. J. Oral Surg., 23:650, 1965.
23. Hayward, J. R.: Oral Surgery. Springfield, Charles C Thomas, 1976, p. 111–127.
24. Hayward, J. R., and Costich, E. R.: The use of elevators. Practical Dental Monographs. Chicago, Year Book Medical Publishers, Inc. 1957.
25. Killey, H. C.: The problem of the tooth or root in the maxillary antrum. J. Oral Surg., Anesthesiol. & Hosp. D. Serv., 22:391, 1964.
26. Krogh, H. W.: Extraction of teeth in the presence of acute infections. J. Oral Surg. 9:136, 1951.
27. Ibid., p. 110.
28. Ibid., p. 177-201.
29. Ibid., p. 288.
30 Lurie, M. H.: Antral infections. Am. J. Orthodont. & Oral Surg., 27:500, 1941.
31. McClung, E. J., and Chipps, J. E.: Tantalum foil used in closing antraoral fistulas. U. S. Armed Forces Med. J., 2:1183, 1951.
32. Mead, S. V.: Diseases of the Mouth. 4th ed., St. Louis, The C. V. Mosby Co., 1933, p. 274.
33. Moorehead, J. J.: A foreign body finder: The locater. J.A.M.A., 121:24, 1943.
34. Noyek, A. M., and Zizmor, J.: The Otolaryngology Clinics of North America. Symposium on the Maxillary Sinus, Philadelphia, W. B. Saunders Co., 1976, p. 213-222.
35. Robinson, I. B., and Laskin, D. M.: Tetanus of oral origin. J. Oral Surg. Oral Med. Oral Path. 10:834, 1957.
36. Robinson, M., and Lytle, J.: The broken needle and other metallic foreign bodies. In McCarthy, F. M.: Emergencies in Dental Practice. 1st ed. Philadelphia, W. B. Saunders Co., 1967, p. 277.
37. Rogers, A. H.: The oral cavity as a source of potential pathogens in local infections. J. Oral Surg. Oral Med. Oral Path. 42:245, 1976.
38. Rossi, D. J.: Controlling hemorrhage in exodontia and oral surgery. Dent. Clin. North Am., Jul., 1957, p. 349.
39. Ryan, R. E., Thornell, W. C., and von Leden, H.: Synopsis of Ear, Nose and Throat Disease. 2nd ed., St. Louis, The C. V. Mosby Co., 1963, p. 194.
40. Schwartz, L. J.: Lingual anesthesia following mandibular odontectomy. J. Oral Surg., 31, Dec. 1973.
41. Segelman, A. E., and Doku, H. C.: Treatment of the complications of leukemia. J. Oral Surg. 35:6:469, 1977.
42. Shira, R. B.: Control of postoperative hemorrhage. J. Oral Surg., 16:144, 1958.
43. Shira, R. B.: Management of operative and postoperative complications in exodontia. J. South. Calif. State D.A., 28:283, 1960.
44. Shira, R. B.: The consultant. J. Oral Surg., 24:181, 1966.
45. Shira, R. B.: Wounds and injuries of the soft tissue. Oral Surgery Syllabus, Walter Reed Army Medical Center, p. 762.
46. Shultz, L. W.: Burns of the mouth. Am. J. Surg., 83:619, 1952.
47. Sprague, W. G.: Personal communication.
48. Stefanini, M., and Dameshek, W.: The Hemorrhagic Disorders. New York, Grune & Stratton, 1955, p. 158.
49. Steiner, R. B., and Thompson, R. D.: Oral Surgery and Anesthesia, Philadelphia, W. B. Saunders Co., 1977, p. 178-199.
50. Thoma, K. A.: Oral Surgery. 5th ed. St. Louis, The C. V. Mosby Co., 1969, p. 307.
51. Ibid., p. 309.
52. Ibid., p. 314.
53. Wakefield, B.: Personal communication.
54. Wessler, S., and Avioli, L. A.: Tetanus. J.A.M.A., 207:6, 1969.
55. Williams, P. E.: Personal communication.

19

MAXILLOFACIAL INJURIES

LOWELL E. McKELVEY*

LIFESAVING MEASURES
  Maintaining the Airway
  Control of Hemorrhage
  Preventing Shock
RELIEF OF PAIN
EVALUATION OF OTHER CONCURRENT
  INJURIES

CONSERVATION OF INJURED TISSUES
  Primary Closure
  Wound Dressing
  Secondary Closure

INTRODUCTION

The purpose of this chapter is to give some of the principal indications for emergency treatment in the early care of those who have sustained injuries to the face and jaws. It will also deal with the rationale and principles of treatment to be followed in such cases.

The majority of maxillofacial injuries affecting the civilian population in the United States are a result of vehicular traffic accidents and acts of physical violence. In a research study at Cornell University (1961) it was found that 72.1 per cent of the victims of automobile accidents suffered facial injuries. For the most part, these same etiologic entities also tend to produce the most damaging and destructive wounds. With the continued increase in traffic congestion, in spite of federalized safety measures, the frequency and severity of injuries to the face are likely to show a persistent rise. Under these circumstances the need to direct greater attention to the safe and effective handling of these patients is most timely.

Statistically a lesser number of maxillofacial injuries, generally of less severity, result from a variety of miscellaneous accidents. Regardless of etiology, each individual case presents respective problems which require the attending doctor to thoroughly evaluate the general condition of the patient, the gravity of the injuries, and the sequential order in which these conditions must be treated.

*I wish to express my appreciation to Dr. Ernesto Arill Miranda, Assistant Professor, School of Dentistry, University of Puerto Rico, and to Mrs. Sharon L. Anderson, Medical Illustrator, University of Texas at San Antonio, Texas, for their contributions of the medical illustration artwork contained in this chapter.

540

Of course, optimum safety in protection of the patient's life is the primary consideration. However, other emergency conditions must receive due attention. The priorities for emergency treatment may be arranged in the following order, based on relative importance in protection of the patient's life and the probable bearing existent injuries may have on further deterioration of the patient's capability for recovery or repair:

1. Life saving measures.
2. Relief of pain.
3. Evaluation of the gravity of other concurrent injuries.
4. Conservation of injured tissues.

In the conscious patient, subjective symptoms may be most helpful in supplementing the objective signs to determine the status of the airway, the likelihood of impending shock, and the extent of concurrent injuries. A brief but astutely directed history of the patient at this point is extremely important to uncover allergies to drugs, physical defects, medications being used, and other factors that may pose a complication to treatment or suggest a modification in treatment. The opportunity for obtaining this information may pass with a change in the patient's sensorium. This opportunity should not be precluded by the premature administration of drugs or anesthetic agents that may mask significant signs or symptoms.

In the unconscious patient subjective symptoms are absent. In such case, the patient's welfare is entirely dependent on the ability of the examiner to meticulously evaluate the extent of damage, to review the vital signs and other objective findings, and then to translate these into a sound plan for emergency treatment. At this point, the chronologic order of treatment must be definitively and rapidly carried out. In severe injuries the treatment sequence may require change at any time, depending on the patient's response to treatment and the unpredictable physiologic effects of the initial trauma. Unknown physical frailties present prior to trauma, plus internal injuries not yet revealed, psychogenic factors, etc., may initiate a sudden change in the patient's response to treatment at any time. One must be alert to observe such change at the earliest possible moment through continued surveillance of the patient until safety is assured. Only by close monitoring can the danger of unexpected developments in the patient's progress be minimized and effectively treated.

The term monitoring refers to initial and continued observations in assessment of the patient's signs and symptoms, including findings obtained in the use of whatever devices may be required to determine his current physiologic status. Part of the monitoring procedure is to initially record "vital signs" which will serve as a baseline from which subsequent possible variations can be related in following the physiologic status of the patient. The vital signs initially recorded are temperature, pulse, respiration, and blood pressure. Establishment of the baseline of vital signs is the first step in monitoring the three principal organ systems: the respiratory system, the central nervous system, and the cardiovascular system. Interpretation of these vital signs is indispensable in patient evaluation. Interpretation is a product of knowledge and experience when applied to the observed characteristics presented by each of the vital signs. The chapters on *physical evaluation*, *physical diagnosis* and *monitoring* provide comprehensive coverage on this subject area.

LIFE SAVING MEASURES

The three prime considerations for emergency treatment are to maintain a patent airway, to control hemorrhage, and to prevent shock or to treat it should shock already be established.

MAINTAINING THE AIRWAY

The airway ranks first in importance because of the very short and critical period that a patient may tolerate anoxia and be expected to recover mentally and physically. With present scientific knowledge, this period is approximately 3 to 5 minutes of complete cerebral anoxia (Hosler, 1954). Therefore, it behooves us to be aware of any sign of airway obstruction, which includes difficulty of expiration as well as inspiration, and of any indications of reduced airway dimension, such as labored breathing, tracheal tug, stridor, etc. The patient's color is important, and in this respect it is well to remember that anoxia is not always characterized by cyanosis. For example, in the patient who has suffered severe blood loss with superimposed anoxia, the skin may become an ashen white. This would be a more serious sign than that of cyanosis. All such signs necessitate immediate attention to the airway, beginning with debridement, proper positioning of the patient, and some means of maintaining airway patency.

Complete sudden airway blockage is easily recognized in that the patient becomes aphonic, will usually clutch at the throat, will show extreme anxiety, and will be incapable of inspiration or expiration. Under this circumstance a quick evacuation of the debris may be accomplished by manipulations proposed by Heimlich.[5] Should the patient be upright, in a chair or standing, the doctor delivers four sharp blows rapidly and forcefully to the spine between the shoulder blades while supporting the patient's chest with the other hand. This may dislodge the debris in the throat (Fig. 19–1). If not, stand behind the patient and wrap your arms around his or her waist, with the thumb side of one fist placed under the diaphragm between the xiphoid process and umbilicus (Fig. 19–2A). Grasp the fist with the other hand and press the fist into the abdomen with a quick upward thrust (Fig. 19–2B and C). Repeat three or four times, if necessary. The sequence of back blows and abdominal thrusts may be more effective than either maneuver used alone. If the patient is supine, roll him to a Sims' (semiprone) position and deliver four sharp blows to the spine as previously described. Turn the patient to the supine position and place yourself on your knees close to his hips or astraddle his legs. Place the heel of one hand between the xiphoid and umbilicus, with the other hand on top, and press into the abdomen with quick upward thrusts. Correct placement of the hands is imperative (Fig. 19–3). Repeat three or four times, if necessary. See also Chapter 17, on the Heimlich maneuver. This lifesaving technique is so vital that two independent presentations are made for emphasis and clarity.

Clots, inspissated mucus, fragments of bone, teeth, or dentures, dirt, and other debris may lodge in the airway. Fortunately, the laryngeal isthmus of the tracheal tree with its epiglottic cover generally serves as an impediment to debris that has entered the oropharynx. It may temporarily

Figure 19–1 The Heimlich maneuver for a patient in an upright position. Four sharp blows are delivered rapidly and forcefully to the spine between the shoulder blades while supporting the chest with the other hand.

Figure 19–2 The Heimlich maneuver. A, When the blows to the spine have not dislodged the obstruction, stand behind the patient and wrap your arms around his or her waist. Place the thumb side of one fist in the midline of the abdomen midway between the umbilicus and the xiphoid process. Grasp the fist with the other hand and press in on the abdomen with quick upward thrusts, as shown in B and C.

Figure 19–3 The Heimlich maneuver. The blows to the spine are delivered to the patient in the prone position in the same fashion as in the upright position. Then, with the patient supine, the heel of one hand is placed halfway between the umbilicus and xiphoid process, with the other hand superimposed. Sharp thrusts are directed downward and upward toward the diaphragm.

Figure 19–4 Modified Sims (or semiprone) position: The underlying forearm and the flexed overlying lower extremity brace the body on a table or litter. The head rests on the underlying arm, mouth turned down, to relieve any pressure on the injured middle face or mandible and to insure dependent drainage.

prevent foreign bodies from falling farther into the tracheal tree. Debridement of these foreign bodies is of first and foremost importance. By grasping the tongue and pulling forward, gross debris may be "raked" out of the oral cavity and oral pharynx by the index finger. Of course, a good suction machine with proper tips, a good light, and some assistance in manipulation are highly desirable. The palate, pharyngeal walls, tongue, and floor of the mouth should be inspected for wounds and ecchymotic areas which may indicate potential or active bleeding areas or sites of imbedded foreign bodies. Palpation, bimanually where possible, may reveal imbedded objects otherwise not evident. Loose teeth, bone fragments, and other debris must be removed. Pendulous soft tissue flaps may require suturing to clear the airway and/or preclude further hemorrhage. When a part has been debrided and hemorrhage controlled, suctioning in these areas should be curtailed and only sponges used to blot any oozing. This will allow the small vessels to be sealed by clot formation within their lumina. Suctioning tends to displace these occluding clots with attendant further bleeding.

Following debridement and suturing of lacerations involving the airway, these passages must be kept clear. To accomplish this the patient should be properly positioned, tongue traction maintained, or a mechanical airway placed. Positioning is very important, particularly in the unconscious or semiconscious patient and when a mechanical airway is not immediately available. When there is collapse of the facial skeleton or the mandible that allows the parts to fall into a position of obstruction, or where for some other reason the patient has lost control of the tongue, patient positioning can improve the airway. Under such circumstances the modified Sims' (semiprone) position is suggested for comfort and to provide optimum natural assistance for airway maintenance. This positioning allows oral secretions, debris, or blood to be evacuated from the mouth by gravitational force (Fig. 19–4). Also, the gravitational pull on the fractured and lacerated parts tends to distract them from occluding the airway. Elevation of the rest of the body above the level of the head (as in the slight Trendelenburg position) assists the gravitational distraction of parts and drainage.

Of course, other concurrent injuries may dictate the positioning of the patient, such as cervical or spinal fractures, intracranial injury or edema, chest injuries, extremity fractures, etc. When there is collapse or loss of control of the airway, as in the unconscious patient, an oropharyngeal or nasopharyngeal tube may be utilized. Either tube must be sufficiently long to pass deep to the base of the tongue into the oropharynx. It also must

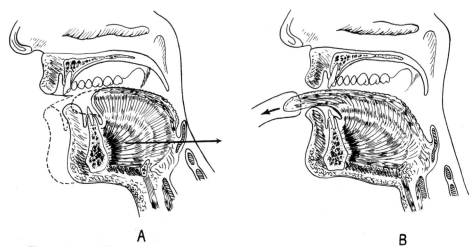

Figure 19–5   Effective tongue traction. *A*, Collapse of the facial skeleton, soft tissue wounds, or loss of muscular control allows tissue mass of lower face and mouth to obstruct airway. *B*, Tongue traction provides an effective distraction force to control this tissue mass and open airway.

have a sufficient aperture to allow optimum air flow for free breathing. Such a tube must be anchored to the nostril, lip or cheek by adhesive tape or some means of fixation to prevent displacement.

Select the better contoured, more patent nasal passage for placement of a nasopharyngeal tube. Septal deviation or enlargement of the inferior nasal concha may dictate which nasal passage is to be utilized. Use the largest tube that can be accommodated. Any sort of flexible rubber or plastic tubing with a sufficient aperture may be used in an emergency. The tube must be rigid enough to maintain its patency. Placement must be carefully accomplished so as not to produce injury to the nasal passage or pharynx. Lubrication of the tube by a water soluble gel or the patient's saliva will ease the passing. Oily lubricants are not desirable because of the possible harmful effects of aspiration.

In severe maxillofacial injuries, in which there is variation in the level of consciousness, in which there is a tendency for the collapse of structures normally fixed to the mandible, or in which there is need for manipulation and better inspection of damage to the tongue and floor of the mouth, a temporary means of tongue traction may be indicated. The passing of a suture of No. 1 black silk through the anterior third of the tongue in the vertical midline provides a good "handle" for traction. This traction suture is easily applied, does not pose a bleeding problem, and is highly effective in distracting not only the tongue but all attached parts of the floor of the mouth and fractured mandible from the upper airway (Fig. 19–5). If necessary, traction can be maintained by anchoring the suture to a button or safety pin on the patient's clothing. This will release a hand for other more urgent use. Of course, a standard tongue clamp, towel clamp, or safety pin may be used to fix the tongue, but these are less flexible and more cumbersome than is the simple tongue suture. Depressed comminuted midface fractures may allow the maxillary structures to be displaced inferiorly and posteriorly to occlude the airway at the base of the tongue (Fig. 19–6). The supine position is especially dangerous for the unconscious patient with

Figure 19–6 Depressed fractures of the midface of the LeForte type, as indicated by the three arrows, may cause airway blockage. A ligature attached to the maxillary process or teeth can be used to distract the collapsed structures and open the airway. A LeForte III fracture, indicated by the uppermost arrow, may involve the floor of the anterior brain chamber and result in the additional problem of cerebrospinal rhinorrhea.

such injuries. A traction ligature tied to maxillary teeth can be used to distract the collapsed structures from the airway. Placement of an artificial airway and/or positioning in a semiprone position will temporarily serve to keep the airway patent.

In case of respiratory arrest a means of artificial respiration must be established at once. If a resuscitation machine is available, oxygen can be administered through a reservoir bag, with intermittent positive pressure and the use of a face mask or endotracheal tube. See chapter on *basic life support*. Where such apparatus is not immediately available, mouth-to-mouth breathing provides the next best method of artificial respiration.

A.   B.

Figure 19–7 Mouth-to-mouth resuscitation. *A*, Patient is supine, head and neck extended in a straight line, chin lifted, and nose pinched shut. The mouth of the operator must form an airtight seal about the victim's mouth as he fills the victim's lungs with his own expired air. *B*, When chest is observed to be fully expanded, quickly move mouth from victim's lips and take another breath. This allows the victim's rib cage to return to the unexpanded position with expulsion of the air previously forced in by the operator. Repeat this sequence at the rate of 12 to 20 times per minute.

This method requires no equipment, can be instituted anywhere, can be applied by anyone with a minimum of experience, and will give positive lung inflation. An outline for the procedure is as follows (Fig. 19–7):

1. Debride the airway.
2. Place patient on back with neck extended, head flexed dorsally, chin lifted up and aligned to straighten airway.
3. Place one thumb in the mouth, at the corner, and grasp the lower jaw firmly between thumb and fingers.
4. With the other hand, pinch nostrils closed to prevent air leak.
5. Then apply your wide-open mouth to the victim's mouth to form an airtight seal.
6. Firmly exhale into the victim's mouth with sufficient force and volume to expand the lungs (the effectiveness can be noted by the magnitude of the chest rise and fall).
7. Remove mouth and take another breath as air escapes from the patient's lungs.
8. Repeat at the rate of 12 to 20 times per minute.
9. Do not release grasp of the mouth between breaths.
10. An oropharyngeal tube should be used if available.
11. Readjust position of chin and neck if air does not flow freely.
12. A compress may be used to assist in sealing a leak due to facial wounds (the mouth may be sealed and resuscitation carried out by mouth-to-nose application).

When the airway cannot be maintained by other means, it may be necessary to make an artificial opening in the tracheal tree. A low tracheostomy is a most effective means of providing such an artificial opening for an indefinite period. It should be considered in the following cases:

1. The unconscious patient.
2. When the airway is jeopardized by collapse of the fractured facial skeleton and the attached soft tissue bulk.
3. Loss of tongue control, swallowing, or cough reflexes.
4. Injuries to the larynx, upper neck, or chest.
5. When vital signs or the sensorium are unstable as a result of cerebral damage.
6. Any flame burn of the face. This condition is perhaps the least obvious indication to most clinicians because of lesser familiarity with such cases. The flame burn that involves the face carries the added danger that an inhalation at the instant of injury may also have seared the mucosal lining of the respiratory tract. Such a patient may appear to be in good condition soon after the accident, with a good airway and little evidence of extensive burns to the face. However, endotracheal edema and excessive secretions can close the damaged airway insidiously or rather abruptly.
7. Any case in which a patent airway is not assured by other means and the probable duration of this uncertainty is undetermined.

When there is a question of the necessity for tracheostomy, choose the plan that holds the greatest assurance for safety to the patient. In other words, in case of doubt do a tracheostomy.

Tracheostomy improves the airway by:

1. Diminishing tidal air dead space. (Tidal air space is the column of air within the tracheal tree that does not come in contact with the lung alveoli and must be displaced before there can be an exchange between alveolar air and the outside atmosphere.)
2. Diminishing airway resistance.
3. Affording ready access to secretions in the tracheal tree.
4. Permitting easy access for insertion of a cuffed tube for positive artificial respiration.

5. Providing an easy access for inhalation general anesthesia and controlled respiration without hampering access to the area for repair of facial injuries.
6. Maintaining it indefinitely.

The surgical procedure for establishing a tracheostomy is not one in which the general practitioner of dentistry is expected to be proficient. However, knowledge of this surgical sequence may provide a valuable assistant to the responsible surgeon at a time when such help is sorely needed. Many of the present day automotive and other severely injured accident cases present a need for efficient and effective teamwork in their emergency attention, as well as in their later care. These circumstances dictate that a broader scope of training in emergency measures is required of all practitioners of dentistry.

In this review of the surgical procedure for tracheostomy, the steps will be presented concisely, stressing the use of a minimum armamentarium. The first consideration is to place the patient in a supine position with the neck in hyperextension with the sagittal plane of the face held in a straight line with the long axis of the neck and perpendicular to the table. Local infiltration analgesia may be used in the conscious patient. The unconscious patient should have an oropharyngeal or oroendotracheal airway during this procedure.

A midline incision about 5 cm long is made through the skin from below the cricoid cartilage to a point just above the border of the sternal notch, as shown in Figure 19–8. This is not as cosmetically desirable as a

Figure 19–8 Vertical midline incision with blunt dissection separates strap-muscles and fascia to expose the trachea.

Figure 19–9 Towel clamps can be effectively used as tissue retractors in emergencies, as illustrated here for tracheostomy.

transverse incision but provides an easier, quicker approach for most. If a transverse skin incision is to be made, the line of incision should be at the level of the fourth tracheal ring. In this plane the incision is carried through the subcutaneous tissues and fascia to the strap-muscles of the neck. From this point the blunt dissection is carried out in the vertical midline plane in the same fashion as through a vertical skin incision. By the use of a curved hemostat or the tips of dissecting scissor blades the deep subcutaneous tissue and the strap-muscles of the neck are bluntly dissected in the vertical midline down to the trachea. This is readily accomplished by placing the closed beaks of the instrument into the depth of the midline incision and then opening the beaks along the vertical plane to separate the muscles along their long axes (Fig. 19–8). As the depth of the wound is developed in this fashion, the walls of the bilateral flaps may be retracted by placement of standard towel clamps in case suitable retractors are not available (Fig. 19–9).

The blunt midline dissection, as described above, usually avoids the nuisance of copious bleeding which would obscure vision and hamper the speed of accomplishment of the procedure. When transverse vessels are encountered they should be clamped and tied. Often the isthmus of the thyroid gland will be encountered. If this cannot be easily by-passed to reach the trachea, it should be clamped and tied on each side of the midline by anchored circumferential sutures of 2-0 cotton or silk. Then the isthmus is severed between the two ties.

Figure 19–10 Excision of a circular window in the trachea to allow insertion of the artificial airway tube.

As the blunt dissection is carried through the strap-muscles, the trachea comes into view. It should be stabilized by the fingers or preferably by a heavy skin hook. With a small scalpel a crescent-shaped incision is made through one or two of the tracheal cartilaginous rings, usually about the level of the fourth and fifth (Fig. 19–10). Through this incision the beaks of a hemostat are inserted to grasp the cut edge of this flap. A circular segment, sufficiently large to accommodate the tracheal tube, is excised and removed. Removal of a circular segment of the trachea, rather than making a simple incision through the tracheal rings, reduces the "buckling effect" on the trachea when inserting the tracheal tube. It also facilitates blind reinsertion of the tracheal tube should it be inadvertently displaced, later. The coughing that may ensue when the trachea is manipulated may be controlled by direct infiltration of a local analgesic solution or by intratracheal use of a topical analgesic spray.

To insert the tracheal tube in the surgical opening of the tracheostomy, the obturator is placed in the outer or larger tube of the set. The tip of the obturator is inserted into the tracheostomy site and dropped into place (Fig. 19–11A). The obturator is promptly removed, and the smaller inner-tube or cannula is inserted in its place (Fig. 19–11B). The outer-tube is secured in place with a cotton tape tie passed behind the neck. This outer-tube remains in position as long as the tracheostomy is required. The wound is loosely approximated on each side of the tracheal tube by several deep skin sutures, and a gauze pad dressing is placed to protect the skin under the wings of the metal tube.

Figure 19-11 *A*, Insertion of the tracheal tube with obturator into the surgical opening of the trachea. *B*, The obturator is immediately removed and the cannula is placed, skin sutured, and dressing placed.

The tracheal tube selected for a specific patient should be the largest diameter that the trachea can accommodate without impingement. The tube length and placement must be such as to prevent tracheal injury, tube occlusion, or contact with the tracheal carina. A tracheal tube that is too long is usually indicated by repeated cough reflex owing to contact with the carina.

The tracheal tube set is a matched set of two metal tubes and an obturator (Fig. 19-12). The parts of one set should not be mixed with another. Even though two sets are marked as the same caliber, their parts may not fit if interchanged.

The cannula may be removed for cleaning and immediately reinserted. The obturator is taped to the head of the patient's bed or attached to the patient's clothing so as to be immediately available for reinsertion of the tracheal tube should it become dislodged.

Figure 19-12 The tracheal tube set.

Tracheostomy may prove inadequate and offer false security if not properly maintained. Maintenance must begin immediately after the tracheal tube is placed. Adequate suction must be at hand to remove any blood or secretions from the cannula and trachea. Secretions usually are increased immediately after placement of the tube and require frequent suctioning until reaction to the stimulation subsides. Whenever inspissated secretions or blood begins to collect in the lumen of the cannula, it must be removed from the outer tube, quickly cleaned, and reinserted. If this aspect of tracheal tube care is neglected, the reduction of lumen size of the cannula may occur so insidiously that progressive anoxia can become well established before it is appreciated by the attending personnel. To illustrate this danger, a layer of secretions adhering to the lumen of a tube reduces the airway passage by an amount greater than three times the square of the thickness of that coating. Thus, a layer of secretions which reduces the diameter of the tube by only one-fourth will reduce the column of air by more than 55 per cent. As successive layers are laid down, the air column size may rapidly become critical.

Occasionally a patient is seen in whom all signs and symptoms point to the necessity for an immediate airway opening. When such urgency will not permit time for the standard tracheostomy, a coniotomy (thyrocricoidotomy, cricothyrotomy, or high tracheostomy) may be performed. The indications for this procedure, the technique for its establishment, and the disadvantages of its use are discussed in the chapter on *establishing an emergency airway*.

Conn et al. (1963), in the study of a series of 1022 automobile accident cases, mentioned that about 25 per cent of traffic deaths result from injuries to the chest. The Cornell report indicated that over 72 per cent of automobile accident victims suffered facial injuries. Therefore, it is apparent that anyone treating facial injuries resulting from automobile accidents should expect a significant number of concurrent chest injuries.

Since chest injuries may present an airway problem in facial injuries, mention is made here of the emergency treatment considerations. Amadeo (1965) states that most emergency treatment measures required in these cases are simple and do not require a specialist to initiate. He suggests:

1. Placement of an airway.
2. Tracheostomy to reduce resistance to respiration, to reduce tidal dead space, and to afford ease of positive respiration, if needed.
3. Give oxygen.
4. Restore blood volume with whole blood or plasma expanders.
5. Splint the flail chest with sand bags.
6. Cover sucking wounds of the chest with a layer of Vaseline gauze and a compress to facilitate reinflation of the lung.

Application of these emergency principles will help maintain the chest injury patient until more definitive help is available.

CONTROL OF HEMORRHAGE

Next in importance of the emergency measures is the control of hemorrhage. Vessels that are easily visualized may be clamped and ligated. Small bleeders may be clamped, sponge-"blotted," and electrocoagulated. This procedure significantly hastens hemorrhage control, thereby reducing treatment time in more extensive injuries. The ligation of large vessels may be made with 3-0 black silk, leaving a 6-inch length of ligature on the tied vessel to identify it at a later stage when more positive hemostasis is undertaken along with debridement and initial treatment of the wound. In tying larger vessels, especially when the tissues are subject to manipulation in debridement and closure, it is wise to use what some call a "stick-tie." This refers to anchoring the ligature in the fascial cover or adventitia of the vessel then tying it on the opposite side. Such anchorage guards against displacement of the tie with subsequent recurrence of hemorrhage.

Many vessels in the loose tissues of the face will have retracted into depths that can be approached only through damaging dissection. With few exceptions, these bleeding areas can be stopped by moderate application of direct pressure. Ligation of the external carotid may be considered only in the most severe wounds. Even then, this procedure is of questionable value because of the excellent collateral circulation of the face. Pressure points in control of hemorrhage about the face are generally of little value. However, in an occasional case, for example, in a large cheek flap, bleeding may be temporarily controlled by compression of the external maxillary artery as it crosses the lower border of the mandible. Areas of generalized oozing are best controlled by direct pressure.

Occasionally it is desirable to circumferentially suture a bleeding soft tissue mass as a temporary measure to allow better vision for location of the principal bleeders. After clamping and ligation the constricting ligature can be released. Direct pressure will then usually control the oozing.

The application of chemical cauterizing agents is never indicated to control bleeding. Such agents will further damage the tissue, hampering the physiologic capability for repair. In addition, the necrotized debris created by the chemical insult offers a favorable medium for bacterial growth.

Topical application of bovine thrombin in saline by a gauze pad or by an impregnated dressing of Gelfoam is an effective tool in stanching oozing areas difficult to control. To be effective, the bovine thrombin must be placed and held directly over the capillary openings so that the resultant clots will seal these vessels. When this compound is placed at a distance from the bleeding source, the rapid action coagulation in the intervening blood mass may form a floating island of coagulum around which bleeding continues. Sometimes the ineffectiveness of this control may not be realized until the patient's blood pressure has been restored to a normal level, at which time the extravascular clots may float free. It is well to remember that even slight elevation of the head will help to curtail venous oozing. This positioning is also desirable in combating cerebral edema. For further information see the chapter on *hemorrhage*.

PREVENTING SHOCK

The third consideration of importance concerning emergency treatment is that of the prevention of shock. Given the choice, it is certainly more desirable, safer, and more simple in all respects to prevent the development of shock than to treat it after it has become advanced. Factors which may precipitate the development of shock are fatiguing and psychogenic factors in addition to the traumatic insult to the body's physiologic processes caused by the maxillofacial and concurrent injuries. Generally, one is inclined to think of hemorrhage and obvious injuries as the only contributors to shock. However, other factors may contribute markedly to its development. To name some of these, we may list dehydration, exposure to the elements, disease present prior to injury, prior therapeutic programs such as corticosteroid administration, anticoagulant therapy, drug addiction, alcoholism, nutritional status, etc. When it is possible to obtain a good history of the patient these important considerations may be uncovered and used advantageously in the treatment.

Psychogenic factors may contribute more to the development of shock in the severe maxillofacial injury than the mechanical traumas themselves or the effects of other injuries. For many patients the possible permanent facial disfigurement that they may suffer is to them the most disturbing consideration in their plight. Contemplation of this unknown by the conscious patient in unfamiliar and frightening surroundings can provide a strong psychogenic component capable of precipitating shock. These patients must have comforting reassurance about their eventual appearance, and should receive understanding, gentle handling and efficient care to allay their fears. The emergency area should emit an aura of quiet efficiency, confidence, and purpose. These homely factors are mentioned since they can be so important to the patient's well-being, yet sometimes they are overlooked by the attending staff.

Changes in the heart rate and rhythm, blood pressure, pulse pressure narrowing, increased respiration rate, shallow respiration, pallor, depression, etc., are danger signs which may point to developing shock. In the conscious patient we may have his personal evaluation of symptoms such as thirst, chills, nervousness, apathy, profuse sweating, etc., to assist in the diagnosis. To provide a base line, vital signs should be checked and recorded upon admission of the patient. Frequent recheck is necessary when there is evidence of instability. An interval of 10 to 15 minutes should be maintained until a stable level is established. The deflated blood pressure cuff is left in place along with a heart monitoring stethoscope to facilitate surveillance.

The prevention of shock and the treatment of shock after its development require similar basic handling. However, for obvious reasons, preventive measures reduce the incidence of morbidity and mortality. Perhaps one of the greatest factors in prevention of shock is time, so preventive treatment must be instituted early.

Positioning is of prime importance and needs no specific equipment or facility other than the ingenuity of the doctor. Elevation of the extremities will assist in moving some of the blood volume to improve the circulation to vital centers. Excessive Trendelenburg elevation usually is undesirable because of the possibility of increasing cerebral edema where a brain injury may be present. Simple elevation of the extremities only will help. Position is dictated by the type and location of the injuries of major consequence. In impending shock, quick positional changes are not well tolerated, whether the changes are made voluntarily by the patient or by someone handling him. Particularly is this true in elevation of the upper part of the body to the vertical or "jack-knifing" the body while positioning. This may cause a precipitous and dangerous blood pressure drop. This is a point of importance to be remembered in moving a patient from one area to another, as during transfer from a litter to a bed or table.

In hypovolemic shock restoration of circulating blood volume is important as an initial consideration in the prevention or treatment of shock. Therefore, intravenous infusion of distilled water with 5 per cent glucose is routine. Starting this infusion is generally one of the initial steps in emergency treatment. The purpose is not only to restore the circulating blood volume but also to ensure a readily usable intravenous route for medications or other supporting fluids. Another safety feature is that it precludes the problem of attempting to establish an intravenous port in event of possible circulatory collapse when suitable veins may be difficult to locate and enter. In trauma, the body tends to conserve and retain sodium, so that the administration of 5 per cent glucose in saline or Ringer's solution usually is withheld until the need for a second or third unit of intravenous fluid, or where there is evidence of considerable electrolyte loss. Excessive electrolyte loss should be suspected when there has been active diarrhea, vomiting or abdominal wounding involving the gastrointestinal tract.

Caution must be exercised in the administration of fluids so as not to overburden injured or diseased parts. For example, in the head injury case fluid administration must be carefully regulated to reduce the possibility of cerebral edema; the heart decompensation case may be pushed to failure or pulmonary edema may develop; glucose solutions may induce a coma or other complications in the diabetic, etc. Vigilance is a constant necessity for adequate treatment and the prevention of an untoward response. Unfortunately, accurate determination of effective blood volume may be difficult and subject to wide variations. There is no simple way to accurately determine the fluid requirements. History and symptomatic response assist guidance. Central venous pressure monitoring and blood volume determinations are valuable only when performed by skilled personnel. Observations of the urinary output are essential. The normal range for urinary output varies from 600 to 2500 ml per 24-hour period. Air temperature, humidity, the patient's reaction to the environment, loss of fluids through injuries, shock, etc., affect urinary output. Urinary output of 50 ml per hour is considered a normal average. Output below 20 ml per hour should alert one to possible dehydration or impaired kidney function. When voiding is unsatisfactory, free bladder drainage should be established by an indwelling Foley catheter.

Whenever the wounding has resulted in severe hemorrhage, replacement should be by whole blood transfusion. Severe blood loss may require more than one intravenous site of administration. The speed of transfusion can be further enhanced by the use of positive pressure induced through a hand bulb pump. In addition, transfusion may be indicated in cases of a low hemoglobin, though hemorrhage may not have been the etiologic factor, as for example in cases of poor nutrition, debilitating disease, anemia, etc.

When there is need for whole blood and the patient's blood type is not readily available, type "O" may be administered. However, in any case it must be checked for compatibility. When whole blood is not readily available, plasma expanders may be used for interim support.

At the time of starting intravenous fluids a blood sample for hematologic studies should be taken. Should blood for transfusion be required, the sample for typing and crossmatching is also taken at that time. Hematology tests should include a red cell and white cell count, differential, hemoglobin, hematocrit, and blood sugar. These items may furnish valuable information, even though a hemoconcentration due to the injury may have affected some of the values.

Normal body temperature should be maintained by coverings and not augmented by artificial means such as heating pads, water bottles, etc. Application of heat tends to increase blood volume in the body surface capillary bed which denies this volume to vital center circulation.

Since cardiac standstill may become a complication in the shock picture, an effective emergency measure for treatment must be considered. A most effective procedure for external cardiac massage as proposed by Kouwenhoven, Jude, et al. (1961) requires no equipment and a minimum of experience. See Chapter 14, on *cardiopulmonary arrest.*

RELIEF OF PAIN

The administration of drugs, particularly opiates, should be carefully controlled in order not to further depress vital centers or lower blood pressure. Barbiturates may be used for control of restlessness when alleviation of pain is not the primary objective. Intramuscular meperidine hydrochloride has a sedative and spasmolytic effect. It is also an effective analgesic when pain is becoming a factor. Many times the trauma of wounding provides some numbing effect in the initial period soon after injury. Institution of treatment early in this period before acute pain and edema have entered the picture is highly desirable when the patient's general condition permits.

When pain is developing, and especially when it is likely to be increased by time, movement, or manipulation of parts, it is desirable to administer suitable medication for its control. Early control of pain requires less medication to provide and maintain comfort than in cases in which severe pain has already developed. As mentioned before, pain is one of the factors that may precipitate shock, but its control is also important to provide the comfort which will encourage cooperation of the patient and expedite necessary treatment. Many present day analgesics may be used in lieu of the opiates. The intravenous route of administration will insure immediate effect and is more efficient. The immediate effect aspect is an important feature of this method of drug administration in the hypotensive patient. The full action of the drug is noted as it is given, so there is less chance of a later untoward reaction developing, as may occur in the use of the intramuscular administration route.

Intramuscular injections provide depository reservoirs which give a longer lasting effect. This mode of administration, however, has a disadvantage in the hypotensive patient in that optimum effect may not be appreciated or easily gauged because of the reduced circulation. Under such conditions, multiple injections of potent drugs may not be effective, but instead will lie in the deposit sites until such time as circulation is improved and then will be flushed into the circulation. This may possibly result in a toxic effect or depression because of the accumulated dosages.

The oral route for drug administration in these cases is not generally used in the emergency treatment phase because of the many disadvantages. The slow assimilation and less predictable effect of a drug is a factor. The orofacial injuries may preclude oral intake or swallowing of drugs. Even though the oral administration of drugs may be physically possible, it is not desirable to subject the already distraught and perhaps nauseated patient to this added discomfort.

EVALUATION OF OTHER CONCURRENT INJURIES

During the course of evaluation of the patient and the initiation of necessary life saving measures, the examiner has generally formed a tentative estimate of the extent of facial damage. However, we must postpone preparations for definitive treatment in our field of interest until the seriousness of concurrent injuries of other parts has been evaluated. It may be that the gravity of concurrent injuries will take priority over early attention to the maxillofacial trauma. It is rather common that maxillofacial injuries are attended by damage to the central nervous system, the eye, possible cervical fracture, etc. Injuries farther afield, such as compound wounds of the extremities, crushing wounds of the extremities or chest, internal injuries, etc., may escape initial notice unless we remember to observe and evaluate the individual as a whole.

Closed wounds resulting from blunt force may cause extensive damage that is difficult to assess. Diagnosis usually requires astute deduction based upon all available clues; how and what forces were applied, the signs and symptoms present, response to manipulation, and appropriate tests including x-ray findings. In addition, there may be "occult damage" present which may require surgical intervention to determine the exact nature of the injury, or the problem may eventually be revealed by changes in physical findings, by x-rays, or by laboratory studies. In this group, surgical intervention may be delayed for hours, days, or weeks dependent upon the patient's physical response.

The method of examining the patient by regions provides an orderly sequence which will tend to preclude an error of omission in overlooking possible serious injuries to parts other than the maxillofacial area. Examination by region seems best in initial evaluation of the trauma patient in that body segments with their contents are covered in turn. For example, the chest would include that body surface plus rib cage, lungs, bronchi, heart, etc. Thus, a region or body segment will contain parts of one or more organ systems, but the sequential examination from one segment to the next offers a good observation pattern in the search for injuries.

Ballinger, et al.[2] suggest an outline for an initial rapid survey of injuries in the traumatized patient. This begins with examination of the head, face, neck, then chest, abdomen, extremities, and back. From the rapid survey findings, a more comprehensive evaluation of observed specific injury areas is then carried out.

During the initial inspection of facial injuries and upper airway the doctor has usually noted any bruises, swellings, lacerations, or asymmetry of the head.

If the patient had experienced a loss of consciousness and/or nausea, or there is currently a decreased level of awareness, intracranial injury is suspected. The extent of damage is uncertain. Shires et al.[9] point out that widespread brain damage can be caused by blows producing relatively little damage to the scalp or skull. Drainage of cerebrospinal fluid from the nose or ear and posterior auricular ecchymosis (Battle's sign) are diagnostic of basilar skull fracture. Hemotympanum or bilateral periorbital ecchymosis may indicate the same. The patient's status of consciousness and motor power can be checked by his response to verbal stimuli. The eyes should be examined for pupil size, reaction to light, and ocular movements. Early development of papilledema is evidence of increased intracranial pressure. A dilated pupil is usually indicative of an acute increase of intracranial pressure on the same side. Other signs suggestive of development of increased intracranial pressure are bradycardia, hypertension, bradypnea, headache, restlessness, impaired awareness, and increasing neurologic deficit.

Examination of the neck has already received some attention when the airway was checked. Care is taken in any manipulation of the neck as one observes for stiffness or tenderness which might indicate a cervical fracture. Engorgement of the veins in the neck should alert one to possible congestive heart failure or tension pneumothorax, although this same picture may be seen in a struggling or straining patient without such conditions. A frothy hemoptysis may indicate a ruptured bronchus or an injury higher in the respiratory tract. In the former there are usually other signs such as respiratory distress and possibly cyanosis.

Some mention was made earlier in the discussion of emergency treatment of chest injuries under the title *Maintaining the Airway*. Rutherford[2] states that whenever "ventilatory and/or circulatory insufficiency (shock) develop soon after chest trauma, initial examination should be quickly directed toward six conditions: open pneumothorax, airway obstruction, flail chest, tension pneumothorax, massive hemothorax, and cardiac tamponade." Open pneumothorax is characterized by the sucking sound of airflow through the chest opening, while airway obstruction (incomplete) is recognized by stridor or coarse rhonchi and a degree of labored respiration with decreased exchange. Tension pneumothorax and massive hemothorax may produce a hemithorax with poor excursion and diminished breath sounds over that side, with a shift of the trachea to the opposite side. "Splinting" of the chest with voluntary restriction of respiratory excursion occurs when ribs are fractured. Sites of fracture are usually easily located by the elicitation of sharp pain on palpation or deep breathing. In cardiac tamponade, ventilation is not usually interfered with, so chest excursions are bilaterally normal. Heart sounds may be muffled, arterial pressure reduced, and venous pressure increased in cardiac tamponade, although this triad is not always present or readily apparent.

The abdomen is examined for bowel sounds, areas of tenderness on palpation, guarding, muscular rigidity, rebound tenderness, distention, and any evidence of urinary or fecal incontinence. Symptoms of damage to the abdominal viscera may not be evident initially but may develop over a period of 24 hours.

The extremities are examined for areas of swelling, discoloration, crepitation, limitation of motion, weakness, absence of pulse, and other possible abnormalities. Reflexes may be tested, but such detail would most likely be done as a secondary procedure by the respective consultant when evidence of injuries exists. A temporary splint or fracture immobilization may be required to reduce discomfort and prevent further injury during the early period when the patient may be subjected to movement in preparation for treatment, x-rays, or other procedures. Examination of the back for possible injuries can be done at the time of observation of the extremities.

Selective x-rays, laboratory tests, and special diagnostic procedures may be required to verify suspected injuries or to uncover conditions not apparent. Initial requests for x-rays and laboratory tests should be kept to a minimum consistent with good patient care but with thought given to reducing the amount of manipulation and movement of an already traumatized patient. X-rays and other diagnostic procedures dealing with injuries and conditions outside our usual professional field are to be accomplished in conjunction with the appropriate consultant services. Combining of diagnostic procedure requests, as for example in the case of x-rays needed for evaluation of injuries concurrent with the maxillofacial problem, will best serve the patient physically and mentally.

In this brief outline it is not possible to offer comprehensive coverage of the numerous and varied injuries that may occur concurrently with maxillofacial traumas. However, the sequence should supply a framework of reference upon which one may structure his individual pattern of evaluation.

Consultation with colleagues in our own and other services is a sign of mature judgment in a practitioner and of his profound interest in the welfare of his patients. Many times a teamwork arrangement can be effected to provide simultaneous treatment of multiple injuries; as, for example, treatment of an extremity injury at the same time as treatment of the facial injuries, under the same anesthetic. Effective and efficient cooperative effort on the part of surgical teams will lessen the anesthesia time and surgical trauma with a concomitant improvement in mortality and morbidity.

CONSERVATION OF INJURED TISSUES

Protective drugs must be a consideration in the initial treatment of the maxillofacial injury patient. Whenever there are deep penetrating wounds, compound fractures or soil contamination, the patient should be protected against tetanus. Patients who have kept current with inoculations of tetanus toxoid should receive a booster dose of the toxoid. Those in which this background is questionable, or who have not received tetanus toxoid, should be skin tested with tetanus antitoxin serum, and if found not to be sensitized should be administered the optimum dose. These cases should also be protected by suitable antibiotic coverage. Penicillin is still the antibiotic of choice in cases in which the patient is not allergic to the drug.

PRIMARY CLOSURE

The most advantageous way to conserve injured tissues is to carefully debride and restore the parts to their proper anatomical relations by primary closure of the soft tissues when possible. The sooner this can be done following injury, the better the chances for restoration of normal physiologic function and aesthetics. Fortunately, the normally copious blood supply of the maxillofacial region usually permits primary closure of wounds in this area within 24 hours post-injury, even though the wounds may be macerated and grossly contaminated. In this sense we may consider primary closure of maxillofacial wounds under emergency treatment where concurrent injuries do not contraindicate.

Assuming that the patient's general condition is stable and there are no concurrent injuries to contradict, the maxillofacial wounds should be treated by primary closure. In the case of severe damage, a general anesthetic may be required. If there are concurrent injuries that may be attended to by another team, treatment may be done under the same anesthetic. If the patient is primarily under the care of the oral surgeon, it is his responsibility to request consultation in arranging such a plan with the other team. When the patient's general condition poses a question of safety for general anesthesia, but is otherwise essentially stable, primary closure of many severe injuries may be carried out under local analgesia.

Debridement is an important initial step in the treatment of all wounds. Many gross contaminants of the skin can be removed by a gentle scrub with cotton pledgets, using a surgical detergent soap, followed by copious flushings of sterile saline. Tar or grease may be removed by benzene (or common lighter fluid) immediately followed by surgical soap and saline. Certain paints may be removed by lacquer thinner followed by surgical soap and saline. During these cleansing procedures, the eyes and deep wounds are to be carefully protected. An ophthalmic ointment should be used in the eyes then covered by an occlusive pad. Deep wounds may be "plugged" with sterile gauze until the superficial contaminants are removed. Gross decontamination procedures are best done in a "prep room," after which the patient can be moved to the operating suite.

Abraded skin should be vigorously scrubbed with a hand brush and surgical soap followed by sterile saline flushings. Larger embedded particles may be removed with small curets or the point of a No. 11 Bard-Parker scalpel. Thorough debridement of the skin is necessary to prevent the so-called "traumatic tattoo," unsightly discolorations which occur when soil or similar debris remains embedded. If the level of skin abrasion does not extend below the rete pegs and the scrub is adequate, scarring is unlikely to occur. Healing without gross infection will usually proceed if the wound is properly dressed.

Deep wounds are debrided last and all deep tissues are carefully examined. One cannot rely on roentgenograms to reveal all foreign bodies. Glass fragments, wood particles, clothing, and other debris may not be found except by inspection or palpation, or both. Therefore, it is mandatory that all areas of deep wounds be directly examined under good lighting. This is facilitated by flushing away all blood clots with a stream of saline. These clot masses often contain secondary projectile debris including bone splinters, tooth fragments, denture fragments, and devitalized tissues in addition to external contaminants.

In gunshot wounds lead particles are often strewn along the missile path after contact with skeletal structures. The larger pieces should be located and removed. Many small particles may not be eradicated without significant extension of the initial damage. Under these circumstances, attempts to retrieve such particles are contraindicated. Fortunately, these usually encapsulate readily, offering little impediment to healing.

One method of clearing loose debris from the tubular path of a bullet wound is to draw through the wound an unfolded gauze sponge of suitable bulk affixed to the eyelet of a tendon passer probe or carried by a long-nosed, bayonet type nasal forceps. This is followed by saline irrigation. "Dead-end" puncture wounds may be debrided in a similar fashion.

Hematomata should be evacuated. The evacuated cavity may be collapsed by application of an occlusive light pressure dressing after closure is completed. However, it is best to attempt to collapse "dead space" by deep suturing of 3–0 resorbable suture. Should a hematoma show signs of continued internal bleeding, which, as in the neck, may endanger the airway or progress into the upper mediastinum, one must open the area and locate and tie the ruptured vessels.

During inspection and debridement of deep wounds, certain severed structures such as salivary ducts, major nerve trunks, and cartilage plates, when identified, may be "tagged" with 3–0 black silk sutures for ease of location and reapposition during later closure procedures. The "tagging sutures" are made by passing the suture on an atraumatic needle through the fascial cover of a duct or other structure, tying, and the suture ends left 4 or 5 inches long.

Closure is usually started in the depth of a wound, coapting deep parts in proper anatomical relations. The apposition is done to restore function and normal physiology and to eliminate dead space. Dead space offers a site for collection of tissue fluids and/or blood, which collection may serve as a medium for bacteria, may mechanically impair proper healing, or may result in an eventual fibrotic scar which may hamper function or produce disfigurement.

It is very important to preserve all mucosal or skin cover to protect the underlying deep tissues from infection or scarring and to restore the normal physiology. Bone and cartilage (particularly cartilage) are most susceptible to infection and necrosis due to the loss of epithelial covering, probably because of their relatively poor blood supply. So, to ensure mucosal covering of deep wounds, such as those involving the nose or mouth, for example, suturing of the mucosa should be accomplished at the most advantageous time — at the start of closure. Because of the constricted areas of the nasal passages and mouth, reapposition of the mucosae many times is best accomplished by "inverted sutures" of 4–0 or 5–0 chromic gut placed through the depth of the wound, with the ties being made on the mucosal surface.

When the general condition of the patient permits, the author prefers to repair skeletal injuries as a part of the primary closure. When the wound already offers some access to the fractures, restoring bone continuity is usually simplified and will provide a supportive framework upon which to restore the overlying tissues. When bone repair cannot be accomplished at this time, a secondary procedure with interim supportive care will be required, which will be mentioned later.

Closure of the soft tissues is then accomplished in layers. Muscle bundles are reapproximated by deep sutures of 3–0 plain gut. The "tagged" parts are picked up and reapproximated as the closure level advances. Severed trunks of major nerves or salivary ducts may be coapted with several axially placed sutures of 6–0 silk on an atraumatic needle anchoring the sutures in the fascial covers. Such sutures should not penetrate the nerve trunk or the salivary duct walls. Insertion of a fine polyethylene catheter, plastic probe, or plastic filament in the coapted salivary duct will maintain patency and allow salivary flow.

The catheter or filament must be held in place by a nonresorbable suture for 10 to 12 days. When one segment of a salivary duct cannot be located for anastomosis, a rubber drain or catheter should be anchored in the wound near the estimated site of the proximal stump and the other end brought into the mouth. This should be retained in place for 14 days to allow for epithelialization of a new functional salivary tract.

Severed cartilages of the nose, ear, or tarsal plates of the eyelids should be accurately coapted with 5–0 silk suture and carefully covered with an epithelial flap. Coaptation of a tarsal plate of an eyelid must be done on the superficial side of the lid.

Closure of a wound must be guided by anatomic landmarks at every level. As closure of the dermal cover is approached, surface anatomical landmarks such as the mucocutaneous junction of the lips, the philtrum, the alae of the nose and nostrils, the eyebrows, convolutions of the ear, and similar structures are important. Even permanent skin creases or folds provide orientation. Sutures placed across the wound at these points of reference serve to orient the flaps for proper reapproximation between the reference points.

Macerated flaps should be carefully and conservatively trimmed with a sharp scalpel to ensure a viable broad, vertical walled dermal flap on each side of the wound for apposition. The "trap-door" flap (one with a thin sloping side opposite an obtuse surface — wound wall angle flap) should have the thin side cut in the vertical to the subcutaneous level and the bulky side cut in a vertical step to accept it. This will help to prevent necrosis of the thin edge and the possibility of a depressed scar.

Buried subcutaneous sutures of 4–0 plain gut should be placed in the subcutaneous tissues to accurately approximate skin edges and relieve tension on skin margins. The skin is then coapted with 5–0 black silk or synthetic nonresorbable sutures. Strategic placement of mattress sutures of the same material may be required to better support large flaps, with the intervals between the mattress sutures coapted by simple approximation sutures. All subcutaneous and skin sutures should be placed to cause a slight eversion of the suture line. This tends to preclude a depressed or widened suture line scar.

As stated earlier, it is urgent that all deep structures be covered with skin or mucosa. In the severely macerated or avulsed wound, soft tissue approximation is likely to be more complicated because of the initial tissue loss or the extent of debridement required to remove devitalized tissues. Under these conditions, the flaps may require wide undermining or surgical modification to effect a proper closure, providing sufficient soft tissue from adjacent areas is available. Local flap transposition should parallel the skin cleavage lines (Langer's lines) to offer the best cosmetic result. Also, the source of innervation, blood supply, and adjacent structures may limit the remedial flap design. When adjacent tissues are not suitable or sufficient to provide a closing cover, as when full thickness soft tissues of the forehead are lost, a split thickness autogenous skin graft or grafts of freeze-dried animal or human skin may be used. The latter only act as temporary bandages to encourage granulation and re-epithelialization of the wound. In primary closure of a large destructive wound into the mouth, it is sometimes necessary to cover the deep tissues by closing skin-to-mucosa. At a later date, revision must be made to correct the residual defect. However, in the interim, the remaining deep tissues have been effectively conserved in a suitable environment which should encourage return to a normal physiologic state necessary to a successful secondary procedure.

WOUND DRESSING

A well planned and executed primary closure of a wound does not completely fulfill the responsibilities for proper treatment of the patient suffering maxillofacial injury. The probability of earlier recovery with reduced morbidity is enhanced by application of an effective wound dressing followed by good supportive care.

In minor abrasions, after debridement, the wound may be left exposed, although it may well be benefitted by a dressing for comfort and protection. On more extensive abrasions, a dressing of scarlet red or Furacin on fine mesh gauze should be placed over the abraded area upon which an absorbent light pressure dressing is applied. The pressure dressing may be removed in two or three days, but the fine mesh gauze over the de-epithelialized area is left to peel and be trimmed away as healing progresses. If surface infection poses a problem in any area, the fine mesh gauze and any crusts may be soaked off with tepid saline compresses.

The need for drainage is many times at question in severe wounds. In primarily closed wounds, drains are placed when there has been deep gross contamination, when there is maceration, where dead-space cannot be eliminated, where a hematoma exists, when infection is already present, or in the deep puncture wound. A Penrose rubber tube of suitable caliber provides an effective drain. The drain is removed as soon as evidence of flow ceases. The drains may be replaced at 48 hour intervals with shorter ones to encourage granulation filling from the wound depth. "Dead-end" puncture wounds are best treated by incremental reduction of the drain length until they granulate to the surface.

Most severe facial injuries benefit from well applied occlusive light pressure dressings. Such a dressing should have absorbent bulk to pick up exuding fluids from the wounds, act as a barrier to possible external contaminants, provide support to damaged parts, act as a compress to collapse dead-space and prevent fluid collection in the wounds, control edema, and provide comfort. Immobilization of fractures is an accepted principle; it should also be recognized that this principle when applied to soft tissue will enhance healing and comfort.

Application of a light pressure dressing is begun with the placing of a single thickness of fine mesh petrolatum gauze over all drains and wound edges. The petrolatum gauze is wrung out in a dry gauze pad to remove the petrolatum from the interstices of the material. This will allow exudates to pass through the gauze cover into an absorbent pad and thereby reduce the possibility of skin maceration. But the dressing still can be easily removed from the wound. Where exudates may be expected to be rather copious the flow from wound to absorbent pad can be enhanced by laying a 1/4 inch thick cotton pad, which has been moistened with glycerin then wrung dry, over the sheet of petrolatum gauze. Over this a thick, dry cotton pad is placed. Then fluffy compresses made from pieces of 36 inch square dry gauze are applied to form a thick cushion over all the areas to be put under the light pressure dressing. This

Figure 19–13 Light pressure dressing. *A* shows the skin dressing in place with the super-imposed gauze "fluffs"; the cotton pads support the ear as the light elastic bandage is to be applied. The first turns of the bandage are wrapped around the forehead and over the occiput to anchor it. *B*, Next, the bandage is brought from around the summit of the head and from the top of the head down over the face, up over the gauze on the other side in a vertical direction. This sequence is repeated until sufficient bandage has been applied to keep the dressing in place. Care must be taken to avoid posterior traction by the bandage that would impinge on the airway.

will not only serve as additionally absorbent bulk but will equally distribute the force of the superimposed light pressure over the covered area. The whole is held in place by wrapping with a 4 inch roll bandage of a semi-elastic gauze, such as Kerlix. Adhesive tape strips are placed over the wrapping in locations where there may be a tendency to slip out of position.

Because of the rounded contours of the face and head, plus the positional changes of the patient in bed, the light pressure dressing for extensive maxillofacial injuries will most often require inclusion of non-injured areas, such as one or both ears, to secure it against displacement. The cartilage of the external ear is quite sensitive to compressing pressure, which can cause pain or even precipitate chondritis. So, when an ear is to be covered, whether injured or not, by a light pressure dressing it must be well supported by a thick cotton pad placed between the ear and skull, the outer cavity of the conchae packed with cotton, and the whole covered by a thick cotton pad. The procedure will allow inclusion of the ear in overall wrapping of the dressing cover to ensure stability of the whole. (Figs. 19–13*A*, *B* and *C* show the sequential steps in securing a light pressure head dressing in place.) When the eye is to be covered, an ophthalmic ointment containing a topical antibacterial agent such as polymyxin B-bacitracin should be used in the eye and the closed lids covered with an eye pad.

SECONDARY CLOSURE

If for some reason initial reparative treatment is not to be immediately instituted, steps should be taken to provide a temporary means of support with splinting of the fractured parts and soft tissue flaps. The objectives of these immediate treatment measures are:

1. To prevent further injury or hemorrhage in the damaged tissues by positional changes of the patient.
2. To guard against aggravation of pain by movement.
3. To assist in the maintenance of a safe airway.
4. To protect the deep tissues from further contamination or damage.
5. To preserve the present physiologic state of the injured parts by maintaining the natural moisture of the tissues.
6. To prevent deterioration of the blood supply to tissue flaps.

Thus, temporary immobilization is of extreme importance for the conservation of injured tissues about the face. The use of a supporting occlusive head-face bandage may serve the purpose. Any loss of tissue bulk, continuity, skin or mucosal covering, blood supply, innervation, or normal landmarks of the face may be irreparably detrimental in eventual functional and esthetic reconstruction. The consideration of esthetics in facial injuries, in most instances, is far more important to the patient psychologically for his re-entry into a normal community life than is the case for patients who have suffered disfigurement or functional loss of other parts of the body.

Finally, there are certain considerations that must be made for the safety of the patient during the time interval between the initial emergency treatment and that for definitive repair of the injuries:

1. Frequency of obtaining and recording vital signs at time intervals as the case may indicate.
2. Positioning of the patient so as to afford comfort, facilitate airway maintenance, allow for ease of observation and care, and to prevent further disruption of the injured parts.
3. Have available at the immediate bedside good suction facilities, a good headlight or flashlight, an emergency tracheostomy tray when indicated, oxygen equipment, and any other resuscitation equipment or drugs for emergency use that might be required in the specific case.
4. Insertion of a nasogastric tube to facilitate feeding and protect against wound contamination by foodstuffs.
5. Request for any consultation services deemed necessary for further diagnosis, treatment, or supportive care.
6. Complete write-up of history, findings, treatment, future treatment plans, doctor's orders, and special nursing care instructions.

It is desirable that all dental practitioners, regardless of their field of interest, should have a sufficient grasp of the serious emergency problems that maxillofacial injuries may present in order to recognize these threatening conditions and be able to give assistance when a situation dictates. Such knowledge would not necessarily qualify every practitioner to treat these cases routinely but would certainly make him or her more capable of initiating adequate treatment in cases of necessity or to become an effective assistant as a member of a team.

REFERENCES

1. Amadeo, J. W.: Emergency management of patients with chest injuries. Journal of the Puerto Rico Medical Association, 57:192, 1965.
2. Ballinger, W. F., et al.: The Management of Trauma. Philadelphia, W. B. Saunders Co., 1973.

3. Campbell, B. J.: The automotive crash injury research program of Cornell University. J. Iowa Med. Soc., *51*:760, 1961.
4. Conn, J. H., et al.: Thoracic trauma: analysis of 1022 cases. J. Trauma, *3*:22, 1963.
5. Heimlich, H. J.: The Heimlich maneuver: Prevention of death by choking on foreign bodies. J. Occup. Med., *19*:208, 1977.
6. Hosler, R. M.: A Manual on Cardiac Resuscitation. Springfield, Ill., Charles C Thomas, 1954.
7. Judge, J. R., Kouwenhoven, W. B., and Knickerbocker, G. G.: Cardiac arrest. J.A.M.A., *178*:1063, 1961.
8. Krupp, M. A., et al.: Physician's Handbook. 18th ed., Los Angeles, Lange Medical Publications, 1976.
9. Shires, G. T.: Care of the Trauma Patient. New York, McGraw-Hill Book Co., 1966.

HEMORRHAGE

LELAND W. REEVE

INTRODUCTION

Almost every day, often several times a day, the dental practitioner is involved in procedures that involve a break in the integrity and balance of the blood-circulating mechanism. This can be a simple matter such as an exposed pulp chamber eliciting a drop or two of blood, or it can be as serious as the accidental severing of a major artery in the mouth, resulting in near disastrous bleeding that is extremely difficult to control. Clinicians have become highly skilled in the management of bleeding difficulties, and yet the ever-present threat of a problem bleeder can become most bothersome and perplexing.

As is the case with so many facets of the health sciences, *prevention* is the keynote to successful treatment. Far and away the large bulk of bleeding problems could be eliminated by the judicious use of preventive management, both prior to surgery and during the immediate postoperative period. In those instances when postoperative hemorrhage occurs, either as a result of surgery or because some preventive measures were overlooked or not detected, the treatment and management of this condition are based on a few fundamentals, well within the usable command of every general practitioner, the employment of which should cause no hesitancy or apprehension, and the application of which will almost inevitably be successful.

CURRENT CONCEPT OF CLOTTING MECHANISM

The clotting mechanism consists of three major components which are rather independent but closely related systems, i.e., *hemostasis, coagulation* and *lysis.* Much of what follows in this chapter will deal with an interpretation of these three systems: their function, their role in diagnosis and the tests related to each of these systems. In a normal healthy individual there is a rather well-balanced interaction between the coagulation system and the clot lysis. Under the stimulus of an insult to the integrity of the system, various factors trigger the hemostatic and coagulation systems to arrest the bleeding. The lysis system further resolves the formation of a clot once it is formed. The following steps describe how the hemostatic, coagulation and lysis systems function to produce the total clotting mechanism.

Hemostasis

1. There is a *vascular contraction* of a varying degree, depending upon the size and nature of the vessel that has been severed or injured, that not only tends to slow down and restrict the flow of blood from the vessel but also sets up a turbulence which causes the platelets to form a platelet plug. Also, in this vascular contraction, a *cement-like substance* from the mesenchymal supporting tissues of the vessel and from the rupture of the endothelial lining of the vessel wall is liberated. This plays an important role in the formation of the platelet plug.

2. A *platelet plug* is formed so as to impede or restrict the further flow of blood from the torn vessel. Platelets (thrombocytes) are small formed elements in the circulating blood about one fourth the size of a red blood corpuscle. They are formed in the reticuloendothelial system, primarily in bone marrow, and they are generally present in numbers between 200,000 and 400,000 per cubic millimeter. Healthy platelets are essential to the effective coagulation of blood. They contain several factors which are integral parts of the coagulation system. Platelets are altered or modified by many dietary, hormonal, drug and mechanical or environmental stimuli. Any of these modifications in normal platelet function or availability would have an effect upon the coagulation system.

Coagulation

The next part of the clotting mechanism is the development of a *fibrin clot* by the coagulation system. This is done in essentially four parts: (a) The activation of thromboplastin. (b) The conversion of prothrombin to thrombin. (c) The conversion of fibrinogen to fibrin. (d) The contraction of the fibrin clot. Each of these steps is controlled by a highly sophisticated and delicate balance mechanism that requires certain catalysts, substances or factors to propagate the various steps.

Clot Lysis

1. Now that a clot is formed, there must be a mechanism that will *inhibit the further formation* of a clot so as not to continue to develop thromboembolic episodes that would run rampant throughout the entire circulatory system.

2. It is further necessary, once the clot is formed, that there be a system which will lyse the fibrin clot and *remove it* from the blood system in a form that is compatible with normal physiology.

Implications

Certainly relevant to any bleeding problem related to physiologic or biochemical factors — whether it be just troublesome oozing or frank primary or secondary hemorrhage — is an underlying fault in some phase of the clotting mechanism.

Thus, one could expect a bleeding problem as a result of any of the following:

a. Interference with any phase of the hemostatic, coagulation or lysis system.

b. The absence of any of these factors necessary for the conclusion of one phase to the next (congenital or acquired defects).

c. Interference with any phase by drug action.

d. The unavailability of any of the substances involved.

We have come a long way from the time of the classic theory of blood coagulation that Morawitz published in 1905 (the same year procaine was synthesized). It could be summarized by the simple equation:

$$1.\ \text{prothrombin} \xrightarrow[\text{ionic calcium}]{\text{thromboplastin}} \text{thrombin}$$

$$2.\ \text{fibrinogen} \xrightarrow{\text{thrombin}} \text{fibrin}$$

Present day knowledge has uncovered so many facets to the blood-clotting mechanism that today it is a highly complex and poorly understood phenomenon. We have in vogue the "waterfall" hypothesis, Quick's hypothesis, Seeger's hypothesis and many more. All these deal in one way or another with the conversion of the plasma factors to activated factors, which, in the presence of certain other substances, create a fibrin clot.

I think the latest "Mayo Clinic simplified scheme" (modified) is the simplest and the most succinct understanding we have of the clotting mechanism at this time.[11] A simplified diagram of this scheme follows:

1. Platelets
   Factor VIII
   Factor IX   Mesenchymal
   Factor XI   vessel substance
   Factor XII } ——————————————→ Intrinsic thromboplastin
   Ionic calcium   +
                                    Platelet plug

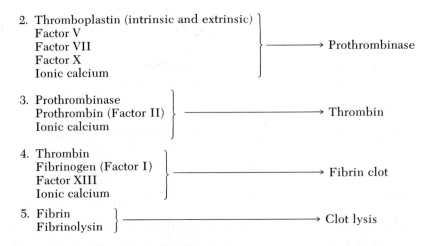

2. Thromboplastin (intrinsic and extrinsic)
   Factor V
   Factor VII   ──────→ Prothrombinase
   Factor X
   Ionic calcium

3. Prothrombinase
   Prothrombin (Factor II) ──────────────────→ Thrombin
   Ionic calcium

4. Thrombin
   Fibrinogen (Factor I)
   Factor XIII   ──────────────────→ Fibrin clot
   Ionic calcium

5. Fibrin
   Fibrinolysin   ──────────────────→ Clot lysis

Coagulation factors are outlined in Table 20–1.

Much could be said and volumes have been written concerning the clotting mechanism, yet as of today all the factors still are not known. I think it is an oversimplification to think of the above scheme or outline per se. Rather a more useful concept is that of the so-called "cascade theory." This approach considers the clotting mechanism resulting in a fibrin clot to take place much like a "cascade" of water tumbling down a rapid series of short falls reaching a calm pool at the bottom. There are many side trickles which will ramify around certain boulders; nevertheless all the water eventually gets down to the bottom, not necessarily at the same rate, not necessarily over the same course, and not necessarily step by step. Any interruption or alteration in the natural confluence of these various pathways, such as an obstruction or dam, or perhaps a tributary taking some of the water away, would naturally have an effect on the total amount of water reaching the bottom pool. To think of the clotting mechanism as a step by step, cut and dried, sequential pattern, is misleading. We are finding that it, after all, is a highly sophisticated, highly integrated, highly effective, and yet easily modified mechanism that serves the purpose of the preservation of the integrity of the individual and his physiologic well being.

CONDITIONS WHICH ALTER NORMAL HEMOSTASIS

Drug-Induced

A. Anticoagulants. The widely popular therapeutic use of anticoagulant drugs for the treatment of people suffering from thromboembolic disease (i.e., coronary heart disease, cerebrovascular accident, pulmonary embolism, venous thrombosis, etc.) is under harsh evaluation currently. Opinion may be in a state of change, but these drugs are still in vogue, and every clinician is constantly seeing and will be treating patients on this medication. It behooves every practitioner whose practice will create a bleeding situation of any type to be completely familiar with the action of

TABLE 20-1 LIST OF COAGULATION FACTORS

Factor	Synonyms	Function	Deficiency Synonym
I	Fibrinogen	Precursor of fibrin	Hypofibrinogenemia Afibrinogenemia
II	Prothrombin	Precursor of thrombin (enzyme which converts fibrinogen to fibrin)	Hypoprothrombinemia
III	Thromboplastin		
IV	Calcium	Necessary for several intermediate reactions	
V	Labile factor Proaccelerin Ac-globulin	Required for activation of tissue thromboplastin	Parahemophilia
VI	No activity assigned this number		
VII	Stable factor Proconvertin SPCA Autoprothrombin I	Required for activation of tissue thromboplastin	Hypoproconvertinemia
VIII	Antihemophilic globulin (AHG) Antihemophilic factor (AHF) Thromboplastinogen	Component of intrinsic thromboplastin generating system	Classic hemophilia Hemophilia A
IX	Plasma thromboplastin component (PTC) Christmas factor Autoprothrombin II	Component of intrinsic thromboplastin generating system	Christmas disease Hemophilia I
X	Stuart factor Prower factor Stuart-Prower factor	Required for activation of tissue thromboplastin	
XI	Plasma thromboplastin antecedent (PTA)	Component of intrinsic thromboplastin generating system	Hemophilia C
XII	Hageman factor Glass factor	Component of intrinsic thromboplastin generating system	Hageman trait
XIII	Fibrin-stabilizing factor (FSF) Laki-Lorand factor (L-L) Fibrinase Serum factor Urea-insolubility factor	Catalyzes normal polymerization of fibrin	

the anticoagulant drugs and their antagonists. Consultation with the physician responsible for the anticoagulant therapy and extreme postoperative vigilance over this patient for a period of six to eight hours following surgery for any possible bleeding complications are absolutely essential.

Basically, anticoagulants come under two major categories: *heparin* and related drugs, and those of the *coumarin* family.

1. *Heparin* is not similar in action to coumarin and is not affected by the administration of vitamin K. It acts as an antithrombic factor to depress the formation of fibrin. Heparin has a tendency to decrease the adhesiveness of the platelets. It also has an action which is mediated through the plasma co-factor, resulting in a substance which inactivates thromboplastin. The drug must be administered by the parenteral route, and its intravenous effect is almost immediate. It is quite expensive, and has gone out of common usage because of these two factors.

2. *Coumarin.* Certainly more popular today is the *coumarin* group, of which these are commonly used: Dicumarol, Tromexan, Coumadin, Hedulin, Sintrom, Danilone, Dipaxin, and Miradon. These drugs act as antimetabolites for vitamin K, or tie up vitamin K so as to depress or prevent prothrombin formation by the liver for the plasma.[4] Therapeutically, coumarin anticoagulants act to reduce the prothrombin levels. Vitamin K has the reversing effect, and is essential for the production of prothrombin by the liver. If the availability of vitamin K is decreased or there is a vitamin K deficiency, or if the vitamin K that is being ingested is not absorbed to where it can be utilized (role of bile), or if liver disease prevents production of prothrombin in the presence of the available vitamin K, *a hypoprothrombinemia* will result. Therefore, the coumarin group induces hypoprothrombinemia.

The onset of action of the coumarin drugs is considerably slower than that of parenteral heparin, being anywhere between 12 and 36 hours. The coumarins may be administered orally or intravenously.

The interaction or competition of the coumarin agents for the available vitamin K, thus producing a decreased prothrombin level, is again an oversimplification of a most complex action involving many facets of the coagulation mechanism, many protein factors, and liver function. A rather simple Lee-White clotting time test is a good indication for the anticoagulant level of heparin. A more complex and technical laboratory procedure of a prothrombin time is necessary to evaluate the prothrombin level of patients on the coumarin drugs. It is generally maintained for adequate therapy in the range of 20 to 30 per cent of normal.

3. Particularly relevant to the alteration of the bleeding and clotting mechanism in patients using coumarin is the use of *aspirin or salicylates* while on this therapy. Salicylates have a depressant effect on the synthesis of prothrombin in the liver, and therefore act in a way somewhat similar to the coumarin anticoagulants. Certainly a clinician should be extremely cautious about the use of salicylates on patients under anticoagulant therapy or maintenance.

Therefore, the overall balance for the treatment of thromboembolic disease becomes a rather complicated interaction of anticoagulant therapy, vitamin K, liver function, vitamin K synthesis and the prothrombin depressant action of salicylates or other drugs.

B. Salicylates. Aside from the aforementioned involvement of aspirin in a patient who is taking anticoagulants, I would like to direct the reader's attention to an excellent chapter in Quick's *Bleeding Problems in Clinical Medicine* (Saunders, 1970, Chapter 2).[13] In beautiful style and most authoritatively, Quick reveals the most important and significant role of aspirin in bleeding problems.

"For many years I have been emphasizing to dental practitioners who use procedures that cause bleeding the significance of aspirin-induced bleeding postoperatively. Recently this has become more and more universally known and accepted. Today, aspirin-induced oral bleeding is common knowledge. Aspirin can produce spontaneous bleeding from the mucosal membranes of the mouth, epistaxis (bloody nose), a prolonged bleeding time, prolonged clotting and/or troublesome postoperative bleeding after surgical procedures in the mouth."

The role of acetylsalicylic acid in the microcirculation appears to be twofold.

1. It acts on the *hemostatic* system in two ways.
    a. It reduces the cohesiveness of the platelets forming the platelet plug, and thereby produces increased bleeding. At the time of injury to a vessel, the platelets have a tendency to adhere to the endotheliocollagen of the vessel wall. These platelets release ADP, which acts as a mediator for the aggregation of other platelets at the site of injury. This forms a hemostatic plug at the site of injury, thus stopping the flow of blood. Aspirin inhibits the release of ADP from the initial group of cells and therefore prevents the formation of the further aggregation of platelets to form a plug. This is the cause of the increased bleeding time which in normal persons can be approximately doubled for three to seven days following the ingestion of 600 mg of aspirin. This tendency can be readily reversed by the infusion of a small number of fresh platelets.[6] This procedure is not recommended for simple troublesome bleeding because of the complication of transfusion difficulties such as hepatitis, etc.
    b. Salicylates also compete for the cholinesterase liberated at the injury of a vessel so that the esterase is not available to hydrolyze the acetylcholine, which dilates the vessel to produce increased bleeding. This competitive inhibition of cholinesterase significantly compromises the effectiveness of a hemostatic plug formed by the platelets due to this dilation effect instead of the normal contraction effect.
2. Aspirin depresses the prothrombin formation, thereby producing a bleeding tendency. It is in this role that aspirin has its effect upon patients taking coumarin anticoagulants and would manifest itself in a decreased prothrombin level.

Many mild and strong analgesics and narcotics available today do not contain salicylates. When an annoying bleeding problem is encountered, the *first thought and the first treatment should be to discontinue all salicylates.* I am convinced that many post-extraction bleeding problems or post-periodontal surgery problems can be traced directly to the use of aspirin taken for pain by the patient prior to presenting to the dental clinician for treatment. Quick has also beautifully portrayed the role of aspirin not only in simple bleeding problems but also in complicated and rare bleeding disorders such as the Minot-von Willebrand syndrome,[14] intrinsic platelet defects, hemophilia, and other related disease.

C. Vitamin C. Vitamin C, particularly the bioflavinoids and rutin compounds, is important for maintenance of the integrity of the capillary walls. Vitamin C deficiencies often cause capillary fragility. Today, true vitamin C deficiencies are rare. Vitamin C is probably more valuable in prophylactic techniques to increase capillary permeability, which, in turn, will somewhat affect the mechanical phase of the blood coagulation mechanism to arrest hemorrhage.

D. Coagulation-Promoting Agents. Drugs dealing with the coagulation-promoting aspect of bleeding, whether for hemorrhagic disorders or for adequate clot formation, would more appropriately be discussed under systemic agents in the treatment of hemorrhagic problems, which follows.

E. Fibrinolytic Agents. It is only within the scope of this topic to discuss in a very brief manner the agents which could be used to dissolve a blood clot that has been formed either within a vessel or extravascularly within various special areas throughout the body. The lytic enzyme *fibrinolysin* is believed to be responsible for the resolution which is spontaneously carried out throughout the body whenever any blood has extravasated from a vessel into a tissue space. There are many enzymes, streptokinase and streptodornase (Varidase) and proteolytic enzymes (Ananase, Papase, trypsin) which have varying degrees of clot liquefying effectiveness. All these drugs would be concerned with the fourth phase of our scheme above.

F. Drug Interactions. There is a virtually endless list of drugs which interact with one another to cause abnormalities in the bleeding and cloting mechanism. These drugs work for and against bleeding and clotting mechanisms in both directions, depending upon the situation. The clinician should become familiar with all drugs that he or she prescribes or that the patient is currently taking in order to prevent these drug interactions from causing bleeding problems. Patients who are on anticoagulants should have their prothrombin time regularly monitored in the presence of other medication or in the presence of any change in the drug regimen. The reader is directed to the book by Martin,[7] *Hazards of Medications,* for an extensive and exhaustive treatise on these coagulation interactions of medication.

Physiologically Induced

We have long been aware that *endocrine imbalances* in the female will have a tendency to prolong the bleeding time and create coagulation problems on *a priori* grounds alone. There seems to be a tendency among women who have prolonged menstruation or who suffer from such disorders as menorrhagia to have a tendency toward prolonged postoperative bleeding. Patients of this type are particularly prone to secondary hemorrhage starting two or three days following the surgery.

Patients with *blood dyscrasias,* such as hemophilia, pseudohemophilia, telangiectasia, thrombocytopenic purpura, any of the anemias, leukopenias, thrombocytopenias, myeloproliferative disorders, or any vascular or hemorrhagic defect, will have coagulation problems that must be managed by the clinician and considered *prior* to any treatment.

Pregnancy generally is no contraindication to a surgical procedure from a bleeding point of view; however, there is often considerable oozing in pregnant patients that would otherwise not be present.

The presence of *infection* brings large quantities of blood to an area. The increased vascular bed will produce an increased bleeding at the time of surgery that should not alter the mechanism of clotting except from the standpoint of quantity alone.

If there has been severe *trauma* in the recent past so that there is a large enough area of ecchymosis or hematoma in the tissues involved in the surgery, the bleeding response will be prolonged and the amount of blood loss will be considerably increased.

Likewise, when there is any *tumor* it is fed by various vessels that normally would not be present. The surgeon may well encounter abnormal bleeding with any areas of this field of operation which would necessitate more careful dissection and considerably more detailed attention to the tributary arteries and veins.

Patients with rather severe *hypertension* pose potential bleeding problems in that the hydrostatic pressure within the vessel itself creates a simple mechanical problem. The fibrin clot that acts as a plug in the capillary or arterial opening is more easily dislodged. The effect of blood pressure is often particularly apparent on a patient who is under a general anesthetic. A clinician should be considerably more prudent in the observation of a patient who has a severe hypertension for the spontaneous recurrence of bleeding in the immediate postoperative period of routine surgery such as dental extraction or dentoalveolar surgery.

There are a large number of pathologic entities (e.g., cavernous hemangioma, aneurysm) involving blood vessels or blood tumors which obviously require careful evaluation prior to surgical intervention because bleeding from these can be extremely serious and at times fatal.

Certain complications may arise following streptococcal infections and certain malignancies, resulting in a *hypofibrinogenemia*. Suitable laboratory procedures for the fibrinogen determination can be conducted; the diagnosis once established will necessitate immediate therapy to prevent circulatory collapse.

EVALUATION OF THE PATIENT

Probably the most significant and essential preventive measures are those taken *before* treatment, and involve the patient's *history, evaluation,* and *required laboratory tests* when any abnormality is suspected. The corrective efforts employed to have the patient in optimal readiness for surgery are self-evident. The information that is revealed during the physical and laboratory evaluation of the patient then can be used to institute preventive treatment for anticipated complications arising from surgery. Whether the surgery is a simple extraction, a minor biopsy, a general curettage, or a complicated extraoral procedure, a potential bleeding patient exists. It is important to make as complete an evaluation for a seemingly innocent and minor surgery as for the patient who is scheduled for a major operation.

History

In every patient history or questionnaire there should be an interrogation made as to *previous bleeding experiences* or results of previous tooth extraction or *previous surgery*. The statement "I am a bleeder," by a patient is a warning which must be considered as predisposing a bleeding problem unless positively ruled out.

Secondly, it is imperative in a questionnaire to inquire into the current or recent *medication* that the patient may be taking, e.g., salicylates, anticoagulants, hormones, iron preparations for anemia, etc. These are related specifically to hemorrhagic difficulties. Other questions in a routine questionnaire may shed light on subtle bleeding difficulties.

A history of leukemia, hemophilia, blood dyscrasias, or any *hemorrhagic diseases* should be thoroughly evaluated, including a consultation with the internist or hematologist currently following the patient. In this manner adequate preparations can be jointly agreed upon prior to the surgical management of the patient with these difficulties. You may want to consider in a questionable history whether the patient has a history of oozing easily or spontaneously, bleeds from minor cuts or wounds for an abnormally long time, or has an familial bleeding history.

Occasionally the *menstrual history* of the woman is important. Metrorrhagia, abnormal uterine bleeding, especially during the intermenstrual period, and menorrhagia, profuse and prolonged menstrual bleeding, may indicate a postoperative bleeding tendency requiring preventive measures.

An inquiry into the patient's *family history* is often very helpful, yet often overlooked.

The use of radiographs is mandatory if surgery on any bone is anticipated. Fatal accidents have been encountered from the seemingly routine extraction of teeth, owing to profuse uncontrollable bleeding from a cavernous hemangioma, terminating in unmanageable shock and death. X-rays will many times give indications of aberrant vessels or pathways of extremely large nutrient arteries in the area of surgery which may possibly be avoided in the procedure.

Physical Examination

The *physical examination* of the patient also should be accomplished. Such things as the nature of the *skin*, appearance of *petechiae*, the color of the *eyes*, and the all too frequently overlooked condition and color of the *gingiva*, *lips* and *nail beds* can reveal liver disease, leukemia, anemia, etc., and might predispose a bleeding tendency. The most casual examination will reveal certain types of purpura and telangiectasia. Jaundice and tenderness of bones or joints may be an indication of a bleeding tendency.

RATIONALE

Upon completion of the history and physical evaluation, any abnormal findings must be followed to a satisfactory conclusion, and the clinician must decide the degree of significance of the bleeding problem detected. Owen et al.[2] classify patients into *four main groups:*

1. Severe bleeding tendency
2. Minor bleeding tendency
3. Equivocal bleeding tendency
4. No bleeding tendency

Before any treatment or surgery is contemplated, the following steps should be taken.

A. Patients in group (1) must be referred to a hematologist for consultation.

B. Patients in groups (2) and (3) should have a simple screening as outlined in the following section. This may be ordered and interpreted by the clinician, or, if he or she prefers, the patient could be referred to a colleague for these tests and the interpretation of the results.

C. If abnormal results are found from these simple screening procedures, the abnormal conditions must be corrected prior to treatment. This can be done either by the clinician, if experienced in this field, or through consultation or referral to a colleague for this correction.

This simple process outlined above should virtually eliminate 95 per cent of the bleeding difficulties *prior* to treatment.

The clinician should not hesitate to request the necessary laboratory tests prior to surgery or any procedure wherein known bleeding will be encountered. They are *simple* and *inexpensive.*

The decision whether the "simple screening tests" outlined later in this section will be all that is necessary to evaluate the bleeding status of the patient, or whether it will be necessary to utilize other specific tests for a specific condition that was detected in the history — i.e., aspirin tolerance test for a patient suspected of having a bleeding problem connected with the use of aspirin, or possibly a rather full gamut of laboratory work which requires a great deal of skill in interpretation to rule out the more serious bleeding problems — *has to be made at this point.* To go on with a procedure that is seemingly minor and innocent has led to patients ending up in the hospital several days later, often requiring multi-disciplined medical management.

Laboratory Tests

Some tests for hemorrhagic disorders have been presented in Table 2 on page 114 of the manual *A Guide to Hospital Dental Procedures*, published by the American Dental Association (1964).[5] This work also lists in Table 1 many of the normal values of blood constituents. Any good recent textbook on hematology will include a section on laboratory tests and their interpretation. The reader is referred to such a source for a complete and exhaustive exposure to this material. The intent is to acquaint the clinician with availability of certain tests and a rationale for their selected use, as the experience of the clinician and the history would dictate.

The selection of any laboratory test must be based upon the nature of the abnormality. The interpretation of the result of the test must be the responsibility of the clinician.

Listed below, as to the system involved, are the currently used laboratory tests for hematologic evaluation.

Hemostatic tests:
   Bleeding time, Ivy method
   Tourniquet test, Rumpel-Leede
   Aspirin tolerance test, Quick
   CBC with platelet count, wet method
   Capillary fragility
   Platelet aggregation
   Platelet adhesiveness
   Clot retraction
Coagulation tests:
   Coagulation test
   Plasma clot time
   Prothrombin time
   Activated partial thromboplastin time
   Prothrombin consumption time
   Stypven time
   Thrombin time
   Thromboplastin generation test
Fibrinolysis tests:
   Euglobulin clot lysis time
   Whole blood clot lysis time
   Fibrinogen lysis
Plasma evaluation tests:
   Fibrinogen
   Prothrombin
   Factor VIII

From this more complete list I would like to select a few of the more commonly used tests to expand upon and describe in more detail.

Bleeding Time (Ivy Method: One to Six Minutes). A bleeding time can be either insignificant, misleading, or extremely valuable, depending upon the degree of accuracy with which it has been done. It is probably one of the least expensive and best screening procedures available to the clinician. Its one fault lies in the fact that it does not positively screen out a small percentage of patients with severe bleeding dyscrasias. It is better thought of as a screening procedure to rule out 95 per cent of the problem bleeders with difficulty in the hemostatic system. A significant abnormal response would be over 15 minutes' bleeding time. This would indicate a capillary defect, thrombocytopenia, acute leukemia, aplastic anemia, liver disease, or a toxic state.

Tourniquet Test (Rumpel-Leede Method). This simple test may be performed in the office with a minimum of equipment. Using a blood pressure cuff on the upper arm, it is inflated to approximately halfway between the patient's systolic and diastolic blood pressures. This is maintained for five minutes. The blood pressure cuff is removed, and five minutes later the forearm is examined for the number of petechiae present. The inside of the elbow region is also a good place to look for these petechiae. A significant result would be more than 20 fresh petechiae in this region after the five minutes' lapsed time. A result such as this would indicate a possible capillary defect, thrombocytopenia, purpuras or telangiectasia. A platelet count would be indicated for further screening.

CBC (Webb Wet Method). Most routine CBCs today consist of the following components:
1. Total number of erythrocytes (RBC)
2. Total number of leukocytes (WBC)
3. Differential count of leukocytes
4. Hemoglobin determination (Hb)
5. Morphologic features and maturity of cells
6. Number of blood platelets

INTERPRETATION OF CBC

1. Erythrocyte count (RBC):
   Normal: 4,000,000 to 6,000,000 cells per mm^3
   Decrease: anemia, pellagra, hemorrhage, liver diseases
   Increase: polycythemia, extreme dehydration
2. Leukocyte count (WBC):
   Normal: 5000 to 10,000 cells per mm^3
   Decrease: anemia, poisons, thrombocytopenia, radiation, massive infections
   Increase: infections, leukemias, overexertion
3. Differential of leukocytes:
   Normal: neutrophils, 60 to 70 per cent; lymphocytes, 20 to 35 per cent; monocytes, 2 to 6 per cent; eosinophils, 1 to 3 per cent
   Decrease: Neutrophils — aplastic anemia, neutropenia, lymphocytic anemia
   Lymphocytes — aplastic anemia, myelogenous leukemia, radiation
   Monocytes — aplastic anemia
   Eosinophils — typhoid fever, aplastic anemia
   Increase: Neutrophils — acute infection, myelogenous leukemia, poisons, erythroblastosis
   Lymphocytes — lymphocytic leukemia, chronic infections, viral diseases
   Monocytes — monocytic leukemia, infectious mononucleosis, malaria, Hodgkin's disease, tuberculosis, Gaucher's disease, subacute bacterial endocarditis
   Eosinophils — allergic diseases, dermatitis, protozoan diseases, Hodgkin's disease, scarlet fever
4. Hemoglobin determination:
   Normal: 12.5 to 17 gm per 100 ml
   Decrease: anemia, hemorrhage, liver disease
   Increase: polycythemia
5. Cellular morphology and maturity:
   Abnormal: nucleation of erythrocytes, leukemia, poisons, parasites, marrow cells, etc.
6. Blood platelets:
   Normal: 200,000 to 400,000 per mm^3
   Decrease: thrombocytopenic purpura, acute leukemia, aplastic anemia, pernicious anemia, acute infections
   Increase: polycythemia, sickle cell anemia, rheumatic fever, hemolytic anemias

Aspirin Tolerance Test. This test has become extremely valuable in diagnosing decreased hemostatic mechanisms in the microcirculation, particularly when there may be an inability to manufacture cholinesterase following an injury, thereby blocking the hydrolytic process of acetylcholine, which dilates vessels. The test has become diagnostic for the Minot-von Willebrand syndrome in which a much greater response to this test occurs than in those not having the condition.

Before taking the test the patient abstains from taking any aspirin for five days. A bleeding time is done and immediately thereafter the patient is given 10 grains of aspirin in a glass of water. The bleeding time is repeated in two hours and four hours. A marked increase in bleeding time would indicate a patient susceptible to having hemorrhagic problems while taking salicylates.

Clot Retraction. This is a very simple test for a laboratory to run. It involves essentially the observation of a clot for an hour and one-half. The inability of a clot to retract or change in size indicates a possible hemostatic problem and may be indicative of a rather annoying bleeding difficulty. It, of course, is predicated upon the formation of an adequate platelet plug and the availability of the elements that the platelets supply in the formation of the clotting mechanism.

Coagulation or Clotting Time (Plastic Tube Method — Normal, 30 to 40 Minutes). An abnormally high clotting time of more than an hour or so will reveal a deficiency or an absence in the factors within the hemorrhagic disorders such as hemophilia, pseudohemophilia, fibrinogen deficiency, etc.

Prothrombin Time (Quick Method, One Stage). This test is generally reported in terms of percentage related to normal control. Twenty to 30 per cent is generally a normal therapeutic level for patients on anticoagulant drugs. This test is extremely significant in discovering abnormalities in the clotting mechanism involving Factors V, VII, X, prothrombin and fibrinogen. It is used to establish and control the level of anticoagulant therapy of the coumarin drugs. The test gives an indication of prothrombin deficiency arising from liver disease, fibrinogen deficiency, and lack of or inability of the body to utilize vitamin K.

Activated Partial Thromboplastin Time. This test is reported generally in percentages, as is the prothrombin time. It is the screening test for Factors VIII, IX, XI, and low levels of V, X, and XII, prothrombin and fibrinogen. It is normal in thrombocytopenia. The test is an excellent screening procedure.

Prothrombin Consumption Time. The normal range is 25 seconds or longer. This test is becoming increasingly widely used as a valid test for indicating deficiencies of Factors V, VIII, IX, X, XI, XII, or platelet Factor III. It would give some indication of a faulty hemostatic system as well as a faulty coagulation system, and is most helpful in differential diagnosis of some of the more difficult and serious bleeding problems.

Euglobulin Clot Lysis Time. This test is becoming very important to indicate an imbalance in the fibrinolytic activity. The euglobulin clot is normally lysed more rapidly than the whole blood clot. If this euglobulin clot will dissolve in less than 90 minutes, it indicates an increase in the fibrinolytic activity which could lead to a bleeding problem.

Plasma Assays. *Fibrinogen, prothrombin,* and several of the *Factors* found in plasma may be tested to indicate whether or not they are present in a normal amount. This information is useful primarily to the hematologist for differential diagnosis of the serious blood dyscrasias.

Type and Cross Match with Rh Factor. If *transfusions* are anticipated, it is necessary to have a type and cross match with Rh determinations prior to surgery, and medical consultation should be utilized before treatment is instituted.

Bone Marrow Studies. These are included for some blood dyscrasias and the leukemias. Interpretation is extremely difficult and involved, and the consultation of a reliable hematologist is mandatory.

SUMMARY OF LABORATORY TESTS

For the clinician the indication, application and practicality of the aforementioned tests are an ever-present dilemma. This need not be the

TABLE 20-2 RECOMMENDED SCREENING FOR BLEEDING PROBLEMS
(GROUPS 2 AND 3)

	Normal
Hemostasis	
1. Bleeding time (Ivy)	1 to 6 minutes
2. Tourniquet test (Rumpel-Leede) – office procedure	Less than 10 petechiae
3. CBC	(See above)
Coagulation	
1. Coagulation time (plastic tube)	20 to 45 minutes
2. Activated partial thromboplastin time	Less than 50 seconds
3. Prothrombin time	100% of normal

case. When a valid and substantiated history and physical evaluation reveal a predisposition to a bleeding tendency (prolonged and heavy menstrual flow, tendency to bruise easily, frequent nose bleeds, spontaneous bleeding from the gingiva without cause, tendency to have recurrent episodes of ecchymosis or a previous problem with a dental or bleeding experience), the clinician is obliged either to obtain a few simple tests in order to screen out a possibly and potentially dangerous bleeding situation, or to refer the patient to a colleague for this screening. A skilled clinician will be able to decide between the subtleties of significant history and the overly apprehensive or hypochondriac patient in relation to bleeding problems.

As we have said, the clotting mechanism involves a threefold system: hemostasis, coagulation and lysis. For the initial screening of these patients whose history and physical evaluation have suggested *possible simple bleeding problems* (groups 2 and 3), the tests shown in Table 20–2 are recommended. These tests will detect 95 per cent of the bleeding tendencies.

The importance of a *consultation* with a competent internist or hematologist cannot be overemphasized when gross abnormalities are found in any of the above hematologic evaluations.

More specific screening profiles for the rare, exotic, and unusual bleeding dyscrasias can be obtained with the cooperation of a competent hematologist. The rationale and interpretation of these screening profiles has become extremely sophisticated, and interpretation, even among the experts, is at best difficult.

DRUG INTERACTIONS

There are several drugs encountered in dentistry which interfere with hematological testing. These include *anticoagulants, tetracyclines, penicillin, salicylates, acetophenetidin,* and *acetaminophen.* Allowances should be made in the interpretation of laboratory values on patients taking any of the above drugs. A complete list of drugs (in addition to those mentioned above) which interfere with hematologic testing has been given by Martin in his book, *Hazards of Medication.*[7]

MODALITIES OF TREATMENT

There is probably a great tendency among clinicians to seek a safe panacea-like drug to give any patient with a bleeding or hemorrhagic problem to promote hemostasis. Such a drug does not exist. In most instances these injectable drugs are used rather empirically, with no sound physiologic rationale. Most of the conditions that they are widely used to treat might well be treated with proper "local" or "topical" applications of hemostatic agents or principles. There is much doubt, and much investigation yet to be accomplished, as to the effectiveness of many of the injectable drugs to produce hemostasis. Treatment can be divided into two groups, systemic and topical.

Systemic Agents

1. Transfusion, Whole Blood. It is necessary to have a type and cross match with Rh. There is a high risk of *allergic reaction* from whole blood, and a high instance of transmission of hepatitis B. Nonetheless, fresh whole blood represents one of the most effective ways of supplying patients with severe coagulation deficiencies, such as pseudohemophilia, true hemophilia, and other deficiency diseases, with the necessary elements lacking to accomplish hemostasis.

2. Plasma. This is used mainly to re-establish circulating blood volume in cases of severe blood loss. There are *no* elements within plasma that are generally effective in hemostasis.

3. Plasma Expanders. These are used solely to develop or recreate a blood volume, and have no direct effect on the clotting mechanism.

4. Fibrinogen. This, with various factors in its total plasma fraction, has been used quite effectively in the treatment of related deficiency diseases. Gamble advocates the use of plasma clottable fibrinogen containing Factor VIII in hemophiliacs.[10] The work of Judith Pool, Research Associate in Medicine, Stanford University, has advanced the useful application of the fibrinogen components for the treatment of specific hemophilic disorders. By freezing fresh whole blood and then fractionally separating the concentration of Factor VIII, she has made it possible to administer in very small quantities (such as 10 ml of this concentrate) as much Factor VIII as would be available in several units of fresh whole blood. This enables the clinician to make high concentrations of Factor VIII antihemophilic globulin available for injection without markedly increasing the circulating volume of the patient.

5. Vitamin K. Vitamin K promotes the formation of prothrombin by the liver. *The use of vitamin K preparations orally or intravenously should be reserved for valid evidence that the prothrombin level is decreased or that there is some deficiency.* The vitamin K deficiency can become significant only when the synthesis of the vitamin K by intestinal bacteria is markedly reduced by altered flora (antibiotics, etc.), or completely absent from the patient's intake. Severe *liver disease* may cause hypoprothrombinemia from the injury to the hepatic cells, and may not respond to the administration of vitamin K. *The use of vitamin K in patients under anticoagulant therapy must be done with consultation.* The prophylactic use of vitamin K for patients with somewhat depressed prothrombin levels who are not on anticoagulant therapy *is* good practice.

Prothrombin deficiencies are both congenital and acquired. The congenital variety does not respond to vitamin K. Acquired hypoprothrombinemias respond well to the therapeutic use of vitamin K. Vitamin K_1 is not water soluble and is available as an emulsion for intramuscular or intravenous use. The water soluble preparations available today, such as Aquamephyton, Synkayvite, and Hykinone, do not require bile salts for their absorption and utilization.

6. Vitamin C. Vitamin C is used to maintain capillary integrity. It is often used in combination with bioflavonoids. Being water soluble it is rapidly depleted if the patient's diet is markedly altered, such as after the removal of four impacted third molars. While not dramatic in its effect, this substance will make noticeable differences in the oozing of the marginal patient. It has an effect upon the availability of the mesenchymal cementin substance, and therefore alters hemostasis. A minimum of 500 mg per day of vitamin C should be prescribed. It is good to start the day before surgery and continue for five days after the procedure is finished or the oozing has terminated.

7. Premarin. The female hormone has been used quite effectively in women — sometimes with dramatic response — to control capillary or mechanical bleeding. It has no effect on deficiency diseases. Sometimes these compounds are used in the management of epistaxis and bleeding from gastrointestinal causes. There is evidence to indicate that intravenous estrogens can produce prompt increase of circulating prothrombin and accelerated globulin and a decrease in the antithrombin activity of the blood. Theoretically, these changes tend to enhance the coagulability of blood, thereby providing a rationale for the current, popular short term use of the estrogens in spontaneous hemorrhage.[9] A single dose of 20 mg of the conjugated estrogen (Premarin) given intravenously is reputed to have a remarkable effect. Therapy should not be continued beyond one dose. Premarin has been favorably employed to control both troublesome oozing over a large area and frank venous bleeding of a rather large magnitude.

8. Adrenosem, Kutapressin, and Koagamin. These drugs occasionally are used to control capillary bleeding. Adrenosem acts by decreasing capillary permeability or increasing capillary resistance. Kutapressin is only effective for capillary oozing. Koagamin is oxalic and malonic acid, and has a tendency to release prothrombin for the formation of thrombin. These drugs are of questionable value and are reported by many to be entirely ineffective. One should not expect these drugs to have dramatic results. They will be most effective if started the day before surgery and continued for three to five days when capillary oozing problems are anticipated in the patient.

Topical Agents

1. Epinephrine. Epinephrine, 1:1000 concentration, applied locally with a piece of cotton or gauze, or injected locally in a concentration of 1:50,000 for hemostasis, is quite effective, but its action is reversible. This technique should not be used on patients with severe hypertension or previous existing cardiovascular disease, as direct absorption of this concentration can be very dangerous. Severe toxic effects can be elicited by the topical use of 1:1000 concentration solution of epinephrine, particularly over wide areas of the mouth. The rationale for its use lies in the temporary arresting of bleeding long enough for a mechanical plug to clot or occlude the vessel. When the vasoconstrictor effect wears off the patient must be watched carefully for further recurrence of the bleeding, as the plug may become dislodged again. Epinephrine, while a physiologic substance, is a very potent drug, and many patients have been known to suffer rather severe hypersensitivities to its topical use.

2. Monsel's Solution. Monsel's solution of ferric subsulfate may be used topically or on an area of capillary bleeding to precipitate the protein. It is relatively harmless to tissue, and is quite applicable and effective for the postextraction bleeding in medullary bone. It should not be applied over large areas. It should be used via a pack.

3. Thrombin. Thrombin may be used the same way, and will act as a precipitating agent for the fibrin clot if there is fibrinogen present in the plasma. The topical (it must never be injected) use of thrombin is favored by many because of its physiologic compatibility to normal processes. It is very kind to tissue and can be quite effective.

4. Russell Viper Venom. Russell viper venom[18] (Stypven), a dry powder constituted with water, made in 5–ml ampules, is a preparation of thromboplastin that can be used similarly in a socket or topically over an area of bleeding to precipitate blood clot formation.

Note: Monsel's solution, Russell viper venom, and thrombin should be used *only* on iodoform or plain gauze, cotton, Surgicel or Gelfoam — *not* Oxycel. The acid formed by the above solutions' reaction with Oxycel inactivates them and makes them completely ineffective. Care should be used when pressure is necessary or desirable. Gelfoam is soft when saturated and is ineffective as a pressure agent, but is absorbable.

5. Tannic Acid. The tannic acid in a tea bag will help precipitate protein and cause clot formation. It is best applied by having the patient bite down on the folded tea bag, dry or very slightly moist, for five minutes, repeating, if necessary, three times. Saliva should not be allowed to pool in the patient's mouth during the treatment. This is more applicable to patients' use for home treatment than in valid office procedures. The tea bag may well be used in conjunction with the folded dry sponge to apply adequate pressure when the mouth is edentulous. Mann Hemostatic is a mixture of tannic acid, alum and chlorobutanol. It is quite effective when applied on either Surgicel or iodoform for the control of a troublesome, oozing type of bleeding.

6. Gelfoam. Gelfoam, which is a gelatin-based sponge that is absorbable in four to six weeks, acts by disrupting the platelets and establishing a framework with the fibrin strands to create a clot.

7. Oxycel. Oxidized cellulose (Oxycel) releases cellulosic acid, which has a marked affinity for hemoglobin, leading to the formation of an artificial clot. It is absorbed in approximately six weeks. The action of Oxycel is not enhanced by the addition of thrombin or other hemostatic agents, for they are destroyed by the high acidity of this material. Oxycel is available as a gauze or as a cotton. It should *not* be moistened prior to use, as the acidity created has a tendency to inhibit epithelialization. This product is not recommended for use over epithelial surfaces.[1]

8. Surgicel. Oxidized regenerated cellulose (Surgicel) offers some improvement over Oxycel in that the gauze pad has more tenacity and resistance, and the poly- and hydroglutonic acids resulting from this product do not inhibit epithelialization. It therefore can be used on surface dressings where epithelium is involved. It is available as bulk ribbon (Fig. 20–1) or individually packaged for single application in sealed glass bottles. The bulk

Figure 20-1.

form can be cut to any size desired, and is very economical. The individual packages are convenient for house calls.

9. Ice. Topical ice application, on five minutes and off five minutes for the first four hours, sometimes will help reduce bleeding. However, some tests have shown this to be totally ineffective. Thermocouple implant studies in skin have shown the insulation properties of skin to be extremely efficient. Patients with ice applications of long duration showed no appreciable change in temperature of the subdermal layers owing to the network of capillaries just below the skin. Tests have shown that ice applied to a local area will increase bleeding time considerably. The flow may be reduced somewhat, but the bleeding duration is increased. The necessity of *keeping the mouth as dry as possible* cannot be overemphasized. It is sometimes advisable to ask the patient to breathe through his mouth to keep the mucosa dry and to keep adequate air traversing over the area for clot formation.

10. Electrocautery. There are many instances when bleeding of some size can be controlled by electrocautery (Fig. 20–2) through two modalities.

a. After securing a moderate-sized vessel with a hemostat, the cautery can be touched to the hemostat, creating a precipitation of the protein elements in the end of the wound and sealing off the vessel through the action of the heat in the hemostat in contact with the occluded vessel.

b. A more common use is to apply the cautery directly to small vessels that are oozing or bleeding. This will coagulate the blood and the protein in the area, and will arrest bleeding from extremely vascular and troublesome sites.

It is not prudent to expect electrocautery to replace ligation of a large vessel, but, used when indicated, electrocautery is a convenient and effective way of controlling hemorrhage.

Figure 20–2.

When used for patients with cardiac pacemakers (fixed-rate *or* demand type), great caution must be exercised. See discussion in Chapter 2.

Mechanical Measures

These include the application of any modality of force that would counteract the hydrostatic pressure within the bleeding vessel until such time as a clot can form and occlude the orifice.

1. Pressure. Usually after an extraction a patient biting down on a *dry* sponge placed directly over the area can control hemorrhage.

2. Pack Socket. Occasionally it is necessary to pack the socket tightly with a sponge or gauze dressing so that the pressure of the packing in the socket will stop the bleeding enough to clot. This is only applicable to bleeding from bone. It may be necessary to use sutures to hold these dressings in place. Packs should not be left in until they are completely saturated with blood and saliva, but changed frequently. This will enhance their effectiveness as a clotting mechanism in stubborn bleeding. It is also important to have any clots wiped clean from the alveolar ridge so that pressure can be applied directly across the alveolar crest itself.

3. Splint. On occasion it is advisable to fabricate a splint prior to surgery than can be wired in place or worn by the patient over the surgical area. This will create pressure over the bleeding area and will stabilize tissues so that the inadvertent motions of eating and swallowing will not reactivate the bleeding in the capillary bed of the flap. Splints are useful in patients who have preexisting blood dyscrasias and hemophilia and in patients who cannot leave the area alone, disrupting the clot following surgery.

4. Ligation and Sutures. The use of absorbable gut for deep ties to ligate large vessels, and of silk or nylon sutures for surface constriction of a bleeding or oozing area, is good surgical practice. However, unless there has been sufficient mobilization of flap or bone removal to allow tight and adequate tissue approximation, sutures in the alveolar crest area only provide additional sites for bleeding. Figure 20–3 shows examples of different types of suture materials commonly available to control hemorrhage. The choice is basically established by the criteria that the bleeding problem presents and the nature of the patient. It is important to use atraumatic needles whenever possible to prevent additional bleeding sites that may become troublesome in their own right. Opinions differ as to the advisability of using absorbable gut sutures for the control of hemorrhage and intraoral bleeding. It is the author's opinion that silk, although it must be removed, affords a more positive control of bleeding when used intraorally. Synthetic or nylon suture material is often irritating to the patient's cheek or tongue. A cut cotton roll affords a rather convenient means of storing a suture which is cut in approximate 12–inch lengths.

5. Bone Wax, etc. Dental practitioners are always dealing with bone which is not compressible, and bleeding many times is very troublesome because of the inability to occlude the vessels that are confined within bony canals. It is sometimes necessary to use bone wax or a stiff substance that will plug the orifice until clotting occurs.

6. Bone Punch. The use of a bone punch to mash and occlude the orifice of the bone canal is often the only means of arresting intraosseous hemorrhage.

Figure 20–3.

Figure 20–4.

Figure 20–4 represents various types of tissue pick-ups, tweezers, hemo-stats, and clamps that are useful in the control of intraoral or extraoral hemor-rhage that a dental practitioner may encounter in routine treatment. Every clinician should have an appropriate hemostat within reach of the dental chair at all times for the unexpected accident resulting in the cutting of a major artery or vein that would require immediate clamping of the vessel to control the bleeding. (This hemostat is also a valuable aid to have at chairside in the event of inadvertent needle breakage.)

TYPES OF BLEEDING

In order to understand and discuss the treatment of dental hemorrhage more thoroughly, it would simplify matters, I think, to arrive at some general grouping of these problems. There are essentially only two types of bleed-ing.

The *first type* comes from minor capillaries, arterioles, and venules. This is many times called *oozing*. It may be primary or secondary. It can occur spontaneously or as a result of trauma, either surgical or otherwise. It is generally mild or troublesome, and only becomes serious upon long duration. It can result from an alteration in the clotting mechanism due to a blood dyscrasia that is acquired, congenital, or drug induced. It can be strictly a result of mechanical difficulties in the vascular bed.

The *second type* of bleeding involves the *major vessels*, both arteries and veins. This can be either primary or secondary, although it generally is of primary nature. It occurs practically always from surgical or accidental trau-ma, and rarely is spontaneous. This bleeding is always severe and will termin-ate fatally if not corrected immediately. It is induced almost invariably by mechanical factors; the underlying cause of its lack of control may be either mechanical or biochemical.

Either of these categories of bleeding can occur within soft tissue, within bone, intraorally, or extraorally.

Oozing

Fortunately, these aforementioned blood dyscrasias and defects are far and away the minority of the bleeding problems seen in everyday practice. It is the troublesome oozing of a postoperative extraction site, third molar flap, or gingival crevice that is the main offender. The need for adequate observation of the patient during the *immediate* postoperative period cannot be stressed too emphatically. Steps taken *at that time* to assure complete hemostasis by employing any of the treatment modalities mentioned above will be rewarding.

There is no set procedure that will work universally, but the following criteria are basic:

1. It is essential that the clot be wiped out of the patient's mouth down to the level of the socket. The bleeding will continue as long as the jelly or liver clot is projecting into the patient's mouth.
2. Immediately withdraw all forms of aspirin from the patient. Prescribe no analgesics containing aspirin or salicylates.
3. It is important to keep the patient's mouth *dry* and as free of saliva as possible. Mouth breathing will help. The use of *dry* gauze packs with pressure over the area of bleeding probably is the best and most effective means of control.
4. If, after frequent and repeated applications of these pressure packs, the bleeding will not subside, one is obliged to use another modality, such as gauze packing, Gelfoam packing, Surgicel, Viper venom, thrombin, cautery, etc.
5. *Suction* is necessary to properly *visualize* the actual bleeding site.
6. Sutures are most valuable when they can be used effectively to apply pressure around a bleeding area so as to mechanically close the orifice of the bleeding vessels or capillaries. It should be remembered, however, that each time a suture is placed two more holes are created that are potential bleeding sites. In many instances in dentoalveolar surgery sutures are employed where they are absolutely useless from a standpoint of effectiveness directly related to a bleeding problem. One main reason for their ineffectiveness is that in relatively few instances in simple dentoalveolar surgery is it necessary to mobilize the mucoperiosteal flap, and without the mobility of this flap a suture merely goes across the open socket, adding to, rather than solving, an existing bleeding problem.

The management of secondary hemorrhage of this type is essentially the same as for primary hemorrhage. It may be necessary to anesthetize the area in order to manipulate the proper dressings in the socket and to achieve the proper pressure to obtain the hemostasis required without causing undue distress to the patient. The vasoconstrictor in a local analgesic injected around the area will have a tendency to reduce the bleeding and cause hemostasis. However, this effect will wear off quickly, and the patient may experience further hemorrhage through the rebound phenomenon of vasodilation.

Profuse Bleeding

For major vessel bleeding of significant proportions there is no substitute for clean and meticulous dissection and the clamping and ligation of these

Figure 20–5.

bleeding vessels with gut. The reader is referred to *Textbook of Oral Surgery*, edited by G. Kruger,[16] where there are numerous illustrations and detailed descriptive explanations of the management of bleeding problems arising from surgical manipulation.

Pressure packing or mechanical closure of the vessel canal is about the only way to stop heavy bleeding in bone.

It must also be said that there can be no substitute for a sound workable knowledge of *anatomy* to avoid the pitfalls of serious hemorrhage or the dangers of massive blood loss from the inadvertent cutting of a major vessel. One must always be prepared to tie off a major vessel if bleeding cannot be locally controlled. Rossi accounts for rather significant blood loss from some routine dental surgery.[15]

Extreme caution must be exercised to avoid the inadvertent involvement of massive blood lesions or *tumors* within bone or soft tissue. The tray in Figure 20–5 contains the following armamentarium: a retractor to gain adequate access to the bleeding area; scissors; a needle holder with a suture, needles of two different sizes; mirror for adequate vision; suction tip for adequate suction of the field to see exactly where the bleeding is arising; analgesic cartridge with epinephrine 1:50,000 or 1:100,000; disposable needles, aspirating syringe; tweezers; gauze packs; curved mosquito hemostat and straight mosquito hemostat; ¼" iodoform gauze; iodoform wax and dispenser; bone wax; medication; and disposable syringe and disposable needle.

It goes without saying that in order to control bleeding the clinician must be able to visualize clearly the exact spot the bleeding is coming from. This means *adequate suction, adequate lighting,* and *adequate anesthesia* to manipulate the tissue. With strict adherence to the above basic concepts and principles, and with this minimum amount of armamentarium, one should approach a bleeding problem with utmost confidence. While there are many and varied causes for bleeding, too numerous to go into in detail, the treatment for all is basically the same. Most often the problem arises from a faulty isolation of the bleeding structure and inability to visualize the bleeding area, poor cooperation of the patient, inadequate preparation of the clinician prior to the operation, or an incomplete armamentarium to implement the above procedures.

It is by no means the intent of the author to ignore or belittle the significance of the *psyche* of the patient, who more often than not is extremely fearful and apprehensive of the slightest amount of innocent bleeding. It may become necessary to sedate these patients in order to maintain a state of equanimity, or to even bring the normal physiologic blood pressure back to the point where adequate hemostasis can be accomplished. Sometimes it is necessary to employ the use of devices such as an ice bag merely to keep a patient immobile and inactive until the bleeding is arrested. Many people feel that there is more usefulness in an ice bag for this purpose than the cooling effect applied to the face. It is extremely important for the clinician to project an air of assurance and confidence that the bleeding is of no consequence and can be arrested simply without any complication.

MANAGEMENT OF SPECIFIC PROBLEMS

Hemophilia

Hemophilia, a disease transmitted by a recessive sex-linked character appearing in many males but transmitted by females, is a problem known to the patient from infancy and not apt to be overlooked in any history. The management of this patient is perhaps one of the most trying that the clinician has to encounter, for despite all modern methods this condition can be extremely difficult to manage, and on occasion will terminate fatally.

Prior to surgery there must be a thorough blood work-up, transfusions, the use of injectable fibrinogen with the factors that are missing in the patient, splints made, and antihemophilic globulin given as indicated. It is essential to keep the surgery to a minimum and conservative. A flap should *not* be used if it is at all possible to avoid it. Any compromise with surgical technique in order to avoid bleeding or trauma would be prudent judgment. Many clinicians have advanced theories, from the use of rubber bands to very radical transfusion schemes, for the prevention of bleeding from the extraction of a tooth in a patient with this disease. When patients with any severe bleeding dyscrasias present, close cooperation between the patient's physician or hematologist and the dental practitioner should be maintained throughout the entire course and management. Most clinicians feel that these patients should only be operated upon in the hospital where supervision for the immediate postoperative period is available.

An outstanding record of success in the treatment of hemophiliacs on an outpatient basis for dental extractions was reported by Mulkey.[10] Briefly, this procedure consists of transfusing the patient with a deficient factor level up to 20 per cent on the day of the surgery. The tooth is extracted as soon as possible after this infusion. The local analgesic is administered by periradicular infusion in the four quadrants around the root. The tooth is removed atraumatically without using a mucoperiosteal flap. After the removal, a piece of Surgicel,* dusted with bovine thrombin,** is placed in the apical portion of the root socket. Sutures are *not* used unless it is necessary to mobilize a flap for the removal of the tooth. An initial dose of epsilon-aminocaproic acid (EACA)† is given immediately after the extraction. This is used to prevent lysis of the initial clot. An initial dose of 5 gm for adults or 2.5 gm for children is used. Subsequent doses of half that amount are given every six hours around the clock for 10 days.

The post extraction diet is extremely important, and for the first 24 hours nothing is taken except a syrup containing the EACA. For the next 48 hours, limited amounts of cold, clear liquids (no dairy products) are consumed. After 72 hours, for the next week, foods with the consistency of applesauce or malted milk are allowed. Chewing of food is not permitted.

Daily contact with the patient is maintained. If bleeding persists, necessitating replacement therapy, then dietary control resumes with a clear liquid for an additional 10 days. Using this technique, Mulkey reports only 5 of 207 patients had to be hospitalized subsequent to the initial procedure.

Surgery for Patients on Anticoagulant Therapy

There is a vast difference of opinion among authorities as to the prothrombin time or level that should be attained prior to surgery. For a long time it was felt that a prothrombin time of 75 per cent might precipitate dangerous episodes of thomboembolic phenomena. The American Heart Association in 1963 recommended that a patient should be brought up to the level of 50 per cent higher than his maintenance level, or one and one-half times the maintenance level, for surgery. In the author's opinion this is a far better approach for everyday dentoalveolar surgery, and to my knowledge there have been no serious complications from operating upon patients at this level. These patients, of course, should have every advantage of the mechanical and topical hemostatic treatment instituted following surgery, and it is essential that they be closely observed for six to eight hours postoperatively. Surgicel should be used routinely on all these patients. Any severe bleeding from a patient on anticoagulants can be reversed with vitamin K. This, again, should be done *only* with the consultation of the patient's physician, as vitamin K may keep the prothrombin level elevated for a period of two weeks or longer.

Many clinicians seem to have an inherent fear of attempting surgical procedures on patients who are on anticoagulant therapy. This seems to be based on superstition rather than fact. It has been the experience of the author that patients who need anticoagulant therapy for the most part seem to have a greater tendency to clot than the average patient to begin with, and therefore, in spite of the fact that they are on anticoagulants, exhibit an almost normal clotting phenomenon. I think a clinician need be more concerned about *elevating a prothrombin level too high* than operating on a patient with a prothrombin level low enough to create some minor bleeding problem. The

---

*Surgicel, Absorbable Hemostat, Johnson & Johnson, New Brunswick, NJ 08901.
**Thrombin, topical, bovine origin, Parlee Davsum, Detroit, MI 48232.
†Amicar, Epsilon-aminocaproic acid, Lederle Laboratories, Pearl River, NY 10965.

rationale for this opinion lies simply in the fact that a low prothrombin time can be elevated very easily by the administration of vitamin K and the bleeding arrested.

CLOT LYSIS

Phase 4 of the coagulation mechanism has been discussed previously. This deals with the inherent capacity for dissolving blood clots by the means of fibrinolysin that will attack fibrin and destroy the clot. *Streptokinase* is one substance that will activate this directly and cause the fibrinolysin to become active against the fibrin clot. The use of streptokinase with streptodornase, a product called Varidase, has been widely suggested for the use of dissolving clots and the dissolution of purulent inflammatory exudates containing fibrin. In the opinion of the author, much investigation is still needed in this field, and the effectiveness of these enzymes must be carefully evaluated. Some of the new enzymes that are of vegetable origin appear to be less allergenic than the previous enzymes of animal origin.

RÉSUMÉ

A simple yet practical explanation of the clotting mechanism has been presented which emphasized three systems: *hemostatic, coagulation* and *lysis*. All bleeding has to come from vessels that have been cut or ruptured. This initiates a stimulus from within the mesenchymal and epithelial parts of a vessel along with the platelets, setting in motion certain mechanisms which lead to the formation of a clot. In the normal patient this process proceeds rapidly and will terminate in the prompt arrest of bleeding, except when major vessels have been involved. The balance between the arrest of the clot formation and the resorption and lysis of the clot has been shown to be a delicate mechanism that can be altered by various drugs, physiologically induced problems and inherent defects in both the coagulation and lysis systems.

A most important and frequently stressed point is the prior evaluation of the patient with an adequate and substantiated medical history and physical examination. When a significant or unusual condition is elicited by the evaluation that has been outlined, a clinician is obliged to obtain the necessary and relevant laboratory tests prior to proceeding with any further treatment. If he feels he does not want to do this, the patient should be referred to a colleague for this laboratory evaluation.

An outline for screening simple hemorrhagic problems elicited in a history has been presented. These can be ordered by the practitioner from a competent laboratory, the results of which are interpreted by the clinician as normal or abnormal. In the absence of abnormal findings with this screening laboratory outline, the clinician can be 90 per cent sure of proceeding without difficulty. Should there be any abnormal findings in the initial screening procedure, the *patient should then be referred to a competent internist or hematologist* for a more sophisticated and complete laboratory evaluation and work-up before treatment is attempted.

The types of problems and modalities of treating each of these problems have been discussed in detail. The systemic and topical agents available for the everyday clinician's use have been described, and specific indications for their use under various conditions have been discussed. The management of specific problems such as hemophilia and blood dyscrasias and major bleeding from large arteries has been presented for those rare emergencies that may occur from either inadequate preoperative evaluation and work-up or unforeseen circumstances.

A current outline for management of the patient who is on anticoagulant therapy emphasizes the danger in taking patients off anticoagulants and raising the prothrombin level to a dangerous high because of a fear of operating upon patients with prothrombin levels of 1.5 times the maintenance dose, which, when proper care is exercised, can be quite safe and often highly advisable for a risk patient.

CONCLUSION

It is not the intent of this chapter to discuss in detail the involved defects of the hemostatic and coagulation mechanisms. The more interested reader is referred to the article on hemorrhagic disorders in Beeson and McDermott's *Textbook of Medicine* for an in-depth study and evaluation of these blood dyscrasias.[2] The intent here is to give the reader a simple, concise and inexpensive means of screening patients with some history of bleeding problems to prevent the occasional rare experience of the serious bleeder.

Throughout this chapter the emphasis has been on *prevention*: (1) prevention arising from the proper evaluation of a patient, (2) prevention based on the intelligent interpretation of laboratory and clinical findings, and (3) prevention based on the proper medical management cooperatively with a competent internist or hematologist, as well as (4) application of sound yet simple techniques in the immediate postoperative period.

It is the clinician's responsibility to detect from an adequate history and through the use of laboratory screening techniques not only the patient with mild and annoying problem bleeding tendencies, but also those that present with severe avitaminosis, hemorrhagic diseases and acquired or hereditary blood dyscrasias that can be life-threatening.

To be sure even the most competent diagnostic clinician today, using all the modern laboratory procedures available to him, realizes that there are many aspects of the blood-clotting mechanism that we do not yet understand. In spite of the most thorough preoperative evaluations, preventive measures, and meticulous surgery, bleeding problems are still going to arise. Any clinician has the responsibility to his patient for the successful completion and management of the complications arising from a procedure that he has undertaken.

The greatly simplified concept of the clotting mechanism and treatment modalities presented here should not create a false sense of security in the clinician; on the other hand, he should not hesitate to proceed if the outlined screening procedures, adequate history and reasonable care have been followed prior to a surgical procedure. For many years dental practitioners have been encountering and dealing successfully with the bleeding patient. It is a common everyday occurrence in clinical dentistry. It is hoped that the material presented in this chapter may be beneficial in renewing a simplified understanding of the current concepts of the bleeding mechanism, and in providing a practical everyday method of preventing or dealing with the bleeding problems that are occasionally encountered so as to be of benefit to both the clinician and the patient.

REFERENCES

1. Accepted Dental Remedies. American Dental Association, 1965, p. 146.
2. Beeson, P. B., and McDermott, W. (eds.): Textbook of Medicine. 13th ed. Philadelphia, W. B. Saunders Co., 1971, p. 1594.
3. Gamble, J. W.: Meeting of American Society for Oral Surgery. November 1964.
4. Goth, A.: Medical Pharmacology. St. Louis, C. V. Mosby Co., 1961, p. 317.
5. A Guide to Hospital Dental Procedure. American Dental Association, 1964, p. 115.
6. Lemkin, S. R., et al.: Aspirin-Induced Oral Bleeding: Correction with Platelet Transfusion. Journal of Oral Surgery, Vol. 37 #4, April 1974, p. 500.
7. Martin, E. W.: Hazards of Medication. Philadelphia, J. B. Lippincott Co., 1971, p. 19.
8. Martin, E. W.: Hazards of Medication. Philadelphia, J. B. Lippincott Co., 1971, p. 470.
9. Modell, W.: Drugs of Choice. 1966–1967. St. Louis, C. V. Mosby Co., 1966, p. 655.
10. Mulkey, T. F., Outpatient Treatment of Hemophiliacs for Dental Extractions. Journal of Oral Surgery, Vol. 34, May 1976, p. 430.
11. Owen, C.: The Diagnosis of Bleeding Disorders. Boston, Little, Brown & Co., 1969, p. 42.
12. Owen, C.: The Diagnosis of Bleeding Disorders. Boston, Little, Brown, & Co., 1969, p. 277.
13. Quick, A.: Bleeding Problems in Clinical Medicine. Philadelphia, W. B. Saunders Co., 1970, Ch. 2.
14. Quick, A.: Bleeding Problems in Clinical Medicine. Philadelphia, W. B. Saunders Co., 1970, pp. 28, 41.
15. Rossi, D. J.: Control of Hemorrhage in Exodontia and Oral Surgery. D. Clin. North America, July 1957, p. 352.
16. Royer, R. Q.: In, Textbook of Oral Surgery (Kruger, ed.). St. Louis, C. V. Mosby Co., 1959, p. 106.
17. Steiner, R. B. and Thompson, R. D. (ed.): Oral Surgery and Anesthesia. Philadelphia, W. B. Saunders Co., 1977, Ch 5.
18. Young, D.: Personal correspondence.

21 | INJURED ANTERIOR TEETH

ROBERT G. ANDREWS

INTRODUCTION

In the practice of dentistry, traumatic injuries[16] constitute one of the emergency situations that every clinician should be prepared to cope with at all times. What the practitioner does in regard to the immediate treatment of the injury may lead to a disfigurement or to a final result that leaves no physical or psychologic scar.

The incidence of injured anterior teeth in children varied from 4 to 13 per cent in surveys done in the United States, England, Japan, and New Zealand.[8]

The first procedure in treatment is for the practitioner, or the receptionist, to assure the parent that everything will be done for the child that it is possible to do. The parent is told to bring the child into the office immediately, and if the tooth was avulsed to place it in a moistened tissue. If the parent is distraught and tends toward hysterical behavior, these feelings will be communicated to the child, thus increasing the problem of treatment. Of course, the opposite is also true: calm the distraught parent.

When the child arrives at the office and the doctor has had the opportunity to assess the problem, sedation should be considered. See chapters on *psychosedation.*

596

GENERAL PROCEDURES FOR ALL INJURIES[4]

1. The patient should be seen immediately. The sooner the injured teeth are treated, the better the prognosis.

2. A thorough history is very important. Insurance usually is involved, and of course there is always the possibility of legal action. The history should include the following:
   a. Time and place of the accident.
   b. How did the accident occur? Were other people involved?
   c. Has the tooth sustained any previous injury?
   d. Record any subjective complaints the patient may express.
   e. Are there any pertinent medical problems?

3. *Clinical examination.* Observe and record the following that are pertinent:
   a. Tenderness to percussion.
   b. Mobility.
   c. Color of the injured tooth in relation to the adjacent teeth.
   d. Crazing of the enamel.
   e. Extent of the coronal fracture.
   f. Extent of displacement.
   g. Soft tissue and alveolar process damage.
   h. Pulp test results on the injured teeth and those that are adjacent.
   i. Check occlusion.

4. *Radiographic examination.* This should include the obviously injured tooth, the adjacent teeth, and the opposing teeth. The following should be observed and recorded if pertinent:
   a. Size of the pulp in relation to the coronal fracture.
   b. Location of root fracture.
   c. Apical radiolucencies and width of the periodontal ligament.
   d. Amount of root formation. Is the apex open or closed?
   e. Immediate postoperative radiographs should be taken for the purpose of future comparison.

5. It is also the doctor's responsibility to be aware of any possible medical complications and to refer the patient for proper treatment. See the chapter on *physical evaluation and treatment modification.*

CLINICAL MANAGEMENT OF SPECIFIC PROBLEMS: PERMANENT DENTITION

The general treatment procedures outlined above are followed in all cases and will not be repeated for each problem.

Many classification systems have been utilized for the various types of injuries. These classifications have been invaluable aids in categorizing the various injuries to facilitate a modus operandi. However, in this chapter no classification will be attempted. The specific problem will be manifest by the clinical description.

Figure 21–1.   Figure 21–2.

Figure 21–1. Coronal fracture involving the enamel.
Figure 21–2. Coronal fracture involving the dentin. The right central incisor has a slight dentin involvement, the left central incisor shows extensive involvement of the dentin.

Coronal Fracture Involving the Enamel (Fig. 21–1)

When only the enamel is involved and it does not extend to the dentino-enamel junction, the treatment is to smooth off any sharp edges with a sandpaper disk. This will prevent laceration of the tongue or lips.

There should be a follow-up examination in approximately six weeks, consisting of radiographs, vitality test, and notation of any color change. The tooth may become nonvital and require root canal therapy. The parent should be advised of this possibility.

Figure 21–3.   Figure 21–4.

Figure 21–3. *Upper right central*, a fracture involving the enamel. *Upper left central*, a fracture involving the dentin.
Figure 21–4. Isolation of the teeth in preparation for an acid etch restoration.

Coronal Fracture Involving the Dentin (Figs. 21–2 to 21–11)

Slight. Exposure of the dentin from the dentino-enamel junction to within one-half the thickness of the dentin. The tooth may be sensitive to touch and thermal changes, such as air passing over the tooth. The exposed dentin may be treated by desensitizing with a solution of stannous fluoride, liquefied thymol, zinc chloride, or any other protein precipitant that will seal the dentinal tubules.

Any sharp enamel may then be smoothed off. Reapply the medicament of choice; then coat the tooth with a cavity liner.

Extensive. If the coronal fracture involves one-half or more of the dentin, it is necessary to treat the tooth in the following manner:
1. Local analgesia
2. Isolate the tooth with the rubber dam if possible.
3. Wash with warm saline solution to cleanse all surfaces.
4. Place CaOH on the exposed dentin to seal from the oral environment.
5. Cement a stainless steel crown, orthodontic band, plastic crown, or acid etch technique crown. It is important to protect the tooth from further trauma.
6. Check occlusion.
7. Follow up examination.

Coronal Fracture Involving the Pulp

Slight (Fig. 21–12). The mesial or distal pulp horn usually is exposed. There may be a slight amount of bleeding which stops quickly owing to the small area in which the clot needs to form. The following procedures should be observed in the treatment:
1. Local analgesia.
2. Isolate the tooth with the rubber dam.
3. Cleanse all surfaces of the tooth with sterile saline solution.
4. Place CaOH over the clot of the exposed pulp and the adjacent dentin.
5. Zinc oxide base over the CaOH.
6. Cement a stainless steel crown or other suitable protective restoration.
7. Follow up examination in 10 to 12 weeks with the following procedure:
   a. X-rays.
   b. Remove the protective crown. Test for vitality and observe the area of pulpal exposure for healing.
   c. If the tooth is vital but the bridging is not complete, establish new bleeding and repeat the procedures as in the initial treatment.
   d. Do endodontic therapy if the pulp is necrotic.

Gross exposure (Figs. 21–13 to 21–21). The pulp usually is hanging and bleeding. Follow these procedures in treatment:
1. Local analgesia.
2. Preparation of a sterile field as in the previous procedure.
3. Sterile pulpotomy kit is opened.
4. The entire coronal portion of the pulp is exposed by using a sterile bur to remove the enamel and dentin.
5. The coronal portion of the pulp is amputated. A pulpotomy is done instead of a pulp cap as there will be a smaller area of the pulp to heal.

Figure 21–5.   **Figure 21–6.**

Figure 21–5.   Placement of CaOH (Dycal) on the exposed dentin.
Figure 21–6.   Placement of the etching material.

6. Place CaOH on the clotted root portion of the pulp.
7. Zinc oxide eugenol base (Fig. 21–14).
8. Protective restoration (Fig. 21–15).
9. See Figures 21–16 to 21–21 for another case of gross pulpal exposure.

Figure 21–7.   **Figure 21–8.**

Figure 21–7.   Teeth after being etched.
Figure 21–8.   Placement of the unfilled resin.

Text continued on page 603

Figure 21-9.

Figure 21-10.

Figure 21-9. Building up the crown with filled resin.
Figure 21-10. The finished restorations.

Figure 21-11.

Figure 21-11. Stainless steel crown placed to protect the fractured incisor.

Figure 21-12.

Figure 21-13.

Figure 21-12. Coronal fracture involving the mesial pulp horn.
Figure 21-13. Coronal fracture involving a gross portion of the pulp.

Figure 21–14.   **Figure 21–15.**

Figure 21–14. The bulbous portion of the pulp has been removed, CaOH placed over the stumps, and sealed with a zinc oxide eugenol cement.
Figure 21–15. Protective restorations placed.

Figure 21–16.   **Figure 21–17.**

Figure 21–16. Coronal fracture of the tooth with gross pulpal involvement.
Figure 21–17. The fractured crown is well attached on the lingual.
Figure 21–18. Fragment is repositioned.

Figure 21–18.

Figure 21–19.

Figure 21–20.

Figure 21–19. A band has been cemented to the tooth to hold the fragment in position.
Figure 21–20. The tooth is opened from the lingual in order to do the CaOH pulpotomy.
Figure 21–21. Follow-up radiograph showing the calyx formation.

Figure 21–21.

Displacement (Figs. 21–22 to 21–30)

Labial or lingual version; intrusion or extrusion. Maintenance of vitality of the tooth will depend on the degree of laceration of the periapical blood vessels and the maintenance of circulation. Treat in the following manner:

1. Under local analgesia realign the tooth to its original position.
2. Splint the tooth with ligature wire, or by any other preferred and suitable means, to stabilize the tooth for six weeks. There should be no movement of the tooth to allow for regeneration of apical tissues and healing of the periodontal ligament and alveolar process.
3. It is advisable to keep close observation of this patient, as most of these pulps become necrotic after a period of time. The patient should be seen every two weeks for the first six weeks until the splint is removed. If the patient has any complaints of swelling, pain, or increased mobility, he should be seen immediately.
4. At the six-weeks examination: take radiographs; note any coronal color change; and do a vitalometer test. If there are any indications of necrosis, root canal therapy is indicated.

Text continued on page 606

Figure 21–22. Labial displacement of the left lateral incisor.

Figure 21–23. Orthodontic ligature wire for splinting.

Figure 21–24. Brass wire for splinting.

Figure 21–25.

Figure 21–26.

Figure 21–27.

Figure 21–25. Placement of orthodontic bands and segmental arch for stabilization.
Figure 21–26. Cold cure acrylic splint.
Figure 21–27. Orthodontic bands and segmental arch.

Figure 21–28.

Figure 21–29.

Figure 21–30.

Figure 21–28. Right central displaced. Left central fractured, porcelain jacket.
Figure 21–29. Right central repositioned.
Figure 21–30. Left central with a temporary crown. Right central stabilized with bands and arch.

Avulsion[10, 13, 14, 17–21] (Figs. 21–31 to 21–44)

When the parent calls to report the accident, the receptionist or the doctor should tell the parent to keep the tooth moist in a clean handkerchief or Kleenex. When the patient arrives, the tooth should be placed in sterile saline solution. Time is of the essence with this problem — not so much because of the clot forming in the socket but because there is an indication that the periodontal fibers that are left on the cementum may proliferate and form a normal attachment of the tooth to the alveolar bone when the tooth is replanted. Recent research indicates that those teeth replanted within 30 minutes have the best prognosis for success. These procedures should be followed:

1. Holding the avulsed tooth in the hand, wrapped in a sterile gauze saturated with sterile saline, do the root canal filling. Use a zinc oxide eugenol sealer and silver point. If root resorption should take place, it is

Figure 21–31. Right central and left lateral avulsed.

much easier to remove a silver point from the alveolar process than gutta-percha points.

2. Leave the periodontal fibers intact and cleanse any debris from the root surface by rinsing with sterile saline solution. Excessive manipulation of the root during root canal therapy will injure the periodontal fibers and should be avoided.

3. Local analgesia.

4. Remove the clot from the socket with a curet or by irrigation. Seat the tooth in the socket, aligning the tooth in its normal position (Fig. 21–32).

5. Splint the tooth with ligature wire, or by any other preferred and suitable means, to stabilize the tooth for six weeks (Fig. 21–18). There should be no mobility of the tooth so as to allow for possible regeneration of the periodontal ligament (Figs. 21–33 and 21–34).

6. Tetanus immunization by the patient's physician should be strongly considered with reimplantation of a contaminated tooth. The danger of serious allergic reactions from the use of tetanus antitoxin (TAT) can almost always be avoided by the use of a tetanus toxoid booster. Authoritative reports recommend the routine use of tetanus toxoid if the patient has had a regular immunization series *or* a toxoid booster

Figure 21–32. The teeth replanted.

Figure 21–33.

Figure 21–33. Cold cure acrylic splint cemented with a zinc oxide cement.

Figure 21–34. An arch bar used for the stabilizing of the avulsed or displaced teeth. (Courtesy, Dr. William Holmes.)

Figure 21–34.

within fifteen years.[1, 2] Few patients would not qualify under this new standard of immunization.

7. Follow up examination in six weeks when the splint is removed: Take radiographs and check for mobility. There should be no radiographic evidence of a thickened periodontal ligament, and no mobility of the tooth. The tooth should be radiographed periodically and watched for external resorption of the root. The average retention of the tooth is approximately ten years. The patient of course should be advised of the prognosis.

Text continued on page 612

Figure 21–35.

Figure 21–36.

Figure 21–37.

Figure 21–35. Radiograph of the alveolus.
Figure 21–36. Radiograph of the replanted tooth.
Figure 21–37. Splinted with orthodontic ligature wire.

Figure 21–38.

Figure 21–39.

Figure 21–38.   Radiograph of the splinted tooth.
Figure 21–39.   Eighteen months after the tooth was reimplanted, the root is completely resorbed.

Figure 21–40.

Figure 21–41.

Figure 21–42.

Figure 21–40.   Histologic section of a replanted tooth of a dog showing active root resorption.
Figure 21–41.   Upper left central avulsed, unable to replant. (Courtesy of Dr. Richard Mungo.)
Figure 21–42.   Teeth acid etched. (Courtesy of Dr. Richard Mungo.)

Figure 21–43. Plastic prosthetic tooth replacing avulsed tooth and bonded with a composite resin to the adacent teeth. (Courtesy of Dr. Richard Mungo.)

Root Fracture

Clinically there may be no evidence of injury. Radiographically it will reveal a fractured root (Fig. 21–44). The prognosis for success depends on the apposition of the fragments,[15] fragments immobilized by splinting, absence of infection, patient's good health, and the position of the fracture on the root. The more apical the fracture the better the prognosis for successful therapy. Treat the root fracture in the following manner:

1. Under local analgesia the fragments are placed in as close approximation as possible (Fig. 21–45).
2. Splint for six weeks.
3. Healing[6, 12] of the injury takes place by the laying down of cementum on the exposed dentin of both fragments. Connective tissue fills in the area between the two fragments. The union is termed a syndesmosis.

Figure 21–44.   Figure 21–45.

Figure 21–44. Radiograph of fractured root.
Figure 21–45. Radiograph of the fracture reduced and stabilized.

4. Periodic radiographs to observe the healing process. These teeth survive very well if the fracture does not communicate with the oral cavity.

Nonvital Teeth

If the patient presents himself with an acute abscess, as seen in Figures 21–46 and 21–47, the infection should be controlled by the use of antibiotics, and the tooth opened for drainage.

After the acute infection is under control, routine endodontic therapy should be instituted, or the tooth should be extracted.

In the case of a tooth that has turned dark (Fig. 21–48) due to pulpal necrosis, but that is not acutely infected, endodontic therapy should be instituted immediately. Should the apex be open (Fig. 21–49) due to incomplete root formation, obtain a sterile canal; then place CaOH in the canal to the apical end to stimulate the completion of the root.[11] Follow the progress of the root formation radiographically until it has closed. The root canal may then be filled (Fig. 21–50).

Figure 21–46. Acute cellulitis of the facial tissues arising from the necrotic tooth.

Figure 21–47. Acute infection of upper left central incisor.

Figure 21–48.

Figure 21–49.   **Figure 21–50.**

Figure 21–48.   The left central incisor has turned dark due to the necrotic pulp.
Figure 21–49.   Open apex of the necrotic central incisor.
Figure 21–50.   The root has completed its formation and the canal has been filled.

CLINICAL MANAGEMENT OF SPECIFIC PROBLEMS: PRIMARY DENTITION

I. Coronal fracture involving enamel (Fig. 21–51).
    A. Treat the same as the permanent tooth.
II. Coronal fracture involving the dentin (Fig. 21–52).
    A. Slight.
        1. Treat the same as the permanent tooth.
    B. Extensive.
        1. Treat the same as the permanent tooth except that no CaOH is placed on the dentin. Use a zinc oxide cement.
III. Coronal fracture involving the pulp (Fig. 21–53).
    A. Slight.
        1. Treat the same as the permanent tooth except that no CaOH is placed over the exposure.
        2. Place formocresol for five minutes; then cover with zinc oxide cement.
    B. Gross exposure.
        1. Do the pulpotomy in the same manner as for the permanent tooth, except that formocresol is placed over the pulpal stumps for five minutes.
IV. Displacement (Fig. 21–54).
    A. Same procedure as with the permanent dentition for labial or lingual displacement.
    B. Intruded tooth (Fig. 21–53). Allow the tooth to re-erupt.
    C. These teeth have to be watched closely. Most of them become necrotic.

Text continued on page 618

Figure 21–51.

Figure 21–52.

Figure 21–51.   Coronal fracture involving the enamel.
Figure 21–52.   Coronal fracture involving the dentin.
Figure 21–53.   Pulpal exposure of the right central incisor. Intrusion of the left central incisor.

Figure 21–53.

Figure 21–54.

Figure 21–55.

Figure 21–54.   Displacement of the maxillary central incisors.
Figure 21–55.   Upper right lateral incisor avulsed.
Figure 21–56.   Radiograph of the root fracture of the right central incisor.

Figure 21–56.

Figure 21–57.

Figure 21–57.   Left central incisor has turned dark from pulpal necrosis. Note the fistulous tract at the apex.
Figure 21–58.   Periapical radiolucency of the left central incisor as a result of the pulpal necrosis.

Figure 21–58.

Figure 21–59.

Figure 21–60.

Figure 21–61.

Figure 21–59. Upper right central, which is necrotic and the labial subperiosteal abscess.
Figure 21–60. Dissection to illustrate the close proximity of the apices of the primary anterior teeth to the developing crowns of the permanent teeth.
Figure 21–61. Hypoplasia of the upper left central incisor as a result of a necrotic primary central incisor.

Figure 21–62.

Figure 21–62. Dilaceration of the right central incisor as a result of an entruded primary incisor.

D. Damage to the permanent tooth may occur in the form of a dilaceration, hypoplasia or hypocalcification of the enamel.

V. Avulsion[22, 24] (Fig. 21–55).

  A. Leave out. Do not replant.

VI. Root Fracture (Fig. 21–56).

  A. Follow the same procedure as for the permanent tooth.

  B. The fragment will resorb with the eruption of the permanent tooth.

VII. Nonvital (Figs. 21–57 to 21–62).

  A. Extract the tooth.

  B. Antibiotic coverage may be necessary.

  C. The pathosis from the primary tooth may cause a hypoplastic or hypocalcific defect of the permanent tooth on the labial enamel surface.

REFERENCES

1. Am. J. Pub. Health, 52:1669, 1962.
2. Bennett, O. T.: Traumatized anterior teeth. Brit. Dent. J., 116:7–9, 52–55, 96–98, 1964.
3. Berman, R. G., and Buch, T. M.: Utilization of a splint combining bracket type orthodontic bands and cold curing resin for stabilization of replaced avulsed teeth. J.A.S.D.C., Nov.-Dec. 1973, pp. 51–54.
4. Bhatia, H., and Emmerson, C. C.: Management of injured anterior teeth. J. South. California Dent. Assoc., 24:165–169, 1961.
5. Binnie, W. H., and Rowe, A. H. R.: A histologic study of the periapical tissues of incompletely formed pulpless teeth filled with calcium hydroxide. J. Dent. R., 35(5):1110–1116, 1973.
6. Blackwood, H. J.: Tissue repair in intra-alveolar root fractures. Oral Surg. Oral Med. Oral Path., 12:360, 1959.
7. Buonocore, M. G., and Davilla, J.: Restoration of fractured anterior teeth with ultraviolet light polymerizing banding materials. J.A.D.A., 86:1349–1354, 1973.
8. Clarkson, B. H., et al.: The prevalence of injured teeth in English school children. J. Int. A.D.C., 4:21–24, 1973.
9. Cutright, D. E.: The reaction of permanent tooth buds to injury. Oral Surg., 32(5):832–838, 1971.
10. Deeb, E., Prietle, P. O., and McKenna, R. C.: Reimplantation of luxated teeth in humans. J. South. California Dent. Assoc., 33:194, 1965.
11. Frank, A. L.: Therapy for the divergent pulpless tooth by continued apical formation. J.A.D.A., 72:87–93, 1966.
12. Garner, A. F.: Trauma and fracture of teeth. South Carolina Dent. J., 20:8–12, 1962.
13. Groper, J. N., and Bernick, S.: A histologic study of the periodontium following replantation of teeth in the dog. J.A.S.D.C., Jan.-Feb. 1970, pp. 25–35.
14. Grossman, L. I., and Ship, I. I.: Survival rate of replanted teeth. J. Oral Surg. Oral Med. Oral Path., 6:899, 1970.
15. Ham, J. W. et al.: Induced apical closure of immature pulpless teeth in monkeys. Oral Surg., 33(3):438–449, 1972.
16. Hare, G. C.: Management of traumatic injuries to children's teeth. J. Canad. Dent. Assoc., 28:114, 1962.
17. Hargraves, J. A., and Davilla, J.: The traumatized tooth. Oral Surg., 34(3):502–514, 1972.
18. Kaqueler, J. C., and Massler, M.: Healing following tooth replantation. J.A.S.D.C., Sept.-Oct. 1969, pp. 303–314.
19. Lewis, T. M., and Dow, P. R.: Replantation of an avulsed permanent central incisor — a case report. J.A.S.D.C., 31:103, 1964.
20. Porteous, J. R.: Vital reimplantation of a maxillary central incisor: Report of a case. J.A.S.D.C., Nov.-Dec. 1972, pp. 11–13.
21. Rabinowitch, B. Z.: Replantation of teeth and management of root fractures. Dent. Clin. North Amer., July 1962, pp. 555–568.
22. Ravn, J. J.: Sequelae of acute mechanical traumata in the primary dentition. J.A.S.D.C., July 1968, pp. 281–289.

23. Sibley, L. C.: Management of root fractures. Oral Surg. Oral Med. Oral Path., 13(12):1475–1487, 1960.
24. Sud, V.: A study of the bacterial flora on the apical portion of the pulp canal of pulpless infected primary teeth. J.A.S.D.C., 4th quarter, 1956, pp. 225–228.
25. Torneck, Calvin P., et al.: Biologic effects of endodontic procedures on developing incisor teeth. Oral Surg., 35(4):541–544, 1973.
26. Via, W.: Enamel defects induced by trauma during tooth formation. Oral Roentgenol., 25(1):49–54, 1968.

Part 4

COMPLEMENTARY TOPICS

22

HOSPITAL DENTISTRY

HERBERT R. PACKARD

INTRODUCTION

Certain high-risk patients and those with behavioral/management di-
lemmas simply cannot be safely and comfortably treated in the office. For
this reason, this chapter on the fundamentals of hospital dentistry has been
included. Through hospitalization, we stress prevention of life-threatening
emergencies by adequate pain/anxiety control and by special medical management; and, should a life-threatening emergency develop during hospitalization, the utmost of treatment modalities, including the cardiac care unit
(CCU), are immediately at hand.

The practice of dentistry in the hospital provides a needed and frequently neglected service. It presents an opportunity for the dental practitioner to broaden the scope of health care delivery by serving the acute or
chronically ill, the mentally retarded, the elderly, and the physically or psychologically handicapped.

The relief of pain and suffering is the greatest contribution any health
professional can offer. Oral disease contributes to systemic disease; elimination of one relieves the other. Good oral health is a prerequisite to
proper nutrition, which, in turn, is directly related to sustaining life to the
highest degree, thereby contributing to the patient's general health and
happiness. To avoid the responsibility of providing this service is to ne-

glect an obligation; to accept this responsibility is to profit those individuals who receive the services of the dental practitioner.

This chapter is designed to help the student and practitioner acquire expertise in the ramifications of hospital dental practice. An understanding of how a hospital functions is essential to the efficient delivery of health care service in the acute and extended care facility.

VISITING THE PATIENT

It is customary and advisable to visit the patient in the hospital the evening before the scheduled procedure. The patient is in a strange place, in unfamiliar surroundings, and is apprehensive about the impending operation. It is recommended that the treatment plan be reviewed with the patient and that it be explained how he or she may expect to feel postoperatively. Reassurance is what the patient needs, and this only the doctor can provide.

For those patients being admitted in the morning for an afternoon procedure, it is virtually impossible to have any degree of contact prior to going to the surgical suite. If time permits, a brief visit 30 to 45 minutes beforehand will offer added assurance and present the practitioner with an opportunity to review the chart for completeness and accuracy.

OBLIGATION OF THE HOSPITAL

The hospital is the center for health care services to the public. It must meet certain state and local criteria to be licensed as an approved health facility. On a national level, the Joint Commission on Accreditation of Hospitals, a voluntary organization composed of representatives from the American College of Surgeons, American Hospital Association, American College of Physicians, and American Medical Association, will approve a hospital provided that it meets guidelines established by that commission. The American Dental Association is represented in an advisory capacity at this time.

AMERICAN DENTAL ASSOCIATION COUNCIL ON HOSPITAL DENTAL SERVICE

The House of Delegates of the American Dental Association in 1948 by their transactions established the Council on Hospital Dental Service. The current duties of the Council, as defined in the bylaws, read as follows:

1. To examine dental services in hospital and patient care units other than hospitals and to issue, in the name of the American Dental Association, certificates of approval to those institutions having dental services which meet the basic standards of requirements established by the House of Delegates.
2. To act on behalf of the Association in the inspection and improvement of dental services in hospitals and dental care units other than hospitals.

3. To study and make recommendations of the effective dental services in the community, state, regional and federal health care programs.

Currently, the Council utilizes the following documents as criteria for approval of dental services in hospitals:

1. *Guidelines for Hospital Dental Services*
2. *Standards for Hospital Dental Services*
3. *Accreditation Manual for Hospitals, J.C.A.H.*

In addition, the Council utilizes the J.C.A.H. *Guidelines for the Formation of Medical Staff Bylaws, Rules and Regulations* as a guide only for recommendations for revisions of bylaws of hospitals.

Today, current and comprehensive medical staff bylaws have become extremely important in view of legal implications and regulations governing all aspects of the medical staff, including the professional medical and dental services. Now that membership on the medical staffs of hospitals has been extended to dental practitioners on a parity with physicians, with equal rights to vote and hold office, it mandates that medical staff bylaws, rules, and regulations be written to apply equally to both medical and dental doctors. The approval program of the Council is voluntary. In preparing for and conducting its evaluation activities, the Council assumes that individual institutions seeking approval and continued approval will adhere to Council standards and requests for progress reports regarding the correction of observed deficiencies of the dental service and of medical staff bylaws, rules and regulations.

In 1957, the American Dental Association requested official representation on the Joint Commission on Accreditation of Hospitals, and reaffirmed their directive in 1959. At its 1969 meeting, the Joint Commission agreed to establish a liaison committee in lieu of full membership for the A.D.A. In 1971, the A.D.A. House of Delegates, at the request of the Joint Commission, approved the appointment of an official Advisory Committee on Dentistry to the Joint Commission to replace the previously functioning liaison committee.

The American Dental Association continues to seek full corporate membership on the Joint Commission so the profession may assume its proper and rightful role in the Joint Commission's voluntary accreditation program.

JOINT COMMISSION ON ACCREDITATION OF HOSPITALS HISTORICAL REVIEW

The Joint Commission on Accreditation of Hospitals developed from the Hospital Standardization Program, which was established by the American College of Surgeons in 1918 to encourage the adoption of a uniform medical record format that would facilitate the accurate recording of the patient's clinical course. By 1951, the American College of Surgeons had determined that it was appropriate to search for ways to broaden the base of support for the accreditation program.

After the formative years, the standards were amended to reflect the intent of the American College of Surgeons to help the program keep abreast of the increasing sophistication and complexity of hospitals. Also in

1951, the College of Surgeons determined that it was appropriate to search for ways to broaden the base of support for the accreditation program. To accomplish this goal, and through a joint effort of North American medicine and hospitals, the founding sponsors of the Joint Commission were the American College of Surgeons, the American College of Physicians, the American Hospital Association, the American Medical Association, and the Canadian Medical Association. The Canadian Medical Association continued its participation in the Joint Commission until 1959, when the Canadian Council on Hospital Accreditation activated its own program.

In 1965, Public Law 89-97 (Medicare) was enacted. The impact of this legislation on hospitals, their financing, the management of their services to the people, and their standards of performance was greater than that of any other single factor. Written into the Medicare Act was the provision that the hospitals participating in that program were to maintain the level of patient care that had come to be recognized as the norm. The standards of the Joint Commission on Accreditation of Hospitals are specifically referred to in the law, and the conditions of participation for hospitals, subsequently promulgated and published by the Social Security Administration, reflected the 1965 standards of the Joint Commission.

The interested reader may review the hospital governing body standards in the reference library of any local hospital. He or she may also review standards for the medical staff and various hospital services.

REQUIREMENTS FOR MEMBERSHIP AND PRIVILEGES

Medical staff membership shall be limited to individuals who are fully licensed to practice medicine, and, in addition, those licensed to practice dentistry. These individuals, after having made a formal application, may be granted membership on the staff in accordance with its bylaws, rules, and regulations and with the bylaws of the hospital.

Clinical privileges granted to dental practitioners should be based on their training, experience, and demonstrated competence and judgment. The scope and extent of surgical procedures that each dental practitioner may perform must be specifically defined and recommended in the same manner as all other surgical privileges. Surgical procedures performed by dental practitioners shall be under the overall supervision of the chief of surgery. All dental patients must receive the same basic medical appraisal as patients admitted for other services. A physician member of the medical staff must be responsible for the care of any medical problems that may be present or that may arise during the patient's hospitalization.

ORGANIZATION OF MEDICAL STAFF

The medical staff organization must provide a framework within which the duties and functions of the medical staff can be carried out. The complexity of the organization will depend upon the size of the hospital and the scope of the activities of the medical staff.

Active Medical Staff

All hospitals must have an active medical staff that should deliver the preponderance of medical services within the hospital and should perform all significant organizational and administrative duties pertaining to the medical staff. Members of the active staff shall be eligible to vote and hold office.

Associate Medical Staff

There may be an associate medical staff, consisting of individuals who are being considered for advancement to the active staff. Members of this category must be appointed and assigned to departments and services in the same manner as are members of the active staff. Although they may not hold office, they may serve on some medical staff and hospital committees.

Courtesy Medical Staff

There may be a courtesy medical staff consisting of those practitioners eligible for staff membership who are given privileges to admit an occasional patient to the hospital. Courtesy staff members may neither vote nor hold office. Because the admission of patients to the hospital is an exercise of a privilege and therefore is accompanied by responsibility, admission of more than an occasional patient should require the practitioner to seek membership on the active medical staff.

Provisional Staff Status. Applicants approved for membership on the active, associate, or courtesy staff should serve an initial provisional staff appointment. During this appointment they must be assigned to department services, where their clinical competence and their ethical and moral conduct may be observed by (a) designated member(s) of the active medical staff, until such time as the probationary requirements established by the medical staff have been fulfilled.

Temporary Staff Privileges. Temporary clinical privileges, at the time of emergency or locum tenens, may be granted to a medical practitioner for a limited and stated period on the recommendations of the chief of the applicable department/service or of the president of the staff, and with the concurrence of the chief executive officer.

Temporary Privileges of an Applicant. Upon receipt of an application for medical staff membership from an appropriately licensed practitioner, the chief executive officer may, upon the basis of information then available, which may reasonably be relied upon as to the competence and ethical standing of the applicant, and with the written concurrence of the department chairman concerned and the chairman of the executive committee, grant temporary admitting and clinical privileges.

Special requirements of supervision and reporting may be imposed by the department chairman concerned on any practitioner granted temporary privileges. Temporary privileges shall be immediately terminated by the chief executive officer upon notice of any failure of practice in the ethical standards of delivering health care services.

Consulting Medical Staff

There may be a consulting medical staff consisting of practitioners of recognized professional ability who are not members of another category of the medical staff and who have signified willingness to accept appointment to the consulting staff. Members of the consulting staff may neither hold office nor vote.

Honorary Medical Staff

There may be an honorary medical staff consisting of former staff members, retired on emeritus, and of other practitioners of outstanding reputation whom the medical staff desires to honor. Those who are members of the honorary medical staff exclusively may neither vote nor hold office.

CLINICAL DEPARTMENTS

The medical staff is subdivided into various clinical departments, the chairperson of each department being the member of the active staff best qualified for the position.

Each department establishes policies for clinical privileges and patient care review.

COMMITTEES

The Executive Committee consists of the officers of the medical staff, chairpersons of each department, and one or more members at large. Various other committees are concerned with applicant credentials, hospital policy, adequacy of medical records, utilization review, drug utilization, and infection control.

PROCEDURE FOR APPOINTMENT AND REAPPOINTMENT

Application for Appointment

All applications for appointment to the medical staff shall be in writing, shall be signed by the applicant, and shall be submitted on a form prescribed by the governing body after consultation with the executive committee. Such an application can be secured through the administrator's office, which requires detailed information concerning the applicant's professional qualifications.

The applicant shall have the burden of producing adequate information for a proper evaluation of his or her competence, character, ethics, and other qualifications, and for resolving any doubts about such qualifications.

The completed application is submitted to the chief executive officer. After collecting the references and other material deemed pertinent, the administrator shall transmit the application and all supporting material to the Credentials Committee for evaluation.

Following review by the Credentials Committee, Executive Committee, and Hospital Governing Body, the application is accepted, rejected, or deferred. A rejected applicant may appeal the decision to the Executive Committee.

MEDICAL EVALUATION PRIOR TO HOSPITAL ADMISSION

It is the responsibility of the dental practitioner to determine the health status of the patient prior to admission. This begins with routine physical evaluation in the dental office, based upon the patient-completed medical history plus dialogue history as indicated, and routine physical examination (see Chapter 2). The practitioner will therefore have a good understanding of the patient's physical status (risk-factor orientation) at the time the decision for hospitalization is made. Consultation with the physician occurs at this time if indicated.

Hospital admission requires that a classic medical history and physical examination (see Chapter 3) be performed and recorded on official hospital forms by a physician who is a member of the medical staff. This may be done either immediately prior to admission or shortly thereafter.

That portion of the medical history and physical examination related to dental disease is the responsibility of the dental practitioner. For example, the chief complaint in the patient's words could be: toothache, wisdom tooth pain and swelling, need fillings and I'm afraid, bad health and need dental care, etc. The practitioner will then analyze this chief complaint in the history of the present illness, which is simply a logically developed story of the current dental disease. Justification for hospital admission will be made under this section, "History of Present Illness."

The dental practitioner is also responsible for recording a relevant history of the dental disease under Past History, including past hospital dental therapy, behavioral problems, and unfavorable experiences with prior dental care or practitioners.

That portion of the head and neck examination which makes up the classic physical examination, and which is within the expertise of the dental practitioner, is performed and recorded by the dental practitioner on the standard hospital form. Depending upon training and experience, this may be a complete head and neck examination or it may be limited to the oral cavity. It is urged that the oral examination be complete and not limited to a narrow presenting complaint. The brief notation "Dental caries" under oral examination is totally inadequate.

The patient's physician will complete the balance of the medical history and physical examination on the hospital form. If the dental practitioner is competent in areas of physical diagnosis beyond a routine dental history and oral examination, *and with the attending physician's concurrence*, it is perfectly proper to complete the form to the level of his or her particular expertise, including complete head and neck (ophthalmoscopic and otoscopic) and heart and lung examination. The physician will simply countersign the history and physical findings if in agreement, or may make pertinent initialed changes or additions.

At present, several thousand dental practitioners in the United States are expert in physical diagnosis. In the future, as dental health professionals gain more knowledge in physical evaluation and physical diagnosis through education and experience, it is probable that hospitals will accept an admission history and physical diagnosis completed solely by the dental practitioner.

The reader may wish to review the chapters on *physical evaluation* and *physical diagnosis*.

SCHEDULING THE OPERATIVE PROCEDURE

Scheduling the Patient

When the dental practitioner has performed the physical evaluation of the patient, he or she is now ready to schedule the proposed procedure. This is done by telephoning the operating room for a time and date. The person scheduling will usually request the name of the patient, age, name of the procedure, amount of time, and type of anesthetic desired.

In many hospitals, this will complete the scheduling procedure; however, in some, the practitioner will be referred to the Admitting Department to make arrangements for admission and accommodations. Be prepared to give the admitting clerk the following information:

1. Patient's full name.
2. Address.
3. Telephone number.
4. Insurance company (medical).
5. Age of patient and date of birth.
6. Name of medical doctor who will be performing the hospital-required classic medical history and physical examination.
7. Type of accommodations patient desires (private, semi-private or ward).
8. Admitting diagnosis.
9. Operative procedure.

Those patients who are scheduled for an early morning procedure should be admitted the night before to secure required laboratory tests and necessary chest x-ray, if indicated, and to allow adequate time for the anesthesiologist to visit the patient for evaluation and to write preanesthesia orders.

It is not uncommon to have early morning admissions (6:30 to 7:00 A.M.) for afternoon cases. The patient must be advised not to take any food or liquids after midnight prior to admission. To minimize delay in early morning admissions, preoperative laboratory tests and x-rays can be done the day before.

Many larger hospitals have established ambulatory care centers or outpatient departments within the hospital to which the patient may be admitted in the morning for a brief procedure under general anesthesia of approximately 20 to 30 minutes and then discharged in the afternoon after recovering from the effects of the anesthetic. Because of increasing hospital costs, this type of service is becoming most useful in the delivery of health care services.

Outpatient general anesthesia has been pioneered by dentistry over the past 100 years, and especially during the past 40 years. Cost savings to the patient are enormous.

Patient's Medical Doctor

After the patient has been scheduled and arrangements for admission have been made, the patient's physician should be contacted for a preoperative medical history and physical examination. This is a requirement of all hospitals to determine if the patient is an acceptable medical risk for the proposed operative procedure and anesthetic. The patient's medical practitioner will be responsible for any medical problems that may occur during the hospital stay. He or she will share the responsibility with the dental practitioner.

A personal telephone call to the patient's physician requesting assistance is made, and a tentative plan of treatment is discussed. If the dental practitioner has performed a complete physical evaluation, an intelligent and meaningful line of communication can be established.

In no case should the patient be advised to secure the service of the medical practitioner for a preoperative history and physical unless the dental practitioner has contacted the physician in advance. It is the practitioner's responsibility to secure this medical service and to make certain the report will be in the patient's chart at the time of admission or shortly thereafter. If not, the case will be canceled by the surgical supervisor.

Notifying the Patient

When all arrangements have been made for admission, the patient should be notified of the date and time of admission in addition to the date and time of the appointment with the medical practitioner for the preoperative physical diagnosis. It is not uncommon for the medical practitioner to examine the patient after admission the night before surgery. Most hospitals require that the preadmission physical diagnosis by the physician be completed within 24 to 48 hours prior to admission. In the majority of cases, the medical practitioner will not see the patient during the hospital stay unless a visit is indicated or a medical complication arises.

In the event the patient develops an upper respiratory infection or fever, the case should be canceled and rescheduled approximately two weeks after all symptoms have subsided.

PREOPERATIVE ORDERS

Admission orders must be placed on an order form provided by the hospital. They may be written at the hospital or delivered to the admissions office prior to the patient's admission. *It is not advisable to send them with the patient.*

The following should be considered in writing preadmission orders:

General Nursing Care

1. Privileges — *Ambulatory:* permits the patient to ambulate in his or her room or on the ward.

Bathroom privileges (BRP): restricts the patient to bed except to use the bathroom.

Bed rest: confines the patient to bed and he or she must use a bed pan.

2. Fluids — *NPO* (nothing by mouth): no fluids, no food.

Fluids ad lib: As desired.

Forced fluids: Nursing staff will encourage the patient to take the amount of fluids ordered.

3. Diet — *Regular:* Permits the patient to eat the menu served by the hospital for this particular day.

Soft: That which is pureed.

Full liquid: A liquid diet containing milk products.

Clear liquid: A liquid diet containing no milk products.

Special: This type is restricted and is usually requested by the patient's physician for a particular reason.
a. Low calorie.
b. Low sodium.
c. Ulcer or low residue.
d. Low fat.
e. High calorie and high protein.

Medications

1. Sleep (hypnotics) — Barbiturates, meprobamate, diazepam, etc.

2. Pain (narcotics) — Codeine, meperidine, acetaminophen, etc.

3. Antibiotics — Penicillin, erythromycin, etc.

4. Special medications as may be required by the patient's physician.

Laboratory

Requirements may vary from one hospital to another.

1. Blood tests
   a. CBC (complete blood count).
   b. Hematocrit or packed cell volume (also reported in a CBC).
   c. Hemoglobin (also reported in a CBC).

2. Urinalysis — Will report the following:
   a. Blood
   b. Glucose
   c. Protein
   d. Acetone
   e. Bacteria
   f. Density
   g. pH
   h. Casts
   i. Mucus
   j. Crystals

3. Special tests   It is not uncommon, when indicated by the patient's physician, to request special laboratory studies on admission; these may consist of the following:
   a. ECG (electrocardiogram)
   b. PBI (protein bound iodine)
   c. FBS (fasting blood sugar)
   d. BUN (blood urea nitrogen)
   e. Electrolyte panel
   f. SMA 12
   g. Prothrombin time
   h. Platelet count
   i. Bleeding and clotting time

X-ray

If an adult patient, 30 years or older, has not had a chest x-ray during the past year, consideration should be given to ordering a PA (posterioanterior) and left lateral film of the chest.

SAMPLE ADMISSION ORDERS

For Patients Admitted Night Before Procedure

1. Admit patient for operative dentistry
2. Treatment consent to be signed
3. CBC and urinalysis
4. PA and left lateral chest x-ray
5. Regular diet
6. Oral fluids ad lib
7. Full ambulation
8. History and physical on patient's chart

_____
Sign your name

For Patients Admitted Morning of Procedure

1. Admit for operative dentistry scheduled 1 p.m.
2. NPO stat.
3. Treatment consent signed
4. CBC and urinalysis
5. History and physical on patient's chart
6. Notify anesthesia department of patient's admission

_____
Sign your name

ANESTHETIST

The anesthesiologist, after reviewing the chart and interviewing the patient, will write orders for preoperative medications. An example of his or her orders for a healthy adult patient may consist of the following:

1. Nembutal 100 mg PO h.s.; may be repeated × 1 p.r.n.
2. NPO past midnight.

3. Nembutal 100 mg IM 6 a.m.
4. Demerol 100 mg IM 7 a.m.
5. Atropine 0.4 mg IM 7 a.m.
6. On call to operating room — 8 a.m.

Dosage and choice of medication will vary with the patient's age, weight, health, and general physical status. Elderly patients and children will, in the majority of cases, receive reduced dosages of premedication agents. The objective of the premedication drugs is to receive the patient in the operating room suite in a state of relaxation, free of apprehension and anxiety. When a patient comes to the operating room suite in a depressed state from the premedicating drugs there is an extra burden on the anesthetist, who must evaluate the patient for the anesthetic agents to be employed.

SURGICAL SUPERVISOR

The surgical supervisor is in charge of the surgical suite. She has the sole authority to cancel cases if, in her judgment, the patient's hospital chart is not complete and the standards of good hospital practice are not followed.

It is recommended that the dental practitioner meet with her several days in advance of the scheduled procedure to discuss the case in regards to special equipment and instruments that the practitioner will furnish and the supplies, materials, and instruments that the hospital is to furnish.

When there is a routine protocol established by the practitioner and the operating room personnel, a card index file is kept in his or her name which contains all of the necessary data to set up future cases.

ARMAMENTARIUM

In planning the case, a careful and detailed study should be given to selecting necessary instruments and supplies. It is not uncommon to take more than is required to complete the procedure. Judgment is related to experience, and after completing several cases and becoming adjusted to hospital practice needs will be amazingly minimized.

REVIEWING THE PATIENT'S CHART

In examining the chart, make certain the treatment consent has been signed by the patient and witness. In the case of a minor, the consent must be signed by a parent or legal guardian.

Examination of the nursing notes will indicate the hour-by-hour condition of the patient and any variation from normal.

Observe the admitting temperature, blood pressure, pulse rate, and respiration. Variations from the normal may indicate an impending acute infection.

Check for the following:

1. Have the orders been properly recorded and signed by the appropriate person?

2. Is the history and physical in the chart?
3. Are the laboratory reports in the chart and are the tests within normal limits? If there are any questions or doubts, consult with the patient's physician or the anesthesiologist.

REPORTING TO OPERATING ROOM

The practitioner should present at the operating room suite 15 to 20 minutes before the case is scheduled. This gives the operating room personnel time to sterilize instruments and allows the practitioner adequate time to change into appropriate surgical dress, to prepare for a surgical scrub, and to be ready to start the case on time. Tardiness leads to operating under tension, delaying cases that are to follow, and disrupting the surgical schedule for the day.

In the event of an unavoidable delay in starting the surgery on time, request that the hospital call your office so that your time can be rearranged to minimize the disruption of the normal schedule.

USE OF AUXILIARY PERSONNEL

Most hospitals will permit the assistance of auxiliary dental personnel, particularly in operative dental procedures not involving the cutting of soft tissues. They may be reluctant to permit the assistance of these personnel in surgical procedures embracing a sterile technique such as oral surgery, periodontic, or endodontic procedures that involve root amputation or curettage unless the personnel have been thoroughly schooled in operating room protocol and sterile procedures.

It is suggested that the dental practitioner make the necessary arrangements with the surgical supervisor to give orientation instruction on operating room protocol to the practitioner's office personnel who will accompany him or her to the hospital and assist in the procedure.

If the practitioner intends to utilize operating room personnel for assistance, a few moments should be spent explaining the routine and how these persons may best serve. Most operating room personnel are highly intelligent and experienced, and will adapt in a short period of time to routine requirements.

OPERATING ROOM ATTIRE

The purpose of changing from street clothing into operating room attire is to help prevent contaminants from entering the surgical area of the hospital. There are strict rules governing the protocol and they are generally clearly marked: *"Do Not Enter Without Appropriate Dress."*

Remove all clothing and jewelry with the exception of underclothes, shoes and stockings.

Appropriate operating room attire consists of:

1. Scrub shirt tucked into scrub pants.
2. Protective shoe covers.

3. Scrub hat or hood. The hood should be worn by all doctors with long hair and beards.
4. Mask. In selecting a suitable mask, make certain it is comfortable and adjusted over the bridge of the nose to prevent fogging of the glasses — not so tight around the head and neck as to create discomfort or restrict breathing.

SCRUBBING ROUTINE

Each hospital has its own rules for a scrubbing technique; these are generally posted in the scrub area and should be followed. Brushes or scrub sponges are available in sterile metal containers or packages. It is optional what the doctor chooses, and those in packages are usually impregnated with a liquid soap. There are also dispensers containing pHisoHex and Betadine soap.

Sterile Scrub. This procedure requires cleaning the fingernails with a file followed by a timed 10 minute scrub with a brush or suitable sponge and soap. Copious lathers should be maintained adding soap and water as necessary. A routine should be followed beginning with the fingers, nails, hands, wrists, and forearms to the elbows, never going from the elbows to the hand, but simultaneously from the right to the left hand.

At the completion of the sterile scrub, the brush or sponge is dropped into the sink with the practitioner having no physical contact with any part of the sink. The hands and arms should be thoroughly rinsed in running water with the elbows bent and the hands held under the nozzle, permitting the water to run from the hands over the arms to the elbows, one arm at a time. At no time should the doctor touch anything following his scrub. Elbows should remain bent with hands held above the waist, making certain that the hands or arms do not contact the clothing.

When the practitioner enters the operating room, the sterile nurse will hand him or her a towel with which to dry in the same order in which he or she scrubbed; hands, wrists, and arms. The towel, held away from the body to prevent contamination, should be dropped on the floor or handed to the circulating nurse. *At no time should the arms or hands be lowered below the practitioner's waist.*

Clean Scrub. In performing operative dentistry, a sterile technique is virtually impossible to maintain and is not required or necessary. The objective is to prevent contaminants from entering the operating room, via the practitioner, the assistant, the instruments, or supplies, which may create a health hazard to the patient or operating room personnel.

A clean scrub is accomplished in the same manner as a sterile scrub, but for a shorter period of time, approximately five minutes.

BASIC EQUIPMENT

It is not necessary to have a fully equipped dental suite in order to accomplish operative procedures in the hospital. Portable equipment that can be utilized in any operating room is desirable and will make scheduling more flexible.

The standard operating table is fully adjustable, allowing flexibility in positioning the patient for the convenience of the practitioner, assistant, and anesthetist.

Basic equipment may include:

1. Portable high-speed air turbine attached to a constant adjustable source of pressure such as a nitrogen tank.
2. Portable x-ray (optional).
3. Large Mayo stands for instruments.
4. Portable cabinet with required supplies for restorations, impressions, etc.
5. Suction and water available for hospital central supply. Additional equipment and supplies can be added as the need arises.

GOWNING AND GLOVING

The operating room team will consist of the surgeon, an assistant or scrub nurse, a circulating nurse (who must be a registered nurse), and the anesthetist.

Oral surgery, periodontal surgery, and other cutting procedures on intraoral soft tissues should be performed using a sterile technique to avoid endangering the patient's cardiovascular or respiratory system by cross-contamination. The operator and assistant in addition to wearing a mask and head dress should be gowned and gloved in sterile attire. The assistant or scrub nurse will gown and glove in the appropriate manner and then assist the practitioner into his or her attire.

The practitioner and assistant should be particularly careful to prevent contamination of themselves by coming in contact with unsterile areas, equipment, instruments, or supplies. The arms should never be lower than the waist; the area below the waist is considered to be contaminated even in sterile attire.

Procedures that embrace restorative dentistry and general operative techniques only require a clean procedure and do not necessitate the use of a sterile gown or gloves. If permissible, and with concurrence of the surgical supervisor and anesthetist, those in the operating room need not wear face masks.

PREPARING THE PATIENT

Preparation of the patient is an important and integral step in following a safe technique for performing the services necessary in the completion of a treatment plan.

The anesthetist will deliver the anesthetic agents intravenously or will employ an endotracheal tube for the administration of inhalation gases. He or she will monitor the patient throughout the procedure by measuring blood pressure, pulse rate, respirations, and temperature and may utilize a cardioscope or other means of monitoring. The circulating nurse will prep the patient's face by appropriate means depending on the type of operative procedure to be performed.

Draping the patient for a sterile procedure requires correct placement of sterile towels and drapes from the head to the feet by the surgeon and the assistant.

In a clean procedure, sterile drapes about the face and chest are all that are necessary for general operative treatment. Care must be taken at all times to protect the patient's eyes from foreign bodies and contamination.

The patient's oropharynx must be protected from foreign body contamination by the use of a throat pack. This is accomplished by placement of a rubber bite block of appropriate size; aspiration of the oral cavity, pharynx, and hypopharyx with a tonsil suction; and placing a moist pharyngeal pack, care being taken not to occlude the endotracheal tube. Placement of a rubber dam is optional and is by choice of the operator.

COMPLETION OF THE OPERATIVE PROCEDURE

At the completion of the operation, the oral cavity should be cleansed of all foreign matter and irrigated with sterile water or saline solution and suctioned. The throat pack should be gently removed with care to prevent injury of the pharyngeal tissues. A cloverleaf retractor or mouth mirror can be utilized to depress the tongue adequately to permit inspection of the posterior pharynx and hypopharynx for any foreign material or mucus that may obstruct the airway. Foreign material should be removed with tonsil suction.

The anesthetist will now prepare the patient for transferring to the postanesthetic recovery area. He or she may extubate the patient by removing the endotracheal tube and insert a nasopharyngeal or oral airway. In many cases, the endotracheal tube is not removed until after the patient has been admitted to the recovery area.

Before the patient is removed from the operating room table to a cart, the vital signs are checked by evaluating the blood pressure, pulse rate, and breathing without assistance from the anesthetist, and the airway is checked to ensure that it is not obstructed.

RECOVERY ROOM

The postanesthetic room, also known as the recovery room, is staffed by trained personnel who monitor the patient's vital signs during the recovery period from the anesthetic. This observation may vary from an hour to several hours, depending on the patient's physical status and ability to metabolize the anesthetic agents and drugs.

Before the patient is released from the postanesthetic recovery area, vital signs, such as blood pressure, pulse rate, and respiration, must remain stabilized and within normal limits.

On rare occasions, it may be necessary to transfer the patient from the postanesthetic recovery area to the intensive care unit for closer observation and monitoring. Patients who may require intensive care may be those with severe cardiovascular, bronchopulmonary, or endocrine disease.

POSTOPERATIVE ORDERS

Postoperative orders should be written and dated immediately following the operative procedure. They should be labeled "Postoperative Orders," keeping in mind they automatically *cancel all previous orders* written on the patient.

In addition to the dental practitioner's postoperative instructions for control of the patient, it is necessary to rewrite any verbal or written orders of the patient's physician for laboratory tests, medications, or special instructions that may be requested postoperatively. If there are any questions or doubts, the physician should be contacted for advice.

When writing postoperative instructions to be carried out for the patient, it is advisable to develop them in an orderly sequence to cover (1) nursing care, (2) diet and (3) medications.

It is not uncommon for the patient to experience nausea following a general anesthetic, usually triggered by oral nourishment the day of the operative procedure. Nausea can frequently be prevented by withholding oral nourishment until the effects of the anesthetic medications have terminated.

To prevent the patient from becoming dehydrated, intravenous fluids may be given until such time that the patient can tolerate oral nourishment without problems.

Sample postoperative orders for a healthy adult patient may consist of the following, keeping in mind they must be altered by dosage of medication or fluid amount for a child or elderly patient, health status and weight:

Postoperative Orders (Example)

1. Vital signs until alert.
2. Bed rest with side rails and head elevated 20 degrees.
3. Oral suction prn.
4. Vaseline to the lips.
5. Continuous ice packs to right and left side of face (for traumatic extraoral or intraoral surgery).
6. May ambulate starting in a.m.
7. NPO today.
8. 1000 cc 5% dextrose/lactate of Ringer's solution q6h. Discontinue after bottle #2.
9. Clear liquid diet starting with breakfast in a.m.
10. Oral fluids ad lib starting at completion of IV fluids.
11. Demerol 50–75 mg IM q3–4h prn pain.
12. Tigan 200 mg IM q6h prn nausea.
13. Valium 10 mg hs, prn. May repeat × 1.

_____

Sign your name

OPERATIVE NOTE

The operative note is a brief résumé of the operation, written by the practitioner on the progress sheet summarizing what was done for the patient.

It need not be in detail, as this will be accomplished in the operative report.

An example of an operative note for a procedure involving the placement of restorations, crown preparations, impressions, and prophylaxis is as follows:

Operative Note

Anesthesia: General with endotracheal intubation.

Operation: 1. Dental prophylaxis with subgingival scaling of all maxillary and mandibular teeth.
              2. Cavity preparations and placement of alloy restorations in 12 maxillary and mandibular bicuspids and molars.
              3. Crown preparations and impressions of the right and left maxillary cuspids.

There were no complications incidental to the procedure. Patient to recovery room in a satisfactory postoperative condition.

_____
Sign your name

OPERATIVE REPORT

The operative report is a dictated, detailed, step by step record of the total operative procedure. It should be developed in an orderly sequence of what was done for the patient. It is advisable to dictate the report at the earliest and most convenient time following the operation and to list the events in the sequence followed in the operating room. This report is an important document which is directed to several areas, for example:

1. Preoperative diagnosis: Dental caries.
2. Postoperative diagnosis: Dental caries.
3. Operation: (Dental restorations, crown preparations and impressions, dental prophylaxis).
4. Anesthesia: General with endotracheal intubation.
5. Procedure: Detailed step by step procedure as it was performed in the operating room:
   a. Facial preparation, how it was accomplished.
   b. Draping the patient—method and type (sterile/clean).
   c. Preparation of the oral cavity—insertion of bite block, removing mucus from posterior pharynx and placement of oropharyngeal pack.
   d. Prophylaxis and subgingival curettage of the maxillary and mandibular teeth.
   e. Placement of rubber dam, if applicable.
   f. Type of restoration, tooth and surface

        (teeth should be identified by name, not by number).

    g. Crown preparation, type, name of teeth, and impressions.

6. Cleansing the oral cavity, removal of throat pack, suctioning posterior pharynx and hypopharynx.
7. Extubation of patient by anesthetist.
8. Complication, if any. If not, indicate. Patient transported to postanesthetic room by whom?

The above information is basically the contents of an operative report. There is no hard and set rule for how the practitioner develops the report; however, it is necessary to include enough detailed information to render it easily understood by any person who may review it.

POSTOPERATIVE VISITS

The doctor should schedule visits so that they can be made during the morning and evening hours.

If a procedure is completed during the morning, a visit to the patient in the evening is necessary to evaluate the postoperative progress and recovery from the anesthetic. Review the chart with particular attention to the "vital signs graph," which plots the patient's pulse rate, blood pressure, temperature, and respirations.

The nursing notes will give the hour-by-hour condition of the patient on a 24 hour basis. In many hospitals the 7 AM to 3 PM shift will record in green ink, and the 11 PM to 7 AM shift will record in red ink. This may vary from hospital to hospital.

Patients completed in the afternoon do not necessarily require a postoperative visit until the following morning. In most cases, they will sleep throughout the day and prefer not to be disturbed. The nursing staff will advise by telephone of any unusual problems that may require the practitioner's attention.

Visitors should be kept to a minimum, namely immediate family. More than a few visitors to a patient who is recovering from an anesthetic will tend to exhaust the patient mentally and physically, requiring excessive and unnecessary medications for comfort.

I always advise the family to keep visits short and to limit them to no more than one or two people. If visiting privileges are being abused, which is frequently the case in young single adults, an order should be written for no visitors or visits should be limited to parents or immediate family.

The practitioner should record on the patient's progress sheet his or her observations concerning the patient's alertness, complaints, general appearance, and pertinent remarks from reviewing the nurses' notes and graphic chart, and his or her impression of the patient's overall condition.

Every visit requires a brief written remark in the chart on the patient's condition. In the event the patient's physician or the anesthetist visits the patient, they will in most cases leave a brief note on the progress sheet, possibly making suggestions or recommendations for follow-up care.

DISCHARGING THE PATIENT

Hospitals vary in their procedure for discharging patients; however, the usual routine is simple and requires:

1. A signed order written by the admitting practitioner.
2. Any special medications or instructions given to the patient, reported on the progress sheet.
3. A note written on the progress sheet and signed by the admitting practitioner that the patient is being released and any special instructions, if applicable, relative to diet, fluids, activities, and follow-up care in the practitioner's office.

The patient is generally released to a responsible person, either family or friend, who accompanies the patient home.

THE HOSPITAL CHART

The patient's hospital chart is a legal document which is protected by the hospital as an important personal health record. It cannot be removed from the hospital or duplicated in any form without the signed permission of the chief administrative officer or designee.

All records and health information are retained for instant recall in the event the patient is readmitted at some future date.

In larger hospitals, where storage of thousands of patients' records becomes a problem, they are destroyed following a specified period of time after being duplicated on microfilm. It is possible to duplicate a complete hospital chart in a matter of minutes from the microfilm if the necessity arises, or the chart can be reviewed by projecting the microfilm on a viewing screen.

When all reports have been transcribed and placed in the patient's hospital chart, the Medical Records Department will inform the practitioner if there is an incomplete record, which must be completed and signed in a specified period of time or admitting privileges will be suspended.

Hospital patient records are basically the same in all institutions; however, there may be slight variations in the development of a record as to structure and content.

TRAINING IN HOSPITAL DENTISTRY

Students and practitioners who are interested in expanding their services to include hospital dental practice should seek a formalized, structured course in orientation to the hospital. Those dental schools which have hospital affiliations may, through the cooperation of the medical staff and oral surgery service, formalize a program to fulfill the needs of the dental student and the general practitioner.

With the cooperation of state or local dental societies, a hospital could structure an excellent program of courses in hospital orientation for those practitioners in the local community interested in hospital dentistry.

Cardiopulmonary resuscitation (CPR) training is an important part of any educational program that deals with the delivery of health care services either in the office or hospital. Formalized six hour basic CPR certification courses should be taken by all health professionals. Arrangements can be made through local Heart Associations and the American Red Cross for approved courses by certified instructors.

COMMENT

While this chapter presents the fundamentals of hospital dentistry for the primary purpose of prevention and treatment of life-threatening emergencies in medically compromised patients, no claim is made for completeness — that must come with experience. Sufficient orientation is given here so that the practitioner will not feel inadequate upon first exposure.

Continuing education in hospital protocol will probably not be available on a structured local basis, but this should not be even a slight deterrent. Approach a dental or medical colleague who is a member of the local hospital medical staff, and accompany or assist that person through several operative cases. Should a dental practitioner not be active on staff, make it your business to meet a medical practitioner; the ideal would be an otorhinolaryngologist (ENT), for a tonsillectomy and adenoidectomy (T & A) presents many of the same constraints faced in dental treatment. The medical staff secretary can assist in identification of and introduction to the proper person.

After you have become familiar with the operating room, as an assistant, schedule a dental case or two, and ask your colleague to assist you. You will soon be a veteran, and will feel completely at ease in what was formerly an unknown and perhaps threatening environment. You will find that hospital dentistry is an exciting, rewarding, and enormously fulfilling facet of comprehensive dental care.

Fully 10 per cent of dental patients are of geriatric age (65 and over), often presenting moderate to high risk medical disease and severe management problems. The contemporary dental doctor is capable of offering comprehensive dental care to such patients because he or she has mastered physical evaluation, treatment modification, and comprehensive pain/anxiety control, including the option of hospitalization when indicated.

Dental practitioners sometimes state that they are not part of the mainstream of health care delivery. It is suggested that you *join* the mainstream by developing competence in hospital dentistry. The trip does not hurt and is very satisfying. It also fulfills a moral obligation to those patients who otherwise would not have the opportunity to enjoy total health care.

REFERENCES

1. American Dental Association: Historical Review in Establishment of The Council on Hospital Dental Service; Transactions of the House of Delegates: Self-Study Report, April 1975.
2. Krupp, M. A., and Chatton, M. J.: Current Medical Diagnosis and Treatment 1979. Los Altos, California, Lange Medical Publishers, 1979.
3. Dunphy, J. E., and Botsworth, T. W.: Physical Evaluation of the Surgical Patient, 3rd ed., Philadelphia, W. B. Saunders Co., 1975.
4. Joint Commission on Accreditation of Hospitals: Accreditation Manual for Hospitals 1970.
5. Nillson, L., and Lindberg, J.: Behold Man; A Photographic Journey of Discovery Inside the Body. (English translation) Boston, Little, Brown and Co., 1974.

23

MAXILLOFACIAL PAIN

GUSTAV O. KRUGER
and
DONALD C. REYNOLDS

INTRODUCTION

One of the most important and time-honored functions of the dental profession is the alleviation of pain. The emphasis on preventive dentistry and maintenance of ideal function in the dental structures has diminished to some extent the need for diagnosis and treatment of pain. Most patients do not have pain, and among those patients who do are many who are able to identify a painful tooth because of proprioceptive nerve involvement.

In many other painful conditions the cause is not readily apparent and often not fully understood. It is easy to say that patients with these conditions can be referred to the neurologist for diagnosis and treatment, and it is true that many painful conditions are eliminated in this manner. However, such referral must be preceded by a careful screening by the dental practitioner in order to eliminate oral causes. There are two reasons: first, referral to specialists is expensive in time and money for the patient; second, if the cause lies in the end-organs of the mouth the patient will be referred back to the dental clinican with considerations in other fields eliminated, but with the primary cause still undiagnosed.

The dental doctor is the expert in the oral structures. He or she must fulfill his or her responsibility by careful analysis of each painful situation and by constant reading. The patient with ill-defined facial pain that is constant and severe is an altogether miserable individual who should be treated as an emergency. Some pains are extremely difficult to diagnose, even by a group of experts in the various specialties — for example, the differentiation of a trigeminal neuralgia and a tumor of the base of the skull. An occasional patient with obscure caries has almost been subjected to intracranial section of the fifth cranial nerve because either he was not referred to dental examination or the cause was not found on routine dental examination.[11] Atypical referred pain originating from derangements of the temporomandibular joint has been misdiagnosed and mistreated for years. It is an oversimplification to state that the main function of the dental practitioner in the field of facial pain is to eliminate the oral structures from consideration., However, if the clinician can refer the patient to the neurologist with a firm and exact statement that no oral structure is involved in the pain, a tremendous contribution has been rendered.

If a primary function of the dental doctor is the elimination of oral structures from consideration, his secondary function is the recognition or suspicion of disease in nearby areas as the cause for facial pain. Nasopharyngeal and other tumors, sinusitis, ear pain, elongated styloid processes, vascular problems in the head and neck, and primary nerve problems such as idiopathic trigeminal and glossopharyngeal neuralgia represent sources of pain which must be eliminated in the search. The problem here is to refrain from removing teeth or surgically exploring the area of referred pain in the jaw, even though the patient points to a specific area. Frequently a patient with an atypical facial neuralgia is referred from one specialist to another, losing one tooth after another, until he becomes a dental cripple in addition to his burden of unrelenting pain.

Psychologic factors can greatly influence the physiologic aspects of pain. The placebo, an innocuous sugar pill made in the form of its corresponding drug and given to the patient as that drug, often can control various pains, including true organic pain, in 33 per cent of all patients. On the other hand a minor discomfort can be distorted into severe pain in a psychologically disturbed patient. The apparently normal individual who develops chronic nervous exhaustion can magnify small disorders or create imaginary ones that are difficult to identify without considering the whole person. The hysterical individual usually has no organic cause for pain, although he may be subjected to surgical biopsy and tooth removal before his psychologic condition is recognized as the cause for his pain. Unfortunately, hysterical people also can have nasopharyngeal tumors or temporomandibular joint derangements, and missing the diagnosis in such situations is disastrous.

Pain is a warning sign to protect against organic disease. Continual, nonending pain can do inestimable damage to a patient's body and mind—it can change an extroverted person into a hermit and a strong man into a coward. There is no one more grateful than the patient whose pain has been relieved. This is an essential and gratifying, although time-consuming, aspect of our work.

HISTORY

It has been said that the patient will tell you the diagnosis if you listen well enough. We are constantly amazed at the excellent diagnoses made by medical trainees in an area about which they know little. They need help to pinpoint the diagnosis, but grossly they are not far off. This is because they have elicited a thorough, orderly history of the ailment. In the field of facial pain the history is more important than the physical examination for two reasons: first, because the nerves themselves are not accessible to direct vision; second, because pain is a subjective phenomenon which the patient must describe.

The wrong approach to the history is to see the patient on a routine half-hour appointment and listen to his complaint while standing next to the chair, hands washed, ready to obtain entrance into the mouth as soon as the patient stops talking. Further snatches of history are obtained by direct questioning during the course of palpation and percussion. With this method, the practitioner tries to recognize and label the condition immediately, and failing to do so, he is unwilling to consider the condition or the patient further except as a nuisance.

The proper approach is to schedule the visit at a time when there is no pressure from a subsequent appointment — preferably at the end of the day. Usually an hour or more is required in order to establish rapport with the patient and to obtain a good history. The patient cannot be asked to pay the fee the office could earn in restorative dentistry during this time, so perhaps the last regular half-hour appointment plus a half-hour or more of "free time" can be used to relieve the feeling of pressure from the practitioner, allowing him to concentrate his thoughts on the patient's problem.

The history should be taken while the practitioner is in a sitting position, preferably away from his usual operating stool, which is too close. The objective is to obtain a complete written history and description of the ailment. The history should be chronological, and it is divided into several portions: chief complaint, present illness, past history, and family history. However, no patient will give the history in chronological order. Order is obtained later, after the patient has finished, although with practice it can be done during the recital. The patient should be allowed to talk on, without guidance or interruption from the practitioner, and certainly without leading questions. Later, specific questions may be asked, but the session is not guided by the practitioner at the early stages. Just having someone at last listen sympathetically to his story provides a sense of accomplishment and well-being to the patient.

The chief complaint is the first portion of the history. It should be written in the patient's own words for later review — not translated into professional terms. For instance, if he says that his lip hurts and then talks for 15 minutes about the terrible dental operations he has had and the automobile accident that injured his neck, it is surprising to note later that he complained of lip pain originally.

The present illness includes both subjective and objective experiences encountered by the patient, including operations, professional examinations and advice, and subsequent trauma related to the problem. It should be recorded in chronological order. The average patient will give an intelligent and fairly comprehensive account of the problem to a sympathetic, unhurried practitioner who listens carefully. The garrulous patient occasionally needs to be guided back to the main stream of thought; the close-lipped patient needs to be drawn out for further details. The extreme extrovert will neglect to recount pertinent points of the history because he may feel that they are not important enough to bother the practitioner— he does not want to be labeled a complainer. These points have to be explored later. The aged will neglect significant points for the same reason, besides those points that are forgotten because of faulty memory. If there is any possibility that age or general incompetence might preclude obtaining a significant history, a second history is obtained later from relatives or friends.

The past history of the patient should be recorded as it relates to the problem at hand. In facial pain a complete medical history often is not relevant, but major operations, illness, and therapy should be made known for their possible impact on the present illness. The family history can be significant in less clear-cut facial pains, particularly in the determination of psychoneurotic tendencies, low pain threshold, some headache problems, and in familial disturbances.

The elicitation of a proper history takes considerable skill and more restraint. After a period in which the patient has had opportunity to recount everything he knows about his affliction, as well as to reveal his emotional make-up and his attitudes about his problem, the healing professions, and society in general, and the practitioner has been able to ask questions that eliminate some syndromes and bring others into consideration, it is time for the laying on of hands in physical examination. During this session the practitioner has had time to reflect on possible diagnoses, and to make mental note of certain specific facets of examination which he wishes to emphasize. The physical examination can then be accomplished in more intelligent and orderly fashion.

PHYSICAL EXAMINATION

The examination is directed toward the symptoms at hand. However, the localized neurologic examination should be part of a complete physical examination and a mental appraisal of the patient, neither of which will be described here. Pain is the first manifestation of many systemic disorders — anemia, vascular disease, neoplasms, toxemias, and metabolic disorders are a few examples — which can be overlooked by a narrow approach. Psychosomatic problems can be suspected by giving attention to the mental make-up of the patient. At times, visceral symptoms may be masked by psychogenic problems. Because there is a relationship between constitutional factors, specific personality patterns, and certain disease syndromes and entities[2] the mental state can be evaluated for personality changes. Appearance and general behavior, the stream of mental activity, the emotional state, content of thought, and intellectual resources are considered.

The general appearance of the patient is noted for such signs as fever, pain, distress, or loss of weight. His posture, general motor behavior, and any unusual mannerisms are noted. The face is noted for flushing, sweating, tears, and for manifestations of anxiety, pain, or depression. Restlessness or lethargy and depression or elation are noted.

The temperature, pulse, and blood pressure are noted. The exposed skin is examined for manifestations of endocrine disturbances. The mucous membranes are noted for color, moisture, or dryness, and for evidences of general or specific pathologic processes. The teeth are examined clinically and radiographically to eliminate the dental structures from consideration in nonspecific pain. Extremely careful evaluation is needed to uncover such obscure causes of pain as a toothbrush bristle embedded in the periodontal membrane parallel to the palatal root of a maxillary molar, or a split tooth. Vitality tests are necessary. Evaluation or elimination of the occlusion as a factor in nonspecific pain often necessitates making casts. The lips, gingival tissues, and tongue are examined, and signs of vitamin deficiency are noted.

The total extent of the pain is mapped to differentiate circumscribed pains from others that are vague. All points of tenderness are examined. The structures are palpated, percussed, and inspected both for disease that can be visualized and for suspected deep-seated disease. The effect of pressure or touch on the area is noted, and a trigger zone is looked for. The muscles of the jaws, mouth, and neck are palpated for spasm and for pressure points that are primarily or secondarily related to the pain. The general nerve distribution of the area is related to the symptoms, if possible. Surrounding structures that may cause pain are examined clinically or radiographically —sinuses, nose and throat, and neck — in order to determine if further detailed examination by specialists is warranted.

The sensory examination is carried out to discover whether areas of absent, decreased, exaggerated, perverted, or delayed sensations are present. One should determine the quality and type of sensation that is affected, the quantity and degree of involvement, and the localization of the change. If abnormalities of sensation are present, the examiner should attempt to determine their type and character, intensity, exact distribution and periodicity, as well as factors that accentuate and decrease them. It should be recalled that pain and numbness may exist together, as they do in the thalamic syndrome.[2]

Sensory sensations are classified by De Jong (after Sherrington) as exteroceptive, proprioceptive, and interoceptive sensations based on the location of the end-organs and the type of stimuli they mediate:

1. The exteroceptive (outside) sensations are those which arise from sense organs in the skin and mucous membranes and respond to external agents and changes in the environment. There are three major types: pain, temperature (hot and cold), and tactile (light touch).[2] The simplest method of testing superficial pain sensation is the use of a common pin. The patient has his eyes closed and alternately the point and the head of the pin are pressed on the tissue. The patient is asked to respond "sharp" or "dull." Temperature sensation is tested with cold or warm metal tubes. There is evidence that the paths for pain and temperature are distinct within the common tract. Tactile sensations are tested with a wisp of cotton or a camel's hair brush. This will reveal anesthesia, hypesthesia, and hyperesthesia. One should observe not only the recognition and discrimination of pain, temperature, and tactile stimulation, but also accuracy in localization. Responses on the two sides of the body should be compared.

2. The proprioceptive sensations are those which arise from the deeper tissues of the body, principally from the muscles, ligaments, bones, tendons, and joints. Deep pain is tested by squeezing the muscles or tendons, or by pressure on those nerves which lie close to the surface. Deep pain is more diffuse and less well localized than superficial pain.

3. The interoceptive sensations are the general visceral sensations which arise from the internal organs. Pain, spasm, or distention in the viscus characteristically results in a feeling of fullness. Visceral pain is often vaguely localized or diffuse, but is described by the patient as being deep-seated. In addition to the pain experienced in the viscus itself, there may be an associated somatic pain of reflex origin known as referred pain. This is referred to the skin and subcutaneous tissues, and the area in which it is felt may be hyperalgesic to stimulation. In general, visceral sensations cannot be adequately evaluated by the routine neurologic examination procedures.

In summation, sensory changes including pain may occur in the presence of lesions at various levels of the nervous system. The end-organs (sensory receptors) are involved in dental pulp disease, skin and mucous membrane burns and abrasions, etc. Local infiltration with an analgesic agent will cause anesthesia. The peripheral nerves may be involved by an irritating lesion to create pain that is either constant or lancinating. The sensory examination is important in the diagnosis of peripheral nerve injuries. Pain in the distribution of a single nerve or a group of nerves can be relieved by injection with procaine or alcohol or by section of the nerves involved.

Disease in the dorsal root ganglia or corresponding ganglia of the cranial nerves gives rise to severe, lancinating pain. The nerve roots are in reality a part of the peripheral nerves, since they constitute a part of the same neuron. The pain may be either constant or intermittent, but it is often sharp and stabbing in character. It is increased by movement, coughing, or straining. It is relieved by injection or section of the roots. If the nerve root is sectioned between the cerebrospinal axis and the ganglion, as in the retrogasserian neurectomy done for the relief of pain in tic douloureux, there will be no regeneration of the nerve. Lesions of the spinal cord and brain stem may cause pain or paresthesias. Lesions of the thalamus may be associated with pain of "central" orgin, usually associated with a diminution of various sensory modalities on the opposite side of the body without loss of sensation.

Examination of the cranial nerves is important to eliminate central involvements which usually affect several adjacent nerves because of their proximity of origin at the base of the brain. Each cranial nerve is examined quickly by standard procedures. The trigeminal nerve, in which we are most interested, is the most important sensory nerve of the face. It is important to find the location of the lesion—peripherally, at the ganglion, or above the ganglion. If the lesion is above or at the gasserian ganglion, all three divisions are affected; if it is peripheral to the ganglion, only isolated divisions are involved. In irritative lesions there is usually hyperesthesia of the peripheral branches at their points of exit from the skull, as at the supraorbital, infraorbital, mental, and alveolar foramina, and stimulation of these "trigger zones" may precipitate attacks of pain. If the painful lesion is a neuritis, there will be evidences of sensory change in the involved branches, together with reflex changes such as absence of the corneal, sneeze, or palatal reflexes. If, however, it is a neuralgia, the routine examination will fail to show objective evidence of nerve involvement.[2]

The end-organs such as the structures of the oral cavity are examined minutely in order to identify the cause of pain or to eliminate them from consideration. Usually, the diffusion of pain from such sources is confined initially to one division, but in cases of severe pain there is radiation over the branches of the other main divisions. There may be associated spasm and contraction of muscles.

MAJOR NEURALGIAS

Trigeminal neuralgia (tic douloureux) is one of the most excruciating pains known to man. This neuralgia can affect any branch of the trigeminal nerve, but most commonly it is associated with the maxillary and mandibular divisions. Because of the location of the pain the dental practitioner is consulted in the belief that the pain may be of dental origin.

The etiology of trigeminal neuralgia is unknown. It is most commonly seen in middle-aged and older people, and in women slightly more often than men. The symptoms are characteristic. The pain is unilateral following the distribution of one division of the fifth cranial nerve, although more than one division may be involved. The pain is described as burning and bright close to the surface with deeper shooting pains which parallel the lower border of the mandible. A trigger zone is characteristic. Touching this zone in any way will trigger the pain, and the patient will go to extremes not to allow anything to come in contact with this area. Trigeminal neuralgia can be an early or late manifestation of multiple sclerosis.

Glossopharyngeal neuralgia is an uncommon disease in which the patient experiences pain similar to that of trigeminal neuralgia. The pain is triggered by eating and swallowing. It is experienced over the distribution of the glossopharyngeal nerve, but does not necessarily extend over the entire distribution of this nerve. Sometimes it is difficult to differentiate glossopharyngeal neuralgia from trigeminal neuralgia, except that the pain is triggered in the throat rather than in the face. Otalgia may be confused with it because pain in the ear may be one of the initial complaints. A trigger zone is present in the tonsillar region or pharynx. Touching this area will trigger the paroxysmal pains associated with the disease, and cocainization will relieve the pain temporarily.

MINOR NEURALGIAS

Over the years many pain syndromes affecting the facial and oral tissues have been described. Some syndromes have a classic anatomic background; others have a pseudoanatomic background ascribed to them by their discoverer but not recognized by present-day neurologists; others have various physiologic backgrounds that are not primarily neurologic. Complicating these factors is the ever-present problem of psychoneurosis which may overlay the main problem or may be the main problem in itself. Treatment in many cases of facial neuralgia is empirical and unsatisfactory.

Whereas the initial work in this field was the separation of as many entities as possible in order to better understand and treat them, recent attempts have been made to combine them in broad categories.

Sphenopalatine (Sluder's) Neuralgia

Perhaps the best known of the minor neuralgias, sphenopalatine neuralgia is an example of the second category. It is recognized and treated by various clinicians, and yet the neurologist is hesitant to ascribe to it a true neurologic background.

It is considered as a headache of the lower half of the head. The patient describes a severe pain centered deep in the base of the orbit, root of the nose, upper jaw and teeth, temple and zygoma, extending to a point about two inches back of the mastoid process, to the neck, shoulder, back, and arm. The diagnosis as well as the treatment consists of anesthetizing the sphenopalatine ganglion by needle injection through an extra-oral second division (trigeminal) approach or through the posterior palatine canal, or by cocainization of the nasal mucosa at the posterior tip of the middle turbinate. Relief of pain is noted immediately. Cure is obtained also by applying a 2 per cent solution of silver nitrate or a 0.5 per cent solution of formaldehyde to the same part of the nose. Sectioning of the nerve is not necessary. Apparently the cycle of impulses is interrupted by the agents, and the pain disappears. Recently, a vasodilation has been recognized in this disease.

Vidian Neuralgia

This is an example of the anatomic variety of pain. It is a rare condition. Pain is characterized by nocturnal, unilateral severe attacks in the nose, face, eye, ear, head, neck, and shoulder. Some people have associated it with nasal (especially sphenoid) sinusitis. It cannot be caused by external stimulation, and is not relieved by opiates. Pain in the ear is a characteristic part of this syndrome, which differentiates it clinically from sphenopalatine neuralgia.

Occipital Neuralgia

Pain begins in the back of the neck below the mastoid process, extends over the side of the head, and often centers behind the eye of the side affected. It is usually unilateral. A procaine block of the second cervical nerve will establish the diagnosis. Cervical traction, nerve injection, or sectioning of the sensory roots of the second and third cervical nerves constitutes the treatment.[1]

Postherpetic Ophthalmic Neuralgia

The supraorbital and supratrochlear branches of the ophthalmic division of the trigeminal nerve are infected by a virus. The pain is excruciating and disabling, and satisfactory treatment is difficult.[1]

Geniculate Neuralgia

"It is rare indeed to encounter a case in which severe pain in the ear and deep structures of the face is the result of disease of the geniculate ganglion, or sensory ganglion of the seventh cranial nerve."[1] This is an involvement of the sensory system of the facial nerve, which usually is not involved in pain. Only a few cases have been authenticated, all of which have been given permanent relief by intracranial section of the nerve of Wrisberg.

Two forms of geniculate neuralgia are recognized — the otalgic form with pain in the ear, and the prosopalgic form with pain deep in the face,

principally in the posterior orbital, palatal, and nasal regions. Deep geniculate prosopalgia is usually accompanied by geniculate otalgia. More recent
observers, however, on the basis of pathologic studies, doubt the presence
of a true geniculate ganglionitis.[2]

Superior Laryngeal Neuralgia

Swallowing or touching the trigger zone with an instrument produces
paroxysms of lancinating pain that extend from the side of the thyroid cartilage or from the trigger area in the pyriform sinus to the angle of the jaw
and occasionally to the ear. This entity may represent an incomplete form
of glossopharyngeal neuralgia. Sectioning of the nerve in the neck is the
treatment.[1]

Tympanic Neuralgia

This is a true incomplete form of glossopharyngeal neuralgia.[1]

Histamine Cephalgia

The patient has intermittent attacks of severe pain, redness, and congestion on one side of the face, with a complete remission and freedom from
symptoms between attacks. He experiences severe pain on one side of the
head ("suicide headache"), eyes, nose, upper jaw, and occasionally lower jaw.
The side affected becomes red, the nose becomes congested on one side, and
the eye waters. The pain does not follow the anatomic distribution of any
cranial nerve. There are no trigger zones. The attack lasts less than an hour,
and occurs several times in 24 hours — usually during sleep, forcing the
patient to get out of bed.

Diagnosis is established by injecting a small amount of histamine into the
tissues. At one time Horton felt that he could cure the affliction by desensitizing the patient to histamine. Progressively large amounts of histamine were
injected until no further exacerbation took place.[12] Unfortunately, the cure did
not last and everyone, including Horton, has abandoned this treatment. The
pain is vascular in origin, associated with dilation of vessels.

Periodic Migrainous Neuralgia

This condition is characterized by attacks, often lasting several weeks, in
which the patient has, once or three times daily, severe attacks of intense
burning pain in and around one eye, persisting one-half to two hours. It often
recurs consistently at the same time of day or night. It is often associated with
watering of the eye and blocking of the nose on the affected side. It is
controlled by prophylactic ergotamine tartrate.[5]

The trend now is to consider many of the nonanatomic facial neuralgias as
"migraine equivalents" related to the true migraine headache.[10, 15] The basis
for pain in migraine is extreme vasodilation of the arteries of the brain. The

migraine equivalents respond to small amounts of ergotamine tartrate, and therefore this drug and similar ones are used for treatment.

Many of the atypical facial neuralgias may be reflex in origin, and others may be secondary to disorders of autonomic nervous system origin; the pain is deep, boring, and agonizing, and it is not relieved by section of the trigeminal nerve. Those of psychogenic origin are called psychalgias.[2]

Other conditions simulate some of the pains described. For instance, the neuroma has not been given enough consideration in jaw pain. Almost all other nerves of the body form neuromas when injured or broken.[6] Every time an extraction takes place one or more peripheral nerves is torn apart. Sometimes the extracted tooth shows a portion of nerve filament extending 1 to 2 mm. beyond the apex. Presumably the nerve filament separates in the middle of the pulp canal in other instances, and the nerve becomes enveloped in the healing granulation tissue of the socket and later in bone. A neuroma developing on a filament of this size would be quite small and difficult to see in a surgical procedure. We do not have neuromas of this size to show, and so this idea is unsubstantiated. There is no reason for a neuroma not to develop on dental nerves, however. Robinson and Slavkin[19] have reported ten cases of intraoral neuromas. Seven cases were visible, palpable tumors; three were not visible until dissected from bone.

For persistent pain in an edentulous area for which no cause can be found, we have taken a bone biopsy of the apical region one chisel-width square. Some patients are relieved of the pain. We are not sure whether relief is afforded because of removal of a pathologic lesion (neuroma) that cannot be demonstrated histologically or radiographically, or because "something was done," which these people want. The laying on of hands would cure the psychoneurotic patient, but the cure would be temporary only, since a similar pain would develop within months or years in the jaw or elsewhere. If the patient did not return to the original practitioner for reevaluation, the continuity of the record would be lost.

The psychiatrist places atypical facial pains in a special category together with intractable headache, backache, and pain in phantom extremities. He feels that an emotional disturbance underlies them. Patients may be entirely undisturbed by their symptoms during the psychiatric interview, but they suddenly complain and grasp at the affected part when their important conflicting personal relationship comes into focus during the interview; at such a time, if the examiner is not distracted by the symptom and pushes on with further inquiries it is common to obtain a clear description of the conflict occurring between the patient and the person of importance to him who has come under discussion.

To summarize the treatment of minor neuralgias, first a complete history of the affliction is elicited, including a map of the subjective extent of the pain. Areas of hypalgesia or anesthesia are tested, and a map is made of objective findings. If indicated, anesthesia blocks are made in an attempt to eliminate the pain. Pain not associated with an end-organ that responds to anesthesia is referred to the neurologist. Response to a test dose of ergotamine tartrate identifies the condition as a migraine equivalent. If no overt evidence of psychoneurosis exists, and the pain is continuous and not consistent with the usual end-organ pain (tooth, sinus, nerve pressure), a bone biopsy can be made. If the mouth and its structures can be eliminated from consideration as the cause of pain (and this is difficult at times), the patient can be referred to the neurologist for evaluation of the entire nerve tract, including the spinal and intracranial connections, and a psychiatric study.

NEURITIS AND OTHER PAINFUL CONDITIONS

Dental Pain

As mentioned earlier, the prime responsibility of the dental practitioner is the alleviation and prevention of dental pain. Dental pain is one of the most severe pains experienced by man, and we have all seen it reduce capable adult patients to ineffective individuals.

Pulpal disease is the most common cause of dental pain. Such pain can vary from intermittent discomfort caused by changes in temperature to a constant throbbing that makes a minute seem like an eternity. Pulpal disease can be divided into three phases: hyperemia, pulpitis, and pulpal necrosis.

In *hyperemia* there is a vascular response caused by an external stimulus such as dental caries or trauma. The patient usually becomes aware of this situation when drinking cold fluids or eating ice cream causes pain. The pain can be severe, but usually subsides shortly after stimulation. In hyperemia the tissues are hypersensitive and give an exaggerated response to any stimulation such as heat, cold, and electric pulp testing. Hyperemia can be a reversible reaction if the cause is removed.

Pulpitis is an inflammatory disease which begins as mild inflammation and may progress to pulpal necrosis. The pain is sharp and throbbing. In the early stages there is moderate pain which is decreased by heat and increased by cold applications. As the condition progresses the opposite reaction is seen in which heat may cause pain. In the early stages of pulpitis there is an above normal response to stimulation as is seen in hyperemia, but as the inflammation progresses the responses decrease, and as necrosis is approached there is less reaction to external stimuli.

Pulpal necrosis is death of the pulpal tissue. The pain experienced by the patient is caused by fluid pressure. If there is no place for this fluid to escape, heat produces pain and cold relieves pain because of relative pressure changes. The tooth does not respond to electric pulp testing, except in the case of the multirooted tooth in which the pulp in one root may have maintained its blood and nerve supply. Care must be taken that a positive electric response is not obtained by transmitting the current to adjacent teeth by metal restorations or to the surrounding gingivae.

Roentgenograms and careful visual examination with a mirror and explorer are invaluable in looking for causes of pulpal disease. Since there are no proprioceptive nerve fibers within the dental pulp, it is often impossible for the patient to localize the pain in a particular tooth. Only when deeper tissues (bone, periodontal membrane) are involved can localization be assured. Heat, ice, and the electric pulp tester should be used to localize and confirm the diagnosis of pulpal disease.

Fractured or cracked teeth can be the source of vague dental pain. The diagnosis of a fractured tooth is difficult to make, for many times the fracture line cannot be seen. The patient may give a history of pain upon biting down on a hard object, but often the onset of pain cannot be associated with any known trauma. Usually the pain is experienced when chewing or when drinking hot or cold liquids. Since only the tooth itself is involved, often the patient cannot localize the pain. Posterior teeth, especially maxillary bicuspids, are most commonly involved. Patients with well developed, plunging cusps are most often affected. The fracture line usually runs in a mesiodistal direction, separating the buccal and lingual segments of the tooth. When a fractured tooth is suspected, the teeth in the area should be dried and examined for a linear crack in the enamel. Each cusp should be percussed in all directions. An explorer should be used in all pits and fissures to wedge fracture segments apart. If restorations are present, an instrument should be wedged between the tooth structure and the filling material to see if a space can be created. Roentgenograms are of little value if the fracture line runs mesiodistally and fracture segments are not displaced enough to be seen on the film.

Patients with persistent dental pain should be examined for hidden *caries*. No matter how much care is taken when placing dental restorations, recurrent decay can occur. Even with good roentgenograms it is difficult to detect caries under existing restorations. Unfortunately, some of the cement bases and pulp capping materials are radiolucent and can be mistaken for caries under a restoration. Patients with obscure dental pain should have all questionable restorations (amalgams, inlays, crowns) removed before any surgical procedure is done.

Although *periodontal disease* in general is not usually noted as a source of acute dental pain, certain periodontal conditions can be painful. Periodontal pain can be differentiated from pulpal and other forms of dental pain by its character. This type of pain usually has a dull, gnawing nature as compared to the sharp, pulsating pain seen in pulpitis, because the inflammation is not confined in an unyielding pulp chamber. The most common form of periodontal pain is the acute periodontal abscess, which is associated with deep vertical periodontal pockets or trifurcation and bifurcation involvement of molar teeth. The gingiva in the area is red and edematous, and purulent material may be expressed with pressure. The pocket depth around each tooth should be measured with a periodontal probe. Roentgenograms will show vertical or horizontal bone loss in that area.

Acute necrotizing ulcerative gingivitis (Vincent's disease) is another periodontal problem that may be presented because of pain. This pain is a dull, burning one. The lower anterior region is most often involved, but it can occur anywhere in the mouth. Examination will show ulceration, loss of the interdental papillae, and redness of the marginal gingivae. This tissue is tender and will bleed easily when irritated. The breath has a characteristic fetid odor.

One of the most difficult periodontal problems to diagnose is the pain associated with a toothbrush bristle or other foreign object lodged in the periodontal structures. As in most cases of periodontal pain the patient can point out the painful area, but unless a fair amount of inflammation is present it is difficult to see the cause of the problem. An explorer should be used to go around the tooth carefully in the hope that the foreign object can be located. Since most foreign objects are radiolucent, roentgenograms are of little help. Unfortunately, the diagnosis is often made after the tooth has been removed and the culprit can be seen in the alveolar socket or clinging to the extracted tooth.

The postextraction *dry socket* is one of the most exasperating and severe forms of dental pain. The pain from a dry socket is constant, sharp, and radiating. Characteristically it begins on the third or fourth postoperative day. On examination the alveolar socket is filled with debris which, when removed by irrigation, reveals underlying exposed bone. This exposed bone is extremely painful.

Pericoronitis, or infection of the soft tissue around the crown of a partially erupted tooth, can be the cause of variable pain. Pericoronitis is most commonly seen in young adults during the eruption of a lower third molar, although it can be associated with any erupting tooth. The amount of pain varies with the severity of the infection. The pain may be well localized or it may radiate up toward the ear and down into the throat and neck in more severe cases. Often the maxillary third molar is one of the causative factors if it occludes on the soft tissue over the partially erupted lower third molar to cause tissue irritation and infection. The edema associated with infection and trauma compounds the problem, causing even more irritation as the teeth are closed together.

Pressure exerted on nerve bundles as they emerge from foramina can result in pain. This is seen when prosthetic appliances exert pressure on the palatal and mental nerves. The mental nerve is most commonly involved. As the alveolar process of the mandible is resorbed, the mental foramen assumes a more superior position and may even be seen on the crest of the ridge. The patient complains of inability to wear a lower denture because of pain over the distribution of the mental nerve during mastication. Pain in the maxilla, especially in the anterior region, may be caused by pressure on the incisive papilla. If the lower posterior teeth are missing and not replaced, the natural lower anterior teeth exert considerable pressure against the anterior portion of a maxillary denture.

Reports of retained root tips and impacted teeth causing neurologic problems have appeared in the literature quite often. Undoubtedly these entities have produced problems, but the number of root tips and impacted teeth that cause pain and neurologic problems is very small. Only after all other possible causes have been eliminated should they be considered.

Causalgia is a form of postextraction neuralgia that can occur two or three weeks after the surgery is performed. It is characterized by burning, throbbing pains ranging from a sharp, piercing type to a sensation of pins and needles, accompanied by a condition of general hyperesthesia and nervousness. The examining finger evokes pain over the socket area, but food does not trigger a response, suggesting an emotional basis for the pain. The patient usually is a tense, busy, efficient individual. There is no evidence of dry socket or inflammation in the area of surgery. The sympathetic nervous system has been implicated as well as the emotions. The only treatment seems to be a sympathetic talk with the patient in which less stress is recommended.[4]

Salivary Glands

Pain of salivary gland origin usually is moderate but increases at mealtime because of stimulation of the gland. The pain from the parotid is centered in the area of the gland, but it may radiate over the entire side of the face and neck as the pain and swelling increase at mealtime. Submaxillary gland pain radiates up toward the ear and downward into the neck. The patient may also experience pain such as that associated with "sore throat." The salivary glands themselves are tender to palpation.

Fractures

Fractures, especially of the mandible, may remain undiagnosed and cause pain. Because of the circumstances under which the trauma was received the patient may be reluctant to seek treatment until all signs of trauma are gone. The patient complains of inability to masticate solid foods and he may notice a slight change in occlusal relationships. Any changes in mandibular function, such as deviation of the jaw upon opening, should be noted. Radiographs of the painful area usually make the diagnosis obvious, but adequate radiographs must be made, and periapical views should be augmented by extraoral films.

Sinusitis

The pain from maxillary sinusitis can be confused with pain of dental origin. The pain involves the posterior teeth on the affected side, but one tooth may be slightly more sensitive than the others when they are percussed. The pain is constant, and it is increased by rapid movement of the head and by lowering the head. The pain can be relieved by lying down on the nonaffected side and allowing the purulent material to drain from the maxillary sinus. The relief is not immediate, but the pain will begin to subside in 30 minutes if drainage is possible. The infraorbital-zygomatic arch areas are tender on palpation. Swelling may occur in the soft tissues of the infra- and periorbital areas. Radiograms of the sinus (Waters view) will show cloudiness of the antrum on the affected side. Periapical radiograms usually are not sufficient to determine cloudiness of the antrum, but an impression may be formed which should be confirmed by a Waters view of the sinuses.

Styloid Process

The elongated styloid process has been associated with bizarre facial pain over the distribution of the third division of the trigeminal nerve. The pain is accentuated by chewing and by opening the mouth. The throat feels swollen, and the patient will swallow frequently in an attempt to alleviate this sensation. Palpation of the soft tissues mesial to the mandible in the tonsillar fossa area is painful, and the elongated styloid process may be felt as a hard, pointed, immobile object. Radiograms will show an elongated styloid process or calcification of the stylohyoid or stylomandibular ligament.[3]

Tongue

Glossodynia is one form of oral pain which has continued to baffle clinicians. Often no definite diagnosis can be reached and a psychoneurosis is suggested. The pain varies in intensity from patient to patient, but it usually is described as a burning one. The tongue should be examined carefully, and areas of redness, ulceration, or induration are noted. The teeth and prosthetic appliances are examined as possible sources of irritation. Local trauma and infection must be eliminated. Fungus infections of the tongue are seen following antibotic therapy and they can be the cause of a burning sensation in the infected area. Galvanic currents caused by dissimilar metals may cause irritation and pain in the tongue in the area contacting the metals. Referred pain from submaxillary salivary glands and temporomandibular joint disturbances may cause glossodynia. Certain systemic diseases such as pernicious anemia, Plummer-Vincent syndrome, and avitaminosis should be considered when no local cause is found.

Otalgia

Otalgia may produce symptoms of pain over one or more branches of the trigeminal nerve. The patient cannot determine from what exact area or teeth the pain arises. This type of pain can be baffling to the clinician because of the absence of disease in the area of pain. The patient usually will give a history of current or previous ear problems, and in a short time generally the pain will localize in the aural region.

Herpes Zoster

Herpes zoster of the trigeminal nerve is an infectious disease caused by a filterable virus.[9] The symptoms are marked by spontaneous pain of a burning and severe nature over the distribution of the nerve affected. There may be a mild systemic effect with malaise, headache, nausea, and low grade fever. The skin in the area affected may become erythematous, and in approximately three days small blisters will form on this base. At this time severe burning, sticking, and often unbearable pain are experienced. The ophthalmic division of the fifth nerve is most often involved. This is in contrast to trigeminal neuralgia, which most often affects the second and third divisions.

REFERRED PAIN

Referred pain is pain in a part other than that in which its cause is situated. It has not been explained satisfactorily. The peripheral connections apparently have nothing to do with reference of pain. Pain referred from a lower molar tooth to the ear is not mediated through the common trunk of the inferior alveolar and auriculotemporal nerves, according to Sicher.

"If the cervical sympathetic chain is exposed, and one pinches the superior cervical ganglion, or the first two thoracic white rami communicantes, or the sympathetic trunk as far up as the middle ganglion — or, if one stimulates electrically these different parts — one causes a short pain in the teeth of the lower jaw, in the mandible, and in the region of the temporomandibular articulation. Again, if the adventitia of the carotid bifurcation, or of the common carotid, is seized with forceps, the same pain is observed. If the capsule of the thyroid gland in front is pinched, the same pain appears. This is not intended to imply that all these nerves share in the innervation of the lower jaw and teeth, and intrude on the fifth cranial nerve area. One explanation is that stimulation of these nerves sets up certain vasomotor phenomena in these areas, and that in this manner facial pain may be brought about, although the trigeminal is not directly affected."[18]

The problem of referred pain in the head and neck is that such pain is not what it seems to be at first contact. A high degree of suspicion is necessary in order to achieve an accurate diagnosis. Pain which is felt in the teeth may not originate in the teeth at all, as illustrated above. Pulpal pain originating in the teeth, however, can be referred to various areas of the face and neck before involvement of the proprioceptive nerves in the periodontal membrane localizes the pain in the tooth.

Suspicion of pain referred to the jaws may be lifesaving to the patient. Coronary heart disease may be represented by pain in the angle of the jaw as its first symptom. In 40 per cent of patients with thyroiditis, preauricular pain is present.[7] Trotter's syndrome consists of neuralgic pain in the lower jaw, tongue and side of head, with middle ear deafness. The soft palate on the affected side is asymmetrical and shows defective mobility. The syndrome is caused by a carcinoma in the nasopharynx. Late in the disease trismus of the medial pterygoid muscle will prevent the patient from opening his mouth. However, the earliest symptoms are headaches on the affected side and middle ear deafness.

Muscle problems have been associated with orofacial pain.[17] Almost all of 24 patients with various orofacial pain problems, the largest group of which was 10 cases of atypical facialgia, had abnormal electromyograms. When electromyography of the temporalis, masseter, and digastric muscles was performed bilaterally, the most common findings were predominance, tetany, or both of one or more muscles, either ipsilateral or contralateral to the origin of pain.

Temporomandibular joint pain can be referred from the muscles of the head and neck to a completely normal articulation. Organic damage to the joint may result if the myofascial pain cycle is not interrupted, or the condition may be classed as psychosomatic.

In a classic article, Travell[16] demonstrated the presence of trigger areas in skeletal muscle in spasm, or in fascia, which refer pain to structures some distance away. Involuntary shortening of one or more of the muscles of mastication or certain neck muscles caused by noxious stimuli creates severe pain in the joint, along with eccentric position of the mandibular condyle, disorientation of jaw movements, and restricted opening of the mouth. The trigger areas must be demonstrated in the muscle.

"In a matter of minutes, local procedures directed at extinguishing trigger areas may abolish the hyperirritable stretch reflex and re-establish normal muscle length and function, even though movement has been painful and limited for months or years. Only a pathophysiologic disorder, analogous perhaps to the discharging focus of paroxysmal cardiac arrhythmia, could be immediately and permanently terminated by such procedures as ethyl chloride spray and local procaine infiltration, which have only transitory pharmacologic effects. Furthermore, biopsy of trigger areas has proved unrewarding. . . ."

Pain reference patterns to the teeth, jaws, and specific areas in the face and head have been mapped for each masticatory muscle as well as the trapezius and sternomastoid muscles. These patterns do not vary from patient to patient, and can be identified readily. Rapid needling of the muscle with procaine (0.25 to 0.5 per cent without epinephrine) may release intracellular potassium, which in turn blocks nerve conduction temporarily, or it may break up fibrous adhesions. Ethyl chloride spray without skin frosting is used for superficial muscles.

Referred pain from pulpitis of the teeth to other areas of the jaws and head has been well documented.[8] An early pulpitis, which is so recent that radiographic evidence of apical bone resorption has not occurred, is difficult to localize. Unerupted teeth, particularly third molars and canines, have given rise to unexplained head pains which have almost caused neurosurgeons to schedule the patient for a cranial operation before the correct dental diagnosis was made.

The intimate relationship of the nasal sinus and the teeth, especially the maxillary sinus, has caused sinus pain to be misinterpreted as dental pain and vice versa. In one study, intentionally rough cavity preparation without anesthesia was followed by severe pain in the same teeth when the nasal orifice of the maxillary sinus was stimulated later; such stimulation was painless when cavity preparations were made gently and under local analgesia.[13]

CENTRAL PAIN

In the back of the mind of the practitioner seeing patients who complain of vague facial and head pains should always be the possibility that these symptoms could arise from central tumors. The symptoms of brain tumors vary greatly and depend on the type of tumor involved and its position within the brain. It is beyond the scope of this article to describe the various types of brain tumors and their diagnosis, but some of the more common symptoms should be noted. Headache is a common symptom of brain tumor, but is not always present. The headache is likely to be constant, and has no specific characteristics. It is not relieved by mild analgesics. The pain is increased by any factor that increases intracranial pressure, such as coughing, sneezing, or straining. Visual disturbances and weakness of one side of the body are seen often. There may be a history of progressive intellectual deterioration. Petit and grand mal seizures may occur as the disease progresses. Slow growing tumors, such as meningioma and astrocytoma, give rise to a long history of symptoms extending over years, whereas tumors such as the medulloblastoma and metastatic carcinoma often develop rapidly.

PSYCHALGIA

A psychogenic facial neuralgia is an idiopathic, nonspecific, nonorganic form of facial pain. This type of pain mimics the major and minor types of facial neuralgias. The pain experienced by the patient is real to him, and it can be severe. It is not affected by the position of the patient, nor is there any area that will elicit pain when touched. The location of the pain is vague, and may shift from time to time. It may be unilateral or bilateral; it follows no clearly defined nerve distribution. Generally some degree of discomfort is experienced by the patient at all times. The severity of the pain varies, and it may be correlated with psychogenic stimuli, such as stress, duress, and tension. The type of patient affected by psychalgias is a nervous individual who may show other symptoms of neurosis or psychopathic disturbances.[14]

Almost any form of treatment will bring about relief of the pain, and placebos are equally effective, but the pain will return. The psychalgia patient often prescribes surgery for himself, but when the surgery does not give permanent relief the patient will condemn the practitioner.

One must be careful when making the diagnosis of psychalgia. The temptation to classify a patient in this category is great, and it may appear to be the easy way out rather than going through an exhaustive history and a series of tests. The diagnosis of psychalgia should not be made until all efforts have failed to arrive at a proper diagnosis and the patient still experiences his pain.

The only effective treatment for psychalgia is psychiatric therapy. The referral of the patient to a psychiatrist may be met with opposition, and must be made in such a way that the patient actually feels that a psychiatric interview might help. The patient should never be told abruptly that his disease is considered a psychogenic one.

REFERENCES

1. Baker, G. S.: Treatment of painful neuralgias of the head. Journal Lancet, 72:525, 1952.
2. De Jong, R. N.: The Neurologic Examination. 2d ed. New York, Harper & Bros., 1958.
3. Douglas, T. E.: Facial pain from elongated styloid process. Arch. Otolaryng., 56:635, 1952.
4. Elfenbaum, A.: Causalgia in dentistry: An abandoned pain syndrome. Oral Surg., Oral Med. & Oral Path., 7:594, 1954.
5. Facial pain (Annotations-Anonymous). Lancet, 7323:30, 1964.
6. Fulcher, O. H.: Personal communication.
7. Gibilsco, J. A.: Unpublished address, 1964.
8. Glick, D. H.: Locating referred pulpal pains. Oral Surg., Oral Med. & Oral Path., 15:613, 1962.
9. Grinker, R. R., Bucy, P. C., and Sahs, A.: Neurology. 5th ed. Springfield, Ill., Charles C Thomas, 1960.
10. Harrigan, W. F.: Facial pain. Oral Surg., Oral Med. & Oral Path., 5:563, 1952.
11. Henny, F. A.: Dentistry and oral surgery in the hospital. J. Oral Surg., Anes. & Hosp. D. Serv., 22:49, 1964.
12. Horton, B. T.: Histamine cephalgia: Differential diagnosis and treatment. Proc. Staff Meet., Mayo Clin., 31:325, 1956.
13. Hutchins, H. C., and Reynolds, O. E.: Experimental investigation of referred pain of aerodontalgia. J. D. Res., 26:3, 1947.
14. Kruger, G. O.: Textbook of Oral Surgery. 3rd ed. St. Louis, C. V. Mosby Co., 1968.
15. Stuteville, O. H., and Levignac, J.: The neuralgias and vascular algias of the face. Oral Surg., Oral Med. & Oral Path., 6:1413, 1953.
16. Travell, J.: Temporomandibular joint pain referred from muscles of the head and neck. J. Pros. Den., 10:745, 1960.
17. Weisengreen, H. H., and Elliott, H. W.: Electromyography in patients with orofacial pain. J.A.D.A., 67:798, 1963.
18. Weisengreen, H. H., and Winters, S. E.: Pathways of referred pain and special reference to head and neck. Oral Surg., Oral Med. & Oral Path., 5:500, 1952.
19. Robinson, M., and Slavkin, H. C.: Dental amputation neuromas. J.A.D.A., 70:662, 1965.

24

ACUTE ORAL LESIONS

DONALD E. COOKSEY

INTRODUCTION

In many instances, patients are spurred to visit their doctor by acute discomfort. Most people in the literate world know that pain, swelling, elevated temperature, and inflammatory or color changes may constitute the first warning signs of more serious underlying problems.

The practitioner of dentistry is often faced with acute oral disease. Frequently the diagnosis and treatment of the problem requires knowledge of the nature of organic disease and of anatomy and physiology of the patient.

A knowledge of how to control disease and to relieve symptoms or produce cures with minimal morbidity is a characteristic all people seek in their doctors. The doctor is also expected to recognize the limitations in his or her scope and therefore be prepared to refer the patient to another competent health professional who is an expert in the specific area.

The teeth, by virtue of their very numbers, themselves are the most prolific producers of acute problems. Most of these problems arise from either the dental pulp or the periodontium.

ACUTE LESIONS OF THE TEETH AND JAWS

ACUTE PULPITIS

Pulpitis occurs as a result of an insult to the dental pulp. The causal agent may be invasion by caries, trauma, caustic agents such as phosphoric acid in cement, or heat such as the heat of polymerization of plastic. In experimental animals, vigorously applied ultrasonic vibrations have produced pulpitis.

Pulpitis represents an inflammatory change in the dental pulp which often results in pulpal necrosis. Necrosis results in toxic changes at the apical foramen and the formation of some apical lesions. Thus, pulpitis is the precursor of periapical disease.

Pulpitis is typified by:

1. Painful response to
   a. Heat
   b. Chemical stimuli
2. Toothache
3. Hypersensitivity to electric stimulation, such as pulp testing
4. Pain remission to cold or chemical obtundants
5. Progression to pericementitis

PERICEMENTITIS

Pericementitis is the next step toward periapical infection and is considered to be present when:

1. The tooth elongates and progresses to a state of "hyperocclusion."
2. The tooth becomes tender to percussion.
3. The first evidence of periodontal membrane thickening occurs radiographically.

Pulpitis may be assuaged by removing the cause, and is treated with obtundants and antimicrobial agents. It may be reversed in the pulp. Pericementitis is usually irreversible in the pulp and represents the next step toward advanced apical periodontitis.

Apical periodontitis represents extravasation of the inflammatory process from the pulp chamber into the periodontal space. Various reactions may transpire:

1. An acute periapical abscess may form.
2. The process may become chronic and an apical granuloma may form.
3. The epithelial cell rests of Malassez may be stimulated to proliferate and a radicular (simple) root cyst may form.

Any such process may become acute, subacute, or chronic depending upon the conditions present. Any such process may exacerbate without apparent cause at any time. An acute abscess may fistulate and drain. A chronic granuloma may increase in size, exacerbate, or disappear under treatment. An apical cyst may remain dormant or increase to giant proportions without apparent explanation.

It follows, then, that the primary responsibility of the dental professional is to respond to the patient's need for help as soon as possible.

Treatment for Pulpitis and Associated Problems.   Early pulpitis may be treated by removal of the cause. Cleaning out a carious lesion threatening the pulp, capping and covering a traumatically injured pulp, removing a noxious restoration, endodontic therapy, or the removal of the tooth may be indicated.

PERIAPICAL LESIONS

Periapical Abscess (Dentoalveolar Abscess)

These are normal sequelae of pulpitis, being the suppurative result of passage of infected material through the apex into the periodontal membrane space.

The use of antibiotics alone is inadequate treatment for dentoalveolar abscess. Treatment should always include some form of drainage, either through the root canal or by incision. The offending tooth may be removed at the time of treatment.

Dentoalveolar abscess does not preclude endodontic therapy but may delay definitive treatment until resolution of the disease.

Not unusually, periapical lesions become cystic and may enlarge to great size and, in turn, become infected.

PERIODONTAL ABSCESSES

When suppurative changes occur gingivally rather than apically, the lesion is termed periodontal rather than periapical (Fig. 24–1). The origin is gingival rather than pulpal. The abscesses may be drained by incision or curettage, or the lesion can be treated by extraction. Antibiotic therapy is indicated when the patient's condition warrants.

Figure 24–1 Periodontal abscess. This abscess may be drained at the gingival cuff by inserting a curette or by incision into the center of the mass.

Figure 24–2 Acute pericoronitis. This acute pericoronitis around a partially erupted third molar has been treated by topical application of aspirin, producing a chemical burn and compounding the patient's symptoms.

PERICORONAL INFECTION

Most pericoronal infections occur with the erupting third molars, although they may occur with any problem of eruption. These infections are typified by swelling of the tissues over and around the erupting crown. Occlusion is frequently interfered with (Fig. 24–2).

The pericoronal space may contain debris which encourages growth of organisms and formation of a local abscess. In lower third molar eruption this is often at the distobuccal angle of the tooth.

Pericoronal abscess and pericoronitis are particularly dangerous because they may spread into surrounding soft tissue spaces quickly, as there is no periosteal barrier involved.

Treatment should be of a combined nature, and antibiotics are most useful in controlling these infections when accompanied by local means.

1. Drainage may be obtained by sliding a thin-bladed plastic instrument between the tooth and the operculum. This maneuver may produce copious drainage.
2. While the pericoronal space is thus held open, it may be irrigated with an oxidizing agent such as hydrogen peroxide, followed by a mercurial such as tincture of merthiolate. These agents remove debris and reduce the activity of the anaerobic organisms present.
3. The opposing maxillary third molar may be removed to reduce occlusal trauma.
4. Incision and drainage may be indicated when fluctuation can be observed.
5. Supportive treatment, including hot saline soaks, may be of some benefit.
6. A decision must be reached whether to retain or sacrifice the tooth.
    a. If the tooth is to be retained, the operculum may be removed surgically either by electrocautery or sharp dissection.
    b. Whether the tooth is to be sacrificed or not, care must be taken to

avoid pushing infected material deeper into the soft tissue by injudicious use of a hypodermic needle.

Operators face this problem with philosophical differences. Many clinicians feel that prompt removal of the tooth is indicated. Others treat the area and wait for several days until the infection subsides. Regardless of the personal differences in management philosophy and regardless of whether the treatment is aimed toward retention or removal of the tooth, a level of antibiotics should be present in the blood stream at the time of the surgical interference. The reason for this is the frequency with which pericoronal infections spread into the pterygomandibular space and other facial spaces, resulting in morbid and occasionally fatal infections of the head and neck (Fig. 24–3).

APPROPRIATE ANTIBIOTIC THERAPY

It is a generally accepted concept that penicillin is the drug of choice in treating oral infection. This is a sound concept, but the therapist should remember that other drugs have been used with great success in the treatment of oral infection and also are appropriate.

Another factor in the successful use of antibiotic drugs is the method of administration. Some drugs, particularly penicillin G, are more effective

Figure 24–3 Multiple fascial space infection from a simple pericoronitis which did not receive early treatment.

when administered parenterally. Many of the depot preparations of pencillin offer protracted levels should the therapist consider the patient to be unreliable or unable to accept oral medication.

Erythromycin, either in the form of hydrochloride, estolate, or stearate, is an excellent drug when taken by mouth, as are potassium penicillin V and the synthetic penicillins.

The cephalosporins are proving to be very effective, but are expensive at the time of this writing. Chloramphenicol has shown itself to be highly effective in vitro but carries a risk which cannot ordinarily be tolerated unless other agents prove ineffective. The tetracycline group, on the contrary, is seldom the specific drug of choice in in vitro studies. This may be due to the widespread use of this drug in animal feeds and other industrial purposes.[6]

The period of time covered by the administration of the drug is important. Whereas three-day courses may be sufficient for prophylaxis in rheumatic heart disease, they are not adequate when dealing with a full-blown infection which genuinely requires antibiotic therapy. No fewer than five days of therapy are adequate to avoid producing a resistant strain which could become refractory.

Most suppurative dental diseases respond very rapidly to incision and drainage and removal of the cause. In many instances it is difficult for the therapist to evaluate the activity of the antibiotic employed because the patient improves in response to the other emergency treatment administered. This experience should in no way deter the clinician from prudent administration of antibiotic agents when the situation demands it.

SPREAD OF INFECTION

When infections of dental origin are untreated or improperly treated, they tend to enlarge and involve tissues distant from the original site of infection. Spread of these infections is by three basic means, or by combinations of these means—specifically, by subperiosteal and fascial space progression, by direct extension, and by hematogenous and lymphatic metastasis. The manner and rapidity of spread of any given infection depend upon the virulence of the organism, the resistance of the patient to the organism, and the location of onset of the infection.

SUBPERIOSTEAL

When infections start within the bony confines of the mandible or maxilla, they tend to become external and drain themselves through the path of least resistance. Since the suppurative material has the physical property of weight, it tends to obey laws of gravity in its progress. When the material leaves the bony confines it encounters periosteal covering which forms the space for the body of the mandible or maxilla. This periosteal cover is dissected away from the bone by expansion of the mass of pus, and an abscess forms between the bone and the periosteal covering. Abscesses at this stage of development are usually easily reached for incision and drainage through the buccal vestibule, either by inserting an instrument beneath the periosteum at the gingival cuff or by making an incision in the bottom of the vertibular fold and directing the dissection down to bone and through periosteum. A drainage portal is then maintained with a flat segment of rubber dam which may be sewn in place to avoid loss. The drain is usually removed within 48 hours. This treatment should at all times be accompanied by appropriate antibiotic therapy.

Should this type of treatment be too long delayed, major complications may ensue.

1. The abscess may break out of the periosteal barrier and burrow to the skin surface, either forming a fistula following spontaneous drainage or requiring that the therapist carry out appropriate external surgical drainage (Fig. 24–4).
2. The abscess may so totally denude areas of bone by raising the periosteum and compromising the blood supply that the bone becomes necrotic and starts sequestration (Fig. 24–5). This unfortunate complication terminates in long and burdensome treatment for osteomyelitis with the need for surgical drainage, long-term antibiotic therapy, surgical removal of sequestra, and, in some cases, pathologic fracture and loss of considerable jaw substance.
3. The abscess material may pass out of the periosteal barrier and involve one or more of the potential fascial spaces of the head and neck. Since these spaces are conveniently connected in many instances by clear-cut anatomic pathways, the number of spaces that may be involved is limited only by the virulence of the organism and the resistance of the patient, until intelligent surgical intervention takes place (Fig. 24–6).
4. The infection may fail to "point" or localize, and progress locally as a phlegmonous swelling without evidence of fluid formation, and with evidence of acute cellulitis. This sort of reaction is common when the patient's resistance to the specific organism is low or when the organism involved is not ordinarily a pus former. It is to be recognized, however, that pus is the evidence of cellular death and is formed when the

Figure 24–4 Active draining fistulae from submasseteric compartment abscess. Cure was obtained by surgically connecting the abscesses, use of antibiotics, and removal of the cause.

Figure 24–5 Removal of bone sequestrum from the inferior border of the mandible resulting from osteomyelitis. Notice the proliferating new bone around the sequestrum.

patient's leukocytic reaction is such that both invading bacterial and invaded cells die along with the leukocytes and phagocytes that are engulfing the organisms.

5. Any or all manifestations of the progress of infection are accompanied by showers of organisms into the blood stream as areas of the vascular system become open to the infection. These showers are usually transient and are overcome by the defensive forces in the blood; therefore, culturing the organism is not always easy. When they are not immediately overcome, they may circulate to distant spots via the blood stream, or take residence in some nearby convenient area. Such metastatic occurrences may be very far reaching in their consequences, and may appear in the form of brain abscess, cavernous sinus thrombosis, bacterial endocarditis, or exacerbation of arthritic or renal disease.

Figure 24–6 Multiple space abscesses. Note the swelling in the submental area and the elevation of the tongue. This can readily lead to airway obstruction. This type of infection was once called Ludwig's angina.

ABSCESSES BENEATH SKIN

When abscesses of dental origin point beneath the skin, little can be done to abort them. Attention should be given to the evacuation of the abscess with as manageable a defect as possible. If left to their own devices, they tend to break through the skin and form fistulae, which may persist as long as the cause remains uncorrected. This situation requires removal of the cause, and excision of the fistula when cosmesis is a factor (Fig. 24–7).

If the abscess can be incised before it bursts spontaneously, and the cause removed, the operator has reasonable assurance of producing a cure. Incision is made at a point lower than the abscess cavity, through the skin (Fig. 24–8). Blunt dissection is then carried out upward into the cavity, and a drain is placed. This technique permits collapse of the abscess cavity without invagination of the drainage portal and formation of an unsightly scar (Fig. 24–9).

SPREAD THROUGH FASCIAL SPACES

Competent descriptions of the anatomic aspects of propagation of infection are available in several text materials.[1, 3, 5, 7] Treatment for these enti-

Figure 24–7 Facial fistula. Suppurative material from a mandibular anterior tooth penetrated bone, periosteum, muscle and subsequently skin in forming this common type of facial fistula. Note the pustule in the center of the contractile scar which forms a dimple. Such scars can be revised surgically after the cause has been dealt with.

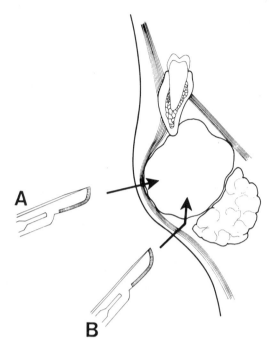

Figure 24–8 The proper and improper approach to incision and drainage. Route A enters unsupported tissues, is not at the most dependent position, and encourages collapse of the abscess cavity with the result shown in Figure 24–9. Route B enters supported tissue, avoiding collapse of the cavity and rollback of the tissue edges. As a consequence, a careful primary closure of the incision can be made and the scar rendered nearly imperceptible. The lower position assists gravity in draining the lesion and places the incision further beneath the shadow of the mandible.

ties universally agrees upon specific courses of action, varying only in details. First, the patient must be protected by adequate antibiotic therapy, and supported by dietary, hydration, and physiotherapeutic agents such as hot, wet applications. At an appropriate time, incision and drainage must be carried out. These patients may be very ill and require hospitalization. Incisions may be intra- or extra-oral, depending upon the location of the problem. The therapist must give full consideration to the evidence presented to make the decision as to where to incise for best results.

Figure 24–9 Retractile scar formed when a very large abscess was incised in the center and the edges collapsed. Cosmetic revision is difficult.

PTERYGOMANDIBULAR COMPARTMENT ABSCESS

These abscesses are usually associated with pericoronitis of the third molar, third molar removal, or administration of mandibular anesthesia. They easily communicate with the submandibular space and the sublingual space. They produce extreme trismus, pain on lateral movement of the mandible, pain at the base of the tongue, and pain on swallowing. They can be palpated by lubricating the examining finger and passing it beneath the tongue posteriorly and lingually and feeling the inferior aspect of the anterior pillar of the fauces. This area is exquisitely tender and bulges into the oropharynx at the tongue base when compared to the opposite side. In addition to the other cardinal signs of infection, swelling, pain, and inflammation, these patients will have a temperature elevation.

Difficulties in treatment lie in obtaining access and anesthesia, so treatment is often done under general anesthesia. Surgery may be done under local analgesia employing the following technique.

A preoperative medication is given; this may be an intravenous combination such as diazepam (Valium) and meperidine (Demerol). Using a ratchet type mouth prop or progressive layers of tongue blades, the jaw is forced open far enough to admit a right angle retractor. The tongue is retracted medially by an assistant, and the bulge of the abscess is exposed, just medial to the ascending ramus and anterior to the anterior pillar, deep in the lingual sulcus. Employing a 28 gauge needle and local analgesia, a series of intramucosal wheals are made. The mucosa should be seen to blanch in the area of the incision. No effort is made to penetrate deeply. Incision should be 2 cm or more, and pass through the mucosa only.

Hemostats are then inserted into the wound and spread. This maneuver produces a quantity of pus, so an aspirator should be present to evacuate the material from the airway. A drain is then placed in the cavity and held with a single suture. Many operators desire assurance of the location and depth of the exudate or wish to obtain uncontaminated samples for culture and sensitivity studies in vitro. This may be done by inserting an 18 gauge needle attached to an aspirating syringe into the abscess and removing some of the contents for transfer to the laboratory. The needle can then be detached and left in place, and dissection can follow the needle to the source of the exudate.

SUBMANDIBULAR COMPARTMENT ABSCESSES

Infections originating in the mandible often spread beneath the periosteum, which forms the space for the body of the mandible, and leave this space to enter other compartments. Lower biscuspids and teeth more anterior may communicate into the sublingual space, producing dysphagia and swelling beneath the tongue. These infections readily spread posteriorly, following the submandibular salivary duct into the submandibular space. They may also migrate into the muscle layers beneath the tongue and cause elevation of the tongue and airway problems. It is simple to find entry into the submental space via this route.

Infections that originate more posteriorly often communicate directly with the submandibular space behind the mylohyoid muscle or from beneath the mylohyoid. Abscesses of the submandibular space are often seen in conjunction with abscesses of other compartments. These infections are typified by swelling beneath the mandible on one side. The patient may have all the other signs and symptoms of infection (Fig. 24–10).

Patients may have some degree of trismus, depending upon the relative myositis of the medial pterygoid and the suprahyoid muscles, but usually not to the extent seen in pterygomandibular abscesses.

Once suppurative material has entered the space, surgical drainage is usually necessary. Antibiotics may halt the spread of the infection and aid in the reduction of swelling and tenderness by their bactericidal action, but only rarely will the suppurative material resorb and the necrotic cavities heal without surgical evacuation. Surgical evacuation in this case usually means incision and drainage through the skin (Fig. 24–11).

Various techniques have been recommended for drainage, all involving the formation of an outlet through the skin to the outside and the placing of a drain. It is important to gain access to all involved spaces and to ensure that all pockets of material are in communication (Figs. 24–11 to 24–13).

INFECTIONS INVOLVING MAXILLARY STRUCTURES

Most acute infections of the maxillary and mandibular dentition which form suppurative material tend to point close to the source of the infection and present themselves as acute dentoalveolar abscesses or parulis in the mucobuccal fold (Fig. 24–14). Occasionally, the course of spread is more obscure and may be very serious.

Figure 24–10 Submandibular space abscess. Note the distortion in the normal relationship of the tissues.

Figure 24–11   Steps in establishing drainage. *A*, Spreading of hemostats in the abscess and the release of pus. *B*, Coalescence of multiple cavities with the exploring finger. This is not necessary in small or unicameral abscesses. *C*, Placing a split Penrose drain into each extremity of the cavity to insure free flow of suppurative material. *D*, Careful closure of the wound around the drain. The drain is sutured to the skin and is easily advanced by cutting one suture. This type of closure has great cosmetic benefits and is possible if the wound is located in supported tissue. (See Fig. 24–8.)

Figure 24–11   *Continued. E,* Submandibular abscess drain. Forty-eight hours after incision and drainage, normal tissue relations can be observed. Note the dependent position of the incision and drain hidden beneath the mandibular shadow and in supported tissue.

Figure 24–12 The dotted line A–B–C represents the course of the digastric muscle which divides the submental and submaxillary spaces. Line A–B represents the anterior belly. B is the location of the pulley at the superior aspect of the hyoid bone. Line B–C represents the posterior belly. Incision D will drain the submental space and the spaces between the suprahyoid musculature of the tongue. The location of the incision hides it beneath the shadow of the mandible. Incision E will drain the submandibular space and will give access to the pterygomandibular compartment and the third molar area of the oral cavity if needed. These areas may be connected by passing above the bellies of the digastric, as seen in Figure 24–13, or may be used as illustrated and shown in Figure 24–3.

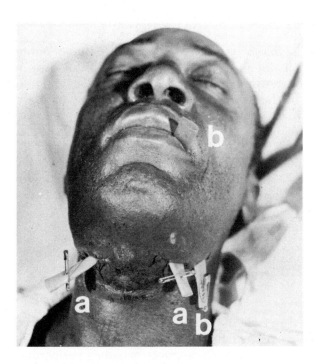

Figure 24–13 Multiple connecting drains. Two drains have been employed to connect five fascial compartments. Drain a–a enters one submandibular space, crosses above the anterior bellies of the digastrics through the submental space and passes through the opposite submandibular space, draining the anterior portion of the huge abscess. Drain b–b enters the submandibular space and ascends beneath the periosteum of the mandible, entering the pterygomandibular space and the sublingual space and emerging in the oral cavity and draining the posterior portion. The safety pins are placed to avoid retreat of the drain beneath the skin. The drains are advanced daily, the intraoral portion being permitted to close first.

Figure 24–14 Parulus. This "gum boil" is associated with a dentoalveolar abscess involving the cuspid and bicuspid.

SPREAD TO MAXILLARY SINUSES

Because of the proximity of the floor of the maxillary sinuses to the maxillary teeth from the first bicuspid posteriorly, maxillary sinus infections of dental origin are not uncommon. These infections may mimic the signs and symptoms of primary maxillary sinus infection, such as pain over the anterior maxilla, headache, postnasal drainage, and positional discomfort. Often the clinician's attention is distracted from an obvious dental cause by the diversity of symptoms.

Dental infections spreading to the maxillary sinus may also tunnel out to the skin surface above the buccinator muscle and produce facial fistulae, or in extreme cases spread by direct extension into other paranasal sinuses and into the anterior or middle fossa of the skull as meningeal infections or brain abscesses. Infections of maxillary teeth that do not respond promptly to treatment should not be taken lightly, and the underlying causes must be clearly understood and managed (Fig. 24–16).

Often, a tooth involving the maxillary sinus is removed and, either at the time of extraction or at a subsequent date, communication is established with the sinus and purulent material will drain from the communication. These oroantral fistulae may close spontaneously with antibiotic therapy or may persist, requiring surgical management of the antrum and plastic closure of the opening (Fig. 24–17).[2]

SPREAD TO BUCCAL FAT PAD

The space in the cheek and in front of the masseter muscle and between the mucosa and the skin contains a pad of fatty tissue and the anterior portion of the parotid duct. Acute inflammation of molar tooth roots, maxillary pericoronitis, or contamination of the space by a dirty needle may induce an abscess of the buccal space.

These abscesses may become very tightly confined if they become large and may be very painful. In addition, they are adjacent to the pterygoid

Figure 24–15 *A*, Pulpally involved maxillary first molar involving the maxillary sinus. Although the dental lesion may be seen on periapical views, the sinal pathosis is not visible. *B*, Sinal radiopacity is often not visible on the Panorex; thus special sinal views are required. *C*, Upright Waters views clearly show sinal clouding in conjunction with infection of dental origin.

Figure 24–16 Facial fistula arising from a dental infection that involved the maxillary sinus. The suppurative material tunneled to the skin surface above the buccinator, rather than pointing in the mucobuccal fold.

Figure 24–17 Sinal disease of dental origin with oroantral fistula. The periodontal lesion seen in the insert (a) required removal of the tooth. An oroantral fistula resulted because of sinal infection associated with the periodontal lesion.

plexuses of vessels, and the possibility of venous thrombosis or hematogenous metastasis from such a neglected abscess is very strong. When such vascular spreading occurs, meningeal infection, brain abscess, or cavernous or other venous structural thrombosis may ensue. For this reason, such lesions must not be neglected, but must be treated promptly by discovery and removal of the cause, with the prompt use of antibiotic therapy, incision, and drainage.

SPREAD TO OTHER FACIAL STRUCTURES

It is important to remember that infections of facial structures, particularly of the maxilla, have the potential of spread to the facial vasculature or to deeper fascial compartments or via sinuses or other routes, eventually invading the cranial cavity in one way or another. The results are always critical, often disabling, and sometimes fatal.

Any dentofacial infection that produces local edema, cellulitis, elevated temperature, redness, or tenderness is worthy of your attention and requires prompt diagnosis and treatment.

Special attention must be given to the periorbital structures. The soft tissues around the eye often manifest early signs of a potent spreading infection. Periorbital edema accompanying other facial edema is common in many minor facial infections and in many postoperative edema responses. Periorbital edema in conjunction with elevated temperature, pain, visual abnormalities, and local inflammation or directly associated with infection is a grave sign and should never be ignored (Fig. 24–18). Periorbital ecchymosis, however, is a frequent response to surgical trauma, and the "black eye," embarrassing as it may be, often accompanies needle insertion trauma or uncomplicated extractions. This is not a grave sign.

Figure 24–18 Cavernous sinus thrombosis. Fortunately, this condition and related life-threatening problems such as brain abcesses and meningitis of dental origin are rare. When they do occur, neglected maxillary abscesses that have metastasized into the pterygoid or orbital circulation are usually involved. The use of antibiotic coverage in all such instances where intracranial involvement is threatened is important. Notice the orbital involvement, common in these problems, and often mimicking dacryocystitis.

MANAGEMENT OF INFECTION IN THE DENTAL OFFICE

Because of the many possibilities of complication, infections are best managed in a defensive manner. The cardinal principles of management are control of spread, removal of cause, drainage of existing reservoirs of suppurative material, and supportive treatment aimed at improvement of the patient's physiology and natural defensive mechanisms.

CONTROL OF SPREAD

The possibility of hematogenic spread is greatly diminished by the introduction of antibiotics into the patient's blood. For this reason, antibiotic therapy should be foremost in the mind of the therapist, regardless of when surgical procedures are contemplated. Many experienced therapists place the patient on antibiotic therapy, treat the infection expectantly, delay the surgery until the acute symptoms diminish, and operate with a high titer of antibiotics in the blood. This approach is reasonable, particularly when circumstances dictate the use of local analgesia and peroral antibiotic medication.

REMOVAL OF CAUSE

Other equally experienced therapists wish to remove the cause at the first possible moment, especially when such a procedure will produce surgical drainage at the same time as the removal of the cause. This approach often requires the use of outpatient general anesthesia or intravenous sedation to control the pain, as local analgesia is often not effective at the site of infection. In addition, it is wise to premedicate this sort of patient with intramuscularly injected antibiotics and await some absorption so that the shower of bacteria that will occur when the infection is disturbed will be met by blood concentrations of bactericide as well as the normal defense mechanisms of the patient.

DRAINAGE OF SUPPURATIVE MATERIALS

Surgical drainage may result from removal of the cause or may require other planned incision and drainage. Many therapists employ a combination of antibiotic therapy and incision and drainage as a preliminary to removal of the cause, delaying extraction until drainage subsides and the infection is subacute.

Regardless of the particular sequential planning of these events, all must be considered as essential to the complete treatment of the patient.

SUPPORTIVE TREATMENT

The ever-present possibility of dehydration and alteration of normal fluid and electrolyte balance accompanies every infection. Patients may not eat or drink properly. They may have taken a wide variety of home or unprescribed remedies before consulting you. They are frequently depressed and often turn to alcohol in combination with other drugs while awaiting some resolution. They often obtain conflicting advice as to the application of heat and cold.

It is necessary to encourage patients to take fluid and to support their diet with high protein foods to help the proliferation of phagocytes. Many therapists feel that the use of antibiotics in treating an infectious process suggests the existence of stress, instrumental in vitamin depletion and, therefore, order vitamin supplements automatically.

Although cold applications have a temporarily palliative effect in controlling post-surgical edema, it is our opinion that cold has little if any place in the treatment of infection, and we tend to employ hot, wet applications inside and outside the mouth during the period of localization, drainage, and resolution.

Pain typical of spreading infection is difficult to control. The use of common obtundants is reasonable; however, overmedication to the point of somnolence or reflex loss, especially when the patient combines therapy with alcohol, is very dangerous because of the triple threat to the airway which might go unnoticed:

1. The abscess might burst while the patient is semicomatose, and suppurative material be aspirated.
2. The patient may vomit if alcohol is taken with strong medication.
3. The swelling may continue to spread, involving the parapharyngeal structures and sublingual structures and producing mechanical obstruction.

The best way to control pain is to control the infection and obtain surgical drainage at the earliest possible practical moment.

LABORATORY TESTS IN INFECTION

Two or three laboratory methods are of importance in the management of infection.

1. Culture and Sensitivity.   This test requires that the therapist obtain an uncontaminated sample of suppurative material from the infected site, transfer it to a growth medium, and transport the contaminated medium to a bacteriological laboratory. Random sampling of oral contamination is not useful. This implies that the therapist has actually opened the infection, and may imply successful or partially successful drainage.

Frequently, the patient will be well on his way to recovery before the results are obtained, and the test will appear futile.

On those occasions when residual problems remain and the patient has not responded well to therapy, the test is of great value in the selection of the appropriate antibiotic. Obtaining such information is an absolute requirement in treating osteomyelitis successfully.

Results are most informative when the sample is obtained before antibiotic therapy has been started. If this is not possible, be sure to include a notation as to the kind and amount of antibiotic therapy the patient has received prior to sampling.

2. Complete Blood Count. A patient's blood constituents reflect his general health and reaction to stressful demands for greater production of certain blood elements. In infection, demand occurs for increases of white blood cells, particularly polymorphonuclear leukocytes. Other phagocytic forms may also increase, but the most notable change will be in the "polys." This change is in the form of an increase in number accompanied by a decrease in maturity. This phenomenon is sometimes called "left shift" because of the position of the keys on the counting machine and implies the presence of stressful demand for greater numbers of phagocytic cells to fight the infection.

Changes from large numbers of immature forms to more mature forms suggest reduction of stress and control of the infection. When accompanied by a drop in temperature, this almost surely signals the presence of pus, which can be drained.

Further changes to the "left" or immature side suggest greater stress and lack of control of the infection. The patient will usually continue to run an elevated temperature, sometimes a severely spiking fever.

Changes from larger numbers in the neutrophil series toward larger numbers of large macrophages and lymphocytes is typical of the recovery phase of infection.

By use of repeated complete blood counts, the therapist can monitor the patient's physiologic response to therapy.

Sedimentation Rate.   Sedimentation rate is the rate at which red blood cells settle as blood stands in vitro and depends upon concentration of substances that aggregate RBC's, particularly fibrinogen and gamma globulin. Stress upon the blood vascular system in disease increases the level of these substances, thus increasing the sedimentation rate. The test is non-specific, and has little value except when compared to other sedimentation rates on the same patient and coordinated with the complete blood count and with the clinical course of the patient. It can usually be done as a part of the complete blood examination.

ACUTE DISEASES OF THE SALIVARY SYSTEM

Although the salivary system is subject to a great many problems, only a few are recognizable as dentally oriented.

Mumps, a viral disease, usually of childhood, may be observed in a unilateral form, rather than bilateral, and as a result be sometimes confused with dental infection.

Acute bacterial infections of the salivary glands usually occur on a unilateral basis. These problems may be acute exacerbations of chronic conditions, in which case the patient may give a history of previous episodes. Acute infection of the parotid capsule may occur as a sequel to buccal space abscess of dental origin. These and other episodes confusing to the practitioner may come through the office. The clinician is well advised to take careful consideration of the anatomic location of the complaints, the history of occurrence, and the results of specific x-rays and clinical findings before sending the patient out for referral or attempting definitive treatment.

ANATOMY

The parotid gland is confined within a parotid capsule, the superior portion of which is anchored to the inferior border of the zygoma. Parotitis should not be confused with superficial temporal pouch infection, as the swelling will not extend above the zygoma. The parotid is bilobular, the deep portion extending behind the mandible, and is tightly confined in the retromandibular space. Swelling of the parotid therefore frequently extends posteriorly past and behind the posterior and inferior border of the mandible, often raising the lobe of the ear (Fig. 24–19). Submasseteric compartment abscesses are confined more laterally and do not tend to extend in a retromandibular direction. Buccal space abscesses are more anterior and can be felt intraorally. The submandibular gland occupies most of the potential submandibular space; thus swelling in this space could be either glandular or dental in origin. Usually glandular swelling offers a history of intermittent occurrence, often associated with eating, and may present itself as a definite discrete oval swelling when submandibular space infection does not change with eating habits and has a more generalized edematous character.

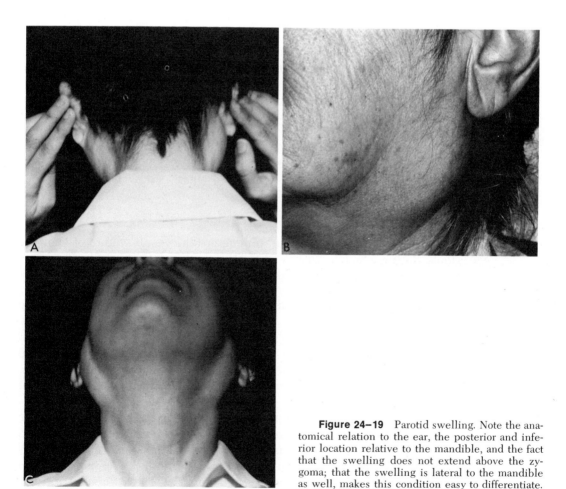

Figure 24–19 Parotid swelling. Note the anatomical relation to the ear, the posterior and inferior location relative to the mandible, and the fact that the swelling does not extend above the zygoma; that the swelling is lateral to the mandible as well, makes this condition easy to differentiate.

By far the most frequent cause of acute swelling of the major salivary glands is acute obstruction. These obstructions may be calcific in character, and therefore easily seen radiographically, or they may consist of non-radiopaque inspissated mucus and be non-radiovisible.

SIALOLITHS

Sialoliths of the submandibular gland and duct may be seen in the Panorex when posterior or on occlusal films when more anterior. They may frequently be seen on both (Fig. 24–20). The absence of a radiopaque object does not preclude the possibility of obstruction.

Sialoliths of the parotid gland are more often relatively radiolucent and difficult to disclose radiographically. They usually occur where the duct curves around the anterior border of the masseter, and thus can be seen best by short exposure of low KVP with the film placed between the teeth and cheek, covering the opening of the parotid duct and the area directly behind and above the opening.

Pain in the glands and ducts is due to buildup of salivary secretions and may be exquisite. This condition is a genuine emergency, as the sequelae are bursting of the duct and formation of a fistula with chronic sialadenitis, or depression of the glandular activity to the point of destruction of the acinic cells, loss of salivary function, and fibrosis and chronic sialadenitis of the gland.

The only satisfactory treatment for such conditions is drainage of the gland through the ductile system. This can be accomplished by the removal of the sialolith when one is present, or by dilation of the duct opening and the expulsion of a soft plug by massage. All treatment should be accompanied by antibiotic therapy, as retrograde infection is likely.[4]

LACERATIONS

Lacerations of oral mucosa and tongue are the result of auto or sporting accidents, during which teeth may be fractured or avulsed, of iatrogenic causes such as the slipping of a sharp instrument or revolving disk, and of a wide variety of other causes.

Not infrequently, these lacerations will be through and through, involving the skin surface as well as the mucosa.

Care must be taken to explore all lacerations and contusions to ensure that no foreign bodies remain in place. Fragments of teeth are especially liable to produce soft tissue reaction. Exploration should take place under anesthesia, when necessary, and the wound carefully washed with repeated lavages of normal saline or sterile water.

Deep and through-and-through wounds should be closed by suturing. The muscularis is closed first with absorbable sutures, when this is necessary. Bleeding must be controlled at this time to prevent hematoma. The mucosa is closed next to halt the entrance of oral fluids into the wound. The skin surface is closed last. If good debridement, lavage, and hemostasis have been carried out, no drain is necessary. When the wound is grossly contaminated, or when debridement cannot be carried out to the satisfaction of the operator, a small flat

Figure 24–20   Stones (sialoliths) in the submandibular duct and gland. *A*, A small stone in the superficial portion of the duct as seen in the occlusal radiograph. *B*, A moderately sized stone at the posterior border of the mylohyoid muscle obstructing the flow of dye into the gland. The lateral oblique radiogram is excellent for this purpose. *C*, A group of very large stones in the superior pole of the gland. They are well demonstrated by Panorex or by lateral oblique radiograms, but may be out of reach of the occlusal radiogram.

drain of rubber dam may be placed in the most dependent portion of the skin surface. Through-and-through injuries to the tongue do not require drainage but do require dependable hemostasis.

Often the clinician sees wounds that are several days old or have become infected before coming to his or her attention. Debridement other than removal of sloughing dead tissue is not advisable at this time. Suturing is usually fruitless and often deleterious. Attention to control of the infection by antibiotics and wound cleanliness and expectant treatment are acceptable and may be reinforced by use of chlorine based solutions or by dilute (1.5 per cent) hydrogen peroxide solutions.

BURNS

Thermal injuries of the oral cavity often occur as a result of taking some overheated food or liquid into the mouth. The patient seldom is able to reject the material in time to avoid blistering, and the resulting bleb soon bursts in the oral cavity. For these reasons, thermal injuries usually consist of a denuded area surrounded by an erythematous border and may be very tender. They may be protected by gelatinous preparations containing a corticosteroid (Kenalog in Orabase) for a reasonable period. The pain may become unimportant in three or four days, although the evidence of the burn may persist much longer, as the surface must completely reepithelialize. Chemical burns may occur from any of many noxious substances, including agents used by the therapist or available at the drugstore for dental application. Toothache poultices and toothache drops are constant offenders, as is aspirin applied directly to the area. These agents usually do not burn as deeply as thermal agents, and often may only result in erythematous tender areas (as in the case of aspirin burns) covered with desquamating epithelium, which appears as a whitish coat. These burns usually recover in a far shorter period than do thermal injuries, depending entirely upon the completeness of the destruction of the epithelial layer (Fig. 24–21). Their treatment is the same as for thermal injuries.

ACUTE VIRAL DISEASE

There are several related manifestations of viral disease of the oral cavity caused by the herpes simplex virus.

Primary Herpetic Gingivostomatitis. This is the first attack of disease caused by the herpes simplex virus; it may appear at any time after the child has lost the immunity gained from the mother, roughly after six months of age (Fig. 24–22). It often appears in young adults who have not previously had any evidence of herpetic disease. The seriousness of symptoms varies as does the age of onset. The important aspect of the disease is that personal immunity is acquired as a result of the episode and that the virus takes residence in the victim as an obligate intracellular parasite, making recurrence possible at a later date (Fig. 24–23).

Lesions of the primary disease may involve any portion of the oral mucosa.

Treatment is confined to comforting the patient and responding to the febrile courses and nutritional difficulties with expectant care. Everything should be done to avoid transferring the serum from the oral lesions to the eye or into cuts or abrasions on the body of either the patient or the operator.

Acute Herpetic Stomatitis and Herpes Labialis. These are secondary or recurrent diseases that depend upon the presence of an obligate intracellular parasite, which abides intraneurally, probably in the sphenopalatine ganglion. The viruses become activated by the lowering of the body's resistance, fatigue, exposure, dietary excesses, or trauma, and an acute episode transpires, triggering prodromal symptoms of pain, sensitivity in the form of tingling and numbness, minor fever, and stiffness of the oral or facial tissue. Subsequently, the area becomes erythematous and vesiculates. Vesicles are often hard to see in the oral cavity but are very apparent in the facial types (Fig. 24–24).

Figure 24–21 Chemical burns. Chemical burns may result from a wide variety of causes. A, Buffered aspirin; B, 180 proof ethanol; C, merthiolate; D, monomer from plastic filling material; E, cotton roll. Note that all have a similar white covering resulting from coagulation of the overlying mucosa. They are usually not as deep as thermal burns and heal more rapidly.

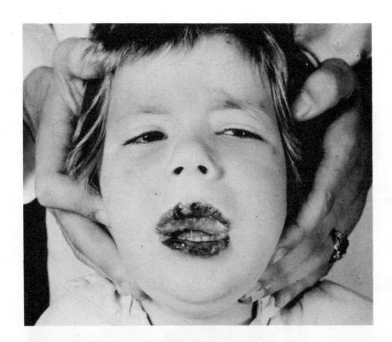

Figure 24–22   Primary herpetic gingivostomatitis in a six-year-old child.

Figure 24–23   Primary herpetic gingivostomatitis. There was no previous history of herpes. *A*, Gingiva; *B*, palate; *C*, lip and tongue.

Figure 24–24 Herpes labialis. This recurrent disease often follows weather trauma or dental treatment.

Serum from the vesicles has been proven to produce the disease experimentally in the conjunctiva of rabbits, and a causal relationship has been established in humans, with transmission of the disease to fingers, conjunctiva, and genital and orofacial areas. It must therefore be considered highly contagious, especially to persons who have never had primary herpetic gingivostomatitis. The disease can be identified microscopically by the size of the virus and the presence of granular inclusion bodies in the nuclei of involved cells. These bodies fill with fluid and burst the cell, releasing the fluid, which is responsible for the vesiculation.

Clinically, the disease is most often seen in intraoral locations where the mucosa is attached to bone (Fig. 24–25). Following rupture of the vesicles, the lesions acquire a crusty appearance on the face or a white ulcerated appearance in the mouth. Healing occurs in 10 days to two weeks when untreated or when ineffectual treatment methods are used.

Treatment may be efficaciously rendered during the prodromal stages and the vesicular stages. Treatment usually consists of topical applications of drugs capable of producing minor tissue destruction in the immediate area. Camphorated phenol, Negatan, and ammoniacal solutions of silver nitrate precipitated by eugenol have produced acceptable results when used early. When the area can be detected early, applications of camphorated phenol may greatly reduce the degree of growth and prevent coalescence of the lesions. Ether applied early to the area of the ruptured vesicle may be effective on the basis of dissolution of the lipid covering of the viruses. The use of any corticosteroid is contraindicated.

Herpes Zoster. Herpes zoster, or shingles, is often associated with an erythematous vesicular eruption around the body trunk related to the distribution of sensory nerves. The same disease occurs on the face and in the oral cavity. The distribution of the lesions is usually rather sharply demarcated, again involving the distribution of sensory nerve branches (Fig. 24–26). This disease is accompanied by pain, discomfort, fever, and often some malaise. To avoid ophthalmic involvement, the eyes must be protected from sera from these lesions.

Figure 24–25   Recurrent herpes. Recurrent disease usually occurs intraorally on surfaces attached to bone.

This virus and the virus of chickenpox have been identified as the same entity, and it is believed that chickenpox constitutes the primary of herpes zoster and the disease previously identified as zoster is secondary and dependent upon the victim previously having had chickenpox. If this is the case, and it seems to be, then herpes zoster represents the neurogenous spread of virus in an individual with humoral immunity, a situation remarkably similar to that produced by the herpes simplex virus.

The use of corticosteroids to treat the itching of zoster is not effectual, and should not be used topically in the oral cavity.

Figure 24–26   *A* and *B*, Herpes zoster. The distribution of the lesions follows neural pathways. Note the abrupt delineation at the midline.

APHTHOUS STOMATITIS

Aphthous ulcers are difficult to differentiate from herpetic ulcers without microscopic assistance. These ulcers may occur anywhere on the mucosal surface, whereas recurrent herpes usually occurs on mucosal surfaces attached to bone (Fig. 24–27). The origin of aphthous ulcers is unknown, with various theories related to stress, some distant source such as stomach upset, and lowered resistance being advanced.

These ulcers are very painful, and are especially so when they involve movable portions of the oral cavity, such as the tip or side of the tongue.

It is safe to apply anti-inflammatory agents such as steroids to these ulcers, and one of the treatments suggested is triamcinolone (Kenalog in Orabase). Another successful treatment is cautery in the center of the lesion by a substance such as ammoniacal silver nitrate precipitated by eugenol, which kills just a few cells lining the ulcer and for some reason brings relief from the pain and, seemingly, more rapid healing.

ACUTE MONILIASIS

Moniliasis, called thrush in infants, is a fungal disease caused by invasion of the oral tissue by *Monilia albicans* (*Candida albicans*). This invasion frequently occurs following alteration of the nature of the mucosa and its inhabitants by long term antibiotic therapy or following irradiation. The orbital, vaginal, and rectal mucosae are subject to the same disease, a point to be remembered when long term antibiotic administration is to be considered.

Persons who have had perioral irradiation with loss of major or minor salivary gland function are subject to this troublesome disease, especially when some form of dental treatment or perioral trauma occurs during the

Figure 24–27 Apthous stomatitis. These ulcers are clinically indistinguishable from herpes except that they occur on surfaces unattached to bone.

Figure 24–28 Acute perioral moniliasis. This patient had received radiation to gingival malignancy followed by dental therapy.

mucositis stage (Fig. 24–28). The disease may manifest as whitish patches. The overlying white membrane may be wiped off to disclose an ulcer beneath. Smears of the lesions readily reveal presence of the fungus. The disease may also manifest itself as a fiery red area, particularly in the perioral area.

The condition responds well to discontinuation of the causal agent, the administration of an antifungal agent such as nystatin, and local application of some dye fixative such as gentian violet. Nutritional support must be emphasized, as the patient's mouth may be too sore to permit proper diet.

ACUTE NECROTIZING ULCEROMEMBRANOUS GINGIVITIS

This disease is also called Vincent's disease, trench mouth, and other appellations such as the acronym ANUG. It is often seen in almost epidemic proportions such as among military troops in adverse circumstances (hence the name "trench mouth" from WW I), among young persons under stress (in universities at exam time, military training camps, etc.), and, as a consequence, has often been believed to be contagious. Bacteriologic examinations reveal the unvarying presence of fusospirillary organisms along with other bacteriologic contaminants. It also is found to be associated with poor oral hygiene.

In the acute phases there may be swelling of the gingival papilla, followed by necrosis and blunting of the tips. This is accompanied by considerable inflammation and pain, producing the common symptom of "pink toothbrush" and discomfort in brushing. The patient tends to avoid this exercise, believing that he is harming himself, resulting in the collection of additional materia alba. The disease is usually accompanied by fetid odor (Fig. 24–29).

Effective treatment may be obtained by the use of three modalities:

1. Penicillin orally or parenterally reduces the bacterial count, temperature, inflammation, and pain, making the patient easier to treat. It does not cure the disease.

2. The use locally of an oxidizing agent which partially debrides the area and kills the obligate anaerobic population that it reaches. The agent may be hydrogen peroxide, sodium perborate, or other proprietary oxidizing agents. The patient should be cautioned about the continued use of the agent after the disease is controlled, as some patients are afflicted with stomatitis medicamentosa following the continued use of oxidizers.
3. Professional physical debridement by scaling and curettage followed by meticulous personal hygiene and professional followup.

The disease should be controlled as early and effectively as possible because the tissue necrosis leads to permanent periodontal problems.

SERIOUS DISEASES OFTEN MISTAKEN FOR OTHER CONDITIONS

There is a wide variety of diseases often mistaken for common conditions in the oral cavity. Among those most frequently seen are various manifestations of serious malignant diseases, which do not respond to the types of therapy that would be expected to be effective.

Early manifestations of leukemia may mimic gingival disease or herpetiform disease. The presence of submucosal hemorrhages is a prominent sign and requires early investigation (Fig. 24–30).

Lymphomata may mimic salivary gland swellings when fortune places the early swellings in the areas of anatomic proximity (Fig. 24–31).

Squamous carcinoma may emerge from a tooth socket, even in young people, and imitate a granuloma of an infected socket (Fig. 24–32).

What appear to be traumatic ulcers, even when the history is disposed to the diagnosis, may easily be a malignant disease (Fig. 24–33).

Certain general systemic disease may mimic abscesses of dental origin (Fig. 24–34).

Special infections of non-dental origin may be present (Fig. 24–35).

The practitioner should be acutely aware of these facts, and should maintain a wary attitude toward any acute condition that does not respond promptly to what he or she considers proper treatment. The use of biopsy and clinical laboratory techniques to formulate an early and accurate diagnosis of any unresponsive or suspicious lesion is desirable and prudent.

Figure 24–29 Acute necrotizing ulceromembranous gingivitis (ANUG).

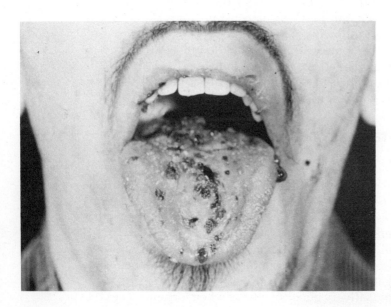

Figure 24-30 Acute leukemia. This was first treated as some form of localized stomatitis.

Figure 24-31   Hodgkins disease. This lymphoma gave the original impression of swelling of the submandibular gland.

Figure 24–32 Squamous carcinoma. This lesion grew from the socket of a fractured lateral incisor. The patient was 19 years old.

Figure 24–33 Squamous carcinoma. This was thought by the patient and the therapist to be traumatic injury. The patient was 26 years old.

Figure 24–34 Tuberculosis of cervical lymph nodes (scrofula). This patient was thought to have dental abscesses. Diagnosis was made by clinical laboratory procedures and biopsy.

Figure 24–35 Peritonsillar abscess (quinsy). This lesion is often thought to be of dental origin. This is seldom true, although maxillary pericoronitis or contaminated needles have been indicted. The usual cause is tonsillar infection. Note the displacement of the uvula at its base, the tip pointing back toward the abscess. These patients are often quite hoarse.

REFERENCES

1. Coller, F. A., and Yglesias, L.: Infections of the lip and face. Surg. Gynecol. Obstet. *60*:277–290, 1935.
2. Cooksey, D. E., and Middleton, R. A.: Management of oral surgical problems complicated by maxillary sinus involvement. J. Oral Surg., *17*:14–36, 1959.
3. Kruger, G. O.: Textbook of Oral Surgery. 4th ed., St. Louis, C. V. Mosby Co., 1974, pp. 170–201.
4. Ibid., pp. 591–619.
5. McKelvey, L. E.: Sugical Anatomy of Oral Infections. Syllabus, USAF and U. Puerto Rico School of Dentistry.
6. Pfizer Laboratories. Antibiotic Therapy for Oral Infection. (Tape) Available through the American Society of Oral and Maxillofacial Surgeons. 211 East Chicago Avenue, Chicago, IL 60611.
7. Sicher, H., and DuBrul, E.: Oral Anatomy. 6th ed., St. Louis, C. V. Mosby Co., 1975, pp. 478–495.

25

LEGAL ASPECTS OF EMERGENCIES

G. A. SHEPPARD

DEFINITION AND EFFECT

When the dental practitioner is confronted with an unforeseen combination of circumstances that calls for immediate action, this is an emergency. This may be bizarre or common, does not arrive gift wrapped, and the degree of severity is widely fluctuating. A word of caution: The law does not allow the operator to falsely proclaim an emergency just so "extra work" can be justified or to "explain away" a mistake.[1] An attempt will be made here to illustrate only the common and frequent happenings and the probable legal consequences that flow therefrom. By airing the various problems, it is intended to encourage the prevention of disastrous dental eventualities.

Many practitioners like to play "ostrich" and place their heads in the sand about being responsible for office emergencies. The time is long past when just a hope and a prayer will shield those clinicians from malpractice litigation. Thinking and acting preventively lets practitioners deliver better quality care to their patients.

698

This chapter is a *very* brief compilation of what the writer understands to be legally accepted standards, gathered from all states. In no way is it meant to be interpreted as a rule of law. Also, each state has its own "standards of care" pronounced through judicial interpretation of specific cases. These change *constantly*.

Let there be no mistake, the writer in no way means that what is cited as a "rule — standard — doctrine" will *always* be true, even when similar facts are litigated. The adequacy of counsel, preparation of the case, selection of dental and medical experts, choice of trial attorney, etc., govern any given result. The "situations" cited are for educational purposes only, in that, from actual experience, we know, with proper records, preparation, etc., that most like situations are defensible and won for the practitioner when tried before a jury.

This chapter presupposes that the reader has already been exposed to and understands the use of such terms as liability, negligence, fault, duty, proof, res ipsa loquitur, malpractice, and standard of care.

This writer also believes that the following commonly known factors have a major influence on the continuing rise in claims and lawsuits against health practitioners for alleged malpractice and lack of informed consent:

A. The pervasive idea that one can get something for nothing.
B. The consumerism vogue, with its obvious attendant philosophy of cheaper prices rather than quality of care.
C. Expanded duties by dental auxiliaries.
D. Third party factors that dilute the true doctor–patient relationship.
E. Contingent fee arrangements between patients and attorneys.
F. Changing public moral and ethical standards.
G. Tax free (not even "reportable" to the IRS) recovery by plaintiff when he or she prevails in trial and receives a monetary judgment or verdict against the clinician.

Dental practice often requires that decisions and actions be taken under circumstances of stress and immediacy, and courts tend to evaluate these decisions and actions less critically than decisions and actions accomplished under "normal conditions."[2]

The above presupposes, of course, that there is a *true* emergency such as a broken needle,[3] or a tooth or foreign object that has been aspirated.[4]

The courts also look most favorably when *immediate* consultation is accomplished.[5]

A "decision," made in an emergency, *not* to attempt the removal of a broken needle so that more damage might be prevented, or because more anesthesia might jeopardize the patient, is praiseworthy and might avoid liability.[6]

The foregoing is most pregnant because of the following legal doctrines:

1. The original "incident" may submit the practitioner to liability for additional harm (even death) resulting from later negligent care and treatment addressed to the original injury.[7]
2. The original "incident" may submit the practitioner to liability for additional harm (even death) resulting from later care and treatment (not negligent).[8]

3. The original "incident" may submit the practitioner to liability for additional harm (even death) resulting from later care and treatment, when an inherent risk, like *infection*, is the aftermath.[9]

Courts recently have become prone to *not* call an emergency an emergency. One leading case stated that even cardiac arrest during the treatment might not be classified as an emergency, owing to the fact that it might be considered a complication that could be and should be foreseen.[10]

EVERYDAY EMERGENCIES

Quite frequently every clinician will be confronted with so-called emergencies that exist, at least in the minds of his patients, in regard to hypersensitive teeth, minor abrasions to the mouth, side effects from drugs, and the like. These, of course, call for specific knowledge as to what product the patient should buy, usually without prescription, and which would be applicable to his particular problem.

If prescriptions are utilized, the amounts must be carefully controlled and the cumulative effects of the drugs known, as a recent case awarding over $1,500,000 in damages was upheld on appeal, where these facts were involved.[11]

More important would be the instant knowledge and use of the correct size and gauge of needles, asepsis, the standard of care in regard to disposable needles, disposable needle with suture, and so forth. Remember that the law is well settled: emergencies can be of any nature, and if there is peril to life and health, then lightning action is required. The clinician must have at his fingertips the exact knowledge of how to treat and with what equipment and products.

Modern "advertising" includes, many times, the information by manufacturers of drugs concerning printed material explaining the product. These data are held to be known by the prescribing doctor and the pamphlet allowed in evidence if distributed with the product.[12] This is why it is so important that the dental practitioner have immediate knowledge of the need for a particular product, know its limitations and any contraindications, antidotes, etc.

Courts usually hold that it is a matter of the doctor's judgment whether a tooth he is attempting to save can be saved or filled. Just because, at a later date, the tooth becomes diseased and has to be extracted is no reason to hold the doctor liable.[13]

The above is based on the presumption that the doctor acted in good faith and had reasonable justification in his attempt to save the tooth in the first instance. To help bolster and prove his judgment, a phone call to another clinician who agrees with the diagnosis and prognosis is most helpful. To the same effect is having another clinician view any x-rays and verify the reading. These precautions should be commonplace, and the results entered on the patient's chart.

What knowledge is known is to be promptly imparted to the patient. Assume there is a finding of a possibility of cancer; the patient must be notified *immediately* if liability is to be avoided.[14] To the same effect is the requirement that if the patient's address is faulty, the doctor is under a high duty to *find* the patient.

One of the most frequent "emergency" areas centers around infection. The doctor must, of course, have an adequate health history to determine how many months pregnant the patient is and to guide her actions accordingly, or else liability ensues.[15] Postoperative care and treatment and "developing" infection always require proof of the methods of sterilization, procedures, etc., and when these are adequately explained there usually is no liability in a later suit even when death ensues following placement of immediate dentures.[16]

Many doctors ignore the seriousness of the legal consequences *subsequent* to an emergency, i.e., that if found liable in court for allowing a broken tooth to become lodged in the lung, the patient's loss of profits, wages, etc., while off work, are part of damages to be awarded.[17]

Because the law looks favorably upon the doctor's efforts during an emergency is no excuse not to proceed with due caution *during* the emergency. Proceeding "blindly" by clamping an artery is contraindicated because of the possible damage to other structures and if done "blindly" liability may lie.[18] Thus the operator cannot panic, but must proceed with the commensurate care due the emergency. Just because, for instance, a fistula later occurs, this can often be explained as an inherent risk of the procedure for which no liability should attach.[19] But if an infection following an operation *cannot* be explained, the jury should have a right to decide the issue of malpractice.[20]

Just because the doctor has an emergency, and there is a fracture, does not excuse him from not having sterile instruments immediately at hand.[21]

The price and availability of disposable needles makes an "old" method of sterilization a problem at the very least. When infection arises after injection and the old "flaming" method of sterilizing the needle was followed, the court can find that the cause of the ultimate infection was an unsterile instrument.[22] It is interesting to note that disposable needles are responsible for an increasing number of post-injection paresthesias (lingual and inferior alveolar nerves), with attendant malpractice allegations.

The basic problem in this area of the law is that the plaintiff-patient need not exclude every possibility that the infection-injury might have been caused by some means other than the doctor's actions,[23] whether the result is cellulitis or osteomyelitis.

As time goes on and more knowledge is gained, it *sometimes* is best in an emergency *not* to operate further. This is especially true when needles break or roots are broken off. Facts now tend to show that more damage is done by attempting to remove broken roots (paresthesia, etc.) than by leaving them alone.[24] Generally it is very difficult not to have malpractice "found" by the jury when foreign bodies are found in the stomach after an operation.[25]

It is imperative that the doctor know the capabilities of the local analgesic utilized, what type of inherent risk is involved, and what percentage of people have reactions. A recent case in which Ravocaine (by aspirating technique) was given as a mandibular block points this up. The patient immediately felt uncomfortable; a headache developed, with rapid pulse and a feeling of faintness. The doctor took her to the recovery room, and thereafter had her husband take her to her physician. The condition did not improve and she was hospitalized. The doctor involved could justify his use of the local analgesic and its capability, and he provided an adequate medical history. The court held that under the circumstances there should be no liability.[26] To the same effect is the doctrine that even when death ensues after a local analgesic (Xylocaine), if the nature and purpose of the analgesic were proper, the injection itself was within the standard of care, and a proper health history and informed consent were gained, no liability is involved.[27] But when paralysis results from a local analgesic and there is *conflicting* evidence as to the standard of care in the case, there is possible liability.[28]

Cases are constantly seen wherein the teeth and gums are so involved that the patient complains of inability to eat. This should warn the doctor to be certain that a correct dietary supplement is utilized. How often we hear from the patient's attorney about the "cruelness" of the doctor's action resulting in severe loss of weight.

A more serious instance would be the action necessary to remedy a cut lip. With high-speed equipment more lacerations of major consequence are seen. (And, you guessed it, the plaintiff's attorney is always there in time to get a color photograph of the swelling and discoloration.) Instant know-how would seem to be mandatory in this type of situation, with immediate referral to a sympathetic plastic surgeon. If the patient is left to his or her "own devices," invariably the plastic surgeon seen by the plaintiff will have a lack of understanding, or keloids will form, etc.

Sometimes even the method of injection (in one particular case, mandibular rather than local infiltration) can be a suspected cause of the infection/osteomyelitis that follows.[29]

To the same effect is the emergency occurrence in which the warning on the label of the local analgesic has not been heeded by the doctor, who did not inquire as to the state of the patient's blood pressure prior to the injection.[30]

Often emergencies arise when too much time elapses while the doctor attempts to perform an unsuccessful extraction, as exemplified by trismus, hospitalization, undue pain, etc.[31] The same emergencies are often present when nerves are severed, when adjacent teeth are broken, or when needles are broken.[32]

The importance of the injection as opposed to the agent injected becomes most important when there is evidence to prove correct skill in making the injection but the product itself may be shown to be the cause of the anaphylactic reaction.[33]

Probably the knowledge of what to do and how to do it would be mandatory if the crown of the tooth broke off and protection were needed for the pulp. The same could be true if a wrong tooth were extracted, making an implant necessary. The examples could be endless in the necessity of proper knowledge of technique and products to be used in such emergencies. The same would be true of procedures that the doctor is required to know and prescribe with regard to home care after any of a variety of accidents imparted to the patient to control bleeding. The courts have held that failure to give a patient proper instructions as to his home care will create liability.[34]

Wrongful *diagnosis* of an emergency type condition "caused" from dental care and treatment can make a practitioner liable.[35] In this situation, after an extraction the doctor failed to diagnose (after local analgesic —

Novocain — and extraction) the swelling and pain. The doctor stated the patient had the mumps. The real cause, though, was acute osteomyelitis and cellulitis. The court was very plain in stating that not only was the diagnosis in error but the doctor also endangered the plaintiff in refusing to acknowledge his error.

Even if the patient is referred to a doctor after an emergency, the receiving doctor must be cognizant of what to do and how to do it, or be held liable.[36] In one instance, after extraction, the patient developed undue trismus. By "missing" the diagnosis (a broken jaw was diagnosed), the "wrong" treatment was prescribed and the patient's condition deteriorated from an *infection,* the true condition. Suppose a root is broken during an extraction. The doctor is held accountable for deciding whether or not it should be removed or left. Suppose further that the cavity shows disease. When death subsequently ensues, the court can hold the doctor liable either for failing to curette or for not referring the patient on.

What can be more common to the doctor than an injection for local analgesia? But the possible consequences are seldom realized.

A patient might appear with complaint of great pain, and the matter may seem an emergency. If in the process, though, the injection is into an infected area, liability might be predicated[38] upon the theory that the invasion of the infected area might have caused the infection to spread.

Suppose under the same circumstances a *wrong* substance is injected, instead of the intended local analgesic. Then of course there would be liability.[39] This latter matter involved a dental practitioner utilizing a local pharmacy to make up the local analgesic, and instead Lysol was prepared and injected.

Doctors often ask about their liability via law to control an infection that occurs after extraction. All that can be stated in a general way is that if an injection is done properly and if the substance is proper, there should not be any problem. But the exception always points up the dilemma. When the injection is intravenous in the arm and the vein is missed, causing pain and swelling, liability might ensue[40] when the condition worsens and a physician's care is required.

The law states that if one does not have the training or equipment to give definitive treatment, he is then inadequate to treat emergencies, and liability will ensue.[41] The matter might not be a major emergency, but even in the care of immediate denture work there may be a limitation of diet. Malnutrtion can be a very serious allegation, and one should be able to suggest the correct supplement.

If the person treating lacks the necessary skill or equipment, he or she is obligated to perform no treatment at all, but rather to immediately refer the patient to the proper person.[42]

X-RAYS AND BIOPSIES

Seemingly, each day, science and the healing arts become more sophisticated in their ability to think of tests, procedures, and so forth, that are to benefit the patient. Dental practitioners must be aware of all these advances and methods, often including x-rays, cultures, biopsies, blood gas tests, warnings via updated PDR, etc.

Failure to diagnose figuratively is "thrown at" the defendant doctor as a cause of the plaintiff's alleged injuries and damage. Realizing that there are recoveries by plaintiff on this ground, the doctor should remind himself that whenever there is the least doubt about any diagnosis, further tests should be considered, and a colleague should review with him all factors and mark this review on the patient's chart.

Jurors have found, on the basis of "failure to diagnose," liability running the gamut from aspirin poisoning[43] to x-ray burn[44] to suspected fractures[45] to nausea[46] to cancer[47] to neuromas[48] to embolism[49] to foreign objects[50] to broken bur[51] to tumor.[52]

Delay in taking x-rays in many cases results in the fixing of liability on the doctor. Each factual situation is unique, but a week's or month's delay often is enough to cause liability.[53] One case in which the doctor was held liable turned on the fact that while treating the patient via an emergency extraction a small root portion was broken off at the time of the surgery; the doctor was unaware of this. Postoperatively the patient complained of pain and remained infected. No postoperative x-ray was taken and several days later the subsequent treating doctor x-rayed the area and easily spotted the small root tip; upon its removal the plaintiff became "well."[54]

In the same vein, failure to initiate tests and failure to take biopsies are "easy grounds" for injuries to find a doctor liable.[55]

Suppose the slides and report from a biopsy are to be forwarded to someone else. Liability has been found when there is a delay in sending them on (death case – 6 week delay).[56]

Jurors have no trouble fixing responsibility on the doctor when infrequent x-rays are taken and the patient has a suspected periodontal problem — that even when x-rays are taken but misread liability follows.[57]

Some very disturbing legal results have involved liability being placed upon the doctor for not following the label instructions on products or the admonitions in the PDR, in cases of:

1. Prescribing a drug without warning of side effects.
2. Improper dilutions of solutions.[59]
3. Use of a product in an abnormal way (doctor used extraoral impression material to obtain fingertip impressions, with resultant loss of fingers).[60]
4. Use of drug that caused tooth discoloration.[61]

Needless to say, any "experimental" use of a product, technique, or equipment should be avoided. Each jurisdiction has its own rules and possibly regulations regarding procedures such as acupuncture and hypnotism. Wherever a doctor practices, he or she should make certain that procedures used are *not* experimental and *are* within the standard of care. This writer, in representing doctors, has had experience in cases involving both acupuncture and hypnotism, including the doctor's failure to gain complete anesthesia, and including not "awakening" the patient following hypnosis. To date, very little record of litigation on these subjects exists, but what there is fixes liability on the doctor.[62]

Most states have recently adopted, or are in the process of adopting, dental radiation laws covering such subjects as exposure, adequate instruction and licensing of operators, shielding, leakage. combs, space frames, timer control, protective barriers, etc. Remember that violation of a law or ordinance is negligence per se, which means, in effect, strict liability.

Adequate x-rays are necessary to show enough of the area to allow one to proceed if there is an emergency. It must be remembered that in the absence of any agreement to the contrary, x-rays form a part of the doctor's records and are his, even though they might be paid for by the patient.[63] X-rays should never be billed separately, as this frequently misleads the patient as to ownership.

In this latter regard, the doctor must never let the patient tell him what to do or how to do it. If the patient refuses to be x-rayed and films are needed for proper diagnosis, then by all means they must be taken or the patient not treated. Remember — doctors by law must practice the proper standard of care, and a patient cannot require a practitioner to do otherwise. The doctor might be consenting to a violation of the law if he or she condescends.

The doctor's assistants, of course, must be adequately trained and be given proper procedures to follow. They cannot act as primary health providers. If the doctor himself wants to use hypnosis, he must certainly be qualified and properly trained, and he must be absolutely certain that it is an accepted technique and the acceptable standard of care.

Often after an emergency some settlement is attempted directly with the doctor by or in behalf of a minor. Be reminded that only the court can approve any release or settlement.[64]

If an emergency occurs, such as a fractured root, root in the antrum, cracked tooth, etc., good judgment and the standard of care seemingly evidence the necessity of postoperative x-rays. The same is true if the patient returns after an operative procedure and has complaints in the area wherein the treatment was rendered. Besides other testing, these x-rays should help to ascertain any possible disease. As mentioned before, the x-rays are the doctor's records and should be kept with his other records at all times and the originals *never* be given to the patient under any circumstances. Not that it isn't advisable to let some other practitioner borrow them under proper circumstances; but the patient should never be the bearer. We have seen lost x-rays, defaced x-rays, stolen x-rays, substituted x-rays, etc., always to the doctor's detriment.

The use of x-rays points up a very pregnant possibility of failing: i.e., failure to use x-rays for diagnostic purposes and, even more important, alleged failure to keep abreast of progress.[65] Courts have also found that it is negligence when the doctor fails to use an x-ray in locating a piece of steel left imbedded, or when he fails to use the x-ray in locating the source of pain, e.g., a broken fragment of tooth.[66] The importance of the use of x-rays and proper equipment cannot be stressed too heavily.

Besides declaring liability in the failure to make use of x-rays for tests,[67] courts state that if the proper x-ray procedures are not followed, liability may be imposed.[68] Many doctors would like to laugh at the problem of overexposure and dental laws, but let me remind you of a decision in which a plaintiff sued for personal injuries allegedly as a result of an overdose of dental x-ray. The court felt that the patient's resulting complaints of nervousness could certainly have been caused by the x-ray exposure.[69] Of course in proved areas wherein there is no dispute as to the requirement that an x-ray be taken, the mere failure to take the x-ray might be malpractice in itself.[70]

The proper attitude of the doctor would thus seem to be dictated by the factual questions involved and by the particular patient's problem. It is probably malpractice to fail to remove a root or a piece of tooth from a jaw, if it may *"easily"* be recovered.[71]

Most doctors like to advise conservative treatment, and generally this is fine. But assume that the patient continues to complain after an extraction. This should raise a red flag in the doctor's mind if the situation persists. X-rays would normally be deemed necessary, and if not taken postoperatively under these circumstances, liability might ensue.[72]

Because an "emergency" occurs is no excuse not to *correctly* diagnose via proper reading of x-rays.[73]

X-rays often give a dental practitioner a basis for his diagnosis-prognosis, and without the film he would be in a most difficult position explaining the reasons for his care and treatment. Thus x-rays are like *gold*. Normally, testimony based on x-rays is *not* admissible when the x-rays are not produced.[74]

Often there is a conflict between a radiologist and the practitioner as to the reading of an x-ray or even as to whether or not the patient was advised of the results learned from the film (fracture).[75] This graphically points to the reason for keeping good records and entering on the chart all findings and advice given to the patient.

Akin to this is the failure to use modern methods for gaining pathologic examinations such as biopsies to determine malignancies. Courts have held that failure to utilize proper procedures and tests may give rise to liability.[76]

A common problem of liability is due to postponement in treatment caused by a delay in recognizing or biopsying the suspicious area. Some cases go so far as to hold that the failure of prompt diagnosis and biopsy might result in the failure of possible cure of a malignancy and thus create liability.[77]

If the laboratory report on the biopsy is in any way ambiguous, the doctor must take further steps for diagnosis, for if not, liability for later death of the patient may be affixed.[78]

EMPLOYEE EMERGENCY

New laws are rapidly being enacted in some jurisdictions granting auxiliary employees varying degrees of activity that traditionally were classified as only being done by the doctor. Each clinician must be cognizant of what these rights and limitations are in his own jurisdiction.

The majority of jurisdictions still do not permit dental assistants or other employees to treat pyorrhea, to fill teeth, to take impressions, to adjust bridges, etc., and declare this to be an unlawful practice of dentistry.[79] An emergency should not change this rule. Prior laws went even so far as to make certain the doctor couldn't have a "manager" who would advise patients as to type of dentures or assist in any "facial correction" or even quote fees.[80]

A dental assistant or dental hygienist also has an independent duty to the patient, and that is to use reasonable skill and care, just as medical nurses need observe their own standard of care.[81]

The dental assistant or nurse should be acting under the direct supervision of the employer.[82] The doctor cannot allow an unlicensed practitioner to perform operations. Doctors' employees cannot examine an appliance in the mouth of the patient with a view to replacement or correction.[83]

Recently, a clinician had his wife in the office helping him. The patient made them *both* defendants, when, during endodontic therapy, a broach slipped and was swallowed by the patient.[84]

What should be done under these circumstances is legal and lengthy, and will not be presented here. The preventive techniques and admonitions are uniform for all jurisdictions and if not taught in all dental schools should be made mandatory. Swallowed objects are a most common emergency, and this writer has personally assisted in legal cases concerning swallowed or aspirated crown, ear ring, denture, x-rays, watch crystal, button, broken glass from lamp, plaster from ceiling, contact lens, clamp, bur, file, tooth; you name it and it has been swallowed or aspirated.

For liability purposes, "volunteers" in the office are classified as employees.[85]

Following are only a few examples in which the employee becomes involved, followed, naturally, by the employer doctor:

1. When the employee dispenses drugs.[86]
2. When the employee fails to relay to the doctor the patient's current health history.[87]
3. When the hygienist employee fails to inform the doctor of the depth of the periodontal pockets.[88]
4. When the employee doctor who assisted without the knowledge of the plaintiff, was unlicensed.[89]
5. When the employee positions the patient "improperly" and injury results therefrom.[90]

EMERGENCY RESTRAINT OVER FEE — NO VISITORS

A doctor had a dispute with the patient over his fee. This of course was to him an *emergency,* and he grabbed the patient, locked her up in a room, and wouldn't let her go until he called the Marshal. The doctor had told the patient, "Leave the teeth or pay the price," and kept the patient from leaving. As fate would have it, the patient-plaintiff later had a miscarriage, and the court was most lenient in granting general damages plus punitive damages.[91] The court was most positive in its approach that there is no excuse for this type of procedure; although even today many doctors' actions parallel this, there is no justification for it.

It has been clear for many years that when a mother suffers mental upset and illness from seeing intentional injury to her child liability on the part of the injurer has been created.[92] This points up a rule most doctors follow: the parents or friends of the patient will not be allowed in the operating room. It is easily seen from newspaper reports of alleged manhandling of children and alleged assault and battery that if "Mama" were allowed to view the treatment, and an untoward incident occurred, there might be an additional cause of action for her supposed mental grievances, besides those that the minor-patient urges for himself.[93] It must be remembered that monetary damages in personal injuries are tax free.

Assault and battery charges will lie against a doctor who takes back the dentures to insure payment of a "debt." What is significant is that the law allows *punitive* damages under these circumstances.[94]

For the uninitiated, punitive damages are those that are assessed against the defendant when he is being "punished" for his actions. They are in addition to the usual "pain or suffering" damages, which are classified as general or compensatory damages. They are "important" in that they are *not* covered by the usual professional liability insurance.

Recovery by the patient's spouse, mother, or father for "their" emotional distress has now been extended to cases in which they are not even present when the alleged "negligent act" by the doctor takes place, but are only in some theoretical "zone of danger," and even when the "act" is negligent, not intentional (injection case).[95]

A word of caution regarding the collection of fees. Judgment should be used as to whether or not it is advisable to collect a fee from a patient who suffered from an untoward incident during dental care and treatment. Also, when attempting to collect fees, courts (usually of monetary jurisdictional limits up to $1000) where we attorneys are not allowed to practice should be the method of choice. Suing through collection agencies usually forces your ex-patient to hire an attorney. So frequently we then see the counterclaim for malpractice as "retaliation" to the collection attempt.[96]

Recently new laws, both federal and state, have been enacted, limiting doctors' rights in collection, and also limiting collection agencies' methods. When there is a violation of the law, we often see countersuits for interference with contract, invasion of privacy, intentional causing of emotional distress, and so on ad nauseam. Be forewarned!

As a corollary, most states have laws making it illegal to record telephone conversations when one party lacks knowledge of the recording. Also, most states allow a cause of action when a person is threatened with criminal actions while attempting to gain advantage in any civil action.[97]

Most jurisdictions have laws regarding who has legal responsibility for dental bills. The writer will not attempt to set forth these rules here, but suffice to say that they involve age, contract, divorce, custody, bankruptcy, etc. To try to collect from a person who doesn't legally owe the debt often leads to a countersuit against the doctor.[98]

PRESCRIPTIONS IN EMERGENCIES

There is a great tendency among doctors to prescribe medicines for patients in emergencies, rather than referring them to a specialist. The danger in not gaining someone else's opinion is that if something goes wrong there is no one to back the doctor up.

Probably in most jurisdictions it is illegal not to write prescriptions for certain drugs. Practice has it that the phone is so easy and some pharmacists are so trustworthy that the law is overlooked. Let me assure you that liability in these regards happens with some frequency; as often as not the doctor will prescribe XYZ over the phone, the pharmacist will write ABC, and the lawsuit follows. The doctor is placed in the position of having no written record, whereas the pharmacist has his written prescription as taken over the phone. The answer to this is, always, whether an emergency or not, write down the prescription, the date and how prescribed on the prescription pad, and place it with the patient's chart. It cannot be stressed enough that if some habit-forming drug is prescribed, extreme caution should be used to avoid being blamed for any addiction that might be formed.

As this chapter is being prepared the FDA has ordered a reassessment of the prescribing practices for Librium and Valium. The "improper" use of a product most certainly may cause liability. The agents, their instructions and contraindications, and the PDR inserts all must be understood and be kept up to date. Recently, the medical doctors who treated Freddie Prinze during his life (he shot himself to death) were sued on the theory that they negligently "prescribed for" him during his life.

More than once a year this writer defends a dental practitioner against the allegation that a prescribed drug caused death, suicide, or addiction.

Science has yet to satisfactorily inform the doctor of all the synergistic and potentiating actions of the various drugs and agents. Therefore, a constant reminder — whatever drug or agent is used, its effect and contraindication should be well known. Lack of tests on the patient, when called for as determined by the health history and/or agent utilized, and when the patient suffers from these tests not being performed, may constitute liability.[99]

It should go without saying that in most jurisdictions it is illegal (a crime) to prescribe certain drugs over the telephone and without seeing the patient. A doctor will usually be held liable for any adverse effects of this practice.

Wrong drugs are often prescribed. Questions also arise as to the site and depth of the injection, allergy, failure to heed the warning of a health history, overdosage, disregard of premedication elements, lack of sterile procedure, no aspiration, unsuitable vasoconstrictor, nonfresh product etc.

The law makes it mandatory that the doctor know the applicable health history of the patient. If the patient is extremely nervous, the doctor is held to know that certain commonly used drugs in dentistry may cause hallucinations, etc. The list of possibilities is endless.

Doctors have been warned about the use of antidepressant drugs and the contraindications of some food such as chicken livers, sherry, etc. The result of not knowing the health history of a patient under these circumstances could well be disastrous — high blood pressure crises. Other common-knowledge drug contraindications are endless, such as aspirin with an anticoagulant, oral contraceptives with an anticoagulant, digitalis drugs with laxatives, etc.

Even a labeled cosmetic may be a "drug" and temporarily affect the skin.[100]

Some dental schools now teach their students to take blood and urine tests to aid in recognizing diseases that influence a person's health. This is important owing to the disease and drug counterparts, such as diabetes, because those afflicted are more susceptible to infections and are slow healers.

When the harmful effects of the drug are not told the patient, and a later injury occurs, the statute of limitations does not run against the patient until the patient discovers the cause of the injury.[101]

Stanford University linked a widely used anesthetic (trade name in the United States, Penthrane) to kidney disturbances. This, of course, again reflects the absolute necessity of knowing the drug's side effects and presupposes the doctor's taking an adequate health history from the patient.

The doctor must be on *constant* alert to be certain that a drug he might be utilizing is not "new" or experimental so as to avoid liability from injury by a patient's use.[102]

A doctor's license may be challenged by the appropriate authorities when he is alleged to have been prescribing without proper prescriptions.[103]

Also, a dental practitioner might be charged with illegally selling narcotics when he dispenses dangerous drugs.[104]

FOREIGN BODIES

Some jurisdictions have held against the doctor for negligence in allowing some particle, tooth, bur, x-ray film, etc., to drop into the patient's throat and be swallowed.[105]

In order to alleviate any possible future aggravation, it would seem best to have the patient referred to an M.D. to be certain of the placement of the foreign body and have the M.D. continue x-raying until the foreign body has been evacuated. If a tooth lodges in an area where it won't pass, consideration must be given to the probabilities and potential danger to the patient. This at all times must be discussed with the patient so that he or she may have an intelligent voice in the proceedings.

The cases of foreign bodies, whether a needle, a broken tooth, or a root, are quite frequent. More often than not the doctor is held accountable for such an experience.[106]

The vital point to realize in such an emergency is that if a standard of care requires proceeding immediately to remedy the situation, then one must either be competent to do so or immediately refer the patient to a specialist. Experiences have shown that with modern disposable needles of proper gauge, length, etc., there are fewer broken needles every year. Difficulty arises when doctors attempt to remove the broken piece when they are not qualified and do not have the equipment to proceed properly. In this latter situation it must be recalled that any prolongation of time in holding the patient's mouth open gives serious rise to possible joint problems, trismus, etc. Often there is more damage done to the joint than could ever possibly be anticipated in the tracing of a needle by too long an operation for the recovery. It appears now that the standard of care would call for a competent operator who has been trained in such procedures as obtaining proper x-rays, using tracer needles, etc., so as to block any later attack on the operator's adequacy.

It must also be stressed that records must evidence what instructions are given the patient following an untoward incident. If the patient was properly instructed to use an antibiotic and has failed to follow the instructions, the court probably will state that there is nothing to show any liability on the part of the defendant.[107]

The law places the burden on the professional person to have his instructions understood. The import is that instructions are no good if not understood, or if there is a language barrier, mental block, minority, etc. If the patient once had difficulty with a procedure, the doctor is accountable to act accordingly later. Recently there was a matter in which all proper instructions and preparations were made for multiple extractions. The patient had not eaten for the prescribed length of time, but yet under the general anesthetic there was great regurgitation, and x-rays evidenced vomitus injected into the lungs. The next time the patient was to return for treatment the doctor would be held to the knowledge that at the prior visit the usual time allowed for eating did not suffice, and this patient must have extra time allowed. In a more precautionary vein, probably prior to any further work there should be an O.K. from an M.D. and if at all possible, a local analgesic should be given.

PRE-EMERGENCY PRECAUTIONS

It used to be thought that in an emergency the standard of care would be that of the community in which one practiced. It recently has become apparent that the courts will not allow anyone to practice below a certain minimum standard of care, no matter what type of practice might be prevalent in any one community. The theory is that the day of the horse and buggy is gone and that everyone has access to written material, seminar courses, etc.[108]

As far as can be determined, the courts seemingly hold that it is a factual question whether there is any malpractice in allowing a patient, when under a sedative or awakening from anesthesia, to climb over restraining bars when there was no safety strap in place.[109]

Malpractice jurisprudence advises that instructions put down in the pamphlet of any drug or antibiotic had better be understood and followed (unless there could be contrary conclusive evidence that the drug usage was a departure from what was the standard of care in the community when utilized), because the instruction pamphlet will be admissible in evidence as setting the standard of care.[110]

It would appear advisable, owing to the seeming liberalization of rules within which doctors are found liable, if a doctor is performing operative work of any kind, and if there might be some emergency later, whether it be reaction to a drug, excessive pain, bleeding, infection, etc., that a telephone exchange be available for patients on a 24-hour basis, seven days a week.

With the ease of answering service communication, it now appears apparent that the doctor should be available (or have another doctor on call) at all times, and when not in the office, be able to be reached by phone. If not, liability may ensue if this causes injury to the patient.[111]

Needless to say, a duty is placed on the general practitioner to refer the patient to a specialist if it is the standard of care to so do.[112] Most states have jury instructions that succinctly state this rule. It is not true that all jurisdictions require the general practitioner, if he is doing the work of a specialist, to practice the standard of care of that specialist when he undertakes that specialty type of work for the patient. It is true, unequivocally, though, that if the doctor holds himself out to be a specialist, he is held to that higher standard of care.[113] In one case, the defendant doctor claimed to be a specialist in endodontia. The reamer was swallowed. Usual conflicting versions followed. The patient stated that the doctor said, at the time of the incident, "I dropped it, I dropped it." The doctor said the patient "moved," causing the problem. "Untoward" statements are so very crucial, as will be pointed out later in more detail.

Once control is assumed over the patient, a duty is owed not only to the patient but to third parties. Recently we have seen premedication at home prior to coming to the office. Owing to the circumstances of an improper health history, the premedication was contraindicated, and such patients had auto accidents which involved injuries to other persons.

A patient should not be allowed to leave the office while still under some sedation or not fully conscious and alert after an anesthetic. A patient might not know what he was doing and cause tragic circumstances to others and himself.

It is appalling to note that in some dental offices oxygen is not readily available. It is common knowledge that there are approximately as many cardiac arrests from apprehension *and emotional upset* when local analgesics are used as when a general anesthetic is given. Oxygen, of course, is standard equipment, and it is felt by many that the failure to have it available or not know how to use it would create liability. The entire office staff should be trained for all emergencies, including cardiac arrest, etc.

Existing or prior health problems will govern as to the choice of local analgesic utilized, its strength, and whether a vasoconstrictor is to be used. The manufacturer's instructions show how to control any unusual sensitivity or convulsions. This alerts the doctor that he must have the knowledge, competence, equipment, and supplies with which to operate. It would seem certain that the standard of care should be such that before any local analgesic is administered, the blood pressure be taken — at least that is the indication of the case of Quanital v. Laurel Grove Hospital.[114]

As will be discussed later in detail, consent (informed) must be gained from the *patient,* not his or her spouse, and medication cannot be forcibly administered without liability.[115]

In some jurisdictions, when you injure one spouse the other may also sue for loss of consortium, i.e., loss of society, companionship, conjugal affections and physical assistance. Damages may run high.[116]

OPERATIVE EMERGENCY

In effect, as discussed before, the "emergency doctrine" allows a different and probably lesser standard of care. In reality, this means that treatment under those circumstances need be accomplished within the "emergency doctrine" standard of care. What is this standard? It is most difficult to describe, because each set of facts is different. In general, though, the doctor in the emergency situation must act as others would under the circumstances and proceed onward if he is competent to so do.[117] Certainly the doctor is not required to stop to gain express consent to proceed,[118] and if the emergency situation clearly calls for referral to a specialist, this must be accomplished. Any unneeded delay might be interpreted as aggravating the original incident and be adverse to the doctor's case.[119]

Cases that go to juries seemingly make it very clear what is expected of practitioners in emergencies. The practitioner should be trained in emergency care itself, with accompanying knowledge as to drug usage and administration, CPR, etc. If a doctor does not have the proper equipment, such as differing size oxygen face masks, laryngoscope, etc., he will certainly be open to criticism by the plaintiff's attorney.

If the doctor knows he does not have the capability to handle the situation, it is quite clear there is a duty for immediate referral.[120]

If a doctor decides to tackle the emergency situation himself, he must be properly equipped, and have trained personnel to give him adequate assistance. Without these precautions he lays himself open to grave criticism.[121] Never give assurances like "everything will be all right," and do not "abandon" the patient.[122]

If this sounds like the dental office in which all employees should act like a team and "drill" on various possible emergencies, that is absolutely correct. These could run the gamut from cuts to respiratory collapse to aspirated foreign bodies.

Most dental practitioners do some oral surgery, i.e., extractions of teeth, etc., and must at all times be cautious with regard to hemorrhage. It is now probably standard procedure that the proper health history is utilized by anyone doing operative procedures when a regional or general anesthetic is used.

If the patient is a bleeder, he must of course be asked if he is taking or has recently taken any drugs. If there is any doubt at all, laboratory tests are in order. Usually, though, the patient knows if he suffers from hemophilia. If major dental surgery is involved, the doctor should be prepared for any emergency and be competent to handle it.

Operative procedure probably demands that the doctor be prepared for the possibility of a cut cheek, floor of the mouth wound, or lip laceration. These highly vascular soft tissues bleed easily, and the operator must be competent to control any hemorrhage. The doctor, for example, is held accountable for knowing that the roots of the mandibular third molars are especially close to the inferior alveolar vessels. When these vessels are ruptured, severe hemorrhage often occurs.

There should be a set routine in the office for periodic inspection of all equipment, running from necessary flashlight batteries to the sterilization of equipment. If not done, the ever-alert plaintiff's attorney will certainly crucify the defendant on his office procedure and training of employees.

The doctor should know, in general, how to diagnose shock and what type of shock is involved. Certain types of shock point to specific action.

When the operative result entails infections, and when there is more than one method to treat this and the wrong selection of method is made and followed, this does not mean there is malpractice.[123] This signifies the importance of never criticizing a prior doctor's care and treatment or result, as perhaps there were different alternatives available that are not known at the present time. Also, seldom is the doctor afforded all the facts from the patient, and even if given "most" of the facts, they are often hazy and/or colored or mistaken.

One doctor should not "cause" the termination of a treatment by another doctor whose treatment would prolong life (cancer case). It might result in murder charges.[124]

DECLARED EMERGENCIES

Jurisdictions that have not provided for the protection of their health practitioners should immediately proceed to give them such immunity during times they render services when there is a state of emergency or disaster or when they have been requested by a state official or agency or local disaster counsel to give treatment.[125]

A like situation is the "Good Samaritan" rule. Most states have such rules; in effect, they state that if a doctor helps a person who is in distress and as an emergency, and if the work is in good faith, there will be no liability.[126] To the same effect, where there is a declared emergency in a hospital, then the dental practitioner is given a waiver of liability for his work.[127]

Of course, if a jury finds that there is *no* emergency, then there is *no* waiver of liability.[128] Thus, the afforded protection is not absolute and is subject to after-the-fact interpretation. Very comforting, eh what!

STATEMENTS IN EMERGENCIES

Doctors are human, like anyone else. When faced with an untoward incident and shaken by a result that might be most disastrous, the doctor often lets certain words slip that he will remember the rest of his life, and would probably give a million dollars to retract and erase. Recall the case of the doctor who, after giving a hypodermic injection and extracting teeth (with alleged unsterilized instruments, for the patient-plaintiff ended up with a severe infection on her arm), told his nurse: "I wonder if Mrs. Dimock will ever forgive me for wrecking her arm."[129]

In the same vein, can you picture the doctor, after extracting a tooth and breaking the patient's jaw, stating to the patient: "I did break your jaw; I guess I hit you a little too hard."[130]

Office personnel should be trained so that when an untoward event occurs, the dental assistant won't be saying, "Oh, what a terrible cut," or, "Gee, you goofed that time, didn't you, Doctor?" The doctor can certainly be sympathetic, and teach his employees to be the same, but statements regarding cause, severity, etc., are to be avoided at all times.

If, after the operation is over, the nurse or dental assistant has to admit that the doctor had charged her with the failure to properly sterilize the instruments (and an infection did develop), the liability will, naturally, be against the doctor.[131]

In the cases in which we talk of admissions or exclamations by the doctor and his employees, and how deadly they may be, courts have permitted these items to be relied upon by the plaintiff in establishing liability.[132]

Often the most devastating evidence of malpractice comes from the lips of the doctor, such as, "Boy, I sure made a mess of things."[133]

To the same effect is an improper expression of regret, such as: "He did not blame her husband for being angry about the occurrence."[134]

Can you imagine the effect on a patient who has suffered postoperative complications to hear a doctor say, after reopening the area, "Well, I'll be darned, it is a piece of cotton." And how much consolation is given a patient who, after seeing the doctor be fidgety and grouchy, is cut and then hears the doctor say, "I'm sorry — but these kids have upset me. They have been in here all afternoon."

If the reader were a patient who had just had a mandible fractured, he or she would not be very happy to hear the doctor say, "It gave me the most difficulty I've had in forty years."

There is always a reverse twist to these situations, and invariably, as Murphy's law so decrees, one is likely to hear a judge say, as in one orthodontic matter being tried, that he "felt the dentist's failure to take certain steps . . . constituted negligence!"

POST-EMERGENCY RAPPORT

After some event has occurred which might tend to upset the rapport of the doctor-patient relationship, if the patient still decides to continue with the dental services, ordinarily the doctor's refusal would constitute malpractice.[139] The general rule of mutual cooperation on the part of the patient and the doctor is that the patient must return for treatment often enough to give the practitioner a reasonable opportunity to give postoperative care.[140] Of course, if the doctor is employed for one item of treatment or for some specific matter, there would be no duty to continue thereafter, if he has satisfactorily treated the patient for the contracted service.[141]

It is also true that if the work is badly done, the patient is not required to allow the doctor a second chance.[142] In this particular case the doctor undertook to fit jackets on the teeth and inferentially promised that the color would match the natural teeth; but they didn't. The patient contended that they were a darker color, and that she was the subject of ridicule by her friends. The doctor stated, yes, they were a different color, but that he expected the patient to return. When the jury saw the jackets and the teeth, they decided that the plaintiff was under no duty to allow the doctor to attempt to continue.

Of course it should be noted that if at any time there is an agreement between the doctor and patient that the treatment would be mutually discontinued, it should be put in writing and entered on the chart.

Assuming that there isn't a minor, or incompetent, etc., involved, the doctor is not always blessed with a patient forever. Probably he can discuss the matter with the patient and suggest that dental services can be provided by another doctor, that the rapport has been ruptured, and give the patient a reasonable opportunity to secure the services of another doctor. This does not mean that when a doctor has the emergency of an infection after an extraction, and when it is proved that there was some failure in the sterilization technique, he could shun the problem and send the patient on. To the contrary, those postoperative services are a necessary part of the originally contracted dental care.[143]

Assume that the emergency is "over" and the "result" lingers on, as for example an oroantral fistula. If healing and closure do not progress right on schedule, the failure to refer might be held against the doctor.[144] The logical "next step" is that the doctor will be liable if, after the emergency is treated, a precautionary referral is not accomplished.[145] Cases representative of this dilemma range from orthodontic "failure" to as little as time lost by failure to telephone.

ADVICE RE MISHAP

It has been held that a cause of action will lie against the doctor for allegedly leaving roots of six teeth in the jaw after extractions when he knew it and didn't tell the plaintiff.[146] Later x-rays showed the condition, and the patient suffered pain and generally rundown health. The court's theory is that the patient has the ability to understand the knowledge imparted by the doctor and that this must be passed to him. This particular case also stands for the proposition that the statute of limitations for any alleged negligent act will not begin to run until the time the patient learns of the condition.

A most intriguing case is Furniss v. Fitchett.[147] In the New Zealand case, a doctor disclosed to the patient's husband the patient's mental condition; thereafter, when the patient learned of this, she suffered a severe reaction. The doctor was held liable. A like case in the United States is the well-known "cancer phobia" case,[148] wherein a patient claimed damages following the disclosure that x-ray burns negligently caused by the defendant might result in cancer. In another case, the patient suffered from a malignant disease which required surgery. The court held the doctor liable for emotional distress because the doctor had advised the patient that the surgery would not be advisable now because of the damage done to her heart through his prior negligence.

In the emergency in which some foreign object is left in a patient's person, whether it be a broken needle, root tip, etc., some courts will permit a jury to infer negligence just by the presence of that foreign object.[149]

A doctor and his assistants' manner after the emergency has occurred will be much more important than the requisite dental skill. Human nature being what it is, the patient expects added attention and personal contact. There is nothing wrong in stating that one is sorry for an incident, but that of course does not mean admitting liability for the act. Public relations and kindness go a long way to alleviate problems which might otherwise arise in the mind of the patient. What with the tendency toward more frequent and larger dental malpractice judgments, the practitioner must do more than just practice dentistry.

EMERGENCY REFERRAL

As stated before, the duty of the doctor in referring a patient to a specialist only arises if, under the same circumstances, a reasonable, careful, and skillful general dental practitioner would so act. Elements that can be given attention in considering the need for a specialist include the patient's mental and emotional condition.[150] If at any time there is an emergency and the doctor realizes his own lack of competence in the particular area, he has the duty to advise the patient to employ someone more skilled and to refer the patient on.[151]

In one case it has been held that the doctor who is making dentures and is so intent that he fails to treat an opening into the antrum will be liable.[152]

LOCAL ANALGESIA

A chapter could be written on the legal aspects of local analgesia. Why? Because thousands of injections are given each working day, and various problems naturally arise from them.

It goes without saying that any "incorrect" method of needle insertion may be a cause for liability.[153]

The doctor is held to know the correct type of local analgesic and its contraindications, the percentage that should be used, whether a vasoconstrictor should be included, the injection amount, the size and gauge of the needle, and so on into infinity. The patient's health, age, weight, etc., are the factors that decide the "correctness," and there certainly can be no "general" or "standard" dosage. For your own edification, read the insert that comes with the product to check the contraindications, the *time* that should be taken to inject the solution, and how aspiration is necessary.

Every year there are many deaths from local analgesia; and there are also many other problems involved in its use, so do not be lulled into a false sense of security by the success and apparent ease of administration you normally enjoy.

Let us assume that a patient is seen as an emergency, swollen and in pain. If the local analgesic is injected into an infected area, liability may be predicated upon the theory that invasion of the infected area might have caused the infection to spread.[154]

In a recent case in which the patient broke his arm during a local analgesic injection, the patient claimed that he probably "held on too tight" and that the doctor was to blame because he improperly positioned the patient's arms.[155]

Although an entire chapter could also be written about nitrous oxide, suffice it to say that, from the author's personal experience, every calamity from death to hallucinations can and does occur with its use. Again, just read the literature to remind yourself of the admonitions concerning health history, extreme nervousness, and so on. *Records* about this subject will be covered later in this chapter.

What is worrisome to those of us who defend in dental malpractice matters is the declaration by some courts that when nitrous oxide is used the patient is considered to be "under the influence" and hence not responsible for his or her acts, thus depriving us of affirmative defenses such as contributory negligence, assumption of risk, comparative negligence, etc.[156]

POST-EMERGENCY TREATMENT

If there has been a prior operation on a patient and a complication of the same or a like condition is now in question, the law requires that, before proceeding, the professional person who last treated the patient must be contacted.[157]

A doctor may not induce the nonhiring of a troublesome patient.[158]

Perhaps every day each doctor sees a patient who has suffered some incident at the hands of a fellow practitioner's. It would appear that a few cardinal rules should govern:

1. Don't attempt to judge the other doctor's efforts — even judges and juries have difficulties in this endeavor.
2. Don't make conclusionary statements about the prior doctor's work; just do the best possible. Tell the truth in a factual and dental way.
3. Don't assume to know the condition of the patient when originally treated, nor the handicaps or instructions given.
4. Always call the other doctor before proceeding.
5. Avoid giving conclusions as to what might have been done or what should have been done. Always explain, and this is true, that there are many different methods and techniques that are proper in regard to the same problem, all of which are acceptable and constitute good practice. The law allows no guarantee to the patient.

If in treating the emergency or treating someone else's emergency, there is some question in mind, by all means call in a consultant or verify, whether it be by phone or otherwise, the plan or procedure.

DEATH

The recent decisions regarding alleged malpractice causing cardiac arrest while under an anesthetic state startling principles.[159] The child who suffered the cardiac arrest was six years old and was normal except that he had a runny nose, he was very apprehensive, his eyes turned inward a bit, and he had a slight temperature. When all vital signs ceased, the doctor knew something had to be done but didn't feel qualified to give resuscitation. Because of this a lengthy interval passed until someone else was found to give open heart massage. The court stressed that there is always a calculated risk of cardiac arrest when a patient is given a general anesthetic. The court stated that there should be qualified personnel immediately available in order to handle emergency resuscitation attempts. It also stated that great attention should be given to the health history, paying special regard to any slight rise in temperature and any slight apprehension. It is known that apprehension is an emotional state which causes epinephrine to be pumped into the circulatory system, which increases the sensitivity of the heart, which in turn can cause a reaction to the vagus nerve. The court stated that both apprehension and temperature increase are danger signals. The time element in regard to being prepared and competent to handle the rescue effort was all important. The court concluded that the doctrine of res ipsa loquitur might well be given to the jury, and if it applied there would be an inference of negligence.

The humane issues at death far outweigh any of the legal issues, but some legal conclusions will be set forth:

1. Do not volunteer to take care of everything, and state that the body will be preserved, etc. If someone else takes care of the remains and directions are not followed, and the next of kin notices this and suffers shock, the doctor will be liable for damages.[160]

2. The next of kin has the right to bury and/or preserve the remains; one cannot allow this to be done by someone else without the next of kin's consent.[161]
3. The surviving spouse is the person who has the right to control the disposition, not other relatives.[162]
4. Probably the fact that the doctor authorized an autopsy without gaining the proper consent would create liability.[163]
5. No arrangement should be made with anyone but the next of kin as to the retention of body organs, brain, etc. Although retention of body parts might enhance the advancement of science, this does not negate the next of kin's rights, and when this right is violated, damages for mental suffering are proper.[164]

The foregoing does not vitiate the instructions in a decedent's will, of course. California has now set out an Anatomical Gift Act, allowing the deceased to dispose of the whole or any part of his body.[165]

A wrongful death action may be brought by a deceased man's illigitimate children.[166]

Failure to promptly attempt to find and tell the next of kin of the death can cause liability.[167]

A false notice of death can create liability.[168]

Allowing undue display of the deceased *body* creates liability.[169]

The "secret" burial of the deceased creates liability.[170]

As a corollary to the foregoing, just because there is an inability to determine the cause of death is no excuse for failing to gain permission for the autopsy.[171]

This section of the chapter is *meant* to be cursory. The reason is that the causes, agents utilized, lack of health histories, types of damages, *who* recovers damages, lack of equipment, inadequacy of training for CPR, and so on, are so extensive that they should not be treated except in *great* depth. Please believe the writer, death or "vegetable cases" do occur, under any and all circumstances and to any and all age groups and under any and all health conditions. Prevention and recognition of the problem, and the legal difficulties and solutions should be taught in every dental school.

At the time this chapter was being prepared a jury awarded the heir 2.8 million dollars in a death case allegedly arising from "contaminated equipment." The latest and largest malpractice verdict noted was 7.6 million dollars in an x-ray radiation case.

RECORDS

The proper preparation and maintenance of records can be a doctor's salvation in a lawsuit. These can include the patient's chart, medical history, x-rays, consent, data, etc. Records—meaning adequate records—are expected of the doctor, and if he does not keep them he may possibly be guilty of malpractice. The reason for this stems from the fact that although the patient does not have property rights to the records themselves, he does have a right to expect that proper records will be kept of his case.

Experience repeats itself many times over as to how a witness' memory will fade with time. Adequate records will refresh a doctor's recollection.

From the writer's own practical experience, a recent lawsuit was won because of detailed records the doctor had kept. The case in question involved a broken needle in the jaw, but more specifically, whether or not the patient was told of the incident. The doctor said yes; the patient said no. The patient claimed he had been discharged and was not told of any problem. The doctor alleged the plaintiff gave a phone number where he could be reached, so as to make the appointment for the plaintiff to go to the hospital for the removal of the needle fragment. The plaintiff denied this, but the records of the defendant showed a phone number written on the x-ray envelope, which, under investigation and proper presentation into the evidence, was proved to be that of the manager of the apartment house wherein the plaintiff resided. This little penciled notation undoubtedly played a major part in gaining a verdict for the defendant.

Records that are offered and accepted into evidence are physical in nature; they are tangible, not illusory. They may be viewed by the jury. The jury frequently will forget or discount what has been said two or three days before, but if they can take the physical evidence into the jury room during deliberation, they cannot ignore those items.

Records, if kept in the usual business of the doctor, need not be personally entered by the doctor, but may be put down by whoever usually does those chores. The importance of this is shown when the patient suffers a cut cheek. If the patient's chart evidences that the patient moved after being warned, this could go a long way toward providing a complete defense. Assume, in the same case, that the patient's chart evidences only that the doctor and the assistant were present. It forecloses the frequent allegation that there was some other witness present. These allegations usually state that a friend of the patient was present who will testify, "Oh, the doctor acted carelessly or fumbled about."

In another instance in the writer's practice, the patient died in the dental chair after having been administered a local analgesic. As luck would have it, the inevitable plaintiff's attorney showed up stating that he represented the widow and that he believed that filing a dental malpractice suit would be a fine idea. He was shown the records of the doctor, and on the plaintiff's chart was a signed health history, including a question asking about prior cardiac conditions. The deceased had lied and stated that he had none, when as a matter of fact, he had been under the constant care of a physician for the past few years. The deceased had signed the health chart, and with that, of course, the claim and threatened litigation ended.

The proper time to prepare records is at or near the time of the emergency itself. At no other time will the doctor have so fresh in his mind the facts to be recorded. At a later date an entry should not be recorded, as there are adequate methods to determine that the entry was not made at or about the time of the treatment. This writer well remembers the doctor whose records were adequate. The defendant-doctor's deposition had been taken and the records properly marked and photostated. Later at the time of trial the doctor appeared with his records for final review. He had "doctored" and changed the records, stating that he thought this would be a truer reflection of the facts and would help his case. A winning case thus became questionable.

The public policy of keeping records even outweighs provisions in a doctor's will to destroy or bury all his patients' records.[172]

When it comes to proof in court about the patient's complaints (opening into sinus), records, when kept properly, can be a good defense.[173]

If a patient refuses help from an employee in sitting down, leaving the office, etc., this should be marked on the chart and would be proof of assumption of risk on the patient's part if an injury later occurs.[174]

The *records* must show the *age* of a minor (assuming a valid informed consent is gained from the proper person), for if the patient is a minor and prescriptions for drugs are provided, the doctor may be guilty of contributing to the delinquency of a minor.[175]

The problems of records and minors are always troublesome to the doctor. California has adopted *modern* laws addressed to the subject. California allows a pregnant minor to seek dental care as if an adult.[176] California also allows a minor over 15, under certain conditions, to give valid consent to the doctor.[177]

An adequate history is of course a most vital and important "record" regarding the patient. It should be signed by the patient and taken before any care and treatment are rendered.[178] A good history will "catch" the use of drugs or the mixing of medications.[179]

An adequate history should allow the doctor a *correct* choice of local analgesic, or *correct* sedation, etc., covering such important considerations as use of vasoconstrictor, aspirin, etc.

False records can be absolutely disastrous and subject the doctor to punitive damages.[180]

When the examination by the doctor might have called for a different type of operative procedure and this was not entered on the record, liability might follow.[181]

Courts have become very strict when any dental surgery is performed without a signed adequate health history. An allegation by plaintiff that the failure to take the history caused an aggravation of a pre-existing cardiac valvular lesion and subacute bacterial endocarditis will allow the jury to determine whether or not this constitutes malpractice.[182]

Some dental practitioners utilize a voluminous medical history such as shown in Figure 25–1. Individual questioning of the patient seems to be an absolute must. The reader is referred to chapter 2 for a discussion of the merits of brief vs. long medical histories.

Adequate records must be kept in order to defend against allegations of fraud in Medicare actions.[183] Records are necessary to show the plaintiff's present health condition and his or her condition before care and treatment was undertaken. In a recent case handled by this author, a postoperative complaint following an injection was involuntary muscle tremors. The patient's health history was utilized to prove that the patient had a long-standing history of alcoholism, and that this condition predated any treatment supplied by the defendant.

Properly and adequately prepared records can show the true cause of a residual foreign body and help prove affirmative defense of the statute of limitations. Records can prove the doctor's acts and reasons in cases of mandatory reporting to the authorities regarding the "battered child" or "contagious disease" patient.

Dental records often reflect and uncover the fact that severe pain in the oral cavity is referred pain from the cardiac area as a result of heart attack.

Text continued on page 727

MEDICAL/DENTAL HEALTH HISTORY

PATIENT NAME _____ AGE _____

DATE OF BIRTH _____ PLACE OF BIRTH _____

HEIGHT _____ WEIGHT _____

DIRECTIONS: ALL QUESTIONS WILL REQUIRE A "NO" ANSWER OR A POSITIVE
             RESPONSE IN ONE OR MORE WORDS. PLEASE FILL IN COMPLETELY
             AND ANSWER ALL QUESTIONS.

EXAMPLES: A. DO YOU HAVE A TOOTHACHE?   YES, FOR 3 DAYS
           B. HAVE YOU BEEN HOSPITALIZED?   1970, APPENDECTOMY
           C. DO YOU HAVE PAIN AT THIS TIME?   NO

MEDICAL

1. Have you been examined by a physician within the past year? _____

   For what reason? _____

2. Has there been any change in your general health in the past year? _____

   _____

3. Are you currently being treated by a physician for a medical problem? _____

   _____

4. Please list any prescribed medications taken within the past year: _____

   _____

5. Have you ever been seriously ill? _____

6. Please list dates and reasons for all hospital admissions: _____

   _____

7. Have you had radiation treatment for any tumor or growth? _____

8. Do you often feel exhausted or fatigued? _____

Figure 25-1

9. Have you ever had any of the following diseases or conditions? Please list dates:

    Hepatitis_____Colitis_____

    Tuberculosis_____Thrombophlebitis_____

    Stomach Ulcers_____Diabetes_____

    Epilepsy_____Arthritis_____

    Porphyria_____Other_____

CARDIOVASCULAR

1. Have you ever had a heart attack or stroke?_____

_____

2. Do you have high blood pressure?_____

3. Have you ever had rheumatic fever?_____

4. Do you have a heart murmur or any heart defect?_____

_____

5. Do you have chest pain (angina) with physical exertion?_____

_____

6. Do you have any blood disorder such as anemia (thin blood)?_____

_____

7. Have you ever had an excessive bleeding problem?_____

_____

8. Do your ankles ever swell?_____

RESPIRATORY

1. Do you have a persistant cough?_____

2. Are you ever short of breath with mild exertion?_____

3. Do you have asthma?_____

4. Do you have emphysema?_____

5. Do you have bronchitis?_____

Figure 25-1 *Continued*

Illustration continued on following page

ALLERGIES

1. Have you ever experienced an unfavorable reaction to any of the following medications? If yes, please indicate type of reaction:

   Valium_____Percodan_____

   Penicillin_____Aspirin_____

   Atropine_____Codeine_____

   Demerol_____Talwin_____

   Erythromycin_____Sodium Pentothal_____

   Sodium Brevital_____Other_____

NEUROLOGICAL

1. Do you have numbness or tingling in any part of your body?_____

   _____

2. Has any part of your body ever been paralyzed?_____

3. Do you ever have convulsions?_____

4. Do you have frequent severe headaches?_____

5. Have you ever had psychiatric treatment?_____

6. Do you have a tendency to faint?_____

7. Do you consider yourself to be a nervous person?_____

8. Have you ever suffered from severe nervous exhaustion (breakdown)?_____

   _____

9. Do you often feel unhappy and depressed?_____

10. Do you often cry?_____

11. Do you have a profound fear of dental treatment?_____

DISABILITY

1. Do you wear contact lenses?_____

2. Do you use a hearing aid?_____

3. Are you disabled in any way?_____

   _____

Figure 25–1 *Continued*

DENTAL

1. Have you ever experienced an unfavorable reaction to a local anesthetic (Xylocaine or Novocain)? _____

2. Have you ever had Sodium Pentothal or Sodium Brevital in an Oral Surgery office? _____

3. Have you ever had an unfavorable reaction to any dental treatment? _____

_____

4. Do you have difficulty in opening your mouth wide? _____

_____

5. Have you ever had an injury to the face, jaws or neck? _____

_____

6. Does your jaw ever "click", "pop", or give you a sharp pain or discomfort?

_____

7. Do you have regular dental care? _____

8. Have you had orthodontic care? _____

9. Would you like a referral to a general dentist for further care? _____

PERSONAL

1. Do you smoke or use tobacco frequently? _____

2. Do you drink alcohol frequently? _____

3. Have you ever been addicted to any drug? _____

FOR THE LADIES ONLY

1. Are you pregnant? _____

2. Have you passed through menopause? _____

3. Have you had a hysterectomy or ovariectomy? _____

GENERAL

1. How do you consider your health to be?

    Excellent_____ Good_____ Average_____ Fair_____ Poor_____

Figure 25–1 *Continued*

Illustration continued on following page

2. Please list all medications that you are now taking:_____

    _____

    _____

    _____

    _____

3. Are you currently experiencing dental pain or swelling?_____

    _____

4. Do you prefer general anesthesia (Sodium Brevital) or local anesthesia

    (Xylocaine or Novocain)?_____

5. Please indicate any important medical or dental information not already

    covered by this questionnaire:_____

    _____

    _____

    _____

    _____

    _____

    _____

PLEASE SIGN AND DATE BELOW:

_____   _____
SIGNATURE (Patient, or parent if minor)   Date

_____   _____
Reviewed by: Nurse   Doctor

Figure 25–1 *Continued*

Within six months of this writing the author has handled eight trial matters for dentists involving local analgesic reaction (epilepsy), mandible fracture, local analgesic fear (cancer), lingual and inferior alveolar paresthesia, root canal-apico, crown and bridge, periodontal operation, and full-mouth reconstruction. In each instance, on each doctor's chart, there were notations regarding advice given and not followed, alternate choices, referral to specialists, offers to redo the work, etc. In *each* trial, after the jury rendered their verdict for the defendant, they related the *huge* influence on their decision by the doctor's records. In *each* instance these records and x-rays were placed in evidence, marked as exhibits, and taken by the jury into their private deliberation chamber.

Some interesting asides:

1. Some jurisdictions hold that an unseated bridge belongs to the patient.[184]
2. Since records are available to the patient, their content is held to be in the knowledge of the patient when the statute of limitations is involved.[185]

Number 2, above, is a most common help in defense of the doctor's claim that the plaintiff knew of the condition at a specific time, in which case the chart may help to convince the plaintiff's attorney not to file suit, or, if suit is filed, the records are concrete evidence for jurors to refer to. Records can also be utilized to show that an emergency was involved, thus calling into effect that particular doctrine.

INFORMED CONSENT

The cocoon of confidence is not embodied in this legal doctrine. This area of law is the fastest growing within malpractice litigation. The reader would do well to confer with the attorney in his own state who specializes in defense of dental malpractice matters, as each jurisdiction is developing its own law on the subject.

In general, *at least,* the patient must be advised concerning projected dental care and treatment as to the following:

1. Reasons for care and treatment
2. Diagnosis
3. Prognosis
4. Alternatives
5. Nature of care and treatment
6. The risks involved (inherent included)
7. Expectancies of success
8. Possible results if care and treatment are not undertaken

The problem confronting the doctor is normally most perplexing in that his guidelines as to gaining informed consent from the patient come from legal language in court decisions — a veritable "professional gap." One of the "early" leading cases[186] used language as follows: ". . . (professional person) violates his duty to his patient and subjects himself to liability if he withholds any facts which are necessary to form the basis of an intelligent consent by the patient to the proposed treatment . . . may not minimize the known dangers of a procedure or operation in order to induce his patient's consent . . . is to explain to the patient any risks attendant . . . no matter how remote. . . ."

Contrast the foregoing with the language of another state court as to all that is needed in informed consent, wherein merely stating "It's a serious operation, not done without risks" was found to be sufficient.[187]

A continuing problem of "decision" lies with the situation of a patient whose psychological and emotional conditions (depressed, nervous, unstable, etc.) are in question. How far should the doctor go? To alarm the patient might generate reactions that increase the hazards to the patient. The law has become most *exacting* in these circumstances and unrelenting in demanding that informed consent be gained even when the patient was "upset, agitated, anxious, depressed, crying, and had been drinking and having marital difficulties."[188] To the same effect the law seems clear that if the risk is "high" of an untoward result, informed consent is mandatory.[189]

Some jurisdictions appear to hold that informed consent need address itself only to "probable" risks and not "possible" risks.[190] Very often there is an "overlap" between informed consent and the question of the balance of surgery as against other treatment, but invariably the issue is still treated as malpractice and liability will be imposed.[191]

The farthest reaching court language on imposing a duty of informed consent to "possible risks" is as follows: ". . . explain every risk to the patient . . . full disclosure of facts. . . ."[192] By the very nature of some treatment (cobalt irradiation), even expert evidence is not necessary to establish liability when there is *silence* as to any risks.[193] To the same effect is the statement by the doctor that "no danger can result."[194]

When a drug (antibiotic) is prescribed that has dangerous side effects, the patient must be "warned" and informed consent gained or the doctor will be liable.[195] Likewise, any "deliberate" misleading of the patient or "playing down" the risk may bring liability.[196]

The courts have become most stringent in stating that the patient must "understand" the informed consent, the meaning of words, etc., and it is incumbent on the doctor to make certain that his warnings are fully comprehended or else liability ensues.[197]

There is one case that gives solace to dental practitioners in Montana. It specifically held under the facts of that case that the doctor was *not* liable for failure to warn the patient that the mandible might fracture on the extraction of a tooth.[198] A word of caution: every case stands or falls on its own peculiar facts, testimony, experts, and judge or jury.

The law is well settled that the patient in order to make an intelligent choice must be informed of the various types of treatment possible and must give *valid* consent to his choice. The courts hold that the patient must be informed when there is offered a more hazardous type of operation so that he might select a less dangerous type of treatment.[199]

It is generally recognized that when the practitioner is confronted by an emergency of an unanticipated condition (and it would be impracticable and impossible to obtain consent) he will be allowed to proceed with what the occasion demands without gaining express consent.[200] The theory is that there is implied consent to go forward.[201]

In a case in which the mandible fractured during an attempted extraction of an infected wisdom tooth, it was alleged that the repair of the fracture was without consent because the patient-plaintiff was still under the anesthetic. In this case[202] the court stated that because of the emergency it would be impractical to bring the patient to consciousness; thus consent was implied. An interesting aside was that the court held as a matter of law that alleged rough method and discourteous manner would not prove malice. Also, the court stated that just because an operation in dentistry is painful does not mean that it is intentionally cruel so that punitive damages will be assessed against the doctor.

In the same vein, many professional people have attempted to formulate a consent that is all inclusive, like a panacea; but in reality it turns out to be a Pandora's box of troubles. The courts have held, when there are utilized the words "consent to any and all surgery," etc., that this is not valid, that it is too broad, and that it will have no more effect than to allow only the operation that was discussed with the plaintiff.[203]

It seems fairly apparent nowadays that informed consent should be gained from a patient before any operative treatment is performed. The courts say that the doctor must disclose to the patient all the facts which mutually affect his rights and interests. If this is not done, there is no intelligent consent, and any consent given is without foundation and *invalid*.[204]

The deadly effect of the informed consent doctrine is most graphically illustrated by the following: (1) If the patient is not given an informed consent and understands same, the performance of the care and treatment constitutes a technical battery.[205] (2) The defendant doctor will be liable for all damages proximately resulting, whether or not they could be anticipated.[206]

Figure 25–2 is an example of the form used for informed consent for surgery, and Figure 25–3 is an example of the informed consent form for orthodontia, formulated by the doctor and this writer. For each specialty or type of treatment we have attempted to do likewise. A word of caution: these forms are only part of the office records and should not be utilized alone. Office procedure and other records are necessary in order to make informed consents effective and practical. They, and the other planning that makes them work, have proved to be very effective in fending off litigation, and, as a bonus, are a great public relations plus for the doctor.

It is impossible in the space allotted to render a complete account of the many facets of informed consent. I *would* like to point out that there are exceptions to the mandatory requirements of informed consent, but they are minor.

Many practitioners still scoff at the legal requirements of the Informed Consent Doctrine. Let me remind you that it has been imposed by law that the patient be fully apprised, in advance of treatment, of information that will allow him or her to make an intelligent decision.

The language of the instruction by a judge to the jury in a dental malpractice case on the subject might give credence to "think preventively," and, as the old Boy Scout motto proclaims, "Be Prepared." In California the law reads as follows:

It is the duty of a dentist to disclose to his patient all relevant information to enable the patient to make an informed decision regarding the proposed operation of treatment.

There is no duty to discuss minor risks inherent in common procedures, when such procedures very seldom result in serious ill effects.

Text continued on page 733

CONSENT FOR SURGERY/ANESTHESIA

This is my consent for Dr. _____ or any dentist or physician who may be employed by Dr. _____, to perform the oral surgery indicated on my examination chart, as previously explained to me, and any other procedure deemed necessary or advisable as a corollary to the planned operation. I also agree to the use of a local and/or ultralight general anesthetic, sedation, and analgesic, depending upon the judgment of the dentists involved with my care.

I have been informed, and understand, that occasionally there are complications of the surgery, drugs and anesthesia, including pain, infection, swelling, bleeding, discoloration, numbness and tingling of the lip, tongue, chin, gums, cheeks and teeth, pain and numbness and tingling, and thrombophlebitis (inflammation of a vein) from intravenous and intramuscular injection, injury to and stiffening of neck and facial muscles, change in occlusion or temporomandibular joint difficulty, injury to the adjacent teeth or restorations in other teeth, or injury to other tissues, referred pain to ear, neck and head, nausea, vomiting, allergic reaction, bone fractures, bruises, delayed healing, sinus complications, and nasal antral fistulas and openings.

Medications, drugs, anesthetics and prescriptions may cause drowsiness and lack of awareness and coordination which can be increased by the use of alcohol or other drugs; thus, I have been advised not to operate any vehicle or hazardous devices, or work, while taking such medications and/or drugs, or until fully recovered from the effects of same. I understand and agree not to operate any vehicle or hazardous device for at least twenty-four (24) hours, or until further recovered from the effects of the anesthetic, medication and drugs that may have been given to me in the office for my care.

I acknowledge the receipt of pre-operative instructions, and understand that I should have nothing to eat or drink for at least six hours prior to receiving a general anesthetic. In addition, I acknowledge the receipt of, and understand, post-operative instructions and have been given a specific appointment date to return to the office. It has been explained to me, and I understand, that there is no warranty or guarantee as to any result and/or cure. *I understand that I can ask for a full recital of possible risks attendant to all phases of my care merely by asking.*

The following were used as an aid in the explanation of the surgery and anesthesia:
Radiographs (x-ray)_____
Drawings_____
Audiovisual media_____

_____   _____
SIGNATURE (Patient, or parent if minor)   Date

When the patient is a minor or incompetent to give consent, signature should be of a person authorized to consent for the patient.

_____
Witness

Figure 25–2

ADDENDUM TO CONSENT FOR SURGERY/ANESTHESIA

I acknowledge that my health history has revealed the following conditions:

1. _____

2. _____

3. _____

4. _____

Because of these medical conditions, it has been thoroughly explained to me, and I completely realize, that any surgical procedure may, therefore, be classified as a risk procedure. The risk involved is defined as a greater *possibility* of experiencing morbidity (the relative incidence of disease) and mortality (the proportion of deaths to population) during the surgical procedure than a person in good health. These complications which can occur during surgery may involve more than the average amount of post-operative discomfort, increased pain and swelling, and delayed healing.

I fully acknowledge that these possible complications have been *EXPLAINED IN DETAIL TO ME.* With clear knowledge of all of these possible complications, I have requested that the surgical procedure be performed in the office environment, rather than a hospital. However, it is my understanding that additional precautions will be made during my surgical procedure that will include the use of oxygen for several minutes prior to the commencement of the procedure, and electronic monitoring of the cardiovascular system by an ECG machine.

I may request further explanations of the *risks involved and possible outcome of the procedure, merely by asking.*

_____   _____
SIGNATURE (Patient, or parent if minor)   Date

When the patient is a minor or incompetent to give consent, signature should be of a person authorized to consent for the patient.

_____
Witness

Figure 25–2 *Continued*

Illustration continued on following page

INFORMED CONSENT

I hereby authorize that all necessary orthodontic treatment be given for_____
_____. This shall include the taking of necessary diagnostic records and the administration of necessary medications. I understand that all records may be used for reproduction in scientific publications and books, for exhibit under the auspices of a scientific group, and for teaching purposes at established dental schools.

I understand that orthodontic treatment cannot succeed through the efforts of the orthodontist alone, but rather through the joint cooperation of all parties involved and together we may achieve the best possible result. In many instances, lack of co-operation in the requested use of headgear, elastics, retainers and positioners will make a successful completion of treatment or maintenance of treatment result impossible.

I understand that treatment time varies with the difficulty of the problem, cooperation of the patient, and individual physiological response to treatment. Treatment time can be prolonged by broken appointments, broken appliances, poor oral hygiene, poor diet. I further understand that for the best orthodontic result progress records may be taken to evaluate treatment and make a progress diagnosis which may involve a change in the treatment plan. Occasionally, due to lack of cooperation and/or the severity of the problem a rediagnosis may require maxillofacial surgery and/or selected teeth to be removed to obtain the best possible treatment result.

I understand that during orthodontic treatment there is a possibility the following may occur: cold sores; canker sores; irritation or injury to the oral mucosa or skin; periodontal involvement; root involvement; decalcification; decay or staining under or around the orthodontic appliances; chipped or broken teeth; tooth sensitivity and mobility; loss of teeth; undesired facial changes; temporomandibular joint problems; allergic reactions to dental materials or medications; possible need for crown and/or bridgework; possible need for endodontic and/or periodontal treatment; aspiration or swallowing of dental materials, appliances or portions of appliances; eye damage; heart involvement; hepatitis.

I understand my responsibility in maintaining a well-balanced soft textured diet which is free of hard, sticky, and high sugar foods as well as maintaining a hygiene program of three brushings a day. I understand that regular dental check-ups are necessary so that the general dentist may check for decay and clean the teeth, if necessary. It is also my responsibility to immediately report any faulty appliances and insure the wearing of any supplemental appliances or retainers as instructed. If it becomes evident that further orthodontic treatment will endanger oral health or if lack of cooperation will prevent completion of a satisfactory result treatment may be discontinued.

I understand that Dr._____ will use his knowledge, skill and training to do his very best but that there is no guarantee of success of treatment and that relapse of treatment results is possible.

I understand what the problem is and the reason for treatment; the alternatives have also been explained to me, one of which is no treatment and the possible results if nothing is done. The treatment plan and the type of appliances to be used have been explained to me.

It has been explained to me, and I understand there is no specific warranty or guarantee as to any result and/or cure, and I understand I can ask for a full recital of all possible risks attendant to phases of _____
orthodontic care and treatment by just asking.

I understand the variables associated with the degree of success to be achieved and have read and understood the above.

_____   _____
(date)   (signature)

Figure 25-3

However, when a procedure inherently involves a known risk of death or serious bodily harm, it is the dentist's duty to disclose to his patient the possibility of such outcome and to explain in lay terms the complications that might possibly occur. The dentist must also disclose such additional information as a skilled practitioner of good standing would provide under the same or similar circumstances.

There is no duty to make disclosure of risks when the patient requests that he not be so informed or where the procedure is simple and the danger remote and commonly understood to be remote.

Also, a dentist has no duty of disclosure beyond that required of dentists of good standing in the same or similar locality when he relied upon facts which would demonstrate to a reasonable man that the disclosure would so seriously upset the patient that the patient would not have been able to rationally weigh the risks of refusing to undergo the recommended treatment.

Notwithstanding the patient's consent to a proposed treatment or operation, failure of the dentist to inform the patient as stated in this instruction before obtaining such consent is negligence and renders the dentist subject to liability for any injury (proximately) (legally) resulting from the (treatment) (operation) if a reasonably prudent person in the patient's position would not have consented to the (treatment) (operation) if he had been adequately informed of all the significant perils.

Recent court decisions have interpreted this requirement to definitely include alternative treatment options.

To translate informed consent into actual practice, let us assume the following has been properly accomplished:

A. Adequate x-rays
B. Complete health history, up to date and signed.
C. The patient is capable of understanding what is to be explained to him.

Let us further assume the doctor's skill and judgment tell him that what is dentally desirable is a deep filling on a lower molar tooth, a crown on an upper first molar, and an extraction of an upper bicuspid. For all three procedures, numbers 1 and 2 of the Informed Consent are almost self-explanatory.

Listed are some possible explanations, as examples, and are not complete, for the *deep filling* with the corresponding numbers from the Informed Consent form numbered items listed on page 727:

No. 3. Crown? Root Canal? Onlay? Inlay? Extraction? etc.
No. 4. A reasonable explanation of the future.
No. 5. A reasonable percentage of usefulness and longevity.
No. 6. A full explanation of what is being attempted.
No. 7. Pain, sensitivity, swelling, possible later root canal and/or apico and/or extraction, etc.
No. 8. The explanation of pain, infection, medical harm possibilities, etc.

Listed are some possible explanations, as examples, and are not complete, for the *crown* with corresponding numbers from the Informed Consent form numbered items listed on page 727:

No. 3. Onlay? Inlay? Extraction? etc.
No. 4. A reasonable explanation of the future.
No. 5. A reasonable percentage of usefulness and longevity.
No. 6. A full explanation of what is being attempted.
No. 7. Pain, swelling, sensitivity, infection, later root canal, later apico, later extraction, later partial or bridge, etc.
No. 8. The explanation of pain, infection, medical harm possibilities, etc.

Listed are some possible explanations, as examples, and are not complete, for the extraction of the *upper first molar*, with corresponding numbers from the Informed Consent form numbered items listed on page 727:

No. 3.   Attempted root canal, apico, etc.
No. 4.   A reasonable explanation of the future.
No. 5.   A reasonable percentage regarding a "good" result.
No. 6.   A full explanation of what is being attempted.
No. 7.   Pain, swelling, bleeding, infection, discoloration, opening into antrum, etc.
No. 8.   The explanation of pain, infection, medical harm possibilities, etc.

Needless to say, the Informed Consent doctrine knows no age limits, whether pediatric or geriatric. Some 15 year olds can comprehend, while some 50 year olds cannot. Proceed with caution.

A signed and dated Informed Consent is needed for *each* different procedure and, like the health history, it must be "up to date."

NO DELAY IN EMERGENCY

The law states generally that when a person is unconscious the operator must take great precaution to see that no injury occurs.[207] Emergency as a defense will do the operator no good if there is any delay or indecision in his actions. By this is meant that if a matter is one that should be referred to a specialist, this must be done immediately, and any delay may be taken into consideration as an aggravation of the original incident and play heavily against the professional person's interest.[208] In the case just referred to, the doctor had left a root in the mandible, and there later developed infection and a joint problem. There was a delay in referring the matter to the proper specialist, which made the doctor liable.

The emergency treatment must be within the standard of care for like emergencies,[209] and if this is not met, then of course liability should lie.

If there is hemorrhage from an extraction, this emergency calls for keeping the patient under constant observation as long as necessary in order to control the problem.[210]

THE FUTURE?

Legal concepts change with great rapidity. It used to be that a patient could be refused treatment, for any reason.[211] Now statutes are being promulgated that under certain circumstances (including an emergency) it becomes obligatory to accept a patient.[212]

Recovery of monetary damages is now becoming "possible" when a parent, seeing her child injured, suffers shock, fright, and emotional trauma.[213] The courts have even gone farther, and it is now "possible" for a child, seeing her sister injured, to recover for "shock, fright, and emotional trauma."[214]

Patient-plaintiffs continually attempt to hold the doctor liable on the theory of *strict liability*, said doctrine, in effect, making the doctor liable even when there is no malpractice, the basis being that the doctor "caused" the injury.[215]

Further attempts are being pressed to hold that supplying items such as blood, drugs, etc., is a sale of a product (and not a service) and if the item is defective, there will be strict liability with no need to show negligence or malpractice.[216]

Can a doctor foresee how long any projected treatment will take with any accuracy? The courts now seemingly hold that the operator is held to know how long he will need the anesthetic, and if he misjudges and it begins to wear off, liability can be predicated on this fact.[217]

The dangers of treating a "mentally disturbed" patient are exemplified by cases that, in effect, state if the patient is not "controlled" and suicide follows, a wrongful death suit may be proper.[218]

An area of concern to most doctors is whether the doctor can sue the plaintiff's attorney and plaintiff for malicious prosecution. Each jurisdiction has its own "rules," but usually, in order to do this, the defendant must first *win* his own malpractice suit. Some doctors now believe they can avoid awaiting this outcome and sue for Abuse of Process and Libel and Slander. Again, each state has its own laws, and attorneys specializing in these matters should be consulted.

Some states now allow a practitioner to be sued when he writes a report about a patient and the patient later complains that it isn't "accurate." This can be true even if the letter by the doctor is to the plaintiff's attorney.

Arbitration is thought of by some health practitioners as relief from the malpractice onslaught. It may well be, but it is *very* technical and is fraught with the danger of we attorneys arbitrating your dental matter, and that may be bad! Jurors seemingly do fine with dental malpractice matters, when the case is prepared properly and thoroughly. Not always so with judges (who are attorneys).

Comparative Negligence is a new doctrine that states, in effect, that there may be some percentage of fault by the patient and some percentage of fault by the doctor. This means, for instance, that in cases where the patient is admonished to sit still, and does not and moves, and is cut, the defense of Contributory Negligence no longer bars the plaintiff from recovery against the doctor. This new doctrine is another way of allowing the plaintiff to prevail, at least in some percentage of his claim for damages, whereas before he would have lost the suit because he was at fault for moving after being warned, as his own actions caused the injury. Woe is me!

Ever encroaching on the doctor-patient relationship are third party influences, whether in dollar allowances, or in what treatment can be done. Please heed the warning: no matter what third party, government or not, allows by way of payment on work to be accomplished, that is *not* the standard of care. It is the doctor's judgment that sets the standard of care and just because it cannot be "paid for" or the work not done more than once a year, or every five years, or whatever, that doesn't excuse the doctor from practicing the proper standard of care and apprising the patient of what is needed. The law does not allow the clinician to practice below the standard of care, *even* if the patient agrees to this in advance, or *even* if the patient gives a "release" to this maneuver. Be forewarned, suits on these facts are being handled now by the writer.

Last, and perhaps most important, is the State Board of Dental Examiners' action in each jurisdiction. This is an increasing hazard to the dental practitioner. It is separate and apart from malpractice. It is disciplinary in nature, is initiated by the governing body or by the patient, and is closely akin to being criminal in nature. Professional liability insurance does not cover this challenge and proceeding, which may end up in a separate time and trial. It is distasteful and embarrassing, and may end up with a loss of the doctor's license. At the first hint of involvement in this type of proceeding, every practitioner should contact an attorney specializing in dental malpractice defense, in that the basis for the State Board involvement, at least ostensibly, is concerned with the standard of care practiced on the patient or patients.

Most jurisdictions are faced with an avalanche of dental malpractice litigation. In order to provide a winning defense, planning is all important. One of the most significant tools to utilize is the protection afforded by law. Different states give varying degrees of protection to the client (dental practitioner) when he makes confidential communications to his attorney. This is highly important in that recent law in most state jurisdictions is to the effect that the plaintiff will have wide latitude in discovering reports, communications, records, etc., while (1) figuring out if he has a case, or (2) planning strategy to prove malpractice against the doctor.

One way to avoid this problem is by the use of all legal and moral defenses and by the discriminating use of the attorney-client privilege. If on the happening of an "incident" or notice of potential problem the doctor contacts an attorney who specializes in dental malpractice defense, the dealings between the two will be clothed with the attorney-client privilege. The proper attorney-client privilege states that all confidential communications from the client to the attorney will be clothed with an absolute privilege so that no one may delve into the private matters at hand.[219]

Malpractice insurance should be arranged so that there is no intermediary between the doctor and the attorney, thus providing the best possible opportunity to prepare a timely defense. The attorney can then notify the insurance company and/or broker.

EDITOR'S COMMENT

To the dental practitioner as yet uninitiated to the courtroom, and to the predoctoral or auxiliary student, the doctrine of informed consent and the various records and suggested policies must appear to be utterly incredible. Yet enormous efforts by the plaintiff's attorney to achieve big-dollar awards must be met by equal effort on the part of potential defendants. The doctor who innocently places his or her faith in total devotion to the highest quality of patient care, and who does not practice defensively, is headed for a very rude awakening. It is unfortunate that the additional time spent by the doctor in defense before the fact must be borne in the final analysis by additional patient costs, but such is the system.

To those health professionals who feel that the full details of informed consent would be shattering to patients, including the risk of death during treatment, may I state that the goriest of warnings rarely faze the patient.

Malpractice *does* occur, and the patient should be compensated in full and proper measure. Until a system of fair compensation is adopted on a "no-fault" or workmen's compensation type basis, we shall have to live with a monster which is vastly increasing costs to the patient, and which is causing a significant number of health professionals in high-risk specialties to seek other employment.

It is the rare reader who will finish this chapter without a sinking feeling regarding his or her choice of the health professions as a life endeavor. However, take heart, most dental malpractice suits are won by the defendant, particularly the doctor-defendant who has had the foresight to follow the three R's: records, rapport, and reason, and who has the courage to prevail.

Further, 691 malpractice claims were filed in California in 1977 against medical and dental practitioners as compared to a high of 874 in 1975. Preventive measures *are* effective.

REFERENCES

So that there be a sense of propriety, the names and citations of the cases will not be included. Only the state from which the decision arose will be listed.

1. Louisiana
2. Delaware–Mississippi
3. Washington, D.C.
4. Louisiana
5. Maine
6. Kentucky
7. California
8. Louisiana–Massachusetts
9. California
10. Massachusetts
11. Florida
12. California
13. California
14. Minnesota
15. Kentucky
16. New Jersey–Michigan–Nebraska
17. Tennessee
18. California
19. California
20. New Mexico
21. Illinois
22. Massachusetts
23. Virginia
24. Washington, D.C.
25. Oregon–Louisiana
26. California
27. California
28. California
29. New Jersey
30. New Jersey
31. Kansas–Minnesota
32. Vermont–Washington, D.C.–California
33. California
34. Wyoming
35. Nebraska
36. New Jersey
37. Georgia
38. California–New Jersey
39. Michigan
40. California
41. California
42. Massachusetts
43. Georgia
44. California
45. California–Illinois
46. Alabama
47. New York–Iowa
48. California
49. California
50. Pennsylvania
51. Michigan
52. California
53. California
54. Florida
55. California–New York–Kentucky
56. Kansas
57. New York
58. Pennsylvania
59. Maryland
60. Minnesota
61. Washington
62. Delaware
63. Michigan
64. California
65. California
66. California–Kentucky
67. Michigan
68. Idaho
69. California
70. Virginia
71. California
72. Louisiana–Oregon
73. Arizona
74. Illinois
75. Michigan
76. November
77. California–Arizona
78. Arizona
79. California
80. California
81. California
82. California
83. Georgia–New York
84. Washington
85. Missouri
86. Arkansas
87. Maryland
88. California
89. Michigan
90. Oregon
91. Utah
92. California
93. California
94. Wisconsin
95. California–New York
96. Louisiana

97. California
98. New York
99. New York–California
100. Washington
101. California
102. Washington, D.C.
103. California
104. Arizona
105. California
106. California
107. California
108. Florida–North Carolina–Washington
109. California
110. Idaho
111. California
112. Washington, D.C.
113. Michigan
114. California
115. Michigan
116. Ohio–Kentucky
117. Ohio
118. California–Louisiana–Washington–Kansas
119. California
120. Maine
121. Arkansas
122. Washington–Florida
123. California
124. California
125. California
126. California
127. California
128. New Mexico
129. California
130. New York
131. California
132. California
133. California
134. California
135. Louisiana
136. New Jersey
137. Washington, D.C.
138. California
139. California
140. Connecticut
141. North Carolina
142. Rhode Island
143. California
144. Washington, D.C.
145. Illinois–California–Montana
146. California
147. New Zealand
148. New York
149. California
150. California
151. Maine
152. Oregon
153. California–Louisiana
154. California–New Jersey–Michigan
155. Louisiana
156. Kansas
157. California
158. California

159. California
160. California
161. California
162. California
163. Oklahoma–Kentucky
164. New York
165. California
166. New Jersey
167. California
168. New York
169. Tennessee
170. Pennsylvania
171. Florida
172. New York
173. Washington
174. Connecticut
175. Utah
176. California
177. California
178. Nebraska
179. Illinois
180. New Jersey
181. Tennessee
182. Ohio
183. Washington, D.C.
184. Louisiana
185. California
186. California
187. North Carolina
188. Missouri
189. North Carolina–Florida
190. Louisiana–Texas–Colorado
191. Georgia
192. California
193. Kansas
194. New Mexico
195. West Virginia
196. Rhode Island–Michigan–California
197. Tennessee–Pennsylvania
198. Montana
199. Massachusetts
200. California
201. Louisiana–Washington, D.C.–Kansas
202. California
203. California
204. California
205. California
206. California
207. Missouri
208. California
209. Ohio
210. Montana
211. Louisiana
212. California
213. California
214. California
215. New Jersey
216. Florida–California
217. California
218. California
219. California

INDEX

Note: in this index, page numbers in *italic* type refer to illustrations; page numbers followed by (t) refer to tables.

Hormones, adverse interactions of, 216
  natural, drug effects of, 201
  synthetic, effects of, 201–203
Hospital, admission to, medical evaluation
    prior to, 629–630
  obligation of, 624
Hospital chart, in hospital dentistry, 642
Hospital dentistry, basic equipment for,
    636–637
  completion of procedure, 638
  discharging patient after, 642
  gowning and gloving for, 637
  hospital chart in, 642
  instruments and supplies for, 634
  notifying patient of, 631
  operating room attire for, 635–636
  operative note in, 639–640
  operative report in, 640–641
  postoperative orders in, 639
  preoperative orders, 631–633
  preparing patient for, 637–638
  recovery room in, 638
  reviewing patient's chart prior to, 634
  role of anesthetist in, 633–634
  role of patient's medical doctor in, 631
  role of surgical supervisor in, 634
  sample admission orders for, 633
  scheduling patient for, 630
  scheduling procedure for, 630–631
  scrubbing routine prior to, 636
  training in, 642–643
  use of auxiliary personnel in, 635
  visiting patient having, 624
Hospital staff, active, 627
  appointment to, procedure for, 628–629
  associate, 627
  clinical departments in, 628
  committees of, 628
  consulting, 628
  courtesy, status and privileges of, 627
  honorary, 628
  organization of, 626–628
  privileges of, 626
  requirements for membership of, 626
Humidity, and sudden death, 6
Hyaluronidase, effects of, 206
Hycodan, 148
Hydrazines, effects of, 199
Hydrocephalus, 90
  head shape in, 69
Hydrogen peroxide, effects of, 208–209
Hydroxystilbamidine, effects of, 194
Hydroxyzine, in oral pharmacosedation, 277
Hydroxyzine/alphaprodine/methohexital
    sedation, 330
Hydroxyzine hydrochloride, 331
Hypercarbia, in general anesthesia, 476
Hyperemia, pain in, 654
Hyperglycemia, 46
Hyperglycemic coma, 413
Hyperinsulinism, 47
Hyperocclusion, in pericementitis, 663
Hyperparathyroidism, 86–87
Hypertension, 41–42
  and anesthesia, 99, 466
  belladonna derivatives and, 334
  bleeding problems in, 575

Hypertension (Continued)
  drugs for, 141, 142
  during analgesia, control of, 441, 446
  stress and, 225
Hypertensive heart disease, 78
Hypertensives, analgesia in, 441, 446
Hyperthermia, in general anesthesia, cause
    of, 471
  clinical signs of, 471
    incidence of, 470
  prevention of, 471–472
  treatment of, 472
Hyperthyroidism, 86
  ASA classification, 49
  facial changes in, 69
Hyperventilation, 57, 411
Hyperventilation syndrome, 71
Hypesthesia, definition of, 43
Hypnosis, in psychosedation, 231
Hypnotic drugs, in pregnant women, 138
Hypofibrinogenemia, 575
Hypoglycemic coma, 413
Hypoglycemics, adverse interactions of,
    211, 215
Hyporeflexia, in psychosedation, 231
Hypotension, 41, 143
  acute, in adrenocortical insufficiency,
    treatment of, 415
  causes of, miscellaneous, 465–466
  in general anesthesia, 476–477
    causes of, 463
    rauwolfia alkaloid therapy of, 463–464
  in vasopressor syncope, 411
Hypothyroidism, 85–86
  ASA classification, 48
  meperidine and, 333
Hypovolemic shock, 80, 555
Hysteria, stress and, 228
Hysterical fainting, 412

Iatrosedation, body distance in, 264
  body orientation in, 263–264
  clinical behavior in, 254–261
    preparatory communication in, 255
  clinical encounters in, 238
    infiltration in, 256–259
  components of process, 238–239
  definition of, 237
  euphemistic language in, 259–260
  eye contact in, 262
  facial expression in, 262–263
  infiltration in, 256–259
  introduction to, 236–237
  nonverbal empathic strategy in, 261
Iatrosedative interview, 238
  model of, 244–245
  physical attending skills in, 261–264
  preparatory interview in, 260–261
  strategies of, 243–244
  technique of, 245–248
  "third ear" and, 248–254
  trunk lean in, 264
  voice in, 263
Ibuprofen, effects of, 152
Ice, in treatment of postextraction bleeding,
    585

Otalgia, 658
Oxacillin, 183
Oxazepam, characteristics of, 276
    usual dose of, 275(t)
Oximeter, 109, *109*
Oxolonic acid, effects of, 195
Oxycel, in treatment of postextraction
    bleeding, 584
Oxycodone, 147
Oxygen, administration of, in heart diseases,
    288
    arterial saturation of, 284
    "available," 284
    body reserves of, 97
    decreased concentration of, during
        general anesthesia, 460
    in nitrous oxide induction, 308
    in treatment of cardiac arrest, 427
    in ventilation of unconscious patient,
        357–358
    positive pressure, in cardiac arrest, 424
Oxygen alarm monitor, 108, *108*
Oxygen cylinder, valve used in, vs. nitrous
    oxide cylinder, *300*
Oxytetracycline, effects of, 186–187

Paget's disease, head size in, 69
Pain, anatomy and physiology of, 200–222
    chest, characteristics of, 30
    CNS states that modify, 230(t)
    control of, balancing negative and
        positive factors in, *221*
        schema for spectrum of, *281*
    dental, causes of, 654
    fear of, 239
    from sinusitis, 657
    guidelines for managing, 233(t)
    in maxillofacial injuries, relief of, 556–557
    in nerve ganglion disease, 649
    in oral lesions, control of, 681
    in sialoliths of glands, 684
    in tongue, 657–658
    maxillofacial, causes of, 644
        central, 660
        control of, role of dental doctor in, 645
        major neuralgias and, 649–654
        nerve ganglion disease and, 649
        neuritis, 654
        psychalgia, 660–661
        psychiatric aspects of, 653
        psychologic factors in, 645
        referred, 658–660
        treatment of, patient history in, 645–647
            physical examination in, 647–649
    nerve pressure, 656
    of angina, management of, 403
        404
    of caries, 655
    of dry socket, 655
    of foreign objects in periodontal structures,
        655
    of fractured or cracked teeth, 654–655
    of herpes zoster, 658
    of hyperemia, 654
    of mandibular fracture, 657
    of otalgia, 658

Pain (*Continued*)
    of pericoronitis, 656
    of periodontal disease, 655
    of pulpal necrosis, 654
    of pulpitis, 654
    originating from salivary glands, 656
    originating in styloid process, 657
    plus anxiety and stress, guidelines for
        management of, 233–234, 233(t)
    interrelationship of, *230*
    postoperative, controlling, 478
    referred. See *Referred pain.*
    relationship of anxiety to, 223
Pain-anxiety-stress experience, controlling,
    229–233
Pain threshold, definition of, 221
Pallor, 53
    in anaphylactic shock, 383–384
    in physical examination, 64
    of anesthetized patient, 95
    of pulse, 98–99
Palpitations, heart, 32
Panic, as cause of sudden death, 6
Pantopon, 149
Papase, effects of, 206
Papules, 67
Paraldehyde, characteristics and effects of,
    160
Paramycin, 187
Parathyroids, physical examination of,
    86–87
Paresthesia, as reaction to local anesthesia,
    436
Parotid gland, description of, 683
    sialoliths of, 684, *685*
    swelling of, *683*
Paroxysmal nocturnal dyspnea, 32
    in congestive heart failure, 34
Paroxysmal tachycardia, 121
Parulis, 673, *676*
Passive transfer test, for allergic response,
    379
Patients, care of during treatment, 336–337
    death of, malpractice liability in, 718–719
    difficult, 236
    fear in, controlling, 236–237
    high risk, and stress, 225–229
        intravenous sedation of, 339–341
            position during, 337
            selection for, 332–334
    medical risk categories of, 24
    postoperative instructions for, 337, *337*
    preoperative instructions for, 335, *335*
    preoperative management of, 334–336
    presurgical visit to, 624
    scheduling hospital surgical procedures
        for, 630
    traumatized, examination of, 557–559
    unconscious, artificial ventilation in,
        atmospheric air, 355–357
            exhaled air, 354–355
        check for airway breathing, 351, *352*
        check for airway patency in, 353
        enriched oxygen ventilation for, *355,*
            357
        forward displacement of mandible in,
            352, *353*

Respiratory rate, ASA classification, 57
Respiratory system, anatomy of, 95
  description of, 95
  monitoring of, 106–110
    by direct observation, 97–98
    carbon dioxide analyzer in, 107, *107*
    oximeter in, 109, *109*
    oxygen alarm monitor in, 108, *108*
    spirometer in, 109
    trace gases in, 110
Rest dyspnea, 29, 399
Resuscitation, in anaphylactic shock, 385
  in cardiac arrest, mouth-to-mouth,
      423–424, *423*
    one-person, 426
Resuscitation apparatus, in intravenous
    sedation, 339
Retina, examination of, 70
Rheumatic fever, chorea in, 79
  classification of, 28
Rheumatic heart disease, 79
  ASA classification of, 42
  treatment modification, 25(t)
Rheumatoid arthritis, 91
Rhinitis, as allergic response, 380
Rifampin, effects of, 189, 191, 195
Rifampin-isoniazid, effects of, 196
Right heart failure, 33
Roentgenography. See also *Radiography*
    and *X-rays.*
  and malpractice liability, 703–706
  in foreign body removal, 29
  in preoperative evaluation, *494*, 495, *495*
Rolitetracycline, effects of, 186–187
R on T phenomenon, and arrhythmias, 461
Roots, breakage of, conditions causing, 515
  removal of, closed, 515, *516*
    open, 517
Root fragments, prevalence in population,
    519
Root tips, removal of, 517–520, *517*
  from maxillary sinus, 525
Rule of Twos, 49
Russell viper venom, in treatment of
    bleeding, 584

Safety equipment, for inhalation
    pharmacosedation, 299–313
Salicylates, adverse interactions of, 216
  and hematologic testing, 581
  as anticoagulants, 573
  effects of, 150
Salicylism, 150
Salivary glands, pain originating from, 656
Salivary system, acute diseases of, 682–684
  anatomy of, 683–684
Scales, on skin, 67
Scars, 67
Scopolamine, effects of, 197
Scrubbing, for hospital dentistry, 636
Seborrheic dermatitis, 67
Secobarbital, in oral pharmacosedation,
    272(t), 273
Secobarbital/meperidine/methohexital
    sedation, 321
  technique of, 329–330

Secondary closure, in treatment of
    maxillofacial injuries, 564–565
Sedation. See also *Analgesia, Anesthesia,*
    Pharmacosedation, and *Psychosedation.*
  conscious patient, definition of, 94
    monitoring in, 93
  diazepam/methohexital, 321
    techniques of, 330–331
  diazepam plus meperidine or
      pentazocine, 321
    technique of, 329
  diazepam plus nitrous oxide, 328–329
  hydroxyzine/methohexital/alphaprodine
      sedation, 330
  in bronchial asthma patient, 399–400
  in patients with bronchopulmonary
      diseases, 399–400
  in pulmonary emphysema patient, 399
  intermittent Althesin, 321, 327–328
  intermittent methohexital, 321, 324–326.
    See also *Intermittent methohexital*
    sedation.
  intravenous. See *Intravenous sedation.*
  Jorgensen technique of, 321, 323
  levels of, mouth breathing to lighten, 293
  of fearful patient, 237
  profound, safety in, 269
  secobarbital/meperidine/methohexital,
      321
    technique of, 329–330
  upright position in chair and, 332
Sedatives, drugs with primary effect, 168
Seizure, grand mal, treatment in, 416–417,
    416, 417
Senile keratosis, 67
Sensations, classification of, 648
Sernylan, 170
Serpentina, 162
Serum hepatitis, 46
Shingles, 689–690, *690*
Shivering, in general anesthesia, 478
Shock, 80
  anaphylactic, 380
  contributing factors, 554
  hypovolemic, 80, 555
  in local analgesia, 446
  in maxillofacial injuries, preventing,
      553–556
  prevention and treatment of, 554–556
  treatment of, administration of fluids in,
      555
    monitoring in, 555
    vital signs in, 554
Sialoliths, 684, *685*
Sickle cell anemia, 87
  ASA classification, 51
Sickle cell trait, 51
Sign reflex, 337
Silver salts, effects of, 209
Sims' position, in maintenance of airway,
    544, *544*
Sino-atrial node, 74
Sinus arrhythmia(s), 120, *120,* 364
Sinus bradycardia, 121, *121*
Sinus tachycardia, 76, 120, *121*
Sinusitis, maxillary, 532
  pain from, 657

Tobramycin, effects of, 196
Tongue, injuries to, in general anesthesia, 474
  lacerations of, 684–685
  pain in, 657–658
  traction of, in airway maintenance, 545, 545
Tooth. See Teeth and specific teeth; e.g., Incisor(s).
Tooth socket, dry, pain of, 655
    therapy of, 502
  granuloma of, squamous carcinoma mimicking, 693, 695
  packing of, in treatment of bleeding, 586
Toothpastes, adverse effects of, 209
Tourniquet, in emergency intravenous drug administration, 368–369, 369, 370
Tourniquet test (Rumpel-Leede), 578
Towel clamps, as tissue retractors in emergency tracheostomy, 549
Toxicity, in local analgesia, 437
Trace gases, monitoring of, 110
Trachea, obstruction of air flow at, 451
Tracheal tube, insertion of, 551
Tracheal tube set, 551
Tracheostomy, high, 552
  in airway maintenance, 547–548, 548
  in maxillofacial injuries, 547–548, 548
  maintenance of, 552
  surgical procedure for, 548–552, 548, 549, 550, 551
Tracheostomy tubes, and oxygen adaptor for, 487, 488, 489
Tracheotomy, 485–489
Training, in hospital dentistry, 642–643
Tranexamic acid, for angioedema, 380
Tranquilization, during dental treatment, sedation levels for, 270
  in psychosedation, 232
Tranquilizers, and intravenous sedation, 333
  classification and actions of, 162
  drugs with primary effect, 168
  in pregnant women, 138
  major, 162–165
  minor, classification of, 168
  moderate, 165–168
  neuroleptic, 176–177
  stimulant, 169–170
Transfusion, in maxillofacial injuries, 555–556
  plasma, in severe blood loss, 582
  whole blood, allergic reactions in, 582
Transient cerebral ischemia, 43
  management of patient following, 44
Trauma, of injection, in local analgesia, 437
Traumatized patient, examination of, 557–559
Treatment record, in intravenous sedation, 340
Tremors, in general anesthesia, 470
  of hands, 53
Triacetyloleandomycin, effects of, 185–186
Triazolam, 166
Trichlorethylene, effects of, 174
Trigeminal neuralgia, 649–650
Trilene, effects of, 174

Trimethobenzamide, actions of, 170
Trimethoprimsulfamethoxazole, effects of, 196
Tripelennamine, effects of, 172
Trismus, prophylaxis for, 444
Troleandomycin, effects of, 196
Trypsin, effects of, 206
Tuberculosis, and Addison's disease, 49
  mimicking dental abscess, 693, 696
Tumor, malignant, involving maxillary sinus, 533, 534
  of lung, 72
Tylenol, 150
Tympanic neuralgia, 652
Type and cross match with Rh factor (blood test), 580

Ulcer(s), peptic, 82
  skin, 67
Ulcerative colitis, 45–46
  ASA classification, 46
Ultralight general anesthesia, definition of, 94
Unconsciousness, airway obstruction in, 349, 349
  monitoring of vital signs in, 361–367
  problems associated with, 349
  treatment of, 349
Ureides, properties of, 168
Urinalysis, 60
Urticaria, definition of, 379
USC physical evaluation system, 24–25

Vaccines, effects of, 206
Valium. See Diazepam.
Vancomycin, effects of, 188, 196
Varidase, in clot lysis, 593
Vasoconstrictors, allergies to, 382
Vasodepressor syncope, causes of, 409
  clinical findings in, 410
  definition of, 409
  differential diagnosis of, 411–412
  in intermittent methohexital sedation, 326
  management of patient in, 412
  summary of findings in, 411
  treatment of, 410–411, 410
Vasopressors, 179–180
  in hypotension, 143
Vastus lateralis muscle, as site of drug administration, 373–374, 373
Venipuncture, in intravenous drug administration, 369, 370
Ventilation, artificial, in unconscious patient, 354–359
  atmospheric air, 355–357
    devices used for, 356–357, 355, 356
  enriched oxygen, 357
  exhaled air, 354–355
  mouth-to-mouth, in airway obstruction, 484–485
    in cardiac arrest, 423–424, 423
  of unconscious patient, adjunctive equipment for, 359–361